AF352065

Cardiovascular Complications of Liver Disease

Editors

Arieh Bomzon, Ph.D., F.R.C.V.S.
Department of Pharmacology
Rappaport Family Institute
Technion
Haifa
Israel

Laurence M. Blendis, M. D., F.R.C.P., F.R.C.P.(C)
Department of Gastroenterology
Toronto General Hospital
Toronto, Ontario
Canada

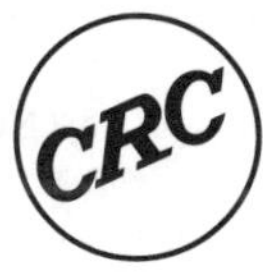

CRC Press
Boca Raton   Ann Arbor   Boston

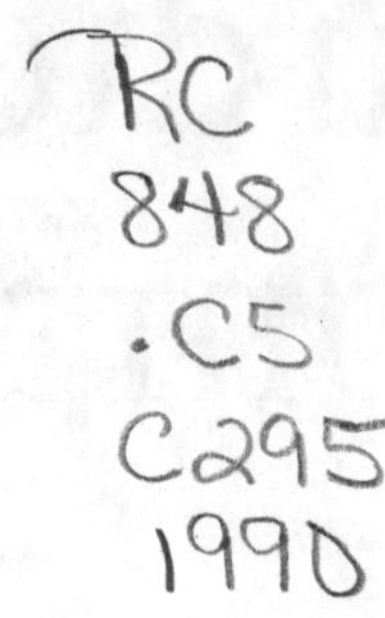

Library of Congress Cataloging-in-Publication Data

Cardiovascular complications of liver disease / editors, Arieh Bomzon,
  Laurence M. Blendis.
      p.   cm.
      Includes bibliographical references.
      ISBN 0-8493-4735-1
      1. Liver—Cirrhosis—Complications and sequelae.
  2. Cardiovascular system—Diseases. 3. Portal hypertension-
  -Complications and sequelae.   I. Bomzon, Arieh, 1947-
  II. Blendis, Laurence M.
      [DNLM: 1. Cardiovascular System—physiopathology.   2. Liver
  Diseases—complications.   WI 700 C267]
  RC848.C5C295   1990
  616.3'62—dc20
  DNLM/DLC   for Library of Congress   90-1318
                                                                          CIP

This book represents information obtained from authentic and highly regarded sources. Reprinted material is quoted with permission, and sources are indicated. A wide variety of references are listed. Every reasonable effort has been made to give reliable data and information, but the author and the publisher cannot assume responsibility for the validity of all materials or for the consequences of their use.

Direct all inquiries to CRC Press, Inc., 2000 Corporate Blvd., N.W., Boca Raton, Florida 33431.

International Standard Book Number 0-8493-4735-1

Library of Congress Card Number 90-1318
Printed in the United States

PREFACE

The idea for this book came as a result of innumerable discussions between ourselves during 1983 and 1984 in Israel. At that time, evidence was accumulating that, far from being an "end stage" disease, patients with uncomplicated cirrhosis had as good a prognosis as those patients with non-cirrhotic liver conditions; and that the reason most patients with cirrhosis developed life-threatening problems, long before liver function started to deteriorate, was the development of complications of the cardiovascular system. We were therefore interested in understanding the cardiovascular changes that occurred with time as cirrhosis and portal hypertension developed. We were unable to answer many of the questions for a variety of reasons. Clinical texts and papers in this area were focused either on the pathogenesis of portal hypertension or on the effects of liver disease on the kidney at one point in time. Some of the questions were addressed in animal experiments, but the results seemed to depend on the species and the experimental designs. For these reasons, we decided to collate the information known on the cardiovascular changes in both clinical and experimental liver disease with the aid of our colleagues at the cutting edge of research in these areas. In so doing, there was little doubt in our minds that overlap between texts would occur. In spite of this, the book has enabled us to answer some of the unanswered questions which we posed in 1983 and 1984 and has assisted us in suggesting possible future research objectives in this area. Whether the reader is a physician or a research scientist with an interest in the liver and liver disease, we hope that this text will save you many hours of searching in libraries, since the information contained herein is a comprehensive collection of currently available information on the effects of liver disease on the cardiovascular system. Finally, we hope that you will find this book as useful as we have, for all the above-mentioned reasons.

Arieh Bomzon
Laurence M. Blendis
Toronto, 1989

THE EDITORS

Arieh Bomzon, Ph.D., is an Associate Professor of Pharmacology in the Faculty of Medicine at the Technion-Israel Institute of Technology, Haifa, Israel.

Dr. Bomzon trained initially as a veterinarian and graduated from the University of Sydney, Australia in January 1969. After spending several years in practice, he obtained his Ph.D. from the Department of Physiology, University of the Witwatersrand, South Africa in 1976. In 1981, he took up a position as a senior research fellow in the Faculty of Medicine and, in 1989, he assumed his present position.

Dr. Bomzon is a member of the European Association for the Study of the Liver, the American Association for the Study of Liver Diseases, and the Israel Pharmacological and Physiological Societies. In 1976, he was awarded a fellowship from the Royal College of Veterinary Surgeons. He was listed in *Men of Achievement* in 1977.

His major research interest is the cardiovascular system in liver disease, with particular emphasis on the regulation of small resistance vessels by the sympathetic nervous system.

Laurence Blendis M.D., F.R.C.P., F.R.C.P.(C.) is a Professor of Medicine at the University of Toronto and a staff physician in the Division of Gastroenterology and Hepatology at the Toronto General Hospital.

Dr. Blendis graduated in medicine from the Middlesex Hospital Medical School, University of London in June 1961. After internships and residences at various teaching hospitals, he undertook a research fellowship in hepatology with Dr. Roger Williams at Kings College Hospital and completed his M.D. thesis for the University of London. He then undertook a post doctoral fellowship in nephrology with Dr. Norman Levinsky at the University of Boston Medical School. After spending three years as a consultant physician in gastroenterology at the Central Middlesex Hospital in London, he took up his present position in Toronto.

Dr. Blendis is a member of several scientific societies in Canada, the U.S., and the U.K., with special interest in hepatology and gastroenterology.

His research interests are in the area of chronic liver disease, especially alcoholic cirrhosis and its major complications, ascites and portal hypertension.

CONTRIBUTORS

Vicente Arroyo, M.D.
Professor of Medicine
Barcelona Medical School
Barcelona
Spain

**Eric D. Bateman, M.D., D.C.H.,
F.R.C.P.**
Head, Respiratory Clinic
Groote Schuur Hospital
Cape Town
South Africa

Harold D. Battarbee Ph.D.
Professor
Department of Physiology and Biophysics
Louisiana State University Medical
 Center
Shreveport, Louisiana

Joseph N. Benoit, Ph.D.
Department of Physiology and Biophysics
Louisiana State University Center
Shreveport, Louisiana

Mauro Bernardi, M.D.
Associate Professor of Pathophysiology
Department of Special Medical Pathology
University of Bologna
Bologna
Italy

**Laurence M. Blendis, M.D.,
 F.R.C.P.(C.)**
Professor of Medicine
University of Toronto
Toronto, Ontario
Canada

**Arieh Bomzon, Ph.D.,
 F.R.C.V.S.(Eng.)**
Department of Pharmacology
Rappaport Family Institute for Research
 in the Medical Sciences
Technion
Haifa
Israel

**P. J. Campbell, M.R.C.P.(U.K.),
F.R.C.P.(C.)**
Department of Gastroenterology
Toronto General Hospital
Toronto, Ontario
Canada

**F. J. Carmichael, Ph.D., M.D.,
 F.R.C.P.(C.)**
Assistant Professor
Department of Anaesthesia and
 Pharmacology
University of Toronto
Toronto, Ontario
Canada

Niels Juel Christensen, M.D., Ph.D.
Associate Professor
Department of Internal Medicine and
 Endocrinology
University of Copenhagen
Copenhagen
Denmark

Murray Epstein, M.D.
Professor of Medicine
Division of Nephrology
University of Miami School of Medicine
Miami, Florida

Daphna Fenyves, M.D.
Research Fellow
Division of Hepatology
Hôpital Saint-Luc
Montreal, Quebec
Canada

Giovanni Gasbarrini, M.D., Ph.D.
Professor of Medicine and Head
Department of Special Medical Pathology
University of Bologna
Bologna
Italy

Pere Ginés, M.D.
Liver Unit
Hospital Clinico y Provincial
Barcelona
Spain

D. Neil Granger, Ph.D.
Professor and Head
Department of Physiology and Biophysics
Louisana State University Medical Center
Shreveport, Louisiana

Jens H. Henriksen, M.D., Ph.D.
Associate Professor
Department of Clinical Physiology
Hvidovre Hospital
University of Copenhagen
Copenhagen
Denmark

Pierre-Michel Huet, M.D.
Professor of Medicine
Division of Hepatology
Hôpital Saint-Luc
Montreal, Quebec
Canada

Wladimiro Jimenez, Ph.D.
Hormonal Laboratory
Hospital Clinico y Provincial
Barcelona
Spain

Ralph E. Kirsch, M.D.
Professor and Executive Director
MRC/UCT Liver Research Centre
University of Cape town
Cape Town
South Africa

Ronald J. Korthuis, Ph.D.
Associate Professor
Department of Physiology and Biophysics
Louisiana State University Medical
  Center
Shreveport, Louisiana

Herbert J. Kramer, M.D.
Professor of Medicine
Medical Poliklinik
University of Bonn
Bonn
Federal Republic of Germany

David Kravetz, M.D.
Liver Unit
Hospital Nacional Posadas
Buenos Aires
Argentina

Didier Lebrec, M.D.
Laboratoire d'Thérmodynamique
  Splanchnique
Unité de Recherches de Physiopathologie
  Hepatique
Hôpital Beaujon
Clichy
France

Samuel S. Lee, M.D., F.R.C.P.(C.)
Department of Medicine
University of Calgary
Calgary, Alberta
Canada

S. S. Louw, M.D.
Senior Lecturer
Department of Medicine
University of Cape town
Cape Town
South Africa

Richard Moreau, M.D.
Service de Réanimation et de Medecine
  d'Urgence
Centre Hospitalier Émile Roux
Eaubonne
France

Hector Orrego, M.D.
Professor
Department of Medicine and
  Pharmacology and Addiction Research
  Foundation
University of Toronto
Toronto, Ontario
Canada

Helmer Ring-Larsen, M.D., Ph.D.
Associate Professor
Department of Hepatology
Hvidovre Hospital
University of Copenhagen
Copenhagen
Denmark

Frank L. Silver, M.D., F.R.C.P.(C.)
Assistant Professor
Department of Medicine
University of Toronto
Toronto, Ontario
Canada

Karl Skorecki, M.D., F.R.C.P.(C.)
Assistant Professor
Department of Medicine
University of Toronto
Toronto, Ontario
Canada

Franco Trevisani, M.D.
Research Fellow
Department of Special Medical Pathology
University of Bologna
Bologna
Italy

Jean-Pierre Villeneuve, M.D.
Associate Professor
Division of Hepatology
Hôpital Saint-Luc
Montreal, Quebec
Canada

Michael D. Voight, M.D., F.C.P., M.Med.
Lecturer
Department of Medicine
University of Capetown, and
Investigator
MRC/UCT Liver Centre
Cape Town
South Africa

TABLE OF CONTENTS

Chapter 1

THE CARDIOVASCULAR COMPLICATIONS OF CIRRHOSIS — A HISTORY

Laurence M. Blendis and Arieh Bomzon

TABLE OF CONTENTS

I. INTRODUCTION

In 1953 Kowalski and Abelman[1] demonstrated that cirrhotic patients had an increased cardiac output and heart rate associated with a low normal arterial blood pressure and thus a decreased systemic vascular resistance. This description of the circulation became known as the hyperkinetic circulation of cirrhosis and was shown to be associated with portal hypertension[2] and to affect all major circulatory regions.[3] In this chapter, we will briefly review the history of the cardiovascular complications of liver disease in order to "set the scene" for the rest of the volume. (See Table 1.)

II. PORTAL HYPERTENSION

Portal hypertension is the major cardiovascular complication of cirrhosis. Until the beginning of the 1980s, it was considered that portal hypertension was due principally to increased resistance to flow as a result of the regeneration nodules in the liver of cirrhotic patients. Despite the introduction of the clinical measurement of portal pressure, first via the intrasplenic pressure[4] and then, with the now established "gold standard", via the hepatic wedged pressure[5] there was little appreciable advance in this area. Even in idiopathic, noncirrhotic portal hypertension, certainly until the late 1950s, investigators were still trying to establish that the pathogenesis of portal hypertension was due to microscopic portal venopathy[6] rather than changes in hemodynamics.

In 1910 Banti[7] had suggested that portal hypertension in noncirrhotic patients might be due to increased splenic blood flow resulting from splenic enlargement. Fifty years later, using sophisticated hemodynamic studies to measure splenic blood flow, Williams and others were able to show that Banti had indeed been correct and that portal hypertension in both noncirrhotic and cirrhotic patients was associated with increased splenic blood flow.[8-10] In addition, splenectomy in noncirrhotic patients resulted in normalization of portal pressure.[11]

III. PORTOCAVAL SHUNTING

Studies of hepatic blood flow in patients with alcoholic liver disease have also shown that portal blood flow is important in the pathogenesis of portal hypertension. In these patients, there is an increased portal component of hepatic blood flow, an incremental increase in portal pressure,[12] and increased portasystemic shunting.[13] It was also clear that the variable postoperative response to portocaval shunting, apart from liver function, was due to the state of the hemodynamics preoperatively.[14-19] Yet, investigators in this area failed to solve this problem and patients shunted for variceal bleeding continued to develop encephalopathy and die from liver failure. The result in randomized controlled trials was that shunting prevented bleeding[20] and rebleeding, but the resultant postoperative deterioration in hepatic function meant no improvement in overall mortality rate.[21-23]

By the late 1970s, it had become obvious that the resistance to portal blood flow was not the principal factor determining portal hypertension or the amount of splanchnic blood being shunted through the varices.[24] In 1982, Groszmann et al.[25] using radiolabeled microspheres both in carbon tetrachloride-induced cirrhotic and partial portal vein-ligated rats, showed that portal hypertension was associated with increased, and not decreased, portal venous inflow. The increase of 50 to 100% was confirmed by Blanchet and Lebrec.[26] Moreover, it was shown to be due in part, in the rat model, to a decreased contractile response to norepinephrine and to the vasodilatory effects of glucagon.[27]

IV. ASCITES

The pathogenesis of salt and water retention in cirrhosis was widely held to be caused

Table 1
The Cardiovascular System in Liver Disease

Blood pressure	Normal or decreased
Pulse pressure	Increased
Peripheral vascular resistance	Decreased
Reactivity to vasoactive agents	Normal or decreased
Cardiac index or output	Normal or increased
Heart rate	Normal or increased
Stroke index	Increased
Plasma volume	Normal or increased
Albumin concentration	Normal or decreased
Hematocrit	Decreased
Red cell mass	Normal or decreased
Portal hypertension	Present
Arteriovenous shunts	Present
Ascites	Present or absent
Renal perfusion	Decreased
Sympathetic nervous system activity	Increased
Renin angiotensin aldosterone system activity	Increased

by a decrease in effective circulating blood volume due to excessive pooling of blood in the splanchnic venous bed—this, despite the fact that ascites developed in the presence of normal renal blood flow, glomerular filtration rates,[28] and increased total blood volume.[29-33]

In addition, there was "third spacing" of fluid out of the intravascular compartment due to hypoalbuminemia as a result of hepatic failure of albumin production.[34] The explanation for the expanded plasma volume was that albumin, including "tagged" albumin, also leaked out of the intravascular space into the lymphatics and ascites so that the measurements were in fact of plasma volume *plus* a third space.[35,36] This "underfilling" of the intravascular volume resulted in elevated plasma renin activity and secondary hyperaldosteronism associated with decreased extraction of para-aminohippurate by the kidney[37,38] which might improve with volume expansion.[38,39]

In the late 1960s, two papers questioned the dogma of a decreased effective circulating plasma volume causing salt and water retention. Lieberman and Reynolds[40] once again confirmed the presence of an increased plasma volume in cirrhotic patients with and without ascites, with functional renal failure, and following portacaval anastomosis. In addition, by measurement of the thoracic lymph space with radioisotopic markers they found that it accounted for a negligible percent of the excess volume. Portal hypertension appeared to be the major factor in the development of the increased plasma volume. In a subsequent paper, these investigators showed that with spontaneous loss of ascites there was no rise in plasma volume, i.e., that third space reduction of effective plasma volume was unlikely to be the cause of sodium retention. Furthermore, portal pressure, a factor in splanchnic volume expansion, remained constant with the loss of ascites.[41] They, therefore, suggested that sodium retention was associated with expansion of the effective circulating volume, i.e., "overfilling".

Thus the "underfilling" vs. "overfilling" controversy began and continues to this day.[42] Animal studies by Levy and co-workers have provided support for the concept that the development of ascites passes through a series of changes from initial overfilling to eventual underfilling of the intravascular volume.[43] Evidence in patients is sparse, but initial "overfilling" was suggested by the finding of normal or low plasma renin activity and serum aldosterone levels in patients with "early" ascites associated with grossly expanded plasma volumes.[44] At the same time, a series of clinical studies utilizing head-out water immersion[45] or the therapeutic procedure of peritoneovenous shunting[46] would superficially appear to support the "underfilling" theory with both maneuvers suppressing highly elevated serum aldosterone levels. However, closer scrutiny would indicate that such studies are performed on patients who have had ascites for some considerable period of time and thus may well have passed through an overfilling period to an underfilling stage.

At the same time, the role of the circulation in the formation of ascites gained increasing importance. Originally, the suggestion had come from the para-aminohippurate extraction studies.[28,37,38] Then came the direct observation of the presence of superficial renal cortical vasoconstriction[47,48] in both early and late stages of fluid retention culminating in the hepatorenal syndrome (HRS). As far as the initial factor in the pathogenesis of ascites is concerned, increasing evidence both in animal[49] and clinical studies[50] pointed to the height of the hepatic sinusoidal pressure.

Thus the concept of an "hepatic nephropathy" was formulated, based on a potentially reversible renal vasoconstriction, associated with hepatic failure and systemic vasodilatation.[51] This was confirmed first, by the transplantation of the kidney from patients dying from HRS, which then functioned normally in the recipient;[52] and second, by the complete reversal of HRS by hepatic transplantation alone, resulting in a return of normal renal function.[53]

V. PERIPHERAL VASODILATATION AND DIMINISHED END ORGAN RESPONSIVENESS

Yet, the renal vasoconstriction occurred in the presence of peripheral vasodilation. The latter was shown to be unresponsive to stimulants of sympathetic nerve activity[54] in spite of highly elevated levels of circulating endogenous catecholamines.[55] Thus, the concept of peripheral vascular unresponsiveness or diminished end organ responsiveness in cirrhosis was identified. This also appears to occur in obstructive jaundice[56-58] and may explain the increased tendency to hypotension and renal failure postoperatively in these patients.[59,60] The mechanism of vascular refractoriness in chronic liver disease remains unexplained, but the resultant expansion of the intravascular volume has now been invoked in the pathogenesis of salt and water retention.[61]

Thus systemic, splanchnic, and renal circulatory changes have lately become recognized to be of major importance in the pathogenesis of portal hypertension and ascites. Well-recognized vasoactive hormones and substances, whose metabolism is deranged in the cirrhotic patient, have been implicated. In addition to those already mentioned, angiotensin II and renal prostaglandin E group[62] have been implicated in maintaining the integrity of the renal circulation until the onset of HRS.[63] The development of renal resistance to the action of atrionatriuretic factor (ANF) discovered in 1981[64], has also recently been emphasized as an important factor. Since ANF is also a vasodilator, elevated levels of this hormone may well contribute to the systemic vasodilatation.

VI. THE PHARMACOLOGICAL THERAPY OF PORTAL HYPERTENSION

With the recognition of the many factors that contribute to the overall changes in the status of the cardiovascular system, the pharmacological treatment of patients with chronic liver disease is a vexing problem. One of the major breakthroughs in the pharmacological treatment of portal hypertension was developed by Lebrec and his colleagues in 1980.[65] They showed that propranolol in sufficient dose to reduce both heart rate, and thus cardiac output, by 25%, and local portal inflow, caused both a significant acute[65] and chronic[66] reduction in hepatic wedge pressure. They postulated that such treatment might prevent rebleeding of esophageal varices and with a carefully performed randomized control trial they confirmed it.[67] However, two subsequent controlled trials failed to confirm this finding.[68,69]

Nevertheless, these observations were of major importance in opening up the possibilities of treating variceal bleeding medically. Since then, many other drugs and combination of drugs have been shown experimentally to lower portal pressure and have resulted in further clinical trials. In addition, the use of propranolol in the prevention of variceal bleeding has been proposed[70] and initial clinical trials look promising.[71]

The treatment of ascites remained problematic despite the appearance of more and more powerful diuretics which were associated with increasing renal and electrolytic complications. Moreover, patients still developed resistance.

All these issues will be discussed in full in this volume. In addition, other new concepts are explored, including the role of the heart itself, circulatory changes in the lungs, the possibility of a role of the cerebral circulation in the pathogenesis of hepatic encephalopathy. We feel that the time is ripe to bring before the scientific community a concise summary of all the various changes in the circulation associated with liver disease so that it may judge for itself whether this topic warrants more attention and to stimulate further investigation in this area.

REFERENCES

1. **Kowalski, H. J., and Abelman, W. H.,** The cardiac output at rest in Laennec's cirrhosis, *J. Clin. Invest.,* 32, 1025, 1953.
2. **Murray, J. P., Dawson, A. M., and Sherlock, S.,** Circulatory changes in chronic liver disease, *Am. J. Med.,* 24, 358, 1958.
3. **Kontos, L. A., Shapiro, W., Mauch, H. P., and Patterson, J. L.,** General and regional circulatory alterations in cirrhosis of the liver, *Am. J. Med.,* 37, 526, 1964.
4. **Atkinson, M. and Sherlock, S.,** Intrasplenic pressure as an index of the portal venous pressure, *Lancet,* 1, 1325, 1954.
5. **Redeker, A. G., Geller, H. M., and Reynolds, T. B.,** Hepatic wedge pressure, blood flow, vascular resistance and oxygen consumption in cirrhosis, before and after end to side portacaval shunt, *J. Clin. Invest.,* 37, 606, 1958.
6. **Tisdale, W. A., Klatskin, G., and Glenn, W. W. L.,** Portal hypertension and bleeding esophageal varices, *N. Engl. J. Med.,* 261, 109, 1959.
7. **Banti, G.,** *Ueber Mortis Banti Folia Nemat,* 10, 33, 1910.
8. **Williams, R., Parsonson, A., Somers, K., and Hamilton, P. J. S.,** Portal hypertension in idiopathic tropical splenomegaly, *Lancet,* 1, 329, 1966.
9. **Williams, R., Condon, R. E., Williams, H. S., Blendis, L. M., and Kreel, L.,** Splenic blood flow in cirrhosis and portal hypertension, *Clin. Sci.,* 34, 441, 1968.
10. **Blendis, L. M., Banks, D. C., Rambeer, C., and Williams, R.,** Splenic blood flow and splanchnic hemodynamics in blood dyscrasia and other splenomegalies, *Clin. Sci.,* 38, 73, 1970.
11. **Hamilton, P. J. S., Richmond, J., Donaldson, G. W. K., Williams, R., Hutt, M. S., and Lugumba, V.,** Splenectomy in "Big Spleen Disease", *Br. Med. J.,* 3, 823, 1967.
12. **Cohn, J. N., Khatri, I. M., and Groszmann, R. J.,** Hepatic blood flow in alcoholic liver disease measured by an indicator dilution technique, *Am. J. Med.,* 53, 704, 1972.
13. **Groszmann, R., Kotelanski, B., and Cohn, J. N.,** Quantitation of portasystemic shunting from the splenic and mesenteric beds in alcoholic liver disease, *Am. J. Med.,* 53, 715, 1972.
14. **Moreno, A. H., Burchell, A. R., and Rousselot, L. M.,** Portal blood flow in cirrhosis of the liver, *J. Clin. Invest.,* 46, 436, 1967.
15. **Fomon, J. J. and Warren, W. D.,** Hemodynamic studies in portal hypertension, *Ann. Rev. Med.,* 20, 277, 1969.
16. **McDermott, W. V.,** Evaluation of the hemodynamics of portal hypertension in the selection of patients for shunt surgery, *Ann. Surg.,* 176, 449, 1972.

17. **Smith, G. W.,** An assessment of validity of preoperative hemodynamic studies in portal hypertension, *Surgery,* 74, 130, 1973.
18. **Reynolds, T. B.,** Promises. Promises. Hemodynamics and portal systemic shunt, *N. Engl. J. Med.,* 290, 1484, 1974 (editorial).
19. **Burchell, A. R., Moreno, A. H., Panke, W. F.,** Hemodynamic variables and prognosis following portacaval shunts, *Surg. Gynecol. Obstet.,* 138, 359, 1974.
20. **Conn, H. O., Lindenmouth, W. W., May, C. J., and Ramsby, G. R.,** Prophylactic portacaval anastomosis, *Medicine,* 51, 27, 1972.
21. **Jackson, F. D., Perrin, E. B., Feux, W. R., and Smith, T.,** A clinical investigation of the portacaval shunt vs. survival analysis of the therapeutic operation, *Ann. Surg.,* 174, 672, 1971.
22. **Resnick, R. H., Iber, F. L., Ishihara, A. M., Chalmers, T. C., and Zimmerman, H.,** A controlled study of the therapeutic portacaval shunt, *Gastroenterology,* 67, 843, 1974.
23. **Ruff, B., Prandi, D., Degos, F., Sicot, J., Degos, J. D., Sicot, C., Maillard, J. N., Fauvert, R., and Benhamou, J. P.,** A controlled study of therapeutic portacaval shunt in alcoholic cirrhosis, *Lancet,* 1, 655, 1976.
24. **Lebrec, D., Kotelanski, B., and Cohn, J. N.,** Splanchnic hemodynamics in cirrhotic patients with esophageal varices and gastrointestinal bleeding, *Gastroenterology,* 70, 1108, 1976.
25. **Groszmann, R. J., Vorobioff, J., and Riley, E.,** Splanchnic hemodynamics in portal hypertensive rats: measurement with labelled microspheres, *A. J. Physiol.,* 242, G156, 1982.
26. **Blanchet, L. and Lebrec, D.,** Changes in splanchnic blood flow in portal hypertensive rats, *Eur. J. Clin. Invest.* 12, 327, 1982.
27. **Benoit, J. N., Barrowman, J. A., Harper, S. L., Kvietys, P. R., and Granger, D. N.,** Role of humoral factors in the intestinal hyperemia associated with chronic portal hypertension, *Am. J. Physiol.,* 247, G486, 1984.
28. **Baldus, W. P., Feichter, R. M., and Summerskill, W. H. J.,** The kidney in cirrhosis, *Ann. Intern. Med.,* 60, 353, 1964.
29. **Perera, G. A.,** The plasma volume in Laennec's cirrhosis of the liver, *Ann. Intern. Med.,* 24, 643, 1946.
30. **Bateman, J. C., Shorr, H. M., and Elgvin, T.,** Hypervolemic anemia in cirrhosis, *J. Clin. Invest.* 28, 539, 1949.
31. **Hiller, G. I., Huffman, E. R., and Levey, S.,** Studies in cirrhosis of the liver, *J. Clin. Invest.,* 28, 322, 1949.
32. **Eisenberg, S.,** Blood volume in patients with Laennec's cirrhosis of the liver as determined by radioactive chromium-tapped red cells, *Am. J. Med.,* 20, 189, 1956.
33. **Blendis, L. M., Ramboer, C., and Williams, R.,** Studies on the hemodilution anemia of splenomegaly, *Eur. J. Clin. Invest.,* 1, 54, 1970.
34. **Sherlock, S. and Sheldon, S.,** The etiology and management of ascites in patients with hepatic cirrhosis, *Gut,* 4, 95, 1963.
35. **Bauer, F. K., Blahd, W. H., Fields, M., and Getchell, G.,** Ascitic fluid and plasma protein exchange in cirrhosis of the liver, *Metabolism,* 3, 289, 1954.
36. **Dumont, A. E. and Mulholland, J. H.,** Flow rate and composition of thoracic duct lymph in patients with cirrhosis, *N. Engl. J. Med.,* 263, 471, 1960.
37. **Baldus, W. P., Summerskill, W. H. J., Hunt, J. C., and Maher, F. T.,** Renal circulation in cirrhosis: observation based on catheterization of the renal vein, *J. Clin. Invest.,* 43, 1090, 1964.
38. **Schroeder, E. T., Shear, L., Sancetta, S. M., and Gabuzda, G. J.,** Renal failure in patients with cirrhosis of the liver, *Am. J. Med.,* 43, 887, 1967.
39. **Tristani, F. E., and Cohn, J. N.,** Systemic and renal hemodynamics in oliguric hepatic failure. Effect of volume expansion, *J. Clin. Invest.,* 46, 1894, 1967.
40. **Lieberman, F. L. and Reynolds, T. B.,** Plasma volume in cirrhosis of the liver. Its relation to portal hypertension, ascites and renal failure, *J. Clin. Invest.,* 46, 1297, 1967.
41. **Lieberman, F. L., Ko, S., and Reynolds, T. B.,** Effective plasma volume in cirrhosis with ascites, *J. Clin. Invest.,* 48, 975, 1969.
42. **Better, O. S. and Schrier, R. W.,** Disturbed volume homeostasis in patients with cirrhosis of the liver, *Kidney Inter.,* 23, 303, 1983.
43. **Levy, M. and Allotey, G. B. K.,** Temporal relationships between urinary salt retention and altered systemic hemodynamics in dogs with experimental cirrhosis, *J. Lab. Clin. Med.,* 92, 560, 1978.
44. **Bernardi, M., Trevisani, F., Santini, C., De Palma, R., and Gasbarrini, G.,** Aldosterone related blood volume expansion in cirrhosis before and during the early phase of ascites formation, *Gut,* 24, 761, 1983.
45. **Epstein, M., Pins, D., Schneider, N., and Levinson, R.,** Determinants of deranged sodium and water homeostasis in decompensated cirrhosis, *J. Lab. Clin. Med.,* 87, 822, 1976.
46. **Blendis, L. M., Greig, P. D., Langer, B., Baigrie, R. S., Ruse, J., and Taylor, B.,** The renal and hemodynamic effects of the peritoneovenous shunt for intractable hepatic ascites, *Gastroenterology,* 77, 250, 1979.

47. **Epstein, M., Berk, D. P., and Hollenberg, N. K.,** Renal failure in the patient with cirrhosis. The role of active vasoconstriction, *Am. J. Med.,* 49, 175, 1970.
48. **Kew, M. C., Brunt, P. W., Varma, P. R., Hourigan, K. J., Williams, H. S., and Sherlock, S.,** Renal and intrarenal blood flow in cirrhosis of the liver, *Lancet,* 2, 504, 1971.
49. **Unikowsky, B., Wexler, M. J., and Levy, M.,** Dogs with experimental cirrhosis of the liver, but without intrahepatic hypertension, do not retain sodium or form ascites, *J. Clin. Invest.,* 72, 1594, 1983.
50. **Greig, P. D., Blendis, L. M., Langer, B., Taylor, B. R., and Colapinto, R. F.,** The renal and hemodynamic effects of the peritoneovenous shunt. Long term effect, *Gastroenterology,* 60, 546, 1981.
51. **Ring-Larsen, H.,** Hepatic nephropathy, related to hemodynamics, *Liver,* 3, 265, 1983.
52. **Koppel, M. H., Coburn, J. W., Mims, M. M., Goldstein, H., Boyle, J. D., and Rubini, M. E.,** Transplantation of cadaveric kidneys from patients with hepatorenal syndrome, *N. Engl. J. Med.,* 280, 1367, 1969.
53. **Iwatsuki, S., Popovitzer, M. M., Corman, J. L., Ishikawa, M., Putnam, C. W., Katz, F. H., and Starzl, T. E.,** Recovery from hepatorenal syndrome after orthotopic liver transplantation, *N. Engl. J. Med.,* 289, 1155, 1973.
54. **Lunzer, M. R., Newman, S. P., Bernard, A. G., Manghani, K. K., Sherlock, S., Ginsburg, J.,** Impaired cardiovascular responsiveness in liver disease, *Lancet,* 2, 382, 1975.
55. **Henriksen, J. H., Christensen, N. J., and Ring-Larsen, H.,** Noradrenaline and adrenaline in various vascular beds in patients with cirrhosis. Relation to haemodynamics, *Clin. Physiol.,* 1, 293, 1981.
56. **Morandini, G. and Spanedda, M.,** Contributo allo studio della reattivita vascolare periferica all'angiotensina ed all noradrenalina in corso di affezioni epatiche, *Minerva Med.,* 57, 2175, 1966.
57. **Morandini, G., Spanedda, M., and Spanedda, L.,** La riposta pressoria all'angiotensina e all noradrenalina in soggetti con affezioni epatiche, *Minerva Med.,* 58, 1794, 1967.
58. **Saito, H.,** Clinical and experimental studies on the hyperdynamic states in obstructive jaundice, *J. Jpn. Surg. Soc.,* 82, 483, 1981.
59. **Pitt, H. A., Cameron, J. L., and Postier, R. G.,** Factors affecting morbidity and mortality after surgery for obstructive jaundice; a review of 373 patients, *Am. J. Surg.,* 141, 66, 1981.
60. **Nixon, J. M., Armstrong, C. P., and Duffy, S. W.,** Factors affecting morbidity and mortality after surgery for obstructive jaundice; a review of 373 patients, *Gut.,* 24, 845, 1983.
61. **Schrier, R. W., Arroyo, V., Bernardi, M., Epstein, M., Henricksen, J. H., and Rodes, J.,** Peripheral arterial vasodilatation hypothesis. A proposal for the inhibition of renal sodium and water retention in cirrhosis, *Hepatology,* 8, 1151, 1988.
62. **Zipser, R. D., Hoefs, J. C., Speckart, P. F., Zia, P. K., and Horton, R.,** Prostaglandin modulations of renal function and pressor resistance in chronic liver disease, *J. Clin. Endocrinol. Metab.,* 48, 895, 1979.
63. **Arroyo, V., Planas, R., Gaya, J., and Rodes, J.,** Sympathetic nervous activity, renin-angiotensin system and renal excretion of PGE_2 in cirrhosis. Relationship to functional renal failure and sodium and water excretion, *Eur. J. Clin. Invest.,* 13, 271, 1983.
64. **deBold, A. J., Borenstein, H. B., Veress, A. T., and Sonnenberg, H.,** A rapid and potent natriuretic response to intravenous injection of atrial myocardial extract in rats, *Life Sci.,* 28, 89, 1981.
65. **Lebrec, D., Novel, O., Corbic, M., and Benhamou, J. P.,** Propranolol, a medical treatment for portal hypertension, *Lancet,* 2, 180, 1980.
66. **Lebrec, D., Hillon, P., Munoz, C., Goldfarb, G., Nouel, O., and Benhamou, J. P.,** The effect of propranolol on portal hypertension in patients with cirrhosis. A hemodynamic study, *Hepatology,* 2, 523, 1982.
67. **Lebrec, D., Poynard, T., Hillon, P., and Benhamou, J. P.,** Propranolol for prevention of recurrent gastrointestinal bleeding in patients with cirrhosis. A controlled trial, *N. Engl. J. Med.,* 305, 1371, 1981.
68. **Burroughs, A. K., Jenkins, W. J., Sherlock, S., Dunk, A., Walt, R. P., Osuaport, O. K., Mackie, S., and Dick, R.,** Controlled trial of propranolol for the prevention of recurrent variceal hemorrhage in patients with cirrhosis, *N. Engl. J. Med.,* 309, 1539, 1983.
69. **Villeneuve, J. P., Pomier-Layrargues, G., Infante-Rivard, C., Willems, B., Huet, P. M., Marleau, D., and Viallet, A.,** Propranolol for the prevention of recurrent variceal hemorrhage. A controlled trial, *Hepatology,* 6, 1239, 1986.
70. **Conn, H.,** Prophylactic propranolol. The first big step, *Hepatology,* 8, 167, 1988.
71. **Pascal, J. P. and Cales, P.,** Multicenter study group. Propranolol in the prevention of first upper gastrointestinal tract hemorrhage in patients with cirrhosis of the liver and esophageal varices, *N. Engl. J. Med.,* 317, 856, 1987.

Chapter 2

ANIMAL MODELS OF LIVER DISEASE

Arieh Bomzon and Laurence M. Blendis

TABLE OF CONTENTS

I. INTRODUCTION

Altered cardiovascular function has been described in patients with cirrhosis and in jaundiced patients, irrespective of the etiology. These cardiovascular complications have been outlined in Chapter 1 of this book.[1] Ethical considerations limit the extent to which these complications can be investigated in patients with liver disease. Hence, animal models of these diseases have been developed to enable clinical investigators to undertake research into these complications. Table 1 summarizes the two principal routes in which cirrhosis and hyperbilirubinemia are induced in laboratory animals. In this chapter, we have chosen to describe and discuss the cardiovascular changes and their sequence of onset in surgically induced and drug-induced cirrhosis. We have also attempted to critically evaluate the appropriateness of these models in their ability to mimic the cardiovascular complications of jaundice, cirrhosis, and portal hypertension as seen in the clinical environment.

II. SURGICALLY INDUCED CIRRHOSIS

A. BILE DUCT LIGATION

Of all the animal models of liver disease, ligation of the common bile duct is the most widely used method in experimental animals to reproduce human cirrhosis. Most of the information which we have obtained using this method has been derived from observations in bile duct of dogs and rats. The popular use of these two animal models is probably attributable to the ease at which the disease process can be induced together with the relative rapid onset of the clinical features of cirrhosis. Since cirrhosis and its complications in these models are preceded by jaundice, the bile duct-ligated animal can also be used to study the effects of jaundice on the cardiovascular system. The jaundice phase is of varying duration and depth both of which are species-dependent as well as being dependent upon whether the bile duct has been only ligated, or ligated and resected.

Figure 1 describes this variability as measured by the plasma total bilirubin concentrations in the bile duct-ligated dog, rat, rabbit and baboon. It can be seen that in the dog, bile duct ligation only results in a moderate hyperbilirubinemia which may not be present after 3 to 4 weeks, by which time the animal is beginning to develop portal hypertension (Figure 2). On the other hand, ligation and resection in the dog induces a more severe hyperbilirubinemia which can persist for at least 10 weeks, by which time the animal has histological evidence of secondary biliary cirrhosis. In the rat, ligation without resection results in a rapid onset of hyperbilirubinemia and hepatocellular damage which reverse themselves completely within 2 weeks (Figures 1, 3). In contrast, ligation and resection in this animal result in secondary biliary cirrhosis with an accompanying jaundice by the end of the 4th week, and is not unlike that seen in the dogs (Figure 3). In the rabbit and baboon, bile duct ligation is associated with the development of hyperbilirubinemia but there are no long-term studies that have demonstrated that these two species ultimately develop cirrhosis.

1. Bile Duct Ligation in the Dog

The sequence of the onset of the primary cardiovascular complications following bile duct ligation in the dog are described in Figure 2. This picture has been derived from numerous investigators who measured some of these parameters in dogs whose bile ducts had been ligated with and without resection of varying duration. This information is summarized in Table 2 and it can be seen that most of the measurements were made in anesthetized animals, which itself can modify cardiovascular function and performance. For example, phenobarbitone-anesthetized bile duct-ligated dogs have heart rates almost twice that of conscious bile duct-ligated dogs.[2]

In the dog, four postoperative phases can be identified. The first phase is of short

TABLE 1
The Animal Models of Cirrhosis
Classified in Accordance with
the Method of Induction

Surgically induced cirrhosis
Bile duct ligation
Portal vein stenosis
Drug-induced cirrhosis
Carbon tetrachloride
Dimethylnitrosamine

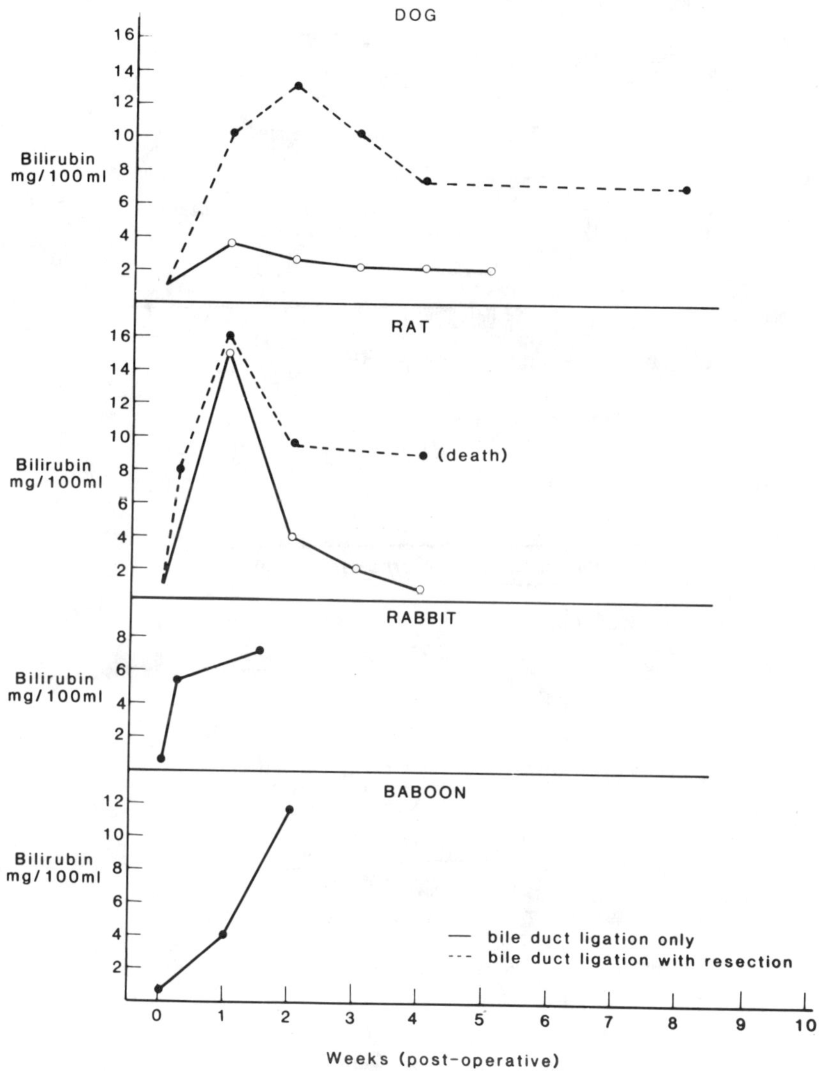

FIGURE 1.   Postoperative changes over time in the serum total bilirubin concentrations in bile duct-ligated dogs (A), rats (B), rabbits (C) and baboons. (From Better, O. S. and Bomzon, A., The effects of jaundice on the renal and cardiovascular systems, in *The Kidney and Liver Disease*, 3rd ed., Epstein, M., Ed., copyright © by Williams & Wilkins, Baltimore, 1988. With permission.)

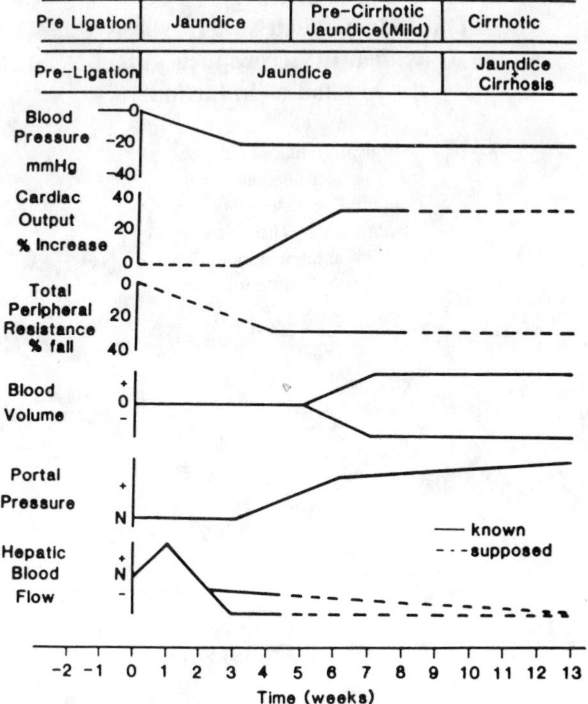

FIGURE 2.   The changes with time of the cardiovascular complications in dogs that underwent bile duct ligation only and bile duct ligation and resection.

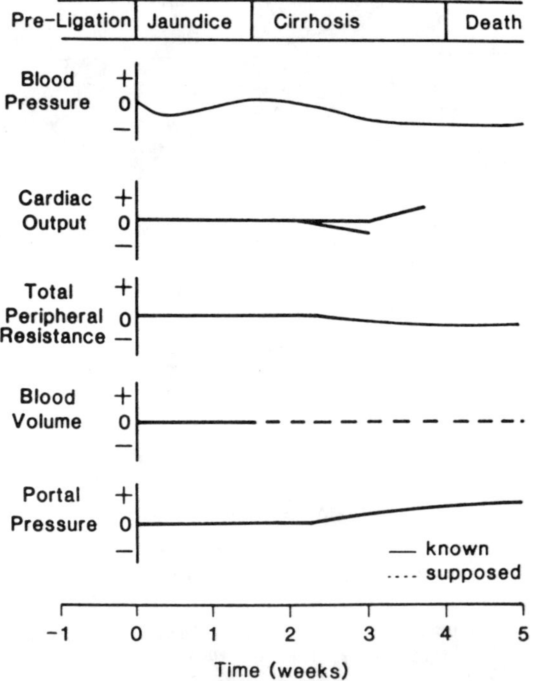

FIGURE 3.   The changes with time of the cardiovascular complications in rats that underwent bile duct ligation and resection.

TABLE 2

The Experimental Conditions under Which Cardiovascular Function Was Measured in Dogs Whose Bile Ducts Were Ligated for Varying Periods

Anesthesia	Ligation only	Ligation with/without division and/ or resection	Duration of the ligation	Ref.
−		+	3—21 d	3
−		+	3—21 d	4
+		+	2 weeks	5
−		+	1—2 weeks	6
−	+		1—2 weeks	7
−	+		1—3 weeks	8
−	+		1—3 weeks	9
+		+	1—4 weeks	10
−	+		1—5 weeks	11
−	+		1—12 weeks	12
+	+		3 weeks	13
+	+		5 weeks	14
+		+	6 weeks	15
+		+	6 weeks	16
+	+		6—8 weeks	17
+	+		6—8 weeks	18
+		+	6—12 weeks	19
+		+	7—13 weeks	20

duration and usually never exceeds 2 days. It is characterized by weight loss and the development of jaundice. Balance studies have not been done, but in our experience, fluid intake appears to be normal although food intake is reduced. The principal cardiovascular change is a tendency to systemic hypotension which appears to be primarily due to a fall in the total peripheral resistance as opposed to altered cardiac function. Hepatic blood flow is increasing although portal hypertension is not evident. This increase in hepatic blood flow is probably a reactive hyperemia to the hepatocellular damage following the extrahepatic obstruction. It should be also noted that over this period, diuresis, associated with a natriuresis and kaliuresis, occurs. A possible explanation of this diuretic response is an increase in renal perfusion with inhibition of the tubular reabsorptive processes by hepatically derived compounds, whose normal excretory route has been blocked, e.g., bile acids. Despite this diuretic response, blood volume is apparently unchanged. While volume status of bile duct-ligated dogs in this phase remains unresolved, it should be noted that the hematocrit of these animals is reduced. Last, it is claimed that there is peripheral arteriovenous shunting in these animals. Although this feature is consistent with clinical cirrhosis, it is difficult to concede that these shunts arise within the first few postoperative days.

The duration of phase 2 is from the 2nd day to the end of the 2nd postoperative week. Fluid and food intake appear to be normal, and there are no further losses in weight. In the dogs whose common bile duct was ligated without resection, the hyperbilirubinemia has almost dissipated. In contrast, in dogs that underwent ligation and resection, hyperbilirubinemia is still evident. The fall in blood pressure is maximal. Hepatic blood flow begins to decline and, if measured during this period, it may even be normal. By the end of the third week, it has dropped to below the normal values. Portal pressure is normal and blood volume is unchanged. The initial diuretic response is no longer evident. A low hematocrit is still present. Arteriovenous shunts have been reported to be present. It is possible that, at this stage, shunts are beginning to develop, since the model is "volatile," as many physical and cardiovascular changes are occurring simultaneously.

Some, but not all, of these aforementioned changes of both phases 1 and 2 have been described in isolated cholemia in which the bile outflow has been diverted directly into the circulation by a choleductocaval anastomosis.[21,22] In this model, the dog has plasma total bilirubin concentrations as high as 60 mg/100 mls (1 mmol/dl) without hepatocellular damage. Information on the cardiovascular system and its function is limited. In addition to the features which are shown in Figure 3, impaired left ventricular performance has been demonstrated in these dogs.[22]

Phase three is best described as the precirrhotic phase, since portal pressure begins to rise in spite of the tendency to or existence of systemic hypotension. The phase is of variable duration and begins from the 3rd postoperative week and extends to about the 10th week, when secondary biliary cirrhosis is histologically established. The early changes in liver histiology are nonspecific with some signs of fibroblast activity around the biliary canaliculi, but by between the 10th to the 16th week, secondary biliary cirrhosis is histologically established. Hepatic blood flow is decreased. The status of blood volume during this phase is controversial since it has variously been reported that blood volume is unchanged, increased, and decreased. Some investigators have reported that ascites may be present as early as the 4th week, but by the end of the 10th week, a measurable proportion of dogs have developed ascites. Renal perfusion has been reported as unchanged during this phase. This contrasts with the elevated renal perfusion of phase 1. One can only assume that, during phase 2, renal perfusion returns to normal and remains so in spite of "fluctuations" in splanchnic capacitance and intravascular volume. As anticipated, peripheral arteriovenous shunts are present.

Phase four is the phase in which all the cardiovascular complications associated with cirrhosis are evident. These include a hyperdynamic circulation, portal hypertension and the presence of ascites. A stable, unaltered renal perfusion appears to be present by this time.

While this picture describes the temporal changes in the cardiovascular parameters following bile duct ligation in the dog and verifies the validity of this model to study the cardiovascular complications of liver diseases, it does not take into account the changes in cardiovascular responsiveness, which have also been described in patients with cirrhosis and jaundiced individuals. Although many of these latter features are described in other chapters, only a few laboratories have undertaken studies in which function was assessed in this model. Furthermore, when these function studies were performed, they were measured at a single time point and it was assumed that the aberration was present throughout the whole postoperative period. For example, Morandini and colleagues[23,24] demonstrated that both jaundiced patients and patients with cirrhosis have blunted pressor responsiveness to the sympathetic neurotransmitter, norepinephrine and angiotensin II. The Haifa group of Bomzon, Better, and others[7-9] have shown that bile duct-ligated dogs of 1 to 3 weeks duration, i. e., in phase 2, have blunted pressor responses to a variety of vasoactive amines such as norepinephrine and isoproterenol. These authors then assumed that this loss of pressor response explained the tendency to hypotension in jaundice as well as in cirrhosis. However, a recent study performed in bile duct-ligated dogs of 12 weeks duration, i.e., in phase 4, by Bomzon et al.,[12] demonstrated that the pressor responses to the same amines was intact. In other words, blunted responsiveness to amines may partly account for the systemic hypotension observed in hyperbilirubinemia, but it cannot be included as part of the explanation for systemic hypotension in this model of cirrhosis. This is certainly not so for angiotensin responsiveness which was found to be blunted at all postoperative times.

Last, it should be noted that the status and role of cardiovascular regulatory systems, viz., the renin-angiotensin-aldosterone and the sympathetic nervous systems is an unknown entity at any one of the four phases. Studies undertaken by Naveh and colleagues[11], and Winaver et al.,[16] in bile duct-ligated dogs of 1 to 5 weeks, and 6 weeks standing, respectively, found that the plasma renin activities were unchanged by the procedure. Saito[13] described a blunted or suppressed rise in blood pressure following carotid occlusion in anesthetized 3- week bile duct-ligated dogs with an intact vagus nerve. However, the response could be

TABLE 3

**The Experimental Conditions under Which Cardiovascular Function Was
Measured in Rats Whose Bile Ducts Were Ligated for Varying Periods**

Anesthesia	Ligation only	Ligation with/without division and/or resection	Duration of the ligation	Ref.
–		+	1—7d	25
–	+		3 d	26
Pithed	+		3 d	27
Pithed	+		3 d	28
–	+		6 d	29
+		+	7 d	30
+		+	7 d	31
+	+		7 d	32
+	+		8 d	33
–	+		8—10 d	34
+		+	14—28 d	35
+		+	15—33 d	36
+		+	21 d	37
+		+	21 d	38
–		+	28 d	39
+		+	28 d	39
Pithed	+		28—40 d	27

restored when the vagus was cut, although basal blood pressure and peripheral resistance were still reduced. This result suggests that there is a defect in the baroreceptor response to hypotension mediated by the vagal component of the carotid sinus nerve.

2. Bile Duct Ligation in the Rat

The sequence of events following bile duct ligation, with and without resection, are quite different from each other, and that observed in the dog. Figure 3 shows the chronological changes in cardiovascular function in this model, and Table 3 summarizes the experimental conditions under which these data have been collected by the various investigators. The important difference between the rat whose bile duct has been ligated without resection and the rat whose duct has been ligated and resected is the ultimate clinical outcome of the procedure itself. In the former instance, the rat does not develop cirrhosis. In fact, the hepatocellular damage induced by the ligation is completely reversible with almost 100% survival. Hence, this animal model is useful to study the cardiovascular complications of acute hepatocellular damage with hyperbilirubinemia. In the latter instance, the rat develops secondary biliary cirrhosis with portal hypertension. As seen in the dog that underwent biliary ligation and resection, hyperbilirubinemia is present in the cirrhotic phase. The mortality rate in this model is high with almost 100% mortality by the end of the 6th week. It is our experience that the onset of mortality can be delayed by performing the ligation and resection in the hilus of the liver as the common bile duct exits from the liver.

In comparing the data obtained from the bile duct-ligated rat to that obtained from the dog, the amount of information is less, and some of the changes are not as striking as that seen in the dog. Moreover, because the time scale is more compressed, and the changes occur rapidly, it is not possible to identify specific phases, especially in the immediate postoperative period.

Irrespective of which surgical procedure is used to obstruct bile flow, in the first few postoperative days, the animal develops hyperbilirubinemia (Figure 1), hypotension (Figure 3) and loses between 10 to 15% of the body weight. As shown in Figure 3, all other parameters appear to be unchanged, with the exception of liver blood flow which is beginning to decrease. The status of renal perfusion is unknown, although it has been suggested that it is reduced. Because of the relatively small magnitude of the cardiovascular changes and the rapidity and enormity at which the physical and "biochemical" changes have occurred, it is difficult to identify which of these changes are attributable to the surgery or the induction of jaundice. Thereafter, the course of the induced disease process is dependent upon the surgical procedure.

In the rat which underwent only ligation of the bile duct, there is a reversal of all the features previously mentioned. In other words, the hyperbilirubinemia, weight loss, and systemic hypotension all disappear and, by the end of the 2nd week, the animal appears clinically normal. In contrast, in those animals that have undergone bile duct ligation with division and/or resection, the animal begins to develop secondary biliary cirrhosis with a hyperdynamic circulation, portal hypertension, splenomegaly and ascites. As seen in the bile duct-ligated dog of long standing, a reduced liver blood flow with intrahepatic shunting is also present. As already mentioned, hyperbilirubinemia is also present.

Almost no data is available on the regulation of cardiovascular function in this model. However, it can be assumed that the activity of the sympathetic nervous system is enhanced since Geoffroy and colleagues[40] found significant elevations in plasma catecholamine concentrations.

3. Bile Duct Ligation in the Rabbit

The biochemical picture immediately following bile duct ligation in the rabbit appears to be identical to that seen in dogs and rats (Figure 1). No studies in rabbits whose bile ducts were ligated longer than 10 days have been reported and hence, the consequences of long-term biliary obstruction are not known. The cardiovascular consequences of surgical-induced extrahepatic obstruction are systemic hypotension, reduced renal blood flow, and an enhanced susceptibility to hemorrhagic shock.[41,41,43] These features are consistent with those that have been described in hyperbilirubinemic states in patients and bile duct-ligated rats, but not in bile duct-ligated dogs. On the basis of these limited data, it would appear that this model is suitable to investigate the cardiovascular complications associated with acute hepatocellular damage and hyperbilirubinemia. Until long term studies are undertaken, one should not consider this animal model suitable to investigate these problems in cirrhosis.

4. Bile Duct Ligation in the Baboon

Evaluation of cardiovascular function in bile duct-ligated baboons were undertaken by Bomzon and his colleagues in the mid 1970s and all of the information has been reviewed by Bomzon and Kew.[44] All the studies were undertaken in the 2-week postligation period during which hyperbilirubinemia and hepatocellular damage associated with normotension were present. The observations from these species are applicable to hyperbilirubinemia and acute hepatocellular damage in man, but not to chronic liver disease. The principal findings of this research group were a time-dependent reduction in renal blood flow and its intrarenal distribution without any change in systemic blood pressure. The reductions in renal perfusion were linked to enhanced responsiveness to norepinephrine due to an increase in the activity of renal α-adrenergic receptors. Additional systemic findings were potentiation of the cerebrovascular responses to norepinephrine and hypocapnea, as well as attenuated responses of the skeletal muscle vasculature to norepinephrine.

Ligation of the bile duct has also been performed in the cat, but there is no information on the cardiovascular consequences of this procedure.[45]

B. PORTAL VEIN STENOSIS

Partial ligation of the portal vein in laboratory animals is the second surgical method in which the cardiovascular complications of liver disease have been studied. The model differs from bile duct ligation in that portal hypertension, without liver pathology, occurs. The other

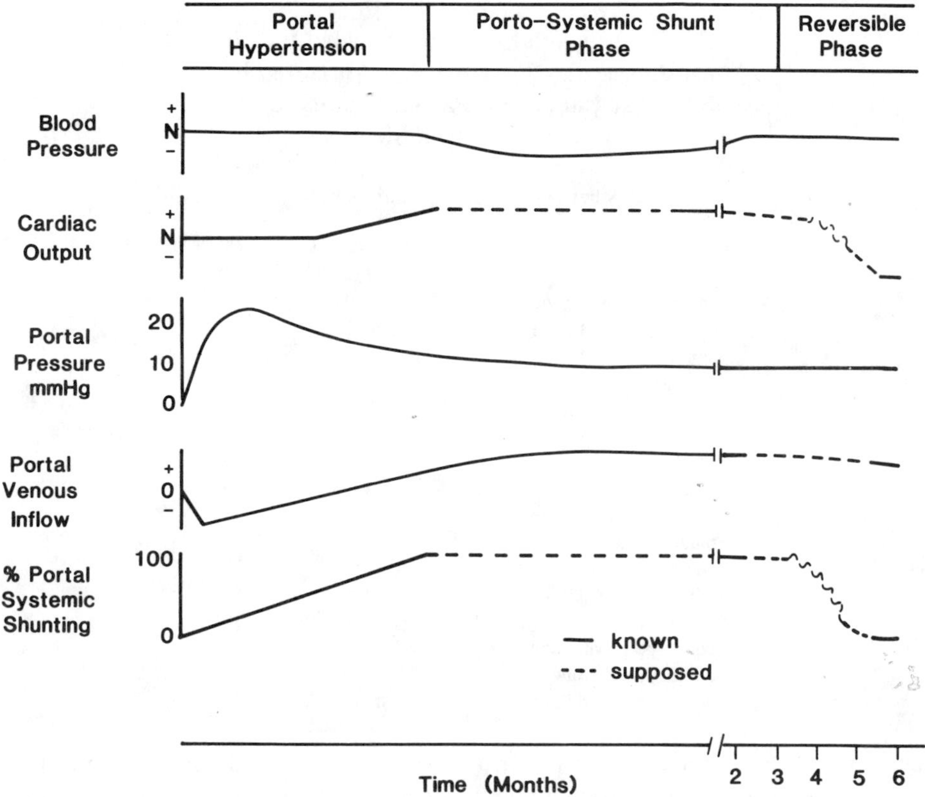

FIGURE 4.   The changes with time of the cardiovascular complications in rats that underwent partial ligation of the portal vein.

obvious differences between these two models are the absence of hyperbilirubinemia, and the more rapid onset of portal hypertension. Of the experimental animals that have undergone partial ligation of the portal vein, most of the cardiovascular data has been collected in the laboratory rat, with some information gleaned from the dog. Before discussing the model in more detail, it should be borne in mind that this model is the one of choice of hepatologists who are concerned with the pathogenesis and treatment of portal hypertension and its consequences. Thus, this model has proved most valuable in understanding the cardiovascular relationships between portal pressure and splanchnic blood flow, as portal hypertension and portosystemic shunting develop, following partial ligation of the portal vein.

1. Portal Vein Stenosis in the Rat

Figure 4 describes the onset of the cardiovascular complications following partial ligation of the portal vein in the rat. The primary sources of this information are listed in Table 4, which details the experimental conditions under which the data has been obtained. It can be seen that all the data, with one exception, have been obtained in anesthetized rats. It should also be noted that all of the investigators used radiolabeled microspheres to obtain their data. Although this technique can give valuable information on systemic hemodynamics and the distribution of cardiac output following the development of portal hypertension, the technique itself imposes certain limitations on the type of data which can be collected. Two of these limitations are (1) that it is customary to do these studies under anesthesia and (2) that time course studies in the same animal are difficult. The untoward impact of anesthesia on splanchnic hemodynamics has been described.[59,63] With regard to temporal studies in the

TABLE 4
**The Experimental Conditions under Which
Cardiovascular Function Was Measured in
Rats That Underwent Partial Ligation of the
Portal Vein (Portal Stenosis)**

Anesthesia	Duration	Ref.
Ketamine	1—14 d	46
Ether	2 d	47
Sodium pentobarbitone	8—10 d	48
Sodium pentobarbitone	10 d	49
Sodium pentobarbitone	10 d	50
Chloralose/urethane	10 d	51
Sodium pentobarbitone	10 d	52
Ketamine	14 d	53
Ketamine	14 d	54
Ketamine	14 d	55
Sodium pentobarbitone	20 d	56
Sodium pentobarbitone	21 d	57
Sodium pentobarbitone	21 d	58
Sodium pentobarbitone	21 d	59
Conscious	21 d	59
Sodium pentobarbitone	21—28 d	60
Sodium pentobarbitone	80—90 d	61
Sodium pentobarbitone	6 months	62

same animal, the determination of regional blood flow involves killing the animal and counting the distribution of radioactivity to the organs. Since the microspheres are trapped in the capillaries, their successive injections can potentially alter organ perfusion by a progressive accumulation of trapped microspheres.

Three postoperative phases can be identified following partial ligation of the portal vein. The first phase is the response to the partial ligation in which there is an immediate increase in portal pressure, and a drop in portal venous inflow with its subsequent recovery. The duration of this phase is about 2 weeks. The return of portal venous inflow is intimately linked with the development of portal systemic shunting, which may be maximal by the end of the phase. The increase in venous return, due to shunt development, causes the cardiac output to increase. There are some reports that hepatic arterial blood flow may increase. Despite these changes in the redistribution of cardiac output and shunt development, systemic blood pressure remains constant.

The second phase begins from the end of the 2nd week but its end has not been established. In its early stages, this phase is characterized by portal hypertension, a marked increase in portal venous inflow and portal systemic shunting. Cardiac output is increased and there is a tendency to hypotension. Groszmann and his colleagues[55] were able to reverse arterial hypertension in spontaneously hypertensive rats, following partial ligation of the portal vein. Using microspheres, they were able to demonstrate that the induction of portal hypertension was associated with a generalized reduction in regional vascular resistance. The degree of portosystemic shunting has been disputed by Blanchet and Lebrec[57] and by Lopez-Novoa and his co-workers.[61] They claim that there is considerable variation in shunting, following partial ligation ranging from 1 to 100%, and this variability influences the cardiac output and its distribution, and individual organ perfusion.

The time point which can be ascribed as the end of this phase is difficult to identify because of the lack of long-term studies in this model. The end may be defined as when portal venous inflow, portosystemic shunting, and cardiac output begin to fall towards normal values, in spite of the persistence of portal hypertension. It appears that it may begin to occur around the end of the 3rd postoperative month when some of the changes begin to fall towards normal values, since in phase 3, some of the parameters are normal.[62]

The third phase can be described as a reversal phase in which the previously increased portal venous inflow and cardiac output have returned to within normal values. The rate of return to normal is unknown, but as noted by Sikuler and Groszmann,[62] the animal no longer has the hemodynamic characteristics of the hyperdynamic circulation. Portal hypertension and portosystemic shunting are still present.

In this model, it can be assumed that there is an increase in the activity of the sympathetic nervous system since plasma catecholamine concentrations[40] and renin activity[61] are elevated in this model. Since there is only a tendency to hypotension, it can be assumed that the compensatory responses of the sympathetic nervous and renin-angiotensin-aldosterone systems are adequate to maintain normotension following the induction of portal hypertension in normotensive rats. In contrast, the induction of portal hypertension in spontaneously systemic hypertensive rats is associated with a reversal of systemic hypertension and generalized reduction in vascular resistance.[55] Furthermore, these investigators suggested that one or more vasodilators may impair the hyperresponsiveness to vasoactive stimuli in these animals. The nature of these vasodilators was not defined although bile acids were implicated as participating in this phenomenon.

2. Portal Vein Stenosis in the Dog

In 1951, Morris and Miller[64] described their attempt to establish a canine model of portal hypertension. In order to establish a successful model, it was necessary to occlude the portal vein gradually. In other words, the induction of portal hypertension in the dog was not a simple one-step procedure but involved, at least, two surgical interventions. In a recent symposium on animal models of portal hypertension, Sharma and Shoennut[64] described their model of portal hypertension in the dog and confirmed that the induction of a satisfactory canine model of portal hypertension is a more difficult undertaking than that in the laboratory rat. All of the publications are oriented towards the different methodologies that have been attempted in order to establish this model. Because the model has been difficult to establish, little information is known about the sequential changes in cardiovascular function. The information contained therein give data on portal pressure and the presence of portosystemic shunts. In the dog, portal pressure rises from a baseline of 12 mmHg to as high as 23 mmHg after 15 weeks and then falls to about 17 mmHg after 28 weeks. There is no information pertaining to systemic hemodynamics.

3. Portal Vein Stenosis in Other Species

Pigs and rabbits have also been used by numerous investigators to establish an animal-model of portal hypertension. While it appears that it is easier to do so in these species, the systemic consequences of the procedure have not been documented.[66,67]

III. DRUG-INDUCED CIRRHOSIS

An alternate method of inducing cirrhosis in experimental animals is by the administration of hepatotoxins. Of all the known hepatotoxins, two such compounds have been successfully used to induce cirrhosis — carbon tetrachloride in the rat and dimethylnitrosamine in the dog. In both instances, the toxin is administered for a period of time and then the evaluation of the cardiovascular system was made. In other words, more often than not, most of the information which has been obtained in these models was at a point when cirrhosis was present. Furthermore, much of the source material, which as been utilized to present the sequential changes in cardiovascular function, has been taken from studies whose primary object was to evaluate sodium retention and ascites formation. In these studies, evaluation of cardiovascular function was only of secondary importance and, as a result, the picture is incomplete.

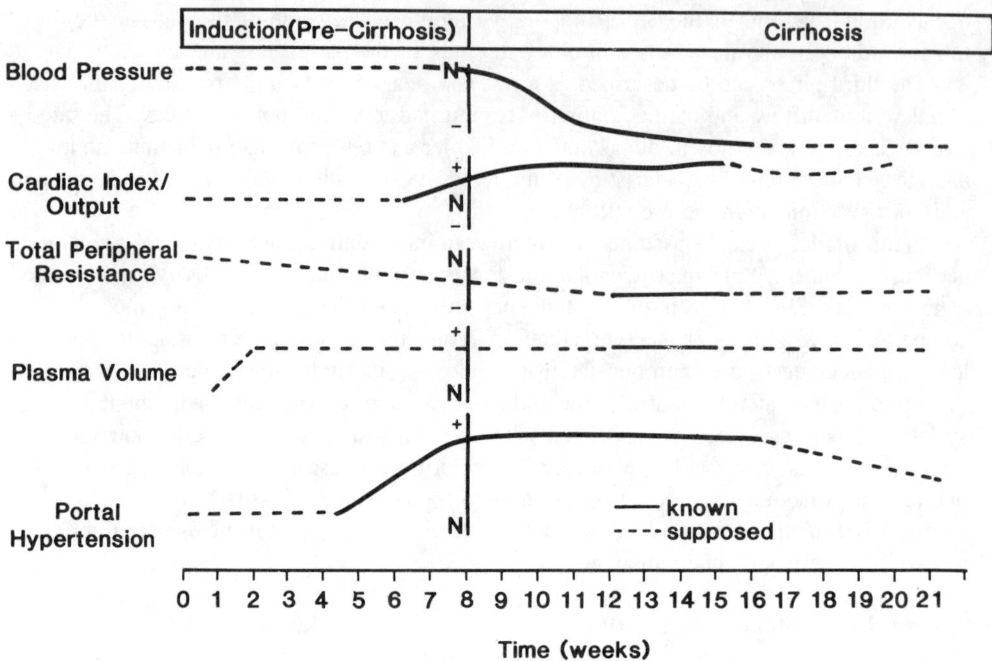

FIGURE 5.   The changes with time of the cardiovascular complications in carbon tetrachloride-induced cirrhosis in rats.

A. CARBON TETRACHLORIDE-INDUCED CIRRHOSIS IN THE RAT

In 1969, McLean and colleagues[68] described the technique for inducing cirrhosis in the laboratory rat, using the toxin, carbon tetrachloride. Since then, the technique has been modified inasmuch that the route of administration of the toxin can be by inhalation, per os, or by subcutaneous or intramuscular injection. Irrespective of the route of administration, successful induction of cirrhosis involves pretreatment with a long acting barbiturate, usually phenobarbitone, for 2 weeks. Phenobarbitone is an inducer of the hepatic cytochrome P450 system and its induction enables the animal to survive the near-lethal doses of administered carbon tetrachloride, often given as frequently as every 4 days for as long as 10 months. Most investigators usually treat the rats for 8 to 12 weeks and report that the histological proven cirrhosis is present after this period. Last, it should be noted that the cessation of administration results in spontaneous reversal of the hepatocellular damage, but it is not known whether the hyperdynamic circulation disappears.

Figure 5 describes the sequence of changes in this model from the time of commencement of the administration of carbon tetrachloride to 22 weeks. The source material for this diagram can be found in References 70 to 82. In this model, all the features of a hyperdynamic circulation can be seen after 8 to 12 weeks of treatment with the hepatotoxin. In addition, it should be noted that portal hypertension preceded the onset of systemic changes. Changes in hepatic microcirculation occur and are characterized by the development of intrahepatic shunts and a reduction in hepatic perfusion. Portosystemic shunting of varying degrees is also present.

The status of the regulatory systems, viz., the renin-angiotensin system and sympathetic nervous system, is poorly defined in this model. Lopez-Novoa[82] reported that plasma renin activity was not elevated whereas Murray and Paller[83] claimed that it was significantly elevated. Both plasma aldosterone concentrations and atrial natriuretic factor concentrations have recently been reported to be elevated in this model.[84] It has been postulated that the basis for the systemic hypotension is due to these elevated concentrations of the atrial peptide and decreased responsiveness to angiotensin II.[82,83]

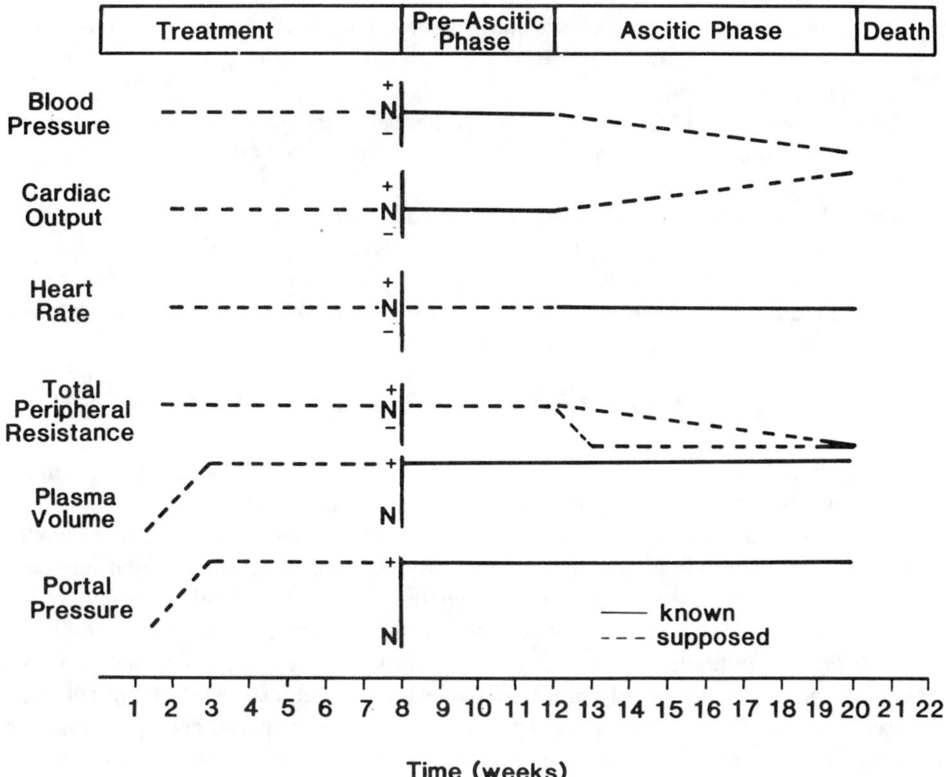

FIGURE 6.   The changes with time of the cardiovascular complications in dimethylnitrosamine-induced cirrhosis in dogs.

The activity of the sympathetic nervous system, especially to the kidney, is enhanced. This has been shown by direct measurement of renal nerve activity[85,86] and indirectly by measurement of urinary catecholamine excretion.[87]

All of these observations on the renin-angiotensin-aldosterone system, atrial natriuretic peptide and renal nerve activity are consistent with what has been observed in patients.[88-90]

B. DIMETHYLNITROSAMINE-INDUCED CIRRHOSIS IN THE DOG

In 1970, Madden and colleagues[91] announced that intermittent oral administration of dimethylnitrosamine for 4 weeks produced hepatic cirrhosis which was stable or progressive for at least 5 months after discontinuing the drug. They reported that the animal developed histological proven cirrhosis with portal hypertension and portosystemic shunts in which a direct correlation between the histological and circulatory abnormalities was present.[92,93] The model was also used by Levy and his colleagues to study the temporal relationships between sodium retention, ascites formation and systemic abnormalities.[95-99]

Using this source material, Figure 6 describes the sequential changes in cardiovascular function as the disease progresses. Four arbitrary phases can be described:

1.   A treatment phase in which the dimethylnitrosamine is administered. During this phase, almost no information is known except that portal hypertension and portosystemic shunting develop soon after the commencement of treatment.
2.   A preascitic phase in which systemic hemodynamics appear to be normal but sodium retention is occurring. Plasma volume is increased and is associated with systemic normotension.

3.   An ascitic phase during which systemic hypotension and elevations in cardiac output can be observed. During this phase, all the cardiovascular features of the hyperdynamic circulation are present.
4.   The fatal phase in which the animal usually dies following gastrointestinal hemorrhage. Often, the animal develops jaundice immediately prior to its death.

Further studies with this toxin have not been undertaken since it is a human carcinogen. Because of the potential danger to the personnel involved in its administration to animals, further studies in this model were discontinued. Hence, no additional information on the regulation of the cardiovascular function in this model is available. However, a recent report describes its use in the laboratory rat to induce cirrhosis.[99]

IV. COMPARISON BETWEEN THE ANIMAL MODELS

Having described the principal cardiovascular features between the animal models, in this section we will attempt to highlight their similarities and differences.

Irrespective of the method in which cirrhosis has been induced, all the animal models develop a hyperdynamic circulation, i.e., systemic hypotension, a decrease in total peripheral resistance, an elevated cardiac output, portal hypertension, portosystemic shunting, and an apparent hypervolemia. The time point at which all these features are present in any of the models differ. Furthermore, the sequence or the order of onset of the elements that contribute to the overall picture of the hyperdynamic circulation differs. This can be seen if one compares the onset times for the appearance of changes in the systemic, portal and splanchnic circulations. In the dimethylnitrosamine-induced cirrhotic dog and the carbon tetrachloride-induced cirrhotic rat, one can see that both models are similar in many respects. It would appear that portal hypertension and hypervolemia precede the onset of systemic hypotension and changes in total peripheral resistance. In other words, altered portal and splanchnic hemodynamics precede the systemic changes. This sequence of onset of change is also observed in the rat which has undergone partial ligation of the portal vein. However, this contrasts with the observations in the animal models of cirrhosis induced by ligation of the bile duct. In these animals, the systemic events occur before the onset of portal hypertension and changes in splanchnic hemodynamics.

Another feature that necessitates some comment is the necessity of hepatocellular damage in the development of the hyperdynamic circulation. Since the portal stenotic rat develops all the features of a hyperdynamic circulation, it would appear that hepatocellular damage is not critical to the development of the cardiovascular complications of liver disease. Indeed this appears to be the case, even if the hepatocellular damage was induced by hepatotoxins or surgical obstruction of biliary outflow. While the histological pictures differ, all the features of a hyperdynamic circulation can be described, indicating that the etiology of the hepatocellular damage per se is also not important for the development of the hyperdynamic circulation.

The third factor that one needs to consider is the influence of jaundice. The studies in the bile duct-ligated animals indicate a cardiovascular depressant role for hyperbilirubinemia. When hyperbilirubinemia is present, the ability of the cardiovascular system to respond is diminished. If one thus compares the models and the presence of jaundice, the severity of the complications is greater when there is coexisting hyperbilirubinemia and portal hypertension.

V. HUMAN CIRRHOSIS AND THE ANIMAL MODELS

In the light of these comments, which of these models are appropriate to study the cardiovascular complications of chronic liver disease? In 1970, Madden and colleagues[91] felt that the appropriate model of human cirrhosis should fulfil the following criteria:

1. The hepatic lesions should duplicate human pathology,
2. The hepatic pathology should not disappear when the inducing agent is removed,
3. The portal circulatory and physiological abnormalities should correlate with the liver histology, and
4. The models should be inexpensive to prepare and the hepatic lesions rapidly produced.

Sherlock[100] defined cirrhosis as "widespread hepatic fibrosis with nodule formation". Moreover, fibrosis is not synonymous with cirrhosis, but nodule formation without fibrosis is not cirrhosis. In the various animal models in which hepatocellular damage has been induced, the histological pictures differ despite the end result being similar. As previously mentioned, the prerequisite for hepatocellular damage is not critical since all the features of a hyperdynamic circulation can be observed in the absence of hepatocellular damage.

The only model that appears to satisfy the second criterion for a successful animal model of cirrhosis is the chronic bile duct-ligated dog since all the features of cirrhosis persist for a long time after ligation of the bile duct. The dimethylnitrosamine-induced cirrhotic dog appears also to be suitable but the hepatoxin is a known carcinogen. The surgically induced rat models are not always suitable since the changes occur rapidly and are often reversible. Cessation of treatment with carbon tetrachloride in the rat results in spontaneous reversal of the micronodular cirrhosis irrespective of the duration of treatment.

In all the models, there is no correlation between the degree of liver pathology and the portal and systemic changes. In fact, an inverse correlation exists in the portal stenotic rat where portosystemic shunting can be as high as 100% in the absence of any hepatic pathology.

Last, Madden and his colleagues felt that the models should be inexpensive to reproduce and the hepatic lesions should be induced rapidly. In the models which we have presented, it can be seen that in the rat the changes can be induced rapidly but the speed at which they occur, especially in the surgical-induced models, is such that it is not possible to separate out the independent effects of surgery and the disease itself. Second, despite the slower onset of the changes such as occur in the bile duct-ligated rat and dog, hyperbilirubinemia is often an unwanted complication.

VI. CONCLUSIONS

As already mentioned, all the features of a hyperdynamic circulation can be observed in all the animal models. This circulation is present, irrespective of the method employed to induce cirrhosis. It is also obvious that the criteria stated by Madden and his colleagues,[90] although useful, cannot be used as the sole guidelines for the selection of an appropriate animal model.

If this is so, is there an appropriate animal model in which to study the cardiovascular complications of cirrhosis? In Table 5, we have attempted to define "the appropriate animal model" by comparing the cardiovascular complications of cirrhosis in man to those described in all the animal models. Using this guide, it can be seen that there is not a single model that is entirely satisfactory. This is partly due to the inherent differences between the models and the patients and partly due to the lack of definition of both. Until such time as both descriptions are made, it will be necessary to utilize all the available animal models in conjunction with clinical observations to validate the use of any one model as "the most appropriate" one in which to study the cardiovascular complications of liver disease.

TABLE 5

Comparison of the Cardiovascular Complications of Cirrhosis in Patients and in the Five Animal Models of Cirrhosis

	Man	BDL Dog	BDL Rat	PHT Rat	CCl$_4$ Rat	DMN Dog
Blood pressure	N or ↓	↓	↓	↓	↓	↓
Pulse pressure	↑					
Vascular indices						
Resistance	↓	↓	↓	↓	↓	↓
Reactivity to vasoactive agents	N or ↓	N or ↓			↑ or ↓	
Cardiac indices						
Index/output	N or ↑		↑	↑	N	
Heart rate	N or ↑	N	N			N
Stroke index	↑					
Plasma						
Volume	N or ↑				↑	↑
Albumin	N or ↓				↓	
Hematocrit	↓	↓	↓			
Red cell mass	N or ↓					
Miscellaneous						
Portal hypertension	+	+	+	+	+	+
Arteriovenous shunts	+	+	+	+	+	+
Ascites	+/−	+/−	−	−	+/−	+
Renal perfusion	↓	N	↑			
Regulatory system activity						
Sympathetic	↑				↑	
Renin-angiotensin	↑				↑	

Note: BDL = bile duct-ligated; PHT = portal stenotic; CCl$_4$ = carbon tetrachloride-induced; DMN = dimethylnitrosamine-induced; N = normal; + = present; − = absent.

ACKNOWLEDGMENTS

The authors wish to acknowledge the secretarial assistance of Joyce Carp and Anita Baker in the preparation of this manuscript, and Ruth Tal who did the graphic work.

REFERENCES

1. **Blendis, L. M. and Bomzon, A.,** Cardiovascular complications of liver diseases, in *Cardiovascular Complications of Liver Disease,* Bomzon, A. and Blendis, L. M., Eds., CRC Press, Boca Raton, FL, 1990, chap. 1.
2. **Lee, S. S. and Bomzon, A.,** The heart in liver disease, in *Cardiovascular Complications of Liver Disease,* Bomzon, A. and Blendis, L. M., Eds., CRC Press, Boca Raton, FL, 1990, chap. 5.
3. **Aronsen, K. F., Nylander, G., and Ohlsson, E. G.,** Liver blood flow studies during and after various periods of total biliary obstruction in the dog, *Acta Chir. Scand.,* 135, 55, 1969.
4. **Aronsen, K. F., Norden, J. G., Nosslin, B., Nylander, G., and Ohlsson, E. G.,** Vascular changes within the liver in biliary obstruction, *Acta Chir. Scand.,* 135, 505, 1969.
5. **Mathie, R. T., Nagorney, D. M., Lewis, M. H., and Blumgart, L. H.,** Hepatic hemodynamics after chronic obstruction of the biliary tract in the dog, *Surg., Gynecol. Obstet.,* 166, 125, 1988.
6. **Ohlsson, E. G., Rutherford, R. B., Haalebos, M. M. P., Wagner, H. N., and Zuidema, G. D.,** The effect of biliary obstruction on hepatosplanchnic blood flow in dogs, *J. Surg. Res.,* 10, 200, 1970.
7. **Bomzon, A., Monies-Chass, I., Kamenetz, L. and Blendis, L. M.,** Anesthesia and cardiovascular responsiveness in chronic bile duct-ligated (CBDL) dogs, *Hepatology,* F, 1392, 1988.

8. **Finberg, J. P. M., Syrop, H. A., and Better, O. S.,** Blunted pressor response to angiotensin and sympathomimetic amines in bile-duct ligated dogs, *Clin. Sci.,* 61, 535, 1981.
9. **Bomzon, A., Rosenberg, M., Gali, D., Binah, O., Mordechovitz, D., Better, O. S., Greig, P. D., and Blendis, L. M.,** Systemic hypotension and decreased pressor response in dogs with chronic bile duct ligation, *Hepatology,* 6, 595, 1986.
10. **Ohlsson, E. G., Rutherford, R. B., Boitnott, J. K., Haalebos, M. M. P., and Zuidema, G. D.,** Changes in portal circulation after biliary obstruction in dogs, *Am. J. Surg.,* 120, 16, 1970.
11. **Naveh, Y., Finberg, J. P. M., Kahana, L., and Better, O. S.,** Renin-angiotensin system in dogs following chronic bile-duct ligation, *J. Hepatol.,* 6, 57, 1988.
12. **Bomzon, A., Binah, O., and Blendis, L. M.,** Temporal changes in pressor and contractile responsiveness in the conscious chronic bile duct ligated (CBDL) dog, *Hepatology,* 8, 1393, 1988.
13. **Saito, S.,** Clinical and experimental studies on the hyperdynamic states in obstructive jaundice *J. Jpn. Surg. Soc.,* 82, 483, 1981.
14. **Sasha, S. M., Better, O. S., Chaimovitz, C., Doman, J., and Kishon, Y.,** Hemodynamic studies in dogs with chronic bile duct ligation, *Clin. Sci. Mol. Med.,* 50, 533, 1976.
15. **Cattell, W. R. and Birstingl, M. A.,** Blood volume and hypotension in obstructive jaundice, *Br. J. Surg.,* 54, 272, 1967.
16. **Winaver, J., Chaimovitz, C., and Better, O. S.,** Natriuretic effect of propranolol on dogs with chronic bile duct ligation *Clin. Sci. Mol. Med.,* 54, 603, 1978.
17. **Melman, A.,** Effect of angiotensin II inhibition in the bile duct-ligated dog *J. Surg. Res.,* 24, 277, 1978.
18. **Williams, R. D., Elliott, D. W., and Zollinger, R. M.,** The effect of hypotension in obstructive jaundice, *Arch. Surg.,* 81, 334, 1960.
19. **Willems, B., Villeneuve, J.-P., and Huet, P.-M.,** Effect of propranolol on hepatic and systemic hemodynamics in dogs with chronic bile duct ligation, *Hepatology,* 6, 92, 1986.
20. **Bosch, J., Enriquez, R., Groszmann, R. J., and Storer, E. H.,** Chronic bile duct ligation in the dog: hemodynamic characterization of a portal hypertensive model *Hepatology,* 3, 1002, 1983.
21. **Alon, U., Berant, M., Mordechovitz, D., Hashmonai, M., and Better, O. S.,** Effect of isolated cholemia on systemic hemodynamics and kidney function in conscious dogs, *Clin. Sci.,* 63, 59, 1982.
22. **Green, J., Beyar, R., Sideman, S., Mordechovitz, D., and Better, O. S.,** The "jaundiced heart": a possible explanation for postoperative shock in obstructive jaundice. *Surgery,* 100, 14, 1986.
23. **Morandini, G. and Spanedda, M.,** Contributo allo studio della reattivita vascolare periferica all' angiotensina e alla adrenalina in corso di affezioni epatiche *Minerva Med.,* 57, 2715, 1966.
24. **Morandini, G., Spanedda, M., and Spanedda, L.,** La riposta pressoria all angiotensina ed alla noradrenalina in sogetti con affezioni epatiche *Minerva Med.,* 58, 1794, 1967.
25. **Hunt, D. R.,** Changes in liver blood flow with development of biliary obstruction in the rat, *Aust. N. Z. J. Surg.,* 49, 732, 1979.
26. **Bomzon, A., Weinbroum, A., and Kamenetz, L.,** Systemic hypotension and pressor responsiveness in cholestasis, *J. Hepatol.,* in press.
27. **Jacob, G., Bashara, B., Hilzenart, N., and Bomzon, A.,** The effect of serotonin on the cardiovascular system in liver disease, unpublished data, 1988.
28. **Jacob, G. and Bomzon, A.,** The effect of jaundice upon adrenergic receptors, unpublished data, 1988.
29. **Heidenreich, S., Brinkema, E., Martin, A., Dusing, R., Kipnowski, J., and Kramer, H. J.,** The kidney and cardiovascular system in obstructive jaundice: functional and metabolic studies in conscious rats, *Clin. Sci.,* 73, 593, 1987.
30. **Aarseth, P., Aarseth, S., and Bergan, A.,** Blood volume partition after acute cholestasis in the rat, *Eur. J. Surg. Res.,* 8, 61, 1970.
31. **Aarseth, S., Bergan, A., and Aarseth, P.,** Circulatory homeostasis in rats after bile duct ligation, *Scand. J. Clin. Lab. Invest.,* 39, 93, 1979.
32. **Finberg, J. P. M., Seidman, R., and Better, O. S.,** Cardiovascular responsiveness to vasoactive agents in rats with obstructive jaundice, *Clin. Exp. Pharmacol. Physiol.,* 9, 639, 1982.
33. **Gillett, D. J.,** The effect of obstructive jaundice on the blood volume in rats, *J. Surg. Res.,* 11, 447, 1971.
34. **Better, O. S., Aisenbrey, G. A., Berl, T. A., Anderson, R. J., Handelman, W. A., Linas, S. L., Guggenheim, S. J., and Shrier, R. W.,** Role of antidiuretic hormone in impaired urinary dilution associated with chronic bile duct ligation, *Clin. Sci.,* 58, 493, 1980.
35. **Franco, D., Gigou, M., Szekely, A.-M., and Bismuth, H.,** Portal hypertension after bile duct obstruction, *Arch. Surg.,* 114, 1064, 1979.
36. **Allison, M. E. M., Moss, N. G., Fraser, M. M., Dobbie, J. W., Ryan, C. J., Kennedy, A. C., and Blumgart, L. H.,** Renal function in chronic obstructive jaundice: a micropuncture study in rats, *Clin. Sci. Mol. Med.* 54, 649, 1978.
37. **Zimlichman, R. R., Kaplanski, J., Genchik, G., and Hanuka, N.,** Evaluation of hemodynamic changes and renal perfusion in experimental liver cirrhosis in rats, personal communication, 1984.
38. **Buchs, A., Kinan, A., Ya'ari, A., and Sikuler, E.,** Hemodynamic characteristics of rats with chronic bile duct ligation and portal hypertension, personal communication, 1988.

39. **Lee, S. S., Girod, C., Braillon, A., Hadengue, A., and Lebrec, D.,** Hemodynamic characterization of chronic bile duct-ligated rats: effect of pentobarbital sodium, *Am. J. Physiol., 251, (Gastrointestinal and Liver Physiology* 14) G176, 1986.
40. **Geoffroy, P., Lhoste, F., Girod, C., Valla, D., and Lebrec, D.,** Impairment of chronotropic response to the β-agonist isoproterenol in rats with portal hypertension due to portal vein stenosis or bile duct ligation, *J. Hepatol.,* 1, S1, S59, 1985.
41. **Hishida, A., Honda, N., Sudo, M., and Nagase, M.,** Mechanisms of altered renal perfusion in the early stage of obstructive jaundice, *Kidney Inter.,* 17, 223, 1980.
42. **Hishida, A., Honda, N., Sudo, M., Kimura, M., and Nagase, M.,** Renal handling of salt and water in the early stage of obstructive jaundice in rabbits, *Nephron,* 30, 368, 1982.
43. **Yamamoto, M., Ozawa, K., Tobe, T., and Isselhard, W.,** Effect of hypovolemic hypotension on plasma proteins and hepatic energy status in jaundiced rabbits, *Eur. J. Surg. Res.,* 14, 45, 1982.
44. **Bomzon, A. and Kew, M. C.,** Renal blood flow in experimental obstructive jaundice, in *The Kidney in Liver Disease,* 2nd ed., Epstein, M., Ed., Elsevier Science, New York, 1983, 313.
45. **Center, S. A., Baldwin, B. H., King, J. M., and Tennant, B. C.,** Hematologic and biochemical abnormalities associated with induced extrahepatic bile duct obstruction in the cat, *Am. J. Vet. Res.,* 44, 1822, 1983.
46. **Sikuler, E., Kravetz, D., and Groszmann, R. J.,** Evolution of portal hypertension and mechanisms involved in its maintenance in a rat model, *Am. Physiol.,* 248, *(Gastrointestinal and Liver Physiology,* 11), G618, 1989.
47. **Belghiti, J., Blanchet, L., and Lebrec, D.,** Effects of general anesthesia on portal venous pressure in the rat, *Eur. J. Surg. Res.,* 13, 285, 1981.
48. **Blanchart, A., Hernando, N., Fernandez-Munoz, D., Hernando, L., and Lopez-Novoa, J. M.,** Lack of effect of indomethacin on systemic and splanchnic hemodynamics in portal hypertensive rats, *Clin. Sci.,* 68, 605, 1985.
49. **Blei, A. T., O'Reilly, D. J., and Gottstein, J.,** Portal-systemic shunting and the hemodynamic effects of nitroglycerin in the rat, *Gastroenterology,* 86, 1428, 1984.
50. **Blei, A. T. and Gottstein, J.,** Isosorbide dinitrate in experimental portal hypertension: a study of factors that modulate the hemodynamic response, *Hepatology,* 6, 107, 1986.
51. **Benoit, J. N., Barrowman, J. A., Harper, S. L., Kvietys, P. R., and Granger, D. N.,** Role of humoral factors in the intestinal hyperemia associated with chronic portal hypertension, *Am. J. Physiol.,* 247 (*Gastrointestinal and Liver Physiology,* 10), G486, 1984.
52. **Korthuis, R. J., Benoit, J. N., Kvietys, P. R., Townsley, M. I., Taylor, A. E., and Granger, D. N.,** Humoral factors may mediate increased rat hindquarter blood flow in portal hypertension, *Am. J. Physiol.,* 249 (*Heart and Circulation Physiology,* 18), H827, 1985.
53. **Kroeger, R. J. and Groszmann, R. J.,** Increased portal venous resistance hinders portal pressure reduction during the administration of B-adrenergic blocking agents in a portal hypertensive model *Hepatology,* 5, 97, 1985.
54. **Cummings, S. A., Groszmann, R. J., and Kaumann, A. J.,** Hypersensitivity of mesenteric veins to 5-hydroxytryptamine- and ketanserin-induced reduction of portal pressure in portal hypertensive rats, *Brit. J. Pharmacol.,* 89, 501, 1986.
55. **Polio, J., Better, O. S., Sterzel, B., Reuben, A., and Groszmann, R. J.,** Portal hypertension reverses arterial hypertension in spontaneous hypertensive rats, *Hepatology,* 7, 1102, 1987.
56. **Hillon, P., Blanchet, L., and Lebrec, D.,** Effect of propranolol on hepatic blood flow in normal and portal hypertensive rats, *Clin. Sci.,* 63, 29, 1982.
57. **Blanchet, L. and Lebrec, D.,** Changes in splanchnic blood flow in portal hypertensive rats, *Eur. J. Clin. Invest.,* 12, 327, 1982.
58. **Lebrec, D. and Blanchet, L.,** Effect of two models of portal hypertension on splanchnic organ blood flow in the rat, *Clin. Sci.,* 68, 23, 1985.
59. **Lee, S. S., Girod, C., Valla, D., Geoffroy, P., and Lebrec, D.,** Effects of pentobarbital sodium anesthesia on splanchnic hemodynamics of normal and portal-hypertensive rats, *Am. J. Physiol.,* 249 (*Gastrointestinal and Liver Physiology,* 12), G528, 1985.
60. **Braillon, A., Cales, P., Girod, C., and Lebrec, D.,** Alteration in response of the portal tributary vascular bed to the B-agonist dobutamine in rats with extrahepatic portal hypertension, *J. Hepatol.,* 2, 267, 1986.
61. **Blanchart, A., Garrido, M. C., Fernandez-Munoz, D., Nuno, J., Hernando, L., and Lopez-Novoa, J. M.,** Splanchnic and systemic hemodynamic alterations in chronic, progressive portal hypertensive rats, *Rev. Esp. Fisiol.,* 40, 493, 1984.
62. **Sikuler, E. and Groszmann, R. J.,** Hemodynamic studies in long- and short-term portal hypertensive rats: the relation to systemic glucagon levels, *Hepatology,* 6, 414, 1986.
63. **Marshall, B. E. and Wollman, H.,** General anesthetics, in *Pharmacological Basis of Therapeutics,* Gilman, A. G., Goodman, L. S., Rall, T. W., and Murad, F., Eds., Macmillan, New York, 1985, 276.
64. **Morris, A. N. and Miller, H. H.,** Chronic portal vein occlusion and portal hypertension in the dog, *Surgery,* 30, 768, 1951.

65. **Sharma, G. P. and Shoenut, J. P.,** The canine model of portal hypertension, in *Animal Models of Portal Hypertension,* Sarin, S. K. and Nayak, N. C., Eds., Kunj Publishing House, New Delhi, India, 1988, 31.

66. **Jensen, L. S., Dybdahl, H., and Juhl, C.,** Experimental prehepatic portal hypertension and esophageal varices in the rabbit, *Scand. J. Gastroenterol.,* 21, 225, 1986.

67. **Jensen, L. S., Krarup, N., Larsen, J. A., Juhl, C., Nielsen, T. H., and Dybdahl, H.,** Chronic portal venous hypertension. The effect of liver blood flow and liver function and the development of esophageal varices, *Scand. J. Gastroenterol.,* 22, 463, 1987.

68. **McLean, E., McLean, A. E. M., and Sutton, D. M.,** Instant cirrhosis: an improved method for producing cirrhosis of the liver in rats by simultaneous administration of carbon tetrachloride and phenobarbitone, *Brit. J. Exp. Pathol.,* 50, 502, 1969.

69. **Linas, S. L., Anderson, R. J., Guggenheim, S. J., Robertson, G. L., and Berl, T.,** Role of vasopressin in impaired water excretion in conscious rats with experimental cirrhosis, *Kidney Int.,* 20, 173, 1981.

70. **Hase, T.,** Development of portahepatic venous shunts and cirrhosis in carbon tetrachloride poisoning in rats, *Am. J. Pathol.,* 83, 1968.

71. **Caramelo, C., Fernandez-Munoz, D., Santos, J. C., Blanchart, A., Rodriguez-Puyol, D., Lopez-Novoa, J. M., and Hernando, L.,** Effect of volume expansion on hemodynamics, capillary permeability and renal function in conscious, cirrhotic rats, *Hepatology,* 6, 129, 1986.

72. **Barrowman, J. A. and Granger, D. N.,** Effects of experimental cirrhosis on splanchnic microvascular fluid and solute exchange in the rat, *Gastroenterology,* 87, 165, 1984.

73. **Lopez-Novoa, J. M., Rengel, M. A., Rodicio, J. L., and Hernando, L.,** A micropuncture study of salt and water retention in chronic experimental cirrhosis *Am. J. Physiol., 232 (Renal and Fluid Electrolyte Physiology* 1), 315, 1977.

74. **Fernandez-Munoz, D., Caramelo, C., Santos, J. C., Blanchart, A., Hernando, L., and Lopez-Novoa, J. M.,** Systemic and splanchnic hemodynamic disturbances in conscious rats with experimental liver cirrhosis without ascites, *Am. J. Physiol.,* 249 (Gastrointestinal and Liver Physiology, 12), 316, 1985.

75. **Alpert, L. I. and Mitra, S. K.,** Anatomic and functional circulatory changes in experimental cirrhosis, *Am. J. Pathol.,* 48, 579, 1966.

76. **Vorobioff, J., Bredefeldt, J. E., and Groszmann, R. J.,** Increased blood flow through the portal system in cirrhotic rats *Gastroenterology,* 87, 1120, 1984.

77. **Chojkier, M. and Groszmann, R. J.,** Measurement of portal-systemic shunting in the rat by using γ-labeled microspheres, *Am. J. Physiol.,* 240 (*Gastrointestinal and Liver Physiology,* 3), G371, 1981.

78. **Khaliq, S. U., Kay, J. M., and Heath, D.,** Porta-pulmonary venous anastomoses in experimental cirrhosis of the liver in rats, *J. Pathol.,* 107, 167, 1972.

79. **Kitano, S., Koyanagi, N., Sugimachi, K., Kobayashi, M., and Inokuchi, K.,** Mucosal blood flow and modified vascular responses to norepinephrine in the stomach of rats with liver cirrhosis, *Eur. J. Surg. Res.,* 14, 221, 1982.

80. **Daniel, P. M., Prichard, M. M. L., and Reynell, P. C.,** The portal circulation in experimental cirrhosis of the liver *J. Pathol. Bacteriol.,* 64, 53, 1952.

81. **Weinbroum, A., Blendis, L. M., Poucell, S., and Bomzon, A.,** Temporal relationships between cirrhosis, portal hypertension and systemic hemodynamics in carbon tetrachloride (CT) induced cirrhosis in rats, *Hepatology,* 6, 1120, 1986.

82. **Lopez-Novoa, J. M.,** Pathophysiological features of the carbon tetrachloride-phenobarbital model of experimental liver cirrhosis in rats, in *The Kidney in Liver Disease,* 3rd ed., Epstein M., Ed., Williams & Wilkins, Baltimore, 1988, 309.

83. **Murray, B. M., and Paller, M. S.,** Decreased pressor reactivity to angiotensin II in cirrhotic rats *Circ. Res.,* 57, 424, 1985.

84. **Jimenez, W., Martinez-Pardo, A., Arroyo, V., Bruix, J., Rimola, A., Gaya, J., Rivera, F., and Rodes, J.,** Temporal relationship between hyperaldosteronism, sodium retention and ascites formation in rats with experimental cirrhosis, *Hepatology,* 5, 245, 1985.

85. **Koepke, J., Jones, S., and DiBona, G.,** Renal nerves mediate blunted natriuresis to atrial natriuretic peptide in cirrhotic rats, *Am. J. Physiol.,* 252 (*Regulatory Integrative and Comparative Physiology,* 21), R1019, 1987.

86. **Zambraski, E. J. and DiBona, G. F.,** Sympathetic nervous system in hepatic cirrhosis, in *The Kidney in Liver Disease,* 3rd ed., Epstein, M., Ed, Williams & Wilkins, Baltimore, 1988, 469.

87. **Alsasua, A., Blanchart, A., Santos, J. C., Lopez-Novoa, J. M., and Rodriguez-Puyol, D.,** Urinary excretion of catecholamine metabolites in three models of portal hypertension in the rat, *Eur. J. Clin. Invest.,* 16, A27, 1986.

88. **Bernardi, M., Trevisani, F., and Gasbarrini, G.,** Renin-angiotensin-aldosterone system in liver disease, in *Cardiovascular Complications of Liver Disease,* Bomzon, A. and Blendis, L. M., Eds., CRC Press, Boca Raton, FL, 1990, chap. 3.

89. **Campbell, P., Skorecki, K., and Blendis, L. M.,** Atrial natriuretic peptide and its role in sodium retention in cirrhosis, in *Cardiovascular Complications of Liver Disease,* Bomzon, A. and Blendis, L. M., Eds., CRC Press, Boca Raton, FL, 1990, chap. 15.

90. **Henriksen, J. H., Ring-Larsen, H., and Christensen, N. J.,** Autonomic nervous function in liver disease, in *Cardiovascular Complications of Liver Disease,* Bomzon, A. and Blendis, L. M., Eds., CRC Press, Boca Raton, FL, 1990, chap. 4.

91. **Madden, J. W., Gertman, P. M., and Peacock, E. E.,** Dimethylnitrosamine-induced hepatic cirrhosis: a new canine model of an ancient human disease, *Surgery,* 68, 260, 1970.

92. **Kreuzer, W., Schueller, E. F., and Schenk, W. G.,** Hemodynamic studies of cirrhosis in the dog, *Sur. Gynecol. Obst.,* 135, 89, 1972.

93. **Mortiz, E., Kreuzer, W., and Schenk, W. G.,** Studies in experimental canine cirrhosis: hemodynamic alterations with emphasis on degree of spontaneous porto-systemic shunting, *Ann. Surg.,* 177, 503, 1973.

94. **Levy, M.,** Sodium retention in dogs with cirrhosis and ascites: efferent mechanisms, *Am. J. Physiol.,* 233, F586, 1977.

95. **Levy, M.,** Sodium retention and ascites formation in dogs with experimental portal cirrhosis, *Am. J. Physiol.,* 233, F572, 1977.

96. **Levy, M. and Allotey, J. B. K.,** Temporal relationships between urinary salt retention and altered systemic hemodynamics in dogs with experimental cirrhosis, *J. Lab. Clin. Med.,* 92, 560, 1978.

97. **Levy, M. and Wexler, M. J.,** Renal sodium retention and ascites formation in dogs with experimental cirrhosis but without portal hypertension or increased splanchnic vascular capacity, *J. Lab. Clin. Med.,* 91, 520, 1978.

98. **Levy, M., Wexler, M. J., and McCaffrey, C.,** Sodium retention in dogs with experimental cirrhosis following removal of ascites by continuous peritovenous shunting, *J. Lab. Clin. Med.,* 94, 933, 1979.

99. **Jenkins, S. A., Grandison, A., Baxter, J. N., Day, D. W., Taylor, I., and Shields, R.,** A dimethyl-nitrosamine-induced model of cirrhosis and portal hypertension in the rat, *J. Hepatol.,* 1, 489, 1985.

100. **Sherlock, S.,** *Diseases of the Liver and Biliary System,* 5th ed., Blackwell Scientific, Oxford, 1975.

Chapter 3

THE RENIN-ANGIOTENSIN-ALDOSTERONE SYSTEM IN LIVER DISEASE

Mauro Bernardi, Franco Trevisani, and **Giovanni Gasbarrini**

TABLE OF CONTENTS

I. THE RENIN-ANGIOTENSIN-ALDOSTERONE SYSTEM: AN ESSENTIAL DRAWING OF SYSTEM REGULATION AND EFFECTS

A. RENIN-ANGIOTENSIN SYSTEM

Renin(s) are peptidases which split the decapeptide angiotensin I from angiotensinogens. They originate primarily in the kidneys, where they are synthesized and stored within the juxtaglomerular apparatus, which is situated within the medial coat of the afferent glomerular arteriole and makes close contact with the macula densa. Renin is secreted chiefly by the afferent arterioles of the outer cortical nephrons.[1] The activity of the system undergoes a circadian fluctuation with higher levels attained at 4 a.m.[2-4]

1. Renin Release Regulation and Metabolism

Renin release is influenced by many kinds of stimuli.[5] Stretching of the afferent arteriole wall results in an inhibition of renin release. Thus, expansion of extracellular fluid, blood pressure elevation, and renal artery vasodilatation are followed by a reduction in plasma renin concentration. On the contrary, vasoconstriction, extracellular fluid contraction, and arterial hypotension of such a degree to impair renal perfusion increase renin release.

The precise mechanism leading to the macula densa-mediated modulation of renin release has not been as yet clarified. It is possible that macula densa cells act as sensors of sodium, chloride, and other solute presentation rates and/or concentrations within the tubular fluid; the tubular fluid osmolality can also be important. As a matter of fact, extracellular fluid volume expansion obtained with large amounts of sodium chloride results in a suppression of renin release which occurs even when afferent arteriole pressure is maintained constant. Extracellular fluid depletion, glomerular filtration rate reduction, and hyponatremia result in an opposite effect. The depression of renin release by potassium loading may in part be mediated by the macula densa.[6]

Renin is also released by adrenergic afferents through vasoconstriction and direct, β_1-adrenergic receptor-mediated, stimulation of the juxtaglomerular apparatus.[7] Other neurotransmitters involved in a central regulation of renin release include serotonin and tryptophan.[8]

Prostaglandins enhance renin release via their hemodynamic effects,[9] and direct stimulation of juxtaglomerular cells.[10] The two systems are interregulated through a positive feedback. The kallikrein-kinin and renin-angiotensin systems are also interrelated.[11]

A panoply of other hormonal factors may enhance or depress renin release. Among the former, adrenal medullary catecholamines, growth hormone, glucagon, and parathyroid hormone are included.[6] The latter are represented by angiotensin II, acting through a negative feedback, antidiuretic hormone (ADH), somatostatin.[6]

It should be underlined that plasma renin activity (PRA) progressively declines with age, due to the reduction of glomerular cell mass.[12] The activity of the renin-angiotensin system is also strongly influenced by diet and posture.[13]

Renin is catabolized by the liver[14] and liver failure can result in an impaired inactivation of renin[15] whose plasma half-life is very short under normal circumstances (from 10 to 65 min).

2. Angiotensin Generation and Metabolism

Once released in the bloodstream, renin cleaves off the decapeptide angiotensin I from the α_2-globulin angiotensinogen. The latter is synthesized by liver cells and is degraded by the kidneys. Its synthesis is enhanced by glucocorticoids, estrogens, progestogens, and insulin.[6] Renin and angiotensin also stimulate angiotensinogen formation.[16]

Angiotensin I is then converted by the membrane-bound angiotensin converting enzymes to the octapeptide angiotensin II. Although angiotensin I is a biologically active peptide, its potency is 5% of the vasoconstrictor potency of angiotensin II.[17] Circulating aminopeptidase produces the heptapeptide angiotensin III by cleavage of angiotensin II. The highest amounts of angiotensin-converting enzymes are located within the pulmonary circulation; their concentration is usually so great that angiotensin II generation is not influenced by the level of enzyme activity.[6]

Angiotensins I, II, and III are then degraded by the ubiquitous angiotensinases, which are mainly produced by the liver.[18,19]

3. Effects of Angiotensins

Angiotensin II and III directly stimulate the zona glomerulosa cells of the adrenal cortex, accelerating aldosterone synthesis within minutes.[20] Such an effect is enhanced by sodium depletion.[21]

Angiotensin II is the most potent known vasoconstrictor: it is 40 times more effective than an equimolar amount of norepinephrine. Angiotensin III is almost devoid of such a property. The sensitivity of the different vascular beds to angiotensin II is variable.[6] The angiotensin II-induced vasoconstriction is enhanced by the hypernatremia by increasing angiotensin receptor population; sodium depletion has an opposite result.[22]

The chronic administration of angiotensin II does not affect the number of its own receptors. In one study, it increased the affinity of vascular receptors and decreased that of adrenal receptors.[23]

The effects of angiotensin II on renal function involve both blood perfusion and sodium handling. Renal vasculature is exquisitely sensitive to angiotensin II. In fact, an amount that is about 3% of that required to elevate blood pressure reduces renal blood flow in sodium-loaded healthy subjects.[24] Such a sensitivity is strikingly reduced by prolonged exposure to elevated angiotensin II levels, both exogenous[25] and endogenous.[24,26] The infusion of pressor doses of the octapeptide enhances both preglomerular and efferent arteriolar resistances, while a subpressor dose only increases the efferent arteriolar resistances: the physiological effect of angiotensin II should then be directed towards the efferent arteriole.[27] This is crucial for the preservation of glomerular filtration rate at the low end of renal blood flow auto-regulation.[28] Moreover, angiotensin can increase filtration fraction through additional mechanisms.[29,30] Such changes lead to a more efficient proximal tubular extraction of ions, by modifying the colloid osmotic and hydrostatic pressures of blood within peritubular capillaries. Whether angiotensin II directly enhances proximal sodium reabsorption or exerts the opposite effect is not clear.[31]

Angiotensin II also stimulates the adrenergic system, by promoting adrenalin release from adrenal medulla cells and potentiating sympathoadrenergic activity through several mechanisms.[13]

Angiotensin II is a potent stimulator of PGE production[32,33] and enhances ADH release.[13]

B. ALDOSTERONE

1. Aldosterone Biosynthesis Regulation and Metabolism

Aldosterone is synthesized within the glomerulosa cells of the adrenal cortex.[34] The healthy adult man secretes 40 to 200 μg of aldosterone daily. The circulating hormone is 36% free, 47% loosely albumin bound, and only 17% linked to corticoid-binding globulin.[35] Aldosterone secretion undergoes circadian fluctuations which account for minimal plasma aldosterone levels (nadir) at night and maximal levels (zenith) in the early morning.[2,3]

The pivotal drive for aldosterone secretion is the renin-angiotensin system. Most studies, but not all, have shown that renin-angiotensin levels and aldosterone secretion change in a parallel fashion following changes in posture, volume, and/or sodium intake.[34] Circadian studies show that plasma aldosterone concentration does not always parallel the renin-angiotensin system activity.[2,3] It may thus be suggested that the renin-angiotenin system in normal humans is involved in the setting of mean secretory level rather than periodicity of aldosterone secretion. Due to the renal sodium retaining effect, and hence extracellular fluid volume expansion, aldosterone secretion is linked to the juxtaglomerular apparatus activity through a negative feedback.

Aldosterone secretion is stimulated by an increase and blunted by a decrease in dietary potassium, an effect which is not mediated by the renin-angiotensin system.[36] Potassium may also be involved with the circadian variation of aldosterone secretion.[37] Whether intracellular[38] or serum[36] potassium drives aldosterone secretion is not known with certainty.

In contrast, sodium effects on adrenal cortex are mainly mediated by the ion influence on renin release. Aldosterone biosynthesis is influenced only by very large changes in plasma sodium concentration.[39]

Adrenocorticotropic hormone (ACTH) modulates aldosterone secretion in normal man when given in pharmacologic doses.[34] Even if aldosterone circadian rhythm closely parallels that of cortisol, dexamethasone administration only flattens cortisol variations.[3] Presumably, other pacemaker(s) than ACTH regulate the aldosterone secretion under physiological circumstances. Whether such a role is played by the recently characterized aldosterone-stimulating factor[40] is not clear as yet.

Dopamine exerts a maximal tonic inhibition on aldosterone secretion.[41]

Other hormones and substances influencing aldosterone secretion include serotonin, growth hormone, somatostatin, and metenkephalin.[6] Finally, atrial natriuretic factor inhibits the aldosterone response to several stimuli.[42]

Aldosterone is mainly metabolized by the liver with production of both tetrahydroaldosterone and aldosterone 18-glucuronide. In addition, about 10% of the hormone is converted to the latter product by the kidney. Hepatic aldosterone extraction is proportional to the hepatic blood flow and clears the non-protein-bound aldosterone in a single pass. Liver and kidney compete against each other as sites for the metabolism of aldosterone, so that hepatic failure gives an advantage to the renal metabolism of the hormone, accounting for the 25% of the degradation.[43]

2. Effects of Aldosterone

The principal target site of aldosterone is the nephron collecting tubule.[44] Tubular receptor stimulation accelerates sodium transfer from the tubular lumen to the tubular cell cytosol and then to the extracellular fluid (and peritubular capillaries) by increasing the activity of Na^+, K^+-ATPase pump. Such an effect occurs within one or more hours from aldosterone presentation to the tubule. The hormone favors hydrogen ion secretion through Na^+/H^+ exchange and, mostly, enhanced NH_3 production.[46] The effect of aldosterone on renal potassium handling is complex, since the latter is also heavily influenced by both urine flow rate and sodium availability at the aldosterone-sensitive portion of the nephron. As a matter of fact, aldosterone causes an acute kaliuresis in the context of either some degree of sodium loading or potassium depletion. In fact, the former minimizes the aldosterone antinatriuretic effect; the latter virtually cancels the flow dependence of urinary potassium excretion.[45]

II. THE RENIN-ANGIOTENSIN-ALDOSTERONE SYSTEM IN CIRRHOSIS

Abnormalites in renal sodium handling (sodium and water retention) and cardiovascular homeostasis (low peripheral vascular resistances, systemic hypotension, reflex increase in cardiac output, and renal ischemia) have long been recognized in patients with cirrhosis.[46-49] As described above, the renin-aldosterone axis is crucial in the regulation of volume homeostasis and resistance vessel tone. Therefore, changes in this system are to be expected in such a context and have been widely investigated.

A. RENIN-ANGIOTENSIN SYSTEM: STATUS AND REGULATION

From the seminal studies dealing with the characterization of the renin-angiotensin system, the first dating back to 1961,[50] the concept arose that in patients with cirrhosis and ascites such a system was activated. Namely either plasma angiotensin concentration[51,52] or plasma renin activity[53-56] were increased. However, the data from these studies often come from anecdotal observations, and little attention has generally been paid to the control of experimental conditions which could affect the results. In fact, posture, sodium intake, administration of diuretics, and other drugs now known to influence the system activity (such as prostaglandin synthesis inhibitors, sympathomimetic amines, etc.), renal function were either not reported or not taken care of. Moreover, the stage of disease was not stated, but usually patients with an advanced disease and ascites were studied. Finally, the common way of assaying the system activity was to evaluate the pressor response of processed samples injected into the rat.

Controlled experimental conditions were fulfilled by Schroeder et al.[57] who evaluated plasma renin by bioassay in cirrhosis with ascites with either preserved renal perfusion and glomerular filtration rate or functional renal failure (? hepatorenal syndrome). All the patients with renal failure showed markedly increased plasma renin. Interestingly, although such a finding was overlooked, eight out of 17 ascitic patients without renal failure had plasma renin within the normal range.

In the late 1970s, with the components of the renin-angiotensin system measured by radioimmunoassay, several new investigations were carried out. Again, methodological differences make a strict comparison between the studies difficult. In fact, the amount of dietary sodium and potassium, previous diuretic treatment, the length of equilibration periods, and the clock time of blood sampling either varied among the studies or were not clearly specified. In any case, it is now evident that the state of hyperreninism emerging from the earliest studies is by no means a rule and it became clear that the ''renin status'' of cirrhotic patients was composite and variable with the stage of the disease.

1. Cirrhosis without Ascites

In 1964, Brown et al.[53] reported that PRA levels were in the normal range in compensated cirrhotics, utilizing a bioassay technique. Subsequent studies documented reduced or low-normal levels of plasma renin concentration[58,59] or activity (PRA).[60-62] (Figure 1) Thus, it can be surmised that cirrhotic patients without ascites usually show a depressed activity of the renin-angiotensin system. Variant results were obtained by Mitch et al.:[63] in their experience, elevated PRA occurred both in compensated and ascitic patients consuming a normal sodium diet. However, caution should be applied in interpreting these results. In fact, all studied patients had alcoholic liver disease and three important pieces of information were lacking: first, whether nonascitic patients had acute or chronic disease; second, how many patients had cirrhosis; and finally, how long before the study had heavy alcohol consumption ceased.

A putative cause of low PRA values in these patients may be a reduction in the hepatic synthesis of renin substrate. In fact, PRA is a measure of *in vitro* angiotensin I generation within the patient's plasma sample. It is then influenced by the amount of both renin and angiotensinogen. However, when plasma angiotensinogen was measured in patients without an advanced disease, it was usually found to be within the normal range[60,61] or only moderately reduced.[58]

''Low renin'' cirrhosis usually shows normal blood pressure, renal perfusion and plasma potassium, and sodium concentrations.[58-64] In contrast, blood and/or plasma volume has been found to be increased in cirrhosis without ascites[58,59,62,65] (Figure 1). These findings fulfill the ''overflow'' theory of ascites formation[66] and have been substantiated by animal studies. In fact, nonportal blood volume expansion took place before the appearance of ascites in dogs with dimethylnitrosamine-induced cirrhosis.[67,68] Therefore it is likely that the

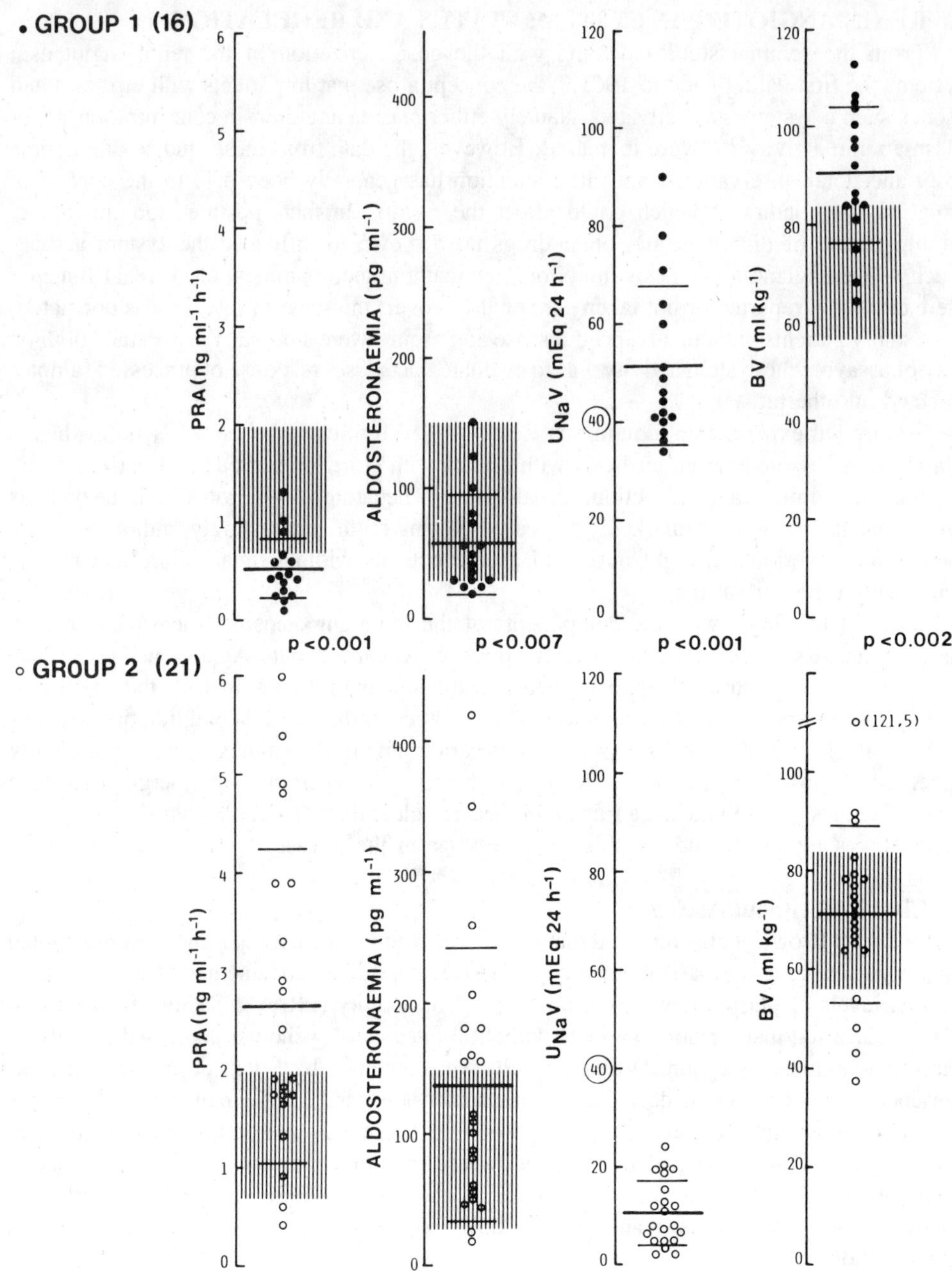

FIGURE 1.   Plasma renin activity (PRA), plasma aldosterone concentration, renal sodium excretion ($U_{Na}V$), and blood volume in liver cirrhosis without (group 1) and with ascites (BV) at the first appearance, untreated by diuretics (group 2). The measurements were carried out after 5 days of equilibration, with a diet providing 40 mEq of sodium and 80 mEq of potassium/daily, and after 2 h of bed rest. The shaded areas represent the range of values observed in a group of healthy subjects maintained under the same experimental conditions.

extracellular fluid (and blood) volume is a major cause of renin-angiotensin system suppression. Interestingly, such a suppression persists even in the face of at least one activating factor. In fact, a direct correlation has been found between both plasma renin concentration and activity and wedged hepatic vein pressure in a group of 52 patients both with and without ascites.[59] In the latter, however, wedge hepatic vein pressure up to 19 mmHg coexisted with normal PRA.

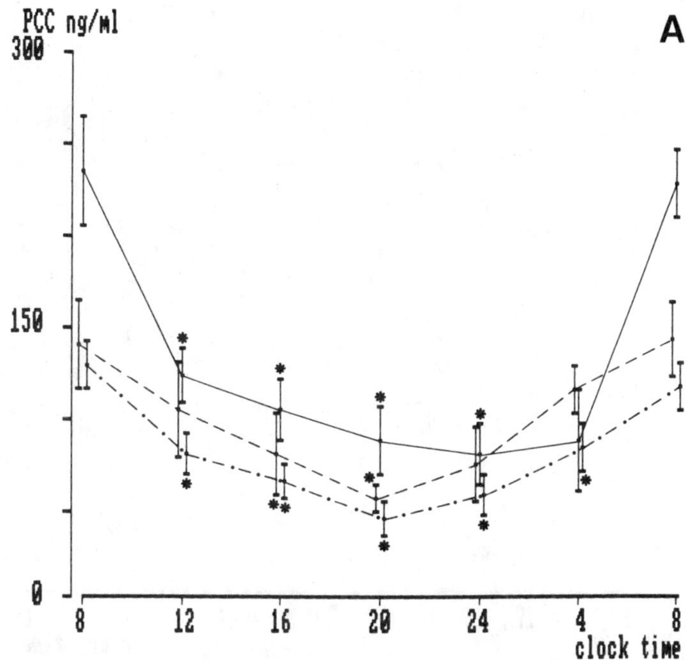

FIGURE 2.   Circadian variations of plasma renin activity (PRA), plasma aldosterone (PAC) and cortisol (PCC) concentrations in healthy subjects (————) and cirrhotics without (----) and with (-·-·-) ascites, maintained supine for 24 h. * = significantly different from baseline values (8 a.m.). (From Bernardi, M., De Palma, R., Trevisani, F., Santini, C., Capani, F., Baraldini, M., and Gasbarrini, G., *Gastroenterology*, 91, 683, 1986. With permission.)

Depression of renin-angiotensin system activity has also been confirmed and further circumstantiated by a circadian study[64] (Figure 2). The chronobiological approach showed that patients without ascites not only had a significantly depressed mesor (rhythm-determined average), but also blunted circadian variations, even maintaining the 4 a.m. zenith. A similar feature was observed during saline infusion in normal volunteers.[4] This indirectly reinforces the hypothesis that, at this stage of the disease, the expanded blood volume is hemodynamically effective, at least in recumbent patients. The lack of correlation between blood volume and PRA, in these circumstances, does not militate against the latter statement, since an unmeasurable fraction of blood volume is obviously compartmentalized within the venous splanchnic bed.[62]

2. Cirrhosis with Ascites

Although "without ascites" patients represent a fairly homogeneous population, the usually made stratification of "with ascites" cirrhotics does not allow us to identify a well-selected group.[69] In fact, along with patients showing fairly preserved nutritional conditions, residual liver function, cardiovascular homeostasis, and renal perfusion, others show severe hepatocellular failure, muscle mass wasting, "hyperdynamic" circulation, and a variably reduced renal perfusion, up to renal failure. In the same way, the status of the renin-angiotensin-aldosterone systems is quite different, ranging from normal activity to marked activation. Therefore, the use of presenting data as averages derived from such a composite population, without providing at least the key to identify the real condition of the single patients, can obscure the meaning of the results and does not allow the comparison between different studies.

Cirrhotics with ascites may show plasma renin concentration and/or PRA within the

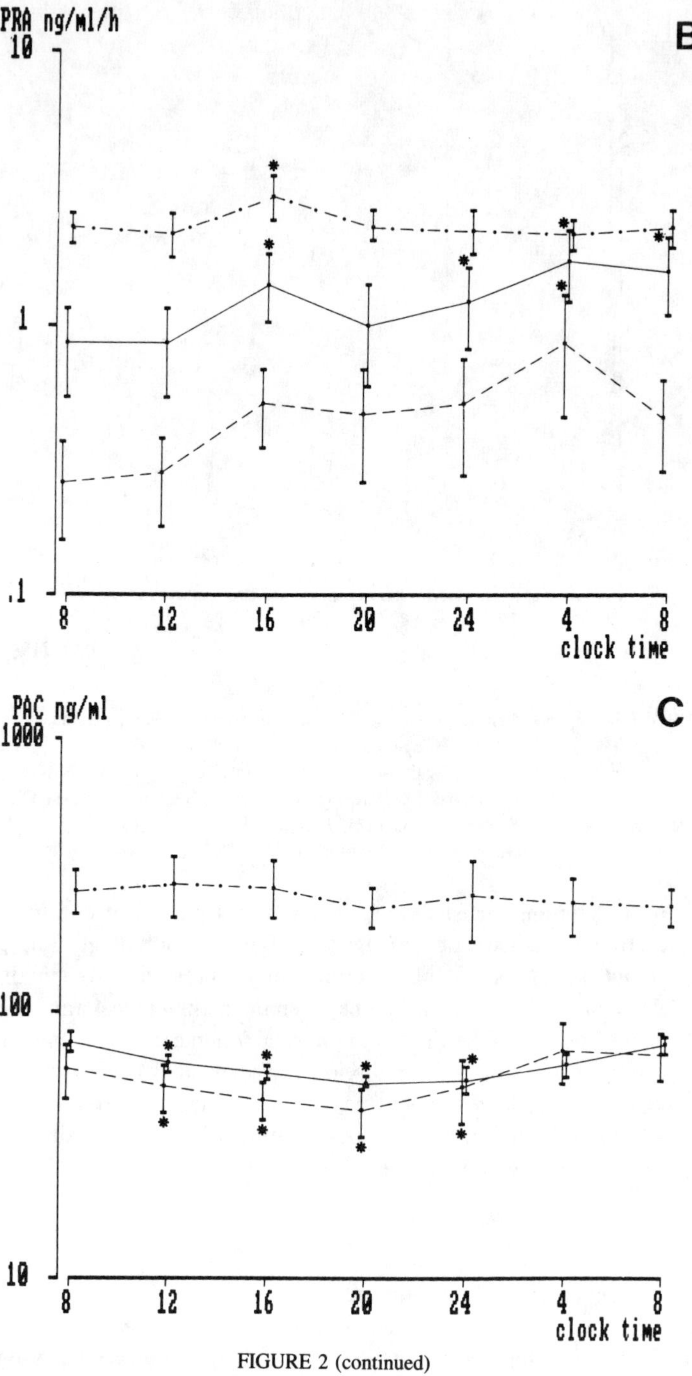

FIGURE 2 (continued)

normal range in at least one-third of cases. When patients with ascites at the first appearance, without previous diuretic treatment, are selectively evaluated, PRA is not elevated in up to 70% of cases, and, in some instances, it may even be reduced (Figure 1). On the contrary, cirrhotics with hyperdynamic circulation and advanced disease, who were previously treated with diuretics, usually present hyperreninism.[56-63,70-72] The importance of previous diuretic treatment in conditioning an activation of the renin-angiotensin system becomes evident from the results obtained in a large series by Wernze et al.[58] In this study, cirrhotics with ascites had increased plasma renin concentration in 22% of untreated cases and in 81% of previously treated cases.

In decompensated patients, the circadian pattern of the renin-angiotensin system activity is completely altered (Figure 2). In fact, in addition to permanently increased levels of PRA, zenith value was rephased by 12 h (4 p.m. instead of 4 a.m.).[64] This finding suggests that a profound derangement in the still unknown pacemaker of renin secretion occurs in these patients. In fact, changes in baseline PRA, serum potassium concentration, salt intake, plasma volume, blood pressure, and mineralocorticoid effect did not alter renin circadian periodicity in humans.[4]

a. Reciprocal Influences between the Renin-Angiotensin System Components and Its Dynamics

Patients with advanced cirrhosis and increased plasma renin concentration or activity usually show depressed levels of plasma angiotensinogen concentration.[56-58,60,61,71] Failure in liver protein synthesis is the most likely explanation for such a finding. Taking into account that renin-angiotensin system activation is followed by an enhanced angiotensinogen production,[16] to find reduced plasma renin substrate associated with increased plasma renin would imply that the system is not allowed to achieve a full-blown response. The addition of excess renin to plasma from patients with cirrhosis led to a complete utilization of renin substrate earlier than in healthy controls.[56] However, in the plasma from patients with an even severely reduced angiotensinogen concentration, the *in vitro* enzyme reaction leading to angiotensin production was of zero-order in most instances, as in controls.[56] Only in one case of cirrhosis with hepatorenal syndrome, after a very rapid initial angiotensin production, the curve became flat.[56] These findings indicate that the amount of angiotensinogen is probably never rate-limiting for the renin enzyme reaction "in vivo" and seldom in the laboratory. As a matter of fact, the renin substrate availability by 5 to 10% of normal is sufficient to ensure a balanced angiotensin production. Further evidence for this also comes from the significant direct correlation between plasma renin and plasma angiotensin II concentration also found in patients with angiotensinogen deficiency.[58] It is noteworthy that an inverse relationship between PRA and substrate was observed.[61] This suggests that consumption of angiotensinogen, secondary to an increased plasma renin concentration, is an important determining factor of the substrate level in cirrhosis, in addition to any reduction in hepatic synthesis.

The dynamics of the renin-angiotensin system can also be influenced by the amount/activity of angiotensin I-converting enzyme and angiotensinases. Serum angiotensin I-converting enzyme has been found to be increased in cirrhosis as measured by bioassay technique.[73] These results have also been observed, using fluorometrical or radiometrical assays, in large series of patients affected by viral hepatitis, fatty liver, granulomatous hepatitis, and cirrhosis.[74-76] The highest levels of plasma angiotensin I-converting enzyme were found in cirrhotics with ascites.[74-76] Such an increase was related to neither the degree of activation of the renin-angiotensin system nor the extent of liver damage. In particular, no relationship was found between serum angiotensin I-converting enzyme and transaminase levels, suggesting that liver cell necrosis was hardly the cause of this alteration. Due to the very high enzyme activity within the lung vasculature, derangements in gas exchange leading to arterial hypoxia, which is known to occur in advanced cirrhosis secondary to intrapulmonary and portopulmonary shunts,[77] is a major candidate.[78] Whether increased serum angiotensin I-converting enzyme levels lead to an accelerated production of angiotensin II in cirrhotics, although possible, has not been proved. In any case, PRA is strictly correlated with plasma angiotensin II concentration in cirrhosis[58,79] and the slope of the regression line does not differ from healthy controls.[80] These features suggest that the normally available amount of angiotensin I-converting enzyme allows the maximal reaction rate. A recent study suggests that the measurement of angiotensin I-converting enzyme may be useful in separating patients with intrahepatic liver disease from those with extrahepatic obstruction. Namely, high serum levels virtually exclude extrahepatic biliary obstruction.[76]

Early studies showed an increase in plasma angiotensinase activity in cirrhosis.[19,81] The actual meaning of angiotensinase measurements in the venous blood is not clear, since a significant proportion of the enzyme activity is localized to the vascular endothelium. In fact, although an accelerated degradation of angiotensin II may be anticipated from the above finding, the ratio between the hepta-/octapeptide and hexapeptide fractions of angiotensin II in cirrhotics has been found to be comparable to healthy controls.[80] This result bears an important methodological message, that is, the measure of PRA in cirrhosis is not only a reliable index of total angiotensin II, but also of its active fractions.

Renin is inactivated by the liver.[14] A reduced hepatic clearance of renin has been described in cirrhosis, being 68% of normal in compensated and 43% in decompensated patients.[82] Similarly, when PRA was determined in both peripheral venous and hepatic venous blood,[15] the highest values were found in the latter. These results not only suggested an inadequate hepatic clearance of renin, but also that a splanchnic source of renin might contribute to the increased PRA. However, Mitch et al.[63] showed that there was a marked discrepancy between PRA elevation and the decrease in hepatic clearance of renin, the former being increased by over 13-fold and the latter decreased by 2.4-fold. Moreover, Bosch et al.[83] not only failed to demonstrate a reduced hepatic extraction of renin in decompensated cirrhosis, but also showed a direct correlation between this parameter and arterial renin concentration as found in normal subjects.[84] Finally, renin secretion rate and plasma renin concentration were closely correlated in these patients.[72] Therefore, it may be inferred that although a reduced renin catabolism can be present in cirrhosis, the enhanced secretion of renin accounts for most of the increased circulating levels of renin and angiotensin.

From the findings reported above, it can be concluded that the disclosed or supposed derangements of the single components may contribute to, but do not determine, the functional abnormalities of the renin-angiotensin system observed in the natural history of the cirrhosis.

b. Renin-Angiotensin System Modulation by Volume Homeostasis

As reported previously, hypovolemia, hyponatremia, hypokalemia, β-receptor- mediated sympathetic activity, arterial hypotension, and renal hypoperfusion are potent stimuli to renin secretion through different mechanisms. All of them can be commonly found, either alone or in association, in patients with advanced cirrhosis.

At this stage of the disease, a reduction in blood volume may occur as a result of diuretic therapy, gastrointestinal bleeding, vomiting, and diarrhea. However, some studies have shown that increased plasma and blood volume are still present in most cases.[58,59,65] Our experience[62] was somewhat at variance (Figure 1): the blood volume at the onset of ascites was most frequently normal (14 out of 21 cases) and even low (4 out of 21). According to our findings it can be assumed that ascites appearance is associated with a "normalization" of blood volume, which would allow an adequate response of the renin-angiotensin system to a variety of stimuli, the first being portal hypertension. Nonetheless, a reduction in circulating (effective) blood volume can easily occur even in the face of an expanded extracellular fluid. In fact, a significant fraction is trapped within the dilated splanchnic venous bed, due to postsinusoidal portal hypertension. A further, and most likely prominent, cause is the impairment of autonomic vascular responses resulting in peripheral arterial vasodilation, and hence systemic hypotension. Whether such a derangement is due to either an impaired reflex response[85] or a vascular receptor sensitivity to endogenous vasoactive agents,[86,87] or both, is not clear at present. As a matter of fact, reduced vascular resistances and altered distribution of cardiac output[49] coexist with increased sympathoadrenergic and renin-angiotensin system activities.[86-89] Therefore, the putative role of reduced effective volemia in the activation of the renin-angiotensin system is not excluded by the lack of correlation between plasma/blood volume and plasma renin concentration/activity.[62] On the contrary, it is supported by the effectiveness of blood volume expansion in reducing an elevated PRA in cirrhosis. In fact, both saline (500 ml/h for 4 h) and salt-poor albumin (25 g/h for 2 h) infusions resulted in a ≈ 45% reduction.[90] Further evidence comes also from different experimental and clinical approaches. Isothermic neck-out water immersion is a reliable tool for inducing central blood volume expansion without concomitant alteration of plasma composition. Such a maneuver produced a profound suppression of PRA as early as 60 min, with maximal suppression (≈ 70%) by 150 min. Recovery from neck-out immersion was associated with a prompt return to prestudy levels.[71] In a clinical setting, retransfusion of ascites[91] and the insertion of a peritoneovenous shunt[92] were followed by a striking decrease in PRA. In the latter condition, PRA reduction persisted up to 29 months after the operation.[93]

Although the volume-dependent stimulation of the juxtaglomerular apparatus may not be the principal factor, it is likely involved in promoting an enhanced renin response to the change in posture by cirrhotics with ascites. In fact, active tilting is associated by a percent reduction in plasma volume and an increase in PRA greater than in healthy controls.[87,94] The former could result from an enhanced loss of protein-free fluid through dependent vascular beds.

c. The Renin-Angiotensin System and Portal Hypertension

As reported above, a direct correlation between wedged hepatic venous pressure and both plasma renin concentration and activity has been reported in one study.[59] In contrast, Mitch et al.[63] did not observe such a finding. The efferent mechanisms connecting altered intrahepatic hemodynamics and juxtaglomerular apparatus function can only be a matter of speculation. As stated above, the unmeasurable ''effective'' blood volume actually drives renin secretion. Thus, the lack of correlation between wedged hepatic venous pressure and systemic hemodynamics and plasma volume[59] does not deny the possibility of portal hypertension-induced activation of the renin-angiotensin system being mediated by changes in systemic hemodynamics. Alternatively, postsinusoidal portal hypertension may lead to the release of a hepatic humoral factor stimulating renin release. In fact, the studies by Orloff et al.[95] demonstrated that thoracic inferior vena cava constriction in the dog was followed by aldosterone hypersecretion independent from any change in plasma volume and systemic hemodynamics. Subsequent cross-circulation studies showed that such a response was possibly mediated by a humoral factor.[96] Finally, experimental postsinusoidal portal hypertension (intrathoracic inferior vena cava constriction in the anesthetized dog) was followed by an increase in activity of renal and cardiac sympathetic efferent nerve activity,[97] possibly mediated through intrahepatic low-pressure baroreceptors.[98]

Conversely, the above-mentioned correlation may imply that the renin-angiotensin system is somehow involved in the development of portal hypertension. Angiotensin infusion to cirrhotic patients was followed by an increase in wedged hepatic venous pressure and a decrease in hepatic blood flow.[99,100] In a model of isolated perfused rat liver, the maximal amplitude of response to angiotensin II perfusion was similar in normal and cirrhotic livers. However, the latter showed a decreased sensitivity to the substance.[101] Angiotensin II blockade by saralasin infusion can help in evaluating the contribution of renin-angiotensin system to cirrhotic portal hypertension. Specifically, this maneuver led to a drop of wedged hepatic venous pressure by ≈20% and a decrease in hepatic sinusoidal vascular resistance, without significantly affecting the hepatic blood flow. The mean arterial pressure also declined significantly and a direct correlation linked its reduction to that in the wedge hepatic venous pressure.[100] Similarly, low oral doses of captopril decreased wedge hepatic pressure by 13% and mean arterial pressure by 15%.[102] Therefore, it would appear that the effects of endogenous angiotensin II on intrahepatic hemodynamics are not independent from those exerted on the systemic circulation. Nonetheless, it cannot be denied that activation of the renin angiotensin system may enhance cirrhotic portal hypertension.

d. The Renin-Angiotensin System and Blood Pressure Homeostasis

An inverse relationship between arterial pressure and PRA has often been found.[62,86,87] Systemic hypotension per se could stimulate renin release. Indeed, a severe reduction in arterial pressure is needed to activate the juxtaglomerular apparatus through a stretch receptor-like mechanism.[5] However, the actual blood pressure value in cirrhotics with hyperreninism is the result of the pathophysiological derangement(s) leading to hypotension and the effect of the compensatory response achieved by the renin-angiotensin system. Therefore, an important role for blood pressure imbalance in prompting renin release cannot be denied. Such an assumption can be backed by experimental findings. When norepinephrine (16 μg/ml solution titrated to raise and maintain mean arterial pressure by 15 to 20 mmHg above baseline) was infused during neck-out water immersion, a greater plasma renin concentration reduction was achieved than with immersion alone.[103] This suggests that both the reduction of effective blood volume and systemic vascular resistance are responsible for renin-angiotensin system activation.

As reported in section I, the sodium status influences the vascular effectiveness of angiotensin II.[22] Although patients with cirrhosis have an increased total exchangeable sodium,[104] they behave as sodium-depleted subjects as far as the renin-angiotensin system activity is concerned. In fact, when angiotensin II was infused to achieve an increment in the mean arterial pressure of about 35 mmHg, a greater amount of the peptide had to be administered in cirrhotics with ascites (mean dose 11.1 μg/min) than in controls (mean dose 3.8 μg/min; duration not specified: ≈hours).[105] Prolonged infusions up to 6 d confirmed a reduced vascular response to angiotensin II.[106] Similar results were obtained when increasing doses of angiotensin II (from 0.25 to 5 μg) were injected as a bolus.[107] However, limb blood-flow changes induced by 2 μg/min infusion for 8 min in cirrhotics did not differ from controls.[85] The different parameter evaluated in the latter study, along with a disease at a less advanced stage (only 9/75 patients in the whole group had clinical evidence of hepatic decompensation; 21 were infused with vasoactive agents, and no information is given about the proportion of decompensated patients in the latter group) can well explain such a discrepancy. More puzzling are the results obtained by Lenz et al.,[108] showing that cirrhotic patients with hepatic encephalopathy and decreased baseline vascular resistance exhibited an enhanced pressor response to 20 ng/kg/min (for 5 min) infusion of angiotensin II with respect to controls. Only differences in the study protocol can be invoked to explain these ''variant'' results. Summarizing, we believe that current evidence support the presence of a reduced systemic vascular sensitivity to angiotensin II in cirrhosis, at least in the advanced stages. This is also confirmed by experimental findings in cirrhotic rats[109] and dogs with bile duct ligation, a model with many similarities to human cirrhosis.[110] Whether the results obtained in humans are due to tachyphylaxis,[79] receptor occupancy by endogenous increased amounts of angiotensin II,[105] or counterbalance to vasodilating substances[108] is not known. In the experimental animal, an important role of endogenous angiotensin II in reducing the vascular responsiveness appeared to be unlikely.[110] Furthermore, pretreatment with converting enzyme or prostaglandin synthesis inhibitors failed to normalize the response to angiotensin II. Although angiotensin II receptor number was increased, their affinity was decreased, leading to an unaltered total angiotensin II binding. A postreceptor defect was therefore the most likely explanation.[109]

In the sodium-depleted status, blood pressure homeostasis is dependent on the renin-angiotensin system to a greater extent than in the normal condition, and the sympathoadrenergic system is progressively less important.[111] The administration of the specific angiotensin II antagonist saralasin (1-Sar, 8-Ala angiotensin II) to cirrhotics with ascites was associated with striking decreases in arterial pressure[100,112] proportional to the baseline levels of endogenous angiotensin II. On the contrary, saralasin does not exert a hypotensive effect in normal subjects. Divergent results were obtained by Saruta et al.[113] In fact, the infusion of another angiotensin II analogue (1-Sar, 8-Ile angiotensin II) did not significantly affect blood pressure. Such a disparity may be explained taking into account that the antagonist used has more agonistic properties than saralasin. Moreover, the patients included in the latter study were not sodium restricted and had increased PRA in a minority of cases. These findings indicate that the renin-angiotensin system, when activated, plays a crucial role in the maintenance of blood pressure homeostasis in cirrhotic patients who may suffer from a functional failure of the sympathetic nervous system.[86,87] Such a pattern has been also confirmed by us through a circadian study.[114]

e. The Renin-Angiotensin System and the Renal Function

Renal underperfusion is generally associated with increased plasma renin concentration/activity, with the highest levels observed in patients with renal failure due to either hepatorenal syndrome[57,61] or acute tubular necrosis.[61] Nevertheless, relative renal ischemia can occur even in patients with preserved total renal blood flow. The evaluation of intrarenal distribution of blood flow can be assessed by different methods. Among them, the measurement of frequency distribution curves of transit times of sodium o-[^{131}]iodohippurate through the kidney allows a noninvasive and reliable approach.[115] Using such a technique, a redistribution of blood flow from the outer cortical to the juxtamedullary nephrons has been found in 8/15 cirrhotics without ascites and in 17/28 patients with ascites. No difference in glomerular filtration rate and renal plasma flow were found between patients with and without redistribution.[60] Since renin is mainly secreted by the afferent glomerular arteries of the outer cortical nephrons,[20] it can be understood why, in that study, the magnitude of blood flow to the outer cortex was inversely related to PRA. It should be noted, however, that in spite of a (moderately) redistributed flow, only one (out of 8) patient without ascites had increased PRA, again suggesting an active suppression of the system, not allowed to respond to activating stimuli. Since effective β-blockade with either propranolol or practolol leading to PRA suppression did not reverse the renal vascular abnormality, the latter is likely the cause, rather than the effect of renin-angiotensin system activation.[116]

As stated above, in patients with cirrhosis and ascites the degree of activation of the renin-angiotensin system correlates inversely with the renal blood flow and glomerular filtration rate.[57,87,117-119] Both reduced glomerular perfusion and filtered load of sodium, the latter by acting through a macula densa-mediated mechanism, can account for increased renin secretion by the juxtaglomerular apparatus. However, when glomerular filtration rate and renal plasma flow were plotted against PRA in patients with preserved renal perfusion, no significant correlation was found. This finding has been considered an argument against a role of renal perfusion as a major determinant of renin secretion in cirrhosis.[72] However, although this may simply be an expected finding in subjects with normal renal perfusion, the above-cited studies demonstrated that intrarenal distribution of flow, rather than total renal perfusion, are related to PRA.[60,116] In any case, extremely high levels of plasma renin concentration or activity may be found in patients with normal renal blood flow and glomerular filtration rate. Moreover, although the suppression of the renin-angiotensin system induced by plasma volume expansion was associated with an increase in glomerular filtration rate, a significant correlation between the increments in creatinine clearance and the reduction in PRA was not disclosed.[71] These findings would suggest that, at least initially, renin release in cirrhosis is mainly related to a systemic circulatory disturbance.

It has been thought that the enhanced intrarenal formation of angiotensin II following the activation of the renin-angiotensin system may play a role in conditioning a poor renal perfusion by renal vasoconstriction. This may ultimately result in functional renal failure. However, the renal circulation in cirrhosis is often refractory to the effects of angiotensin II. In fact, the infusion of angiotensin II necessary to raise arterial blood pressure by 35 mmHg depressed the renal plasma flow (as evaluated by para-amino-hippurate clearance) by 51% in normal subjects and by 23% in 5/6 cirrhotics, the remaining patient undergoing no change.[105] Similar results have been confirmed in later studies.[106,120]. Moreover, the suppression of renin secretion by β-adrenergic blockade had no consistent effect on intrarenal hemodynamics[116] and the infusion of the angiotensin II antagonist saralasin into the renal artery of patients with hepatorenal syndrome was not followed by an improvement in renal function.[176] It is worth noting that converting enzyme inhibition by captopril, although it neither affected[121] nor depressed[122] renal blood flow, always reduced glomerular filtration rate.[121,122] This would suggest that in such patients angiotensin II is crucial in maintaining filtration pressure, by increasing postglomerular resistances, as happens at the lower end of renal autoregulation.[28] When dealing with such issues, some considerations have to be taken into account. First, measuring PRA in the peripheral venous (or arterial) blood does not necessarily give an exact picture of the system activity within the kidney. Second, every pharmacological manipulation of an activated renin-angiotensin system would affect systemic hemodynamics, which ultimately influence renal perfusion, obscuring the net effect of angiotensin II antagonism. Such aspects will be discussed elsewhere (see Chapter 18, Section IV). In any case, current evidence suggest that renal perfusion impairment in cirrhosis appears to be the cause rather than the effect of the increased renin release. This view is strengthened by the results obtained by Barnardo et al.[117] These authors found that an elevated PRA associated with a reduced renal plasma flow could be corrected when the latter was improved by the infusion of subpressor dose of dopamine. For example, all 13 patients treated underwent an increase in total renal plasma flow and PRA declined in 10 instances.

Nevertheless, it should be remembered that under certain circumstances the renin-angiotensin system activation can be responsible for renal ischemia. In fact, in diuretic-induced uremia without volume depletion, the use of β-blocking drugs managed to lead to the suppression of PRA and the normalization of the renal function.[123] Moreover, prostaglandin synthesis inhibitors can precipitate renal failure in cirrhosis with ascites, usually showing an increased renal excretion of PGE_2. The most likely mechanism would be the suppression of the counterbalance by renal prostaglandins on the vasoconstrictor effect of angiotensin II (and other vasopressor substances/systems).[124-126] The predominant role played by endogenous angiotensin II in renal function impairment due to cyclo-oxygenase inhibition in liver disease is further suggested by experimental studies. The decline in glomerular filtration rate and renal plasma flow induced by indomethacin in dogs with experimental cirrhosis was prevented by prior administration of saralasin or converting enzyme inhibitors.[127] These and other studies[128] led to the hypothesis that the development of hepatorenal syndrome may be the result of an impairment of renal prostaglandin synthesis, allowing the full intrarenal vasoconstrictor effect of the renin-angiotensin and other systems. A definite proof of this is, however, still lacking.[128]

Angiotensin II infusion to cirrhotics with ascites usually result in natriuresis.[105,120] Contrary to normal subjects, who underwent antinatriuresis under angiotensin II infusion, patients with cirrhosis and ascites showed an enormous increase in sodium and chloride excretion, up to a hundredfold.[105] This was the effect of a net increase in the clearance of sodium/ clearance of inulin ratio, leading to a change in tubular rejection fraction from 0.23 to 12.1%. The mechanism by which angiotensin promoted sodium excretion in cirrhosis is not clear. Since glomerular filtration rate was not significantly affected, an action on tubular transport seemed to be prevalent. A more recent study[129] demonstrated that ≈50% of cirrhotics with ascites receiving angiotensin II show natriuresis, the remaining undergoing antinatriuresis. The two groups were indistinguishable, taking into account the clinical picture, the baseline renal function, and renin status. The divergent behavior in renal sodium excretion appeared to be associated with that of renal prostaglandin excretion. In fact, the changes in excretion of sodium and PGE_2 were parallel, and after prostaglandin synthesis blockade the initial response to angiotensin II, whether natriuretic or antinatriuretic, was altered.

f. Other Factors Influencing the Renin-Angiotensin System

Dilutional hyponatremia, a frequent finding in advanced cirrhosis, has often been inversely correlated with PRA in cirrhosis with ascites.[58,60,62,64] The reduced filtered load of sodium due to hyponatremia and/or low glomerular filtration rate alters the delivery of sodium and chloride to the macula densa.[6] Furthermore, in our experience, the decrease in filtered sodium following acute changes in posture by ascitic patients was inversely related to the increase in PRA.[94] Thus, in addition to the altered volume homeostasis (see above), the hyperreactivity of the juxtaglomerular apparatus following changes in posture can be also related to the exaggerated modifications of renal function induced by tilting.

Hypokalemia can lead to increased renin secretion.[6] We have generally not found a correlation between plasma potassium concentration and PRA. Similar results have been obtained by others.[58,130] This absence of correlation should not be unexpected. In fact, it is the intracellular potassium content, rather than the plasma level of the ion, which appears to influence the juxtaglomerular apparatus, and the latter does not precisely correlate with the former.[131]

A direct correlation between PRA and plasma norepinephrine concentration, which is believed to reflect the activity of the sympathetic nervous system,[132] has recently been found in different studies, at least in recumbent patients.[87-89] This suggests that enhanced sympathoadrenergic activity can stimulate the renin-angiotensin system in cirrhosis, although the importance of such a mechanism is still unsettled. Thus, the above findings may simply represent the running-in-parallel responses of two systems which are activated by the same pathophysiological disturbance such as effective hypovolemia. β-Blocking drugs induced a suppression in PRA proportional to the height of its initial value[116] and this tends to support a role for the sympathetic nervous system in the hyperreninism of cirrhotics.

As reported above (see Section I.A.1), a panoply of further factors can either enhance (adrenal medullary catecholamines, growth hormone, glucagon, parathyroid hormone, prostaglandins of the E and I_2 types, prostacyclins, and thromboxanes) or depress (antidiuretic hormone) the activity of the renin angiotensin system. All of them have been reported to be possibly altered in cirrhosis. Their role in the renin-angiotensin pathophysiology in such a context is not known, but it is unlikely to be a major one.

B. ALDOSTERONE: STATUS AND REGULATION

In 1951 an increased renal excretion of a sodium retaining substance with the characteristics of aldosterone was described in cirrhotics.[133] Two years later, an increased urine excretion of aldosterone in patients forming ascites was reported by Chart and Shipley.[134] This finding was confirmed by others within the 1950s.[135-139] From these seminal studies and from those performed in the mid-1960s, cirrhosis with ascites was conceptually linked to secondary hyperaldosteronism.[140-144] Due to the changes in aldosterone metabolism in cirrhosis (see Section B.2.a) urine aldosterone measurements in these patients may not be entirely reliable. As soon as plasma aldosterone measurements became available, many studies were then devoted to its characterization.

As happened for the renin-angiotensin system, more recent investigations have shown that patients without ascites have normal or, even more often, low-normal/reduced plasma aldosterone concentration. It can be also found within the normal range in patients accumulating ascites, and is usually very elevated in the advanced stages of the disease.[58,59,62-64,70-72,145,146]

1. Cirrhosis without Ascites

Plasma aldosterone concentration has been always found to be in the low normal range or reduced[58,59,62,64,146] (Figure 1). An exception to these findings comes from the study by Mitch et al.,[63] where elevated plasma aldosterone concentration occurred also in patients with alcoholic liver disease without ascites. However, the same considerations concerning patient selection reported for PRA (see Section II.A.1) should be applied also in this context.

The plasma aldosterone circadian rhythm in such patients is slightly deranged[64] (Figure

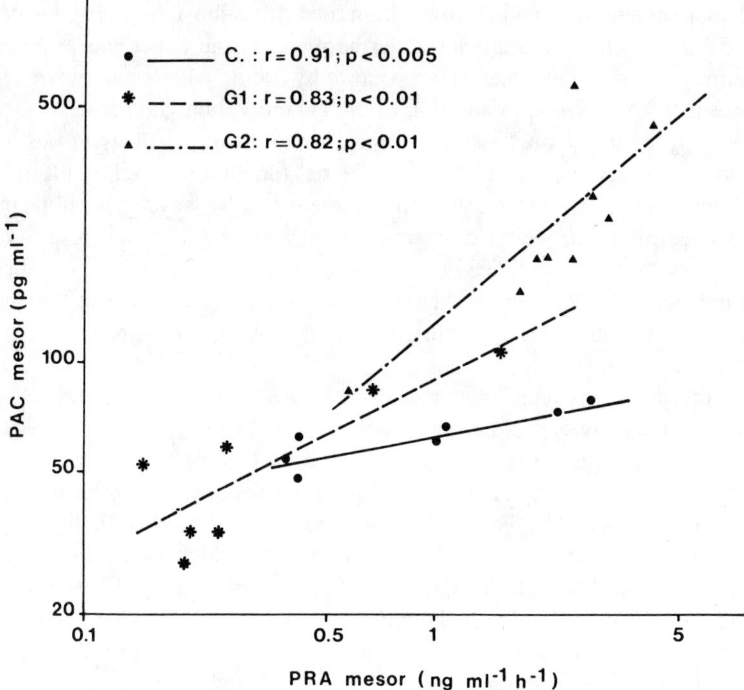

FIGURE 3.   Correlation between rhythm adjusted averages (mesors) of plasma renin activity (PRA) and plasma aldosterone concentration (PAC) in healthy controls (C) and cirrhotics without (G1) and with (G2) ascites. The slope of the regression line is progressively steeper in patients: C vs. G1, p <0.05; C vs. G2, p <0.01; G1 vs. G2, not significant. (From Bernardi, M., De Palma, R., Trevisani, F., Santini, C., Capani, F., Baraldini, M., and Gasbarrini, G., *Gastroenterology*, 91, 683, 1986. With permission.)

2C). Specifically, the achronia (no detection of a statistically significant rhythm) was mainly due to an increased individual variability with respect to healthy controls. In fact, a statistically significant circadian rhythm was recovered when data were evaluated as percent change from the mesor (average daily level). In this study, chronic diseases not developing hyperreninism or secondary hyperaldosteronism in their natural histories did not affect the plasma aldosterone circadian rhythm. Thus, the abnormalities found in cirrhotics without ascites could be considered specific harbingers of future major perturbations present in the advanced stages (see Section B.2.b). Since plasma cortisol levels were normal and its rhythmicity preserved (Figure 2), it is very unlikely that ACTH played some role in the described aldosterone alterations.[64]

PRA did not correlate with plasma aldosterone concentration in a group of compensated patients when such parameters were measured through spot samplings at 10 a.m.[62] Moreover, their values were less frequently correlated than in healthy controls when sequential evaluations during the day were performed. However, when mesors were considered, a direct significant correlation was found, as in the normal subjects and cirrhotics with ascites[64] (Figure 3). Therefore, it is also likely that in compensated patients, as in the normal man, the renin-angiotensin system is the most important determinant of aldosterone secretion level. Therefore, it can be understood why plasma aldosterone concentration is often reduced.

Plasma potassium and aldosterone daily rhythmicity are closely associated in normal subjects.[37] Such a correlation was not found in compensated cirrhotics.[64] Such a finding does not necessarily exclude a regulatory role of the ion on hormone secretion, since intracellular rather than serum potassium is likely to influence aldosterone secretion.[38]

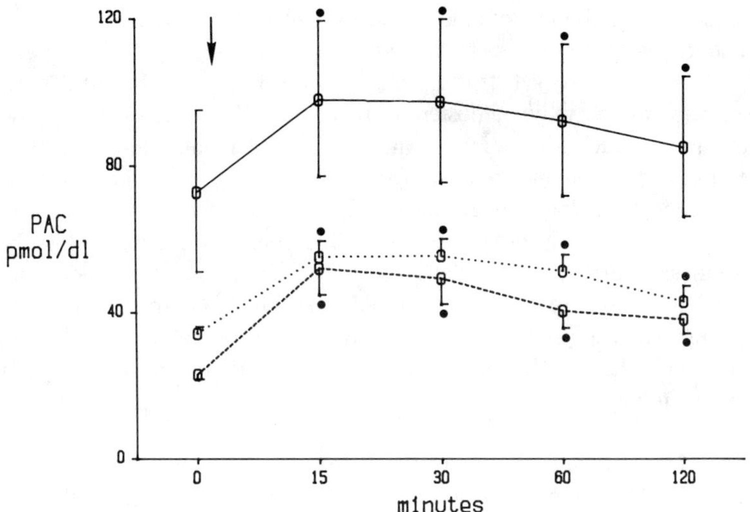

FIGURE 4. Changes in plasma aldosterone concentration induced by metoclopramide administration (10 mg i.v.) in healthy controls (····) and cirrhotics without (----) and with (———) ascites. The incremental areas under the curves were not significantly ● = statistically different from baseline.

As reported (see Section I.B.1), glomerulosa cell secretory activity is modulated by dopaminergic afferents. Derangements in dopaminergic activity have been emphasized as an important pathogenetic factor under certain circumstances in primary and secondary hyperaldosteronism.[41] We have examined the relationship between aldosterone secretion and dopaminergic activity in cirrhosis by evaluating the plasma aldosterone response to an intravenous bolus of 10 mg of the dopamine receptor blocker metoclopramide.[147] In 10 cirrhotics without ascites, the aldosterone response did not differ from that obtained in normal subjects (Figure 4), suggesting that derangements in dopaminergic modulation of the hormone secretion were unlikely.

2. Cirrhosis with Ascites
a. Aldosterone Metabolism

In the presence of increased plasma levels or urinary excretion of aldosterone, the effect of a reduced hepatic metabolism of the hormone has to be taken into account. Coppage et al.[142] showed that the $t_{1/2}$ of intravenously administered 7-^{3}H-d-aldosterone to cirrhotics was prolonged (43 to 81 min) with respect to healthy controls (26 to 39 min). Differences in volume distribution did not justify such an alteration. A reduced metabolic clearance rate of aldosterone in cirrhosis has been confirmed by other studies.[63,70,139,148] However, the aldosterone secretion rate has also been found to be increased.[70,139,142,149] Values reported in one study ranged from 248 to 2,080 μg/24 h in cirrhotics (most being on low sodium diet). Values of normal subjects ranged from 95 to 249 μg/24 h on a sodium unrestricted diet and from 284 to 528 μg/24 h under sodium restriction.[142] Rosoff et al.,[70] by comparing the magnitude of the derangement in aldosterone metabolic clearance (1072 ± 157 1/d vs. 1620 ± 85 1/d in normal controls) and secretion rates (1281 ± 534 μg/d vs. ≈100 μg/d) came to the conclusion that marked aldosterone hypersecretion is the predominant factor in producing very elevated hormone blood levels in ascitic patients. An indirect support to such a statement is given by the marked, rapid decreases in supine plasma aldosterone concentrations (from 282, 126, and 88 ng/dl to 20, 8, and 7 ng/dl, respectively) produced in three patients by oral administration of 1 to 2 g/d of aminoglutethimide (a drug which reduces aldosterone production by the adrenal cortex) plus dexamethasone.

An altered liver metabolism of aldosterone also accounts for a modification of the renal excretory pattern of the hormone metabolites. In fact, a greater proportion of the 18-glucuronide form (3-oxo-conjugated) is excreted with respect to tetrahydroaldosterone, which, in any case, remains the major aldosterone metabolite.[142] It has been proposed that the reduction of ring A, leading to tetrahydroaldosterone formation within the liver, is a rate-limiting step in the hormone metabolism. Thus, 18-glucuronide production, which does not require ring A reduction, could be enhanced.[142] However, also an increased compensatory renal metabolism, which only produces the 18-glucuronide form, is most likely involved. According to these findings, the correlation between measurements of aldosterone secretion rate and the excretion rate of the 18-glucuronide metabolite in cirrhosis was shifted to the left, when compared with predicted values derived from normal subjects.[149] Unless this is taken into account, values for 18-glucuronide excretion will give misleadingly high absolute values for the secretion rate.[149]

b. Aldosterone Hypersecretion: Role of the Renin-Angiotensin System

As noted for PRA, plasma aldosterone concentration is often within the normal range in patients with cirrhosis and ascites. Up to 74% of untreated patients may show normal plasma aldosterone, whereas this percentage falls to 15% in cirrhotics with previous diuretic administration.[58] In the majority of the other studies, such a stratification has not been made, and the frequency of hyperaldosteronism in ascitic cirrhotics is found between the above values[59,62-64,71,72,145,146] (Figure 1).

Increased plasma aldosterone concentration, when present, has usually been attributed to the enhanced activity of the renin-angiotensin activity. In fact, a positive correlation between plasma aldosterone concentration or 18-glucuronide excretion and PRA or plasma angiotensin II concentration has been reported by many authors.[58,59,62,63,72,79,94,116] The same conclusion was reached when the aldosterone secretion rate was studied in relation to PRA.[149]

The most convincing evidence for a key role of the renin-angiotensin system in producing aldosterone hypersecretion comes from dynamic studies, where the activity of the system was suppressed through different means. Neck-out water immersion disclosed that these two variables were reduced in a parallel manner.[71] Analogously, PRA depression by either albumin or saline infusions was followed by a reduction in plasma aldosterone concentration.[90] By plotting arbitrarily the Log PRA and plasma aldosterone mean values observed under basal conditions and at different times during the infusions, a highly significant correlation can be obtained (r = 0.96 after albumin; r = 0.98 after saline). Moreover, ascites retransfusion[91] and LeVeen shunt insertion[93] led to reductions in PRA and plasma aldosterone concentration which were roughly parallel. Finally, when neck-out water immersion failed to reduce PRA, plasma aldosterone concentration also underwent a nonsignificant reduction. Both variables were significantly suppressed when immersion was coupled with norepinephrine infusion.[150] Conversely, the magnitude of the rise in plasma aldosterone concentration stimulated by active tilting correlated significantly with that of PRA.[94]

Pharmacological suppression of renin-angiotensin system activity is usually followed by a decrease in plasma aldosterone concentration. For example, in our experience, PRA suppression by propranolol was associated with plasma aldosterone reduction in 15 out of 16 cases (Figure 5). Similarly, angiotensin II blockade with the angiotensin analogue saralasin was usually followed by a fall in plasma aldosterone concentration.[151] However, the results of some studies appear to be at variance with those reported above. Effective β-blockade leading to PRA suppression was not followed by consistent changes in aldosterone 18-glucuronide excretion.[116] Also, in patients given saralasin, plasma aldosterone did not always decrease. This happened in one study in one case out of five.[112] In a further experience, plasma aldosterone decreased in 4/12 patients, increased in 6, and remained virtually unchanged in the remaining 2. However, as stated above, the angiotensin II analogue used in this study (1-Sar, 8-Ile angiotensin II) possesses more agonistic property than saralasin.[113]

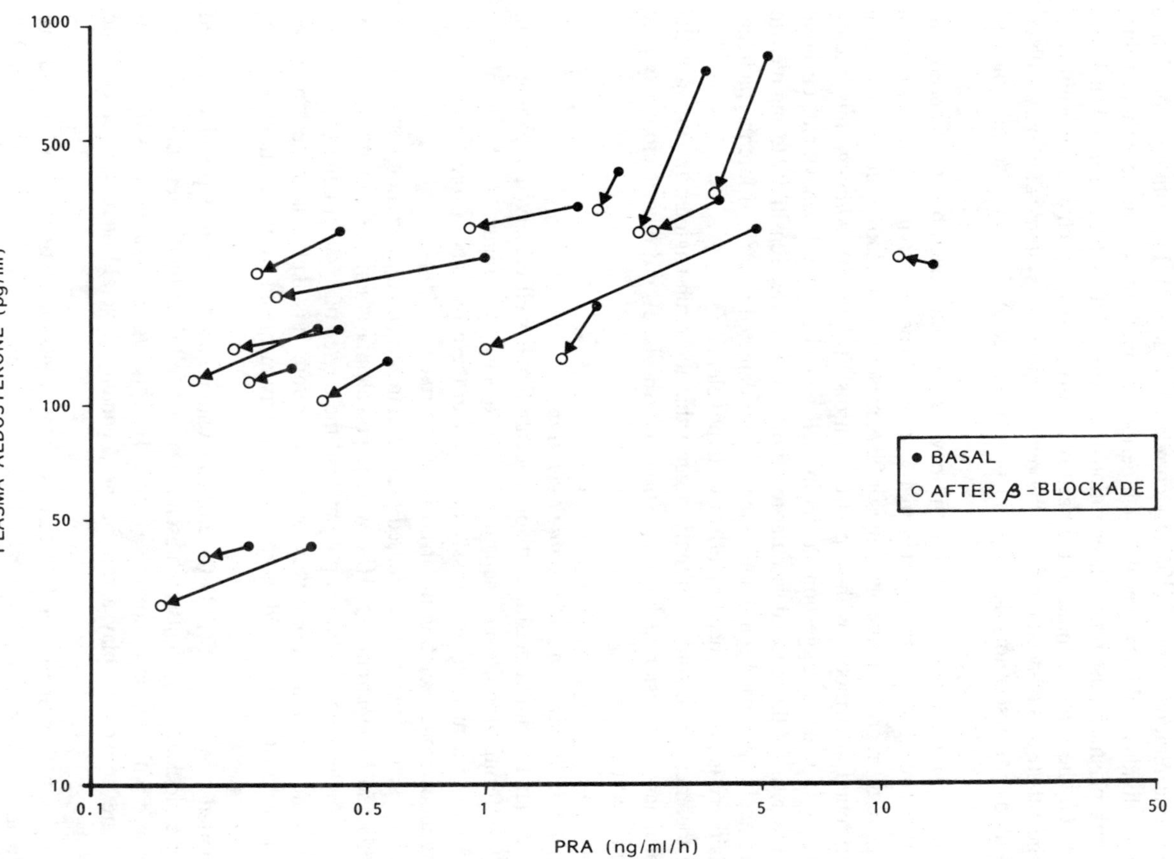

FIGURE 5. Relationship between plasma renin activity (PRA) and aldosterone concentration before and after effective β-blockade (≥20% reduction in resting heart rate) achieved with oral propranolol in cirrhotics with ascites. Arrows show the direction of change.

Moreover, baseline plasma aldosterone concentration was not markedly increased in most cases. It is conceivable that the impact of the suppression of the renin-angiotensin system activity on aldosterone secretion is influenced by the degree of the activity itself. In fact, when plasma aldosterone reduction was attempted with captopril the results were relevant mainly in patients with increased baseline levels.[113]

We have recently reexamined the issue of angiotensin-mediated secretion of aldosterone by a chronobiological approach. The rhythm adjusted averages (mesors) of PRA and plasma aldosterone concentration were significantly correlated (Figure 3). Interestingly, correlation analysis for individual subjects over the 24-h period obtained by plotting sequential values of PRA against plasma aldosterone concentration disclosed significant results in 5/9 cirrhotics with ascites. On the contrary, none of the healthy controls showed such a relationship. This would suggest that, in advanced cirrhosis, the renin angiotensin system is not only a determinant of aldosterone secretory level (as in normal subjects), but can also influence its secretory periodicity.[64]

The role of the renin-angiotensin system may also be potentiated by an enhanced sensitivity of the adrenal cortex to angiotensin II. Such a hypersensitivity is suggested by a steeper slope of the regression line of the mesor PRA/mesor plasma aldosterone concentration relationship found in cirrhotics with respect to controls[64] (Figure 3). Although this finding only allows us to make a suggestion, it fits in well with the general behavior of cirrhotic patients. In fact, as for the reduced vascular reactivity, an increased sensitivity to angiotensin II by the adrenal cortex has been found in the sodium-depleted man.[21,22] Moreover, adrenal cortex sensitivity is also enhanced by effective hypovolemia.[22]

Taken together, these studies strongly suggest that the renin-angiotensin system is the major determinant of aldosterone hypersecretion in cirrhosis, even if other factors may play a role in this setting.

c. Other Factors Involved in Aldosterone Secretion

The circadian rhythm of plasma cortisol concentration is well-preserved in patients with ascites not suffering from severe hepatic encephalopathy[64,152] (Figure 2). Since plasma aldosterone daily fluctuations are grossly deranged in these patients, a role for ACTH in determining aldosterone secretion in cirrhosis can be ruled out.[64]

Additional factors leading to increased plasma aldosterone concentration could include hyperkalemia and hyponatremia.[149] However, hyperkalemia is not often found in patients with cirrhosis, unless renal failure is present, and the degree of hyponatremia necessary to affect aldosterone secretion per se is very large.[39] Therefore, it is likely that in most instances the effect of hyponatremia on aldosterone secretion is mediated by the renin-angiotensin system activation.

As reported (see Section II.B.1) for cirrhosis without ascites, metoclopramide-induced dopaminergic blockade in patients with ascites was not followed by different plasma aldosterone response with respect to controls (Figure 4). This suggests that changes in dopaminergic tone are unlikely to play a role in the secondary hyperaldosteronism of cirrhotic patients.[147]

Other recently identified factors, such as aldosterone-stimulating factor of pituitary origin[40] and atrial natriopeptides[42] (see also Chapter 15) modulate aldosterone secretion, but their importance in cirrhosis is not yet known.

C. ALDOSTERONE: EFFECTS ON RENAL FUNCTION
1. Aldosterone and Sodium Metabolism in Cirrhosis with Ascites

As reported in section 1.2. the site of aldosterone action on the nephron is the collecting tubule, with the final portion of the distal convoluted tubule possibly being also involved. Thus, a first consideration to be approached concerns the segment of the nephron which is responsible for the increased sodium absorption. Such an item is the subject of continuing controversy. Most authors agree that the diluting segment is not involved.[146,153-155] On the contrary, Chaimovitz et al.[156] suggested an enhanced sodium reabsorption at the water-clearing segment. However, the analytical methods used in their study only allowed them to evaluate the fractional reabsorption of sodium "distal" to the proximal tubule, hence including both the ascending limb of Henle's loop and the distal and collecting tubules. Convincing evidence is available for an exaggerated proximal tubular reabsorption.[146,153,-155] In some studies, however, either the distal absorption was not investigated,[153,154] or the renal perfusion was significantly depressed, accounting for a mean glomerular filtration rate ≈ 60 ml/min.[155] In such a circumstance, the hemodynamic-induced proximal absorption would have easily been expected to be enhanced. Wilkinson et al.,[146] demonstrated in a group of cirrhotics showing positive sodium balance (glomerular filtration rate ranging from 63 to 254 ml/min) that sodium retention also occurred at the portion of the nephron distal to the loop of Henle, the latter being quantitatively more important. As a whole, these studies suggest that the main site for the abnormal sodium retention in the cirrhotic patient is the distal nephron, with the proximal also being involved. A reduced renal perfusion may account mostly, even if not entirely, for the latter. Indirect evidence for a distal hyperabsorption also comes from the failure of furosemide (up to 160 mg/d) in inducing diuresis in 10 out of 21 cirrhotics with ascites and preserved glomerular filtration rate.[157]

An enhanced distal sodium reabsorption recalls the presence of an excess of mineralocorticoid hormones. An inverse statistically significant correlation between plasma aldosterone concentration and renal sodium excretion has generally been found in cirrhosis.[59,62,72,94,119,146] However, a correlation does not imply a cause-effect relationship between the two variables. Furthermore, the results of several studies have cast doubts about a main role played by aldosterone in mediating sodium retention in cirrhosis. The administration of aminoglutethiamide to three cirrhotics with positive sodium balance did not increase sodium excretion, in spite of the reduction of previously elevated plasma aldosterone concentration.[70] Unfortunately, the glomerular filtration rate of such patients was not reported, but they were described as having "long-standing, diuretic-resistant ascites". In our and others' experience, such a condition is associated with a poor renal perfusion; in this case sodium retention would continue independently of suppressed aldosterone. Suppression of aldosterone secretion has also been attempted with captopril. Although natriuresis was achieved in two reports,[113,158] captopril administration was usually followed by no response or reduction of sodium excretion.[121,122,159] However, since in the latter studies such a drug lowered glomerular filtration rate by both reducing mean arterial pressure and filtration fraction,[121,122] its failure as a natriuresis-inducer even in the presence of aldosterone suppression can be explained.

Isothermic neck-out water immersion, in spite of the reported significant reduction of plasma aldosterone did not increase renal sodium excretion in a number of cirrhotics.[71] Similarly, plasma aldosterone suppression achieved by dietary sodium loading resulted in an inappropriately low natriuresis.[145] However, such a dissociation is only apparent. In fact, it should be noted that "nonresponders" to water immersion had a strikingly elevated baseline plasma aldosterone and the aldosterone/sodium excretion relationship has the form of a rectangular hyperbole (Figure 6). Thus, in the presence of marked hyperaldosteronism, reductions in aldosterone have to be very marked to result in significant increases in renal sodium excretion. Taking into account the shape of this relationship, the changes in urinary sodium excretion are exactly as would have been predicted, based on the changes that occur in both aldosterone 18-glucuronide excretion after propranolol or practolol administration.[116] Moreover, we were able to disclose this relationship also by plotting plasma aldosterone concentration and renal sodium excretion under basal conditions and after effective β-blockade achieved by propranolol[159a] (Figure 6). Further evidence comes from the finding that negative sodium balance following head-out water immersion plus norepinephrine in-

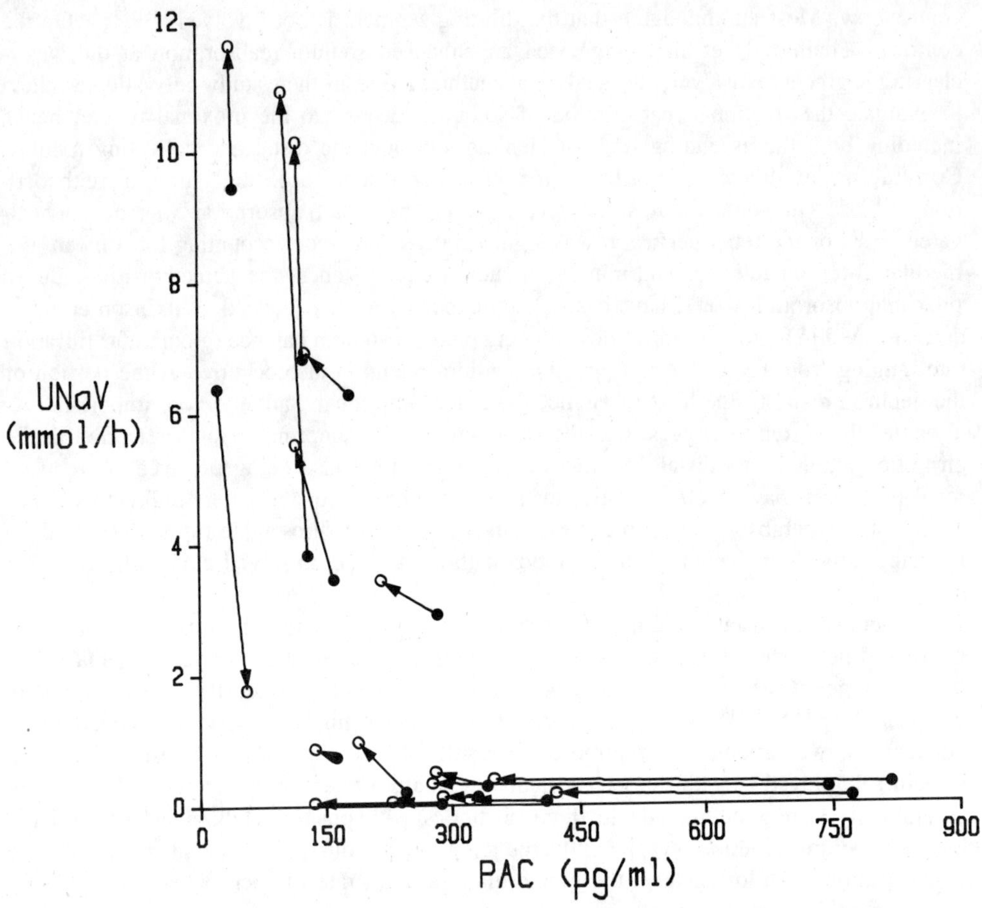

FIGURE 6.   The correlation between plasma aldosterone concentration and hourly renal sodium excretion ($U_{Na}V$) has the shape of a rectangular hyperbole. The $U_{Na}V$ changed as would be predicted from the changes induced in plasma aldosterone concentration by effective β-blockade ($\geq$20% reduction in resting heart rate) achieved with oral propranolol in cirrhotics with ascites (glomerular filtration rate -55 ml/min). Arrows show the direction of change. (From Bernardi, M. et al., *J. Hepatol.*, 8, 279, 1989. With permission.)

fusion ensued only in patients whose plasma aldosterone was suppressed to levels below 50 ng/ml.[150]

Other findings appear to support the concept of a primary role of aldosterone in promoting sodium retention in cirrhosis. The decrease in tubular rejection fraction of sodium due to the change in posture of cirrhotics with ascites, was inversely related to the increase in plasma aldosterone concentration.[94] When spontaneous diuresis develops, the majority of patients show a reduction of elevated plasma aldosterone down to normal levels.[70] Finally, the natriuretic efficacy of spironolactone[157] has traditionally been considered as evidence for a sodium retaining role of aldosterone in cirrhosis. This has been further strengthened by our finding that the daily dosage of spironolactone necessary to promote a negative sodium balance in cirrhotics with ascites was directly correlated with the plasma aldosterone concentration[160] (see also Chapter 18).

Besides extrinsic modulations, such as those cited above, hormonal system impact on targets can be studied by the chronological approach, which allows detection of dynamic interrelationships between variables undergoing time-related fluctuations. In our experience,[161] a significant inverse correlation between plasma aldosterone and urine sodium excretion was present throughout the whole day (divided into 4 h periods) in ascitic patients,

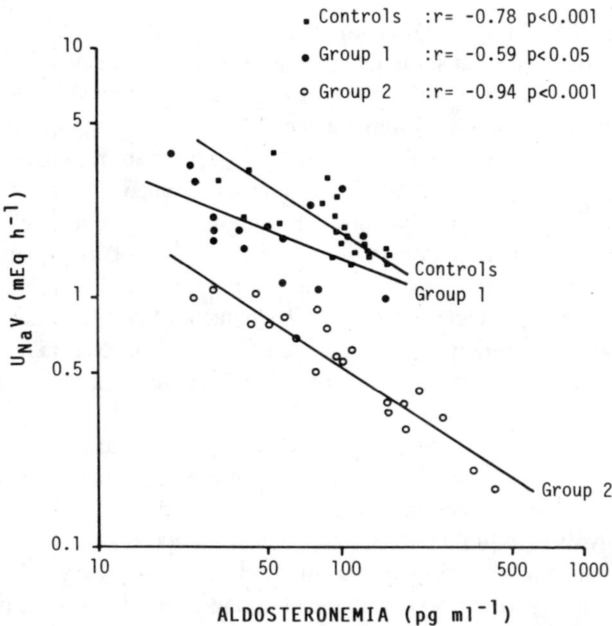

FIGURE 7.   Correlation between plasma aldosterone concentration and hourly urinary sodium excretion
($U_{Na}V$) in healthy subjects and cirrhotics without (group 1) and with (group 2) ascites. The experimental
conditions are the same as those reported in Figure 1. There is a progressive significant shift to the abscissa
of the regresssion line from groups 1 and 2 compared with controls (controls vs. group 1, p <0.01; group
1 vs. group 2, p <0.001). (From Bernardi, M., Trevisani, F., Santini, C., De Palma, R., and Gasbarrini,
G., *Gut*, 24, 761, 1983. With permission.)

whereas it appeared erratically in healthy controls. These findings suggest that in healthy
humans, under steady state conditions, aldosterone seldom reaches a prominent position
among the various factors governing renal sodium handling. On the contrary, in cirrhosis
with ascites the relationship between aldosterone and tubular sodium handling is not only
closer than normal, but also extended throughout the whole day. Thus, the impact of the
hormone on this function is remarkably amplified.

Further doubts arose when recent studies showed that a large number of cirrhotics with
active salt retention actually had plasma aldosterone concentration within the "normal"
range (see section II.B.2). This feature can be explained by an abnormal aldosterone/renal
sodium excretion relationship, first suggested by Wilkinson et al.[146] We pushed forward
such studies and showed also that the abnormality precedes ascites formation and worsens
as the disease progresses.[62] Namely, we observed that, for any given value of plasma
aldosterone, patients with ascites were excreting about one fourth and compensated cirrhotics
about two thirds of the amount of urinary sodium excreted by healthy controls (Figure 7).
Such findings have been subsequently confirmed by others[162] and by us through a chronobiological study.[161] The same abnormality can also explain the need for spironolactone
administration to counteract positive sodium balance in ascitic patients with normal plasma
aldosterone concentration.[157,160]

This would seem to imply an increased sensitivity of the renal tubules to mineralocorticoid
activity, as described in dogs having constriction of the thoracic segment of the inferior vena
cava.[163] Another explanation, which should not exclude the suggested tubular hypersensitivity, would be that of a deficiency of natriuretic factor(s) synthesis and/or release (see next
paragraph).

In conclusion, either plasma aldosterone concentration or renal excretion of its metabolites and sodium excretion have been found to be inversely correlated over a wide range
of experimental conditions, provided that renal perfusion is preserved.

2. Aldosterone and Sodium Metabolism in Cirrhosis without Ascites

Major derangements in renal sodium handling, leading to clinically evident abnormalities are not present in cirrhotics without ascites. However, experimental evidence showing that such patients cannot attain proper sodium balance is available. First, as reported above, they have expanded plasma or blood volumes (Figure 1). Such a feature suggests incontrovertibly that sodium retention somehow occurs before the appearance of ascites and that sodium homeostasis is "reset" at a higher than normal sodium pool. Second, they may not succeed in escaping the sodium retaining effects of exogenous mineralocorticoids[164] or in disposing of a saline load.[165] Finally, an abnormal relationship between aldosterone and renal tubular sodium handling is already detectable[66] (Figure 7). Sequential studies in experimental animals confirmed that sodium retention, in the absence of changes in renal hemodynamics, occur in cirrhotic dogs (dimethylnitrosamine-induced)[67] and rats (carbon tetrachloride-induced)[166] before ascites formation.

Has aldosterone any role in the deranged sodium excretion at this stage of the disease? Renal hemodynamics and glomerular filtration rate are usually unaltered, thus only factors acting directly at the tubular handling should be considered. Systems other than the renin-aldosterone axis involved in sodium retention in the ascitic stage, such as sympathoadrenergic activity[167] and renal PGE_2[128] are in the normal range, as well as atrial natriopeptides.[168] Therefore, it is tempting to attribute a major importance to the reported tubular hypersensitivity to aldosterone. It is worth noting that a significant relationship between the two variables has also been found in cirrhosis without ascites[62] (Figure 7). Furthermore, a direct correlation between plasma aldosterone concentration and blood volume was seen in patients either with or without ascites (Figure 8), suggesting that the mineralocorticoid activity is a major determinant of extracellular fluid volume, by way of renal sodium retention, even before ascites formation.[62] This hypothesis is further supported by the observation that in cirrhotic dogs, preascitic sodium retention occurs at the distal nephron level.[169] Of course, a deficiency or, in any case, a reduced activity of natriuretic factor would lead to the same final result.

All these studies do not clarify which mechanism(s) protect sodium-retaining compensated patients from ascites formation. Alternatively, either volume receptors blunt the efferent mechanisms at a given, higher than normal, level, or most patients are still able to undergo periodic equilibration through an escape phenomenon. Indirect evidence for this may be derived from our recent findings. In seven nonascitic patients maintained supine for 24 h after 6 d of low sodium diet (40 mmol/d) the mesor of sodium excretion was significantly higher than seven normal subjects undergoing a similar protocol, so that natriuresis exceeded by threefold the daily salt intake. Moreover, in such patients the urinary volume was not enhanced with respect to controls and renal sodium excretion never correlated with plasma aldosterone level throughout the day.[161] Taken together, these findings suggest that factor(s) selectively influencing tubular sodium handling have been entrained. Such a feature recalls that seen in compensated patients undergoing "mineralocorticoid escape".[164] Unfortunately, sequential studies protracted over a large time span, which alone would be able to bring light to these aspects, are not presently available in humans.

3. Aldosterone and Renal Potassium Handling

Although the occurrence of potassium deficiency in cirrhosis has likely been overemphasized, reduction in total body, exchangeable and intracellular potassium have been reported.[170] When "false positive" results due to diuretic treatment, excess of total body water, and muscle mass wasting could be ruled out, it is tempting to ascribe to aldosterone the responsibility for such a depletion, due to its effects on renal potassium handling. However, if we assume that absolute or relative hyperaldosteronism is always present in cirrhosis accumulating ascites, the rarity of actual potassium deficiency first raises doubts

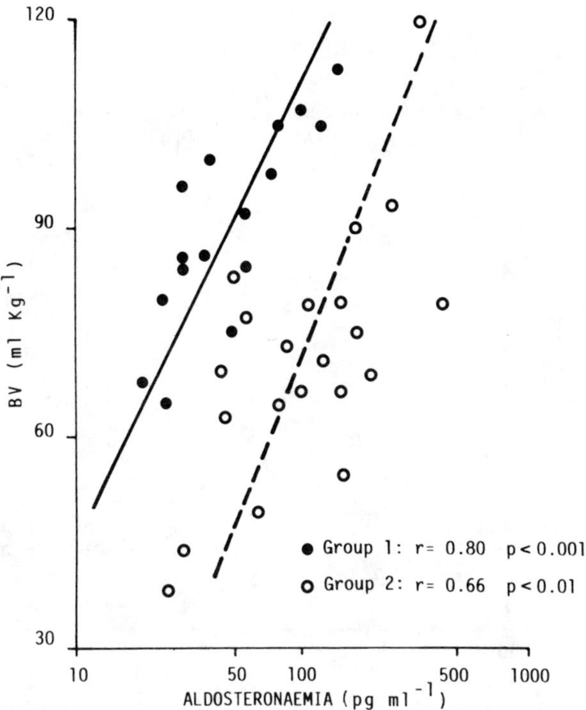

FIGURE 8. Correlation between plasma aldosterone concentration and blood volume in cirrhosis without (group 1) and with (group 2) ascites. The experimental conditions are the same as those reported in Figure 1. (From Bernardi, M., Trevisani, F., Santini, C., DePalma, R., and Gasbarrini, G., *Gut*, 24, 761, 1983. With permission.)

about such an assumption. Moreover, an increased renal potassium excretion should have been found. On the contrary, patients with cirrhosis and ascites tend to have urine potassium excretion lower than control groups.[104,142,171]

We have focused this problem in cirrhotics with ascites and positive sodium balance[172] by evaluating renal potassium circadian excretion, in relation to plasma aldosterone concentration, urine sodium excretion, and flow rate, the latter being the intratubular modulators of potassium output.[173] A circadian rhythm for renal potassium excretion was only found in healthy controls. In agreement with the cited works,[104,142,171] the mesor value of urine potassium excretion was marginally lower in cirrhotics than in controls, in spite of the fact that the former group had a significantly higher mesor of plasma aldosterone concentration. However, taking into account that patients' urine flow and, by a greater extent, sodium excretion were reduced, it can be stated that kaliuresis was inappropriately elevated. In fact, aldosterone contribution to potassium excretion, as evaluated by calculating the kaliuresis corrected by distal tubular sodium delivery[174], was more than twofold higher in cirrhotics. Moreover, plasma aldosterone concentration was extensively correlated with ''corrected kaliuresis'' throughout the whole day only in patients (Figure 9). Finally, neither aldosterone nor ''corrected kaliuresis'' nor renal potassium output displayed the physiological circadian pulsatility. Evidence was thus provided that the contribution of aldosterone to set renal potassium excretion is enhanced in cirrhosis with ascites, so that it may be the main factor responsible for the disruption of the normal circadian profile of kaliuresis. Potassium wasting, however, is effectively prevented by the reduction of urine and renal sodium outputs, until events increasing urine flow and sodium delivery to the distal nephron, such as diuretics, allow aldosterone to exert a full blown kaliuretic activity.

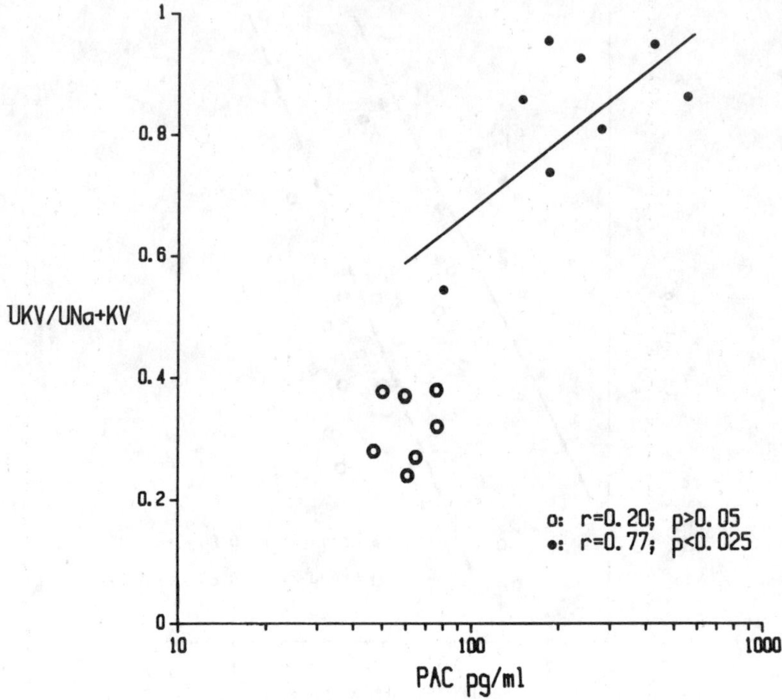

FIGURE 9.   Correlation between rhythm-adjusted averages (mesors) of plasma aldosterone concentration (PAC) and the kaliuresis corrected by the distal tubular sodium delivery ($U_K V/U_{Na+K}V$), which is an index of the aldosterone contribution to renal potassium excretion, in cirrhotics with ascites (•) and healthy control subjects (○). (From Trevisani, F. et al., *Gastroenterology*, 96, 1187, 1989. With permission.)

III. THE RENIN-ANGIOTENSIN-ALDOSTERONE SYSTEM IN ACUTE LIVER DISEASE

Only a limited experience is available on the status of the renin-angiotensin-aldosterone system in acute liver disease, and it is mainly due to anecdotal reports. A comprehensive study on the system activity and dynamics has been carried out in patients with fulminant hepatic failure.[175] The most striking finding was a marked activation of the system, with plasma renin concentration increased up to 200-fold above the 95% confidence limits for healthy controls. Angiotensinogen levels were severely reduced, being at times close to zero. This recalls the report by Ayers,[56] who found the lowest renin substrate concentration in two patients with severe hepatitis. Interestingly, plasma renin and angiotensinogen were inversely correlated, suggesting that, in addition to a reduced hepatic synthesis, an active consumption contributed to lower angiotensinogen (Figure 10). The reduced availability of substrate would possibly prevent the "full expression" of the activation of the renin-angiotensin system. In fact, arterial hypotension often coexisted with elevated angiotensin hepta-/octapeptide levels. In addition to any presumable reduction of vascular sensitivity, an inadequate angiotensin I generation may be involved. This may have therapeutic implications in that, in cirrhosis, a deficit of substrate can be partially corrected by fresh frozen plasma.[176] Another factor limiting the efficacy of the system was also an accelerated degradation of angiotensin II, since the percentage of active hepta-/octapeptides was actually reduced, although both peptides were often increased in their absolute values. This finding was likely due to an enhanced release of angiotensinases from necrotic hepatocytes.

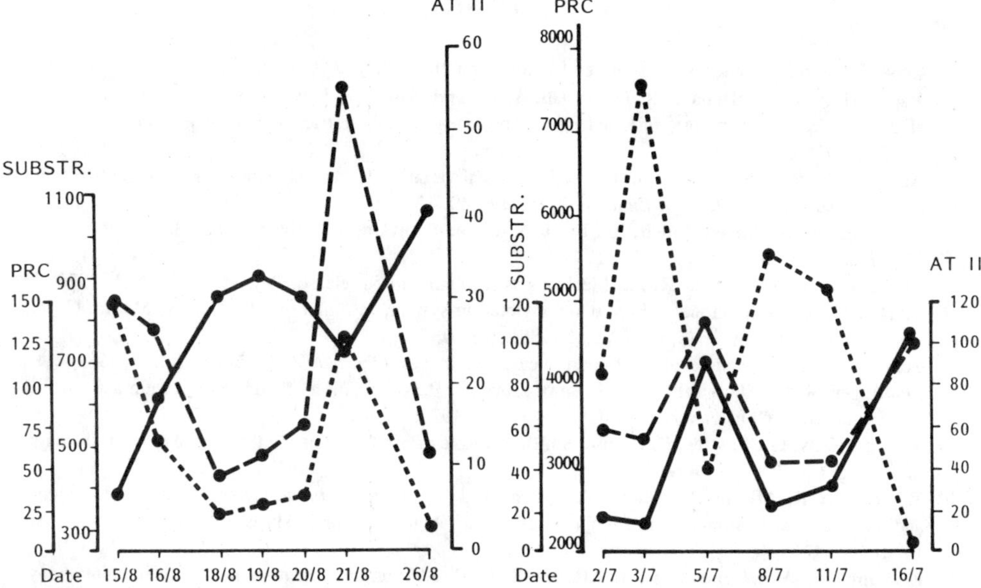

FIGURE 10. Left. Sequential measurements of plasma renin (PRC; ····), total angiotensin II (ATII; ----) and angiotensinogen (substr.; ----) concentrations in one patient with fulminant hepatic failure. The changes in plasma angiotensin II concentration closely paralleled those in plasma renin concentration, whereas plasma angiotensinogen concentration changed reciprocally. System activation led to ATII production and angiotensinogen consumption. Right. Sequential studies in one patient with subacute hepatic necrosis. The changes in plasma angiotensinogen, which was strikingly reduced, paralleled those of ATII. In this case, ATII generation was not a function of PRC, but was conditioned by the amount of substrate available. PRC changed reciprocally to ATII, suggesting either feedback inhibition of renin release or compensation of the activating stimulus(i) by ATII.

As in cirrhosis, arterial hypotension appeared to be a major stimulus to renin release: blood pressure was inversely related to plasma renin concentration. However, a reduced hepatic degradation would have likely contributed to hyperreninism in a more significant degree than in cirrhosis. A reduced renal perfusion, up to renal failure, was found in many patients. Again it is difficult to state with certainty whether increased renin-angiotensin system activity has to be considered its determinant or consequence. Although an inverse correlation between creatinine clearance and angiotensin hepta-/octapeptide would support a role of the system in reducing renal perfusion, it could equally indicate that the reduced renal perfusion responsible for the development of renal impairment was a stimulus to activating renin-angiotensin system. In support of the latter explanation, a statistically significant relationship between creatinine clearance and arterial pressure was also demonstrable.

Plasma aldosterone concentration was also nearly always increased, reaching values up to 14-fold higher than the upper normal limit. Plasma aldosterone was correlated with hepta-/octapeptide angiotensin II, suggesting that also in this context the renin-angiotensin system was an important factor for the increased plasma aldosterone levels. As for renin, however, it is likely that a reduced hepatic degradation could play an important role. The fact that creatinine clearance was often severely reduced, can explain why no relationship between plasma aldosterone concentration and renal sodium excretion was found in these patients.

REFERENCES

1. **Cook, W. and Pickering, G.**, Location of renin within the kidney, *J. Physiol. (London)*, 143, 78, 1958.
2. **Vagnucci, A. H., McDonald, R. H., Drash, A. L., and Wong, A. K. C.**, Intradiem changes of plasma aldosterone, cortisol, corticosterone, and growth hormone in sodium restriction, *J. Clin. Endocrinol. Metab.*, 38, 761, 1974.
3. **Katz, F. H., Romfh, P., and Smith, A. J.**, Diurnal variation of plasma aldosterone, cortisol and renin activity in supine man, *J. Clin. Endocrinol. Metab.*, 40, 125, 1975.
4. **Modlinger, R. S., Sharif-Zadeh, K., Ertel, N. H., and Gutkin, M.**, The circadian rhythm of renin, *J. Clin. Endocrinol. Metab.*, 43, 1276, 1976.
5. **Davis, J. O. and Freeman, R. H.**, Mechanisms regulating renin release, *Physiol. Rev.*, 56, 1, 1976.
6. **Martin, C. R.**, Aldosterone and the renin angiotensin system, in *Endocrine Physiology*, Martin, C. R., Ed., Oxford University Press, New York, 1985, chap. 9.
7. **Torretti, J.**, Sympathetic control of renin release, *Annu. Rev. Pharmacol. Toxicol.*, 22, 167, 1982.
8. **Modlinger, R. S., Shonmuller, J. M., and Arora, S. P.**, Stimulation of aldosterone, renin and cortisol by tryptophan, *J. Clin. Endocrinol. Metab.*, 48, 599, 1979.
9. **Yun, J., Kelly, G., Bartter, F. C., and Smith H.**, Role of prostaglandins in the control of renin secretion in the dog, *Cir. Res.*, 40, 459, 1977.
10. **Whorton, A. R., Misono, K., Hollifield, J., Frolich, J. C., Inagami, T., and Oates, J. A.**, Prostaglandins and renin release: I. Stimulation of renin release from rabbit renal cortex slices by PGI_2, *Prostaglandins*, 14, 1095, 1977.
11. **Flamenbaum, W., Gagnon, J., and Ramwell, P.**, Bradikinin-induced renal hemodynamic alterations: Renin and prostaglandin relationships, *Am. J. Physiol.*, 237, F433, 1979.
12. **Tsunoda, K., Abe, K., Goto, T., Yasujima, M., Sato, M., Omata, K., Seino, M., and Yoshinaga, K.**, Effect of age on the renin-angiotensin-aldosterone system in normal subjects: simultaneous measurement of active and inactive renin, renin substrate, and aldosterone in plasma, *J. Clin. Endocrinol. Metab.*, 62, 384, 1986.
13. **Ciér, J. F.**, La physiologie du système rénine-angiotensine, *J. Physiol. Paris*, 75, 179, 1979.
14. **Heacox, R., Harvey, A. M., and Vander, A. J.**, Hepatic inactivation of renin, *Circ. Res.*, 21, 149, 1967.
15. **Barnardo, D. E., Strong, C. G., and Baldus, W. P.**, Failure of the cirrhotic liver to inactivate renin: evidence for a splanchnic source of renin-like activity, *J. Lab. Clin. Med.*, 74, 495, 1969.
16. **Nasjletti, A. and Masson, G. M. C.**, Stimulation of angiotensinogen formation by renin and angiotensin, *Proc. Soc. Exp. Biol. Med.*, 142, 307, 1973.
17. **Carrière, S. and Biron, P.**, Effect of angiotensin I on intrarenal blood flow distribution, *Am. J. Physiol.*, 219, 164, 1970.
18. **Leary, W. P. and Ledingham, J. G.**, Removal of angiotensin by isolated perfused organs of the rat, *Nature*, 222, 959, 1969.
19. **Biron, P., Baldus, W. P., and Summerskill, W. H. J.**, Plasma angiotensinase activity in cirrhosis, *Proc. Soc. Exp. Biol. Med.*, 116, 1074, 1964.
20. **Braley, L. M. and Williams, G. H.**, The effect of angiotensin II and saralasin on 18-OH-11-deoxycorticosterone production by isolated human adrenal glands, *J. Clin. Endocrinol. Metab.*, 49, 600, 1980.
21. **Oelkers, W., Brown, J. J., Fraser, R., Morton, J. J., and Robertson, J. I. S.**, Sensitisation of the adrenal cortex to angiotensin II in sodium-depleted man, *Circ. Res.*, 34, 69, 1977.
22. **Hollenberg, N. K., Chenitz, W. R., Adams, D. F., and Williams, G. H.**, Reciprocal influence of salt intake on adrenal glomerulosa and renal vascular responses to angiotensin II in normal man, *J. Clin. Invest.*, 54, 24, 1974.
23. **Douglas, J. G. and Brown, G. P.**, Effects of prolonged low dose infusion of angiotensin II and aldosterone on rat smooth muscle and adrenal angiotensin II receptors, *Endocrinology*, 111, 988, 1982.
24. **Hollenberg, N. K., Williams, G. H., Burger, B., Ishikawa, I., and Adams, D. F.**, Blockade and stimulation of renal, adrenal and vascular angiotensin II receptors with 1-sar, 8-ala angiotensin II in normal man, *J. Clin. Invest.*, 57, 39, 1976.
25. **Kiil, F., Kjekshus, J., Löyning, E.**, Renal autoregulation during infusion of noradrenalin, angiotensin and acetylcholine, *Acta Physiol. Scand.*, 76, 10, 1969.
26. **Hollemberg, N. K., Solomon, H. S., Adams, D. F., Abrams, H. L., and Merrill, J. P.**, Renal vascular responses to angiotensin and norepinephrine in normal man, *Circ. Res.*, 31, 750, 1972.
27. **Myers, B. D., Deen, W. M., and Brenner, B. M.**, Effects of norepinephrine and angiotensin II on the determinants of glomerular filtration rate and proximal fluid reabsorption in the rat, *Circ. Res.*, 37, 101, 1975.
28. **Hall, J. E., Guyton, A. C., Jackson, T. E., Coleman, T. G., Lohmeier, T. E., and Trippodo, N. C.**, Control of glomerular filtration rate by renin-angiotensin system, *Am. J. Physiol.*, 233, 366, 1977.

29. **Hornich, H., Beaufils, N., and Richet, G.,** The effect of exogenous angiotensin on superficial and deep glomeruli in the rat kidney, *Kidney Int., 2,* 336, 1972.
30. **Sraer, J. D., Sraer, J., Ardaillou, R., and Mimoune, O.,** Evidence for renal glomerular receptors for angiotensin II, *Kidney Int., 6,* 241, 1974.
31. **Harris, P. J. and Young, J. A.,** Dose-dependent stimulation and inhibition of proximal tubular sodium reabsorption and angiotensin II in the rat kidney, *Pfluegers Arch., 367,* 295, 1977.
32. **Frolich, J. C., Wilson, T. W., Sweetman, B. J., Smigel, M., Nies, A. S., Carr, K., Watson, J. T., and Oates, J. A.,** Urinary prostaglandins: identification and origins, *J. Clin. Invest., 55,* 763, 1975.
33. **Gimbrone, M. A., Jr. and Alexander, R. W.,** Angiotensin II stimulation of prostaglandin production in cultured human vascular endothelium, *Science, 189,* 219, 1975.
34. **Williams, G. H. and Dluhy, R. G.,** Aldosterone biosynthesis. Interrelationship of regulatory factors, *Am. J. Med., 53,* 595, 1972.
35. **Zipser, R. D., Meidar, V., and Horton, R.,** Characteristics of aldosterone binding in human plasma, *J. Clin. Endocrinol. Metab., 50,* 158, 1980.
36. **Dluhy, R. D., Axelrod, L., Underwood, R. H., and Williams, G. H.,** Studies of the control of plasma aldosterone concentration in normal man. II. Effect of dietary potassium and acute potassium infusion, *J. Clin. Invest., 51,* 1950, 1972.
37. **Bernardi, M., De Palma, R., Trevisani, F., Santini, C., Capani, F., Baraldini, M., and Gasbarrini, G.,** The serum potassium circadian rhythm. Relationship with aldosterone, *Horm. Met. Res., 17,* 695, 1985.
38. **Baumber, J. S., Davis, J. O., Johnson, J. A., and Witty, R. T.,** Increased adrenocortical potassium in association with increased biosynthesis of aldosterone, *Am. J. Physiol., 220,* 1094, 1971.
39. **Blair-West, J. R., Coghlan, J. P., Denton, D. A., Goding, J. R., Wintour, M., Wright, R. D.,** The direct effect of increased sodium concentration in adrenal arterial blood on corticoid secretion in sodium deficient sheep, *Aust. J. Exp. Biol. Med. Sci., 44,* 455, 1966.
40. **Saito, I., Bravo, E. L., Zanella, S., Sen, S., and Bumpus, F. M.,** Steroidogenic characteristics of a new aldosterone-stimulating factor isolated from normal human urine. *Hypertension, 3,* 1065, 1981.
41. **Campbell, D. J., Mendelsohn, F. A. D., Adam, W. R., and Funder, J. W.,** Is aldosterone secretion under dopaminergic control?, *Circ. Res., 49,* 1217, 1981.
42. **Chartier, L., Schiffrin, E., Thibault, G., and Garcia, R.,** Atrial natriuretic factor inhibits the stimulation of aldosterone secretion by angiotensin I, ACTH and potassium *in vitro* and angiotensin II-induced steroidogenesis *in vivo, Endocrinology, 115,* 2026, 1984.
43. **Liddle, G. W.,** The adrenals, in *Textbook of Endocrinology,* Williams, R. H., Ed., W. B. Saundeis, Philadelphia, 1981, 249.
44. **Marver, D.,** Receptors in rabbit cortex and red medulla, *Endocrinology, 106,* 611, 1980.
45. **Horisberger, J. D. and Diezi, J.,** Effects of mineralocorticoids on Na^+ and K^+ excretion in the adrenalectomized rat, *Am. J. Physiol., 245,* F89, 1983.
46. **Murray, J. F., Dawson, A. N., and Sherlock, S.,** Circulatory changes in chronic liver disease, *Am. J. Med., 24,* 358, 1958.
47. **Lancestremere, R. G., Davidson, P. L., Earley, L. E., O'Brien, F. J., and Papper, S.,** Renal failure in Laennec's cirrhosis. II. Simultaneous determination of cardiac output and renal hemodynamics, *J. Clin. Invest., 41,* 1922, 1962.
48. **Epstein, M., Berk, D. P., Hollemberg, N. K., Adams, D. F., Chalmers, T. C., Abrams, H. L., and Merrill, J. P.,** Renal failure in the patients with cirrhosis. The role of active vasoconstriction, *Am. J. Med., 87,* 822, 1970.
49. **Better, O. S., and Schrier, R. W.,** Disturbed volume homeostasis in patients with cirrhosis, *Kidney Int., 23,* 303, 1983.
50. **Hartroft, V. S. and Hartroft, P. M.,** New approaches in the study of cardiovascular disease: aldosterone, renin, hypertension and juxtaglomerular cells, *Fed. Proc., 20,* 845, 1961.
51. **Genest, J., Boucher, R., De Champlain, J., Veyrat, R., Chretien, M., and Biron, P.,** Arterial angiotensin blood levels in hypertensive and edematous diseases, *Exc. Med. Int. Cong. Series, 67,* 129, 1963.
52. **Massani, Z. M., Finkelman, S., Worcel, M., Agrest, A., and Paladini, A. C.,** Angiotensin blood levels in hypertensive and nonhypertensive disease, *Clin. Sci., 30,* 473, 1966.
53. **Brown, J. J., Davis, D. L., Lever, A. F., and Robertson, J. I. S.,** Variations in plasma renin concentration in several physiological and pathological states, *Can. Med. Assoc. J., 90,* 201, 1964.
54. **Fasciolo, J. C., De Vito, E., Romero, J. C., and Cucchi, J. N.,** The renin content of the blood of humans and dogs under several conditions, *Can. Med. Assoc. J., 90,* 206, 1964.
55. **Pickens, P. T., Bumpus, F. M., Lloyd, A. M., Smeby, R. R., and Page, I. H.,** Measurement of renin activity in human plasma, *Circ. Res., 17,* 438, 1965.
56. **Ayers, C. R.,** Plasma renin activity and renin-substrate concentration in patients with liver disease, *Circ. Res., 20,* 594, 1967.
57. **Schroeder, E. T., Eich, R. H., Smulyan, H., Gould, A. B., and Gabuzda, G. J.,** Plasma renin level in hepatic cirrhosis. Relation to functional renal failure, *Am. J. Med., 49,* 186, 1970.

58. **Wernze, H., Spech, H. G., and Muller, G.,** Studies on the activity of the renin-angiotensin-aldosterone system (RAAs) in patients with cirrhosis of the liver, *Klin. Wochenschr.,* 56, 389, 1978.

59. **Bosch, J., Arroyo, V., Betriu, A., Mas, A., Carrilho, F., Rivera, F., Navarro-Lopez, F., and Rodés, J.,** Hepatic hemodynamics and the renin-angiotensin-aldosterone system in cirrhosis, *Gastroenterology,* 78, 92, 1980.

60. **Wilkinson, S. P., Smith, I. K., Clarke, M., Arroyo, V., Richardson, J., Moodie, H., and Williams, R.,** Intrarenal distribution of plasma flow in cirrhosis as measured by transit renography: relationship with plasma renin activity, and sodium and water excretion, *Clin. Sci. Mol. Med.,* 52, 469, 1977.

61. **Wilkinson, S. P., Smith, I. K., and Williams, R.,** Changes in plasma renin activity in cirrhosis: a reappraisal based on studies in 67 patients and "low renin" cirrhosis, *Hypertension,* 1, 125, 1979.

62. **Bernardi, M., Trevisani, F., Santini, C., De Palma, R., and Gasbarrini, G.,** Aldosterone-related blood volume expansion in cirrhosis before and after the early phase of ascites formation, *Gut,* 24, 761, 1983.

63. **Mitch, W. E., Whelton, P. K., Cooke, C. L., Walker, W. G., and Maddrey, W. C.,** Plasma levels and hepatic extraction of renin and aldosterone in alcoholic liver disease, *Am. J. Med.,* 66, 804, 1979.

64. **Bernardi, M., De Palma, R., Trevisani, F., Santini, C., Capani, F., Baraldini, M., and Gasbarrini, G.,** Chronobiological study of factors affecting plasma aldosterone concentration in cirrhosis, *Gastroenterology,* 91, 683, 1986.

65. **Lieberman, F. L. and Reynolds, T. B.,** Plasma volume in cirrhosis of the liver: its relationships to portal hypertension, ascites and renal failure, *J. Clin. Invest.,* 46, 1297, 1967.

66. **Lieberman, F. L., Denison, E. K., and Reynolds, T. B.,** The relationship of plasma volume, portal hypertension, ascites and renal sodium retention in cirrhosis. The overflow theory of ascites formation, *Ann. N. Y. Acad. Sci.,* 170, 202, 1970.

67. **Levy, M.,** Sodium retention and ascites formation in dogs with experimental portal cirrhosis, *Am. J. Physiol.,* 233, 572, 1977.

68. **Levy, M. and Allotey, J. B. K.,** Temporal relationships between urinary salt retention and altered systemic hemodynamics in dogs with experimental cirrhosis, *J. Lab. Clin. Med.,* 92, 560, 1978.

69. **Bernardi, M. and Trevisani, F.,** Cirrhosis with ascites: a heterogenous population, *Hepatology,* 7, 199, 1987 (letter).

70. **Rosoff, L., Jr., Zia, P., Reynolds, T. B., and Horton, R.,** Studies of renin and aldosterone in cirrhotic patients with ascites, *Gastroenterology,* 69, 698, 1975.

71. **Epstein, M., Levinson, R., Sancho, J., Haber, E., and Re, R.,** Characterization of the renin-aldosterone system in decompensated cirrhosis, *Circ. Res.,* 41, 819, 1977.

72. **Arroyo, V., Bosch, J., Mauri, M., Viver, J., Mas, A., Rivera, F., Rodés, J.,** Renin, aldosterone and renal hemodynamics in cirrhosis with ascites, *Eur. J. Clin. Invest.,* 9, 69, 1979.

73. **Anderson, J. B.,** Converting enzyme activity in liver disease, *Acta Pathol. Microbiol. Scand.,* 71, 1, 1967.

74. **Schweisfurth, H. and Wernze, H.,** Changes of serum angiotensin I converting enzyme in patients with viral hepatitis and liver cirrhosis, *Acta Hepato-Gastroenterol.,* 26, 207, 1979.

75. **Matsuki, K. and Sakata, T.,** Angiotensin converting enzyme in diseases of the liver, *Am. J. Med.,* 73, 549, 1982.

76. **Johnson, D. A., Diehl, A. M., Sjogren, M. H., Lazar, J., Cattau Jr., E. L., and Smallridge, R. C.,** Serum angiotensin converting enzyme in evaluation of patients with liver disease, *Am. J. Med.,* 83, 256, 1987.

77. **Karetzky, M. S. and Mithoefer, J. C.,** The cause of hyperventilation and arterial hypoxia in patients with cirrhosis of the liver, *Am. J. Med. Sci.,* 254, 797, 1967.

78. **Molteni, A., Zakheim, R. M., Mullis, K. B., and Mattioli, L.,** The effect of chronic alveolar hypoxia on lung and serum angiotensin I converting enzyme activity (38323), *Proc. Soc. Exp. Biol. Med.,* 147, 263, 1974.

79. **Saruta, T., Kondo, K., Saito, I., and Nakamura, R.,** Characterization of the components of the renin-angiotensin system in cirrhosis of the liver, in *The Kidney in Liver Disease,* Epstein, M., Ed., Elsevier, New York, 1978, 207.

80. **Spech, H. J.,** Total immunoreactive angiotensin II, its hepta-octapeptide fraction, and its hexapeptide in patients with liver disease, *Klin. Wochenschr.,* 56, 399, 1978.

81. **Kokubu, T., Ueda, E., Fujmoto, S., Hiwada, K., and Yamamura, Y.,** Plasma angiotensinase activity in liver disease, *Clin. Chim. Acta,* 12, 282, 1965.

82. **Wernze, H., Seki, A., Schneider, K. W., and Jesse, R.,** Hepatische Extraktion und Clearance von Renin bei Lebercirrhosen. *Klin. Wochenschr.,* 50, 302, 1972.

83. **Bosch, J., Arroyo, V., and Rodés, J.,** Hepatic and systemic hemodynamics and the renin-angiotensin-aldosterone system in cirrhosis, in *The Kidney in Liver Disease,* 2nd ed., Epstein, M., Ed., Elsevier, New York, 1983, 423.

84. **Hesse, B., Andersen, E. D., and Ring-Larsen, H.,** Hepatic elimination of renin in man, *Clin. Sci. Mol. Med.,* 55, 377, 1978.

85. **Lunzer, M. R., Manghani, K. K., Newman, S. P., Sherlock, S., Bernard, A. G., and Ginsburg, J.,** Impaired cardiovascular responsiveness in liver disease, *Lancet,* 2, 382, 1975.

86. **Bernardi, M., Trevisani, F., Santini, C., Ligabue, A., Capelli, M., and Gasbarrini, G.,** Impairment of blood pressure control in patients with liver cirrhosis during tilting: study on adrenergic and renin-angiotensin systems, *Digestion,* 25, 124, 1982.

87. **Bernardi, M., Trevisani, F., Santini, C., Zoli, G., Baraldini, M., Ligabue, A., and Gasbarrini, G.,** Plasma norepinephrine, weak neurotransmitters, and renin activity during active tilting in liver cirrhosis: relationship with cardiovascular homeostasis and renal function, *Hepatology,* 3, 56, 1983.

88. **Ring-Larsen, H., Hesse, B., Henriksen, H., and Christensen, N. J.,** Sympathetic nervous system activity and renal and systemic hemodynamics in cirrhosis: plasma norepinephrine concentration, hepatic extraction and renal release, *Hepatology,* 2, 304, 1982.

89. **Bichet, D. G., Van Putten, V. J., and Schrier, R. W.,** Potential role of increased sympathetic activity in impaired sodium and water excretion in cirrhosis, *N. Engl. J. Med.,* 307, 1552, 1982.

90. **Wong, P. Y., Carrol, R. E., Lipinski, T. L., and Capone, R. R.,** Studies on the renin-angiotensin-aldosterone system in patients with cirrhosis and ascites: effect of saline and albumin infusion, *Gastroenterology,* 77, 1171, 1979.

91. **Burmeister, P., Schölmerich, J., Diener, W., and Gerok, W.,** Renin, aldosterone and arginine vaso-pressin in patients with liver cirrhosis: the influence of ascites retransfusion, *Eur. J. Clin. Invest.,* 16, 117, 1986.

92. **Blendis, L. M., Greig, P. D., Langer, B., Baigrie, R. S., Ruse, J., and Taylor, B. R.,** The renal and hemodynamic effects of the peritoneovenous shunt for intractable hepatic ascites, *Gastroenterology,* 77, 250, 1979.

93. **Greig, P. D., Blendis, L. M., Langer, B., Taylor, B. R., and Colapinto, R. F.,** Renal and hemodynamic effects of the peritoneoveous shunt. II. Long term effects, *Gastroenterology,* 80, 119, 1981.

94. **Bernardi, M., Santini, C., Trevisani, F., Baraldini, M., Ligabue, A., and Gasbarrini, G.,** Renal function impairment induced by change in posture in patients with cirrhosis and ascites, *Gut,* 26, 629, 1985.

95. **Orloff, M. J., Ross, T. H., Baddeley, R. M., Nutting, R. O., Spitz, B. R., Slopp, R. D., Neesby, T., and Halasz, N. A.,** Experimental ascites. VI. The effects of hepatic venous outflow obstruction and ascites on aldosterone secretion, *Surgery,* 56, 83, 1964.

96. **Orloff, M. J., Lippman, C. A., and Noel, B. M.,** Hepatic regulation of aldosterone by a humoral mediator, *Surgery,* 58, 225, 1965.

97. **Kostreva, D. R., Castaner, A., and Kampine, J. P.,** Reflex effects of hepatic baroreceptors on renal and cardiac sympathetic nerve activity, *Am. J. Physiol.,* 238, R390, 1980.

98. **Sawchenko, P. E. and Friedman, M. I.,** Sensory functions of the liver — A review, *Am. J. Physiol.,* 235, R8, 1979.

99. **Chiandussi, L., Vaccarino, A., Greco, F., Muratori, F., Cesano, L., and Indovina, D.,** Effect of drug infusion on the splanchnic circulation. I Angiotensin infusion in normal and cirrhotic subjects, *Proc. Soc. Exp. Biol. Med.,* 112, 324, 1963.

100. **Arroyo, V., Bosch, J., Mauri, M., Rivera, F., Navarro-Lopez, F., Rodés, J.,** Effect of angiotensin II blockade on systemic and hepatic hemodynamics and on the renin-angiotensin-aldosterone system in cirrhosis with ascites, *Eur. J. Clin. Invest.,* 11, 221, 1981.

101. **Ballet, F., Chretien, Y., Rey, C., Poupon, R.,** Differential response of normal and cirrhotic liver to vasoactive agents. A study in the isolated perfused rat liver, *J. Pharmacol. Exp. Ther.,* 244, 283, 1988.

102. **Eriksson, L. S., Kagedal, B., and Wahren, J.,** Effects of captopril on hepatic venous pressure and blood flow in patients with liver cirrhosis, *Am. J. Med.,* 76, 66, 1984.

103. **Shapiro, M. D., Nicholls, K. M., Groves, B. M., Kluge, R. K., Ching, H., Bichet, D. G., and Schrier, R. W.,** Interrelationship between cardiac output and vascular resistance as determinant of effective arterial blood volume in cirrhotic patients, *Kidney Int.,* 28, 206, 1985.

104. **Roberti, A., Traverso, H., Vesin, P., Viguie, R., Blanchon, P.,** Étude du Na et du K échangeables et des liquides extra-cellulaires dans les cirrhoses éthyliques, *Sem. Hôp. Paris,* 42, 1714, 1966.

105. **Laragh, J. H., Cannon, P. J., Bentzel, C. J., Sicinski, A. M., and Meltzer, J. I.,** Angiotensin II, norepinephrine, and renal transport of electrolytes and water in normal man and in cirrhosis with ascites, *J. Clin. Invest.,* 42, 1179, 1963.

106. **Ames, R. P., Borkowski, A. J., Sicinski, A. M., and Laragh, J. H.,** Prolonged infusions of angiotensin II and norepinephrine and blood pressure, electrolyte balance, and aldosterone and cortisol secretion in normal man and in cirrhosis with ascites, *J. Clin. Invest.,* 44, 1171, 1965.

107. **Johnston, C. I. and Jose, A. D.,** Reduced vascular response to angiotensin II in secondary hyperaldos-teronism, *J. Clin. Invest.,* 42, 1411, 1963.

108. **Lenz, K., Hörtnagl, H., Magometschnigg, D., Kleinberger, G., Druml, W., and Laggner, A.,** Function of the autonomic nervous system in patients with hepatic encephalopathy, *Hepatology,* 5, 831, 1985.

109. **Murray, B. M. and Paller, M. S.,** Decreased pressor reactivity to angiotensin II in cirrhotic rats. Evidence for a postreceptor defect in angiotensin action, *Circ. Res.,* 57, 424, 1985.

110. **Naveh, Y., Finberg, J. P. M., Kahana, L., and Better, O. S.,** Renin-angiotensin system in dogs following bile-duct ligation. Relation to vascular reactivity, *J. Hepatol.,* 6, 57, 1988.
111. **Barger, A. C.,** Regulation of blood pressure: interaction of the renin-angiotensin-aldosterone system, the autonomic nervous system, and sodium balance, *Angiology,* 29, 326, 1978.
112. **Schroeder, E. T., Anderson, G. H., Goldman, S. H., and Streeten, D. U. P.,** Effect of blockade of angiotensin II on blood pressure, renin and aldosterone in cirrhosis, *Kidney Int.,* 9, 511, 1976.
113. **Saruta, T., Eguchi, T., and Saito, I.,** Angiotensin antagonists in liver disease, in *The Kidney in Liver Disease,* 2nd ed., Epstein, M., Ed., Elsevier, New York, 1983, 441.
114. **Bernardi, M., Trevisani, F., Santini, C., Baraldini, M., Ligabue, A., and Gasbarrini, G.,** Derangement in intradiem activity of adrenergic and renin-angiotensin system in cirrhosis. Relationship with cardiovascular homeostasis, *Ital. J. Gastroenterol.,* 16, (Abstr.), 318, 1984.
115. **Wilkinson, S. P., Bernardi, M., Britton, K. E., Brown, N. J. G., Pearce, P. C., Jenner, R., and Williams, R.,** Validation of "transit renography" as a method for determining intrarenal distribution of blood flow, *Clin. Sci. Mol. Med.,* 55, 277, 1978.
116. **Wilkinson, S. P., Bernardi, M., Smith, I. K., Jowett, T. P., Slater, J. D. H., and Williams, R.,** Effect of β-adrenergic blocking drugs on the renin-aldosterone system, sodium excretion, and renal hemodynamics in cirrhosis with ascites, *Gastroenterology,* 73, 659, 1977.
117. **Barnardo, D. E., Summerskill, W. H. J., Strong, C. G., and Baldus, W. P.,** Renal function, renin activity and endogenous vasoactive substances in cirrhosis, *Dig. Dis.,* 15, 419, 1970.
118. **Pérez-Ayuso, R. M., Arroyo, V., Camps, J., Rimola, A., Costa, J., Gaya, J., Rivera, F., and Rodés, J.,** Renal kallikrein excretion in cirrhosis with ascites: relationship to renal hemodynamics, *Hepatology,* 4, 247, 1984.
119. **Bernardi, M., Trevisani, F., Capelli, M., Bugiardini, G., and Gasbarrini, G.,** Study of renal function, renin-aldosterone axis and plasma electrolytes during diuretic treatment of patients with cirrhosis of the liver, *Ital. J. Gastroenterol.,* 14, 199, 1982.
120. **Gutman, R. A., Forrey, A. W., Fleet, W. P., and Cutler, R. E.,** Vasopressor-induced natriuresis and altered intrarenal hemodynamics in cirrhotic man, *Clin. Sci. Mol. Med.,* 45, 19, 1973.
121. **Pariente, E. A., Bataille, C., Bercoff, E., and Lebrec, D.,** Acute effects of captopril on systemic and renal hemodynamics and renal function in cirrhotic patients with ascites, *Gastroenterology,* 88, 1255, 1985.
122. **Wood, L. J., Goergen, S., Stockigt, J. R., Powell, L. W., and Dudley, F. J.,** Adverse effects of captopril in treatment of resistant ascites, a state of functional bilateral renal artery stenosis, *Lancet,* 2, 1008, 1985 (letter).
123. **Wilkinson, S. P., Bernardi, M., Wheeler, P. G., Smith, I. K., and Williams, R.,** Diuretic-induced renal impairment without volume depletion in cirrhosis: changes in the renin-angiotensin system and the effect of β-adrenergic blockade, *Postgrad. Med. J.,* 55, 862, 1979.
124. **Boyer, T. D., Zia, P., and Reynolds, T. B.,** Effect of indomethacin and prostaglandin A_1 on renal function and plasma renin activity in alcoholic liver disease, *Gastroenterology,* 77, 215, 1979.
125. **Zipser, R. D., Hoefs, J. C., Speckart, P. F., Zia, P., and Horton, R.,** Prostaglandins: modulators of renal function and pressor resistance in chronic liver disease, *J. Clin. Endocrinol. Metab.,* 48, 895, 1979.
126. **Arroyo, V., Planas, R., Gaya, J., Deulofeu, R., Rimola, A., Pérez-Ayuso, R. M., Rivera, F., and Rodés, J.,** Sympathetic nervous system activity, renin-angiotensin system and renal excretion of prostaglandin E_2 in cirrhosis. Relationship to functional renal failure and sodium and water excretion, *Eur. J. Clin. Invest.,* 13, 271, 1983.
127. **Levy, M., Wexler, M. J., and Fechner, C.,** Renal perfusion in dogs with experimental hepatic cirrhosis: role of prostaglandins, *Am. J. Physiol.,* 245, F521, 1983.
128. **Arroyo, V., Ginés, P., Rimola, A., and Gaya, R.,** Renal function abnormalities, prostaglandins, and effects of nonsteroidal anti-inflammatory drugs in cirrhosis with ascites. An overview with emphasis on pathogenesis, *Am. J. Med.,* 81 (Suppl. 2B), 104, 1986.
129. **Lianos, E. A., Alavi, N., Tobin, N., Venuto, R., and Bentzel, C. J.,** Angiotensin-induced sodium excretion patterns in cirrhosis: role of renal prostaglandins, *Kidney Int.,* 21, 70, 1982.
130. **Epstein, M.,** The renin-angiotensin system in liver disease, in *The Kidney in Liver Disease,* 2nd ed., Epstein, M., Ed., Elsevier, New York, 1983, 353.
131. **Oparil, S. and Haber, E.,** The renin-angiotensin system, *N. Engl. J. Med.,* 291, 446, 1974.
132. **Lake, C. R., Ziegler, M. G., and Kobin, I. J.,** Use of plasma norepinephrine for evaluation of sympathetic neuronal function in man, *Life Sci.,* 18, 1315, 1976.
133. **Bongiovanni, A. M., and Eisenmenger, W. J.,** Adrenal cortical metabolism in chronic liver disease, *J. Clin. Endocrinol.,* 11, 152, 1951.
134. **Chart, J. J. and Shipley, E. S.,** The mechanism of sodium retention in cirrhosis of the liver, *J. Clin. Invest.,* 32, (Abstr.), 530, 1953.
135. **Luetscher, J. A., and Johnson, B. B.,** Observations on the sodium retaining corticoid (aldosterone) in the urine of children and adults in relation to sodium balance and edema, *J. Clin. Invest.,* 33, 1441, 1954.
136. **Axelrad, B. J., Cates, J. E., Johnson, B. B., and Luetscher, J. A., Jr.,** Aldosterone in urine of normal man and of patients with edema, *Br. Med. J.,* 1, 196, 1955.

137. **Dyrenfurth, I., Stacey, C. H., Beck, J. C., and Venning, E. H.,** Aldosterone excretion in patients with cirrhosis of the liver, *Metabolism*, 6, 544, 1957.

138. **Wolff, H. P., Koczorek, K. R., and Buchborn, E.,** Aldosterone and antidiuretic hormone (adiuretin) in liver disease, *Acta Endocrinol. (Copenhagen)*, 27, 45, 1958.

139. **Ulick, S., Laragh, J. H., and Lieberman, S.,** The isolation of a urinary metabolite of aldosterone and its use to measure the rate of secretion of aldosterone by the adrenal cortex of man, *Trans. Ass. Am. Phys.*, 71, 225, 1958.

140. **Peterson, R. E.,** Adrenal cortical steroid metabolism and adrenal cortical function in liver diseases, *J. Clin. Invest.*, 29, 320, 1960.

141. **Cope, C. L., Nicolis, G., and Fraser, G.,** Measurement of aldosterone secretion rate in man by the use of a metabolite, *Clin. Sci.*, 21, 367, 1961.

142. **Coppage, W. S., Island, D. P., Cooner, A. E., and Liddle, G. W.,** The metabolism of aldosterone in normal subjects and in patients with hepatic cirrhosis, *J. Clin. Invest.*, 41, 1672, 1962.

143. **Laragh, J. H., Cannon, P. J., and Ames, R. P.,** Interactions between aldosterone secretion, sodium and potassium balance, and angiotensin activity in man: studies in hypertension and cirrhosis, *Canad. Med. Assoc. J.*, 90, 248, 1964.

144. **Wolff, H. P., Bette, L., Blaise, H., Düsterdieck, G., Jahnecke, J., Kobayashi, T., Krück, F., Lommer, D., and Schieffer, H.,** Role of aldosterone in edema formation, *Ann. N. Y. Acad. Sci.*, 139, 285, 1966.

145. **Chonko, A. M., Bay, W. H., Stein, J. H., and Ferris, T. F.,** The role of renin and aldosterone in the salt retention of edema, *Am. J. Med.*, 63, 881, 1977.

146. **Wilkinson, S. P., Jowett, T. P., Slater, J. D. H., Arroyo, V., Moodie, H., and Williams, R.,** Renal sodium retention in cirrhosis: relation to aldosterone and nephron site, *Clin. Sci.*, 56, 169, 1979.

147. **Bernardi, M., De Palma, R., Trevisani, F., Malatesta, R., Baraldini, M., Cursaro, C., and Gasbarrini, G.,** Unaltered dopaminergic modulation of aldosterone secretion in cirrhosis, *Clin. Sci.*, 74, 137, 1988.

148. **Vecsei, P., Dusterdieck, G., Jahnecke, J., Lommer, D., and Wolff, H. P.,** Secretion and turnover of aldosterone in various pathological states, *Clin. Sci.*, 36, 241, 1969.

149. **Wilkinson, S. P., Wheeler, P. G., Jowett, T. P., Smith, I. K., Keenan, J., Slater, J. D. H., and Williams, R.,** Factors relating to aldosterone secretion rate, the excretion of aldosterone 18-glucuronide, and the plasma aldosterone concentration in cirrhosis, *Clin. Endocrinol.*, 14, 355, 1981.

150. **Nicholls, M. N., Shapiro, M. D., Kluge, R., Chung, H., Bichet, D. G., and Schrier, R. W.,** Sodium excretion in advanced cirrhosis: effect of expansion of central blood volume and suppression of plasma aldosterone, *Hepatology*, 6, 235, 1986.

151. **Anderson, G. H., Jr., Anderson, T., Streeten, D. H. P., and Schroeder, E. T.,** Acute effects of saralasin on plasma aldosterone in different pathophysiological conditions, *J. Clin. Endocrinol. Metab.*, 50, 529, 1980.

152. **Ventura, E., Zeneroli, M. L., Tampieri, A., Pinelli, G., Licari, F., Gollini, C., Cremonini, C., Ricci, P., Casalgrandi, G., Baraghini, G., and Marrama, P.,** Chronobiological study of circadian variations of plasma free tryptophan and cortisol in liver cirrhosis with severe degree of encephalopathy, *Ital. J. Gastroenterol.*, 16, 1, 1984.

153. **Schedl, H. P. and Bartter, F. C.,** An explanation for and experimental correction of the abnormal water diuresis in cirrhosis, *J. Clin. Invest.*, 39, 248, 1960.

154. **Vlahcevic, Z. R., Adam, N. F., Jich, H., Moore, E. V., and Chalmers, T. C.,** Renal effects of acute expansion in plasma volume in cirrhosis, *N. Engl. J. Med.*, 272, 387, 1965.

155. **Chiandussi, L., Bartoli, E., and Arras, S.,** Reabsorption of sodium in the proximal renal tubule in cirrhosis of the liver, *Gut*, 19, 497, 1978.

156. **Chaimovitz, C., Szylman, P., Alroy, G., and Better, O. S.,** Mechanism of increased renal tubular sodium reabsorption in cirrhosis, *Am. J. Med.*, 52, 198, 1972.

157. **Pérez-Ayuso, R. M., Arroyo, V., Planas, R., Gaya, J., Bory, F., Rimola, A., Rivera, F., and Rodés, J.,** Randomized comparative study of efficacy of furosemide vs. spironolactone in nonazotemic cirrhosis with ascites, *Gastroenterology*, 84, 961, 1983.

158. **Jorgensen, F., Badskjaer, J., and Nordan, H.,** Captopril and resistant ascites, *Lancet*, 2, 405, 1983 (letter).

159. **Espiner, E. A. and Nicholls, M. G.,** Hormones and fluid retention in cirrhosis, *Lancet*, 2, 501, 1982 (letter).

159a. **Bernardi, M., De Palma, R., Trevisani, F., Tamé, M. R., Ciancaglini, G. C., Pesa, O., Ugabue, A., Baraldini, M., Gasbarinni, G.,** Renal function and effective β-blocade in cirrhosis with ascites. Relationship with baseline sympathoadrenergic tone, *J. Hepatol.*, 8, 279, 1989.

160. **Bernardi, M., Servadei, D., Trevisani, F., Rusticali, A. G., and Gasbarrini, G.,** Importance of plasma aldosterone concentration on natriuretic effect of spironolactone in patients with liver cirrhosis and ascites, *Digestion*, 31, 189, 1985.

161. **Trevisani, F., Bernardi, M., De Palma, R., Pancione, L., Capani, F., Baraldini, M., Ligabue, A., and Gasbarrini, G.,** Circadian variation in renal sodium and potassium handling in cirrhosis. The role of aldosterone, cortisol, sympathoadienergic tone, and intratubular factors, gastroenterology, 96, 1187, 1989.
162. **Décaux, G., Hanson, B., Cauchie, P., Bosson, D., and Unger, J.,** Relationship between aldosterone and sodium, potassium and uric acid clearance in cirrhosis with and without ascites, *Nephron*, 44, 226, 1986.
163. **Davis, J. O., Holman, J. E., Carpenter, C. C., Urquart, J., and Higgins, J. T.,** An extra-adrenal factor factor for chronic sodium retention in presence of increased sodium retaining hormone, *Circ. Res.*, 14, 17, 1964.
164. **Wilkinson, S. P., Smith, I. K., Moodie, H., Poston, L., and Willians, R.,** Studies on mineralocorticoid "escape" in cirrhosis, *Clin. Sci.*, 56, 401, 1979.
165. **Naccarato, R., Messa, P., D' Angelo, A., Fabris, M., Messa, M., Chiaramonte, M., Gregolin, C., and Zanon, G.,** Renal handling of sodium and water in early chronic liver disease, *Gastroenterology*, 81, 205, 1981.
166. **Jiménez, W., Martinez-Pardo, A., Arroyo, V., Bruix, J., Rimola, A., Gaya, J., Rivera, F., Rodés, J.,** Temporal relationship between hyperaldosteronism, sodium retention and ascites formation in rats with experimental cirrhosis, *Hepatology*, 5, 245, 1985.
167. **Henriksen, J. H., Ring-Larsen, H., and Christensen, N. J.,** Sympathetic nervous activity in cirrhosis. A survey of plasma catecholamine studies, *J. Hepatol.*, 1, 55, 1984.
168. **Burghardt, W., Wernze, H., and Diehl, K. L.,** Atrial natriuretic peptide in hepatic cirrhosis: relation to stage of disease, sympathoadrenal system and renin-aldosterone axis, *Klin. Wochenschr.*, 64 (Suppl. 6), 103, 1986.
169. **Levy, M.,** Sodium retention in dogs with cirrhosis and ascites: efferent mechanisms, *Am. J. Physiol.*, 233, F586, 1977.
170. **Perez, G. O. and Oster, J. R.,** Altered potassium metabolism in liver disease, in *The Kidney in Liver Disease*, 2nd ed., Epstein, M., Ed., Elsevier, New York, 1983, 183.
171. **Goldman, R.,** Studies in diurnal variations of water and electrolyte excretion: nocturnal diuresis of water and sodium in congestive cardiac failure and cirrhosis of the liver, *J. Clin. Invest.*, 30, 1191, 1951.
172. **Trevisani, F., Bernardi, M., Pancione, L., De Palma, R., Capani, F., Baraldini, M., Ligabue, A., and Gasbarrini, G.,** Renal potassium metabolism in cirrhosis. The role of aldosterone, cortisol, sympathoadrenergic tone and intratubular factors, submitted.
173. **Brenner, B. M. and Berliner, M. W.,** The transport of potassium, in *Handbook of Physiology, Section 8: Renal Physiology*, Orloff, J. K. and Berliner, R. W., Eds., American Physiological Society, Washington, D.C., 1973, 497.
174. **Hené, R. J., Koomans, H. A., Boer, P., Roos, J. C., and Dorhout Mees, E. G.,** Relation between plasma aldosterone concentration and renal handling of sodium and potassium, in particular in patients with chronic renal failure, *Nephron*, 37, 94, 1984.
175. **Bernardi, M., Wilkinson, S. P., Wernze, H., Spech, H. J., Müller, G., Poston, L., and Williams, R.,** The renin-angiotensin-aldosterone system in fulminant hepatic failure, *Scand. J. Gastroenterol.*, 18, 369, 1983.
176. **Berkowitz, H. D., Calvin, C., and Miller, L. D.,** Significance of altered renin substrate in the hepatorenal syndrome, *Surg. Forum*, 23, 342, 1972.
177. **Wilkinson, S. P.,** unpublished observations.

Chapter 4

AUTONOMIC NERVOUS FUNCTION IN LIVER DISEASE

Jens H. Henriksen, Helmer Ring-Larsen, and Niels Juel Christensen

TABLE OF CONTENTS

I. INTRODUCTION

The autonomic nervous system, or the involuntary nervous system, influences many of the functions of visceral organs (i.e., the cardiovascular system, glands, and smooth muscles) throughout the body, and the activities of this system are coordinated with those of the somatic nervous system. Reflex pathways at different levels integrate these functions. Impulses initiated in visceral receptors are relayed through afferent autonomic nerve fibers to the central nervous system and transmitted via efferent pathways to visceral effectors. The peripheral portions of the autonomic nervous system are made up by the preganglionic and postganglionic neurons. Based on the transmitter in axon terminals of postganglionic fibers, the autonomic nervous system has traditionally been divided into the cholinergic or parasympathetic nervous system, where acetylcholine is the transmitter, and the adrenergic or sympathetic nervous system, where norepinephrine is the transmitter. However, recent investigations have shown that a number of other substances like, e.g., vasoactive intestinal polypeptide and substance P are transmitters or neuromodulators within the peripheral part of the autonomic nervous system[1]. The present survey will mainly include adrenergic and cholinergic functions of the autonomic nervous system, since our knowledge of the role of the "new" neuromodulators in human pathophysiology is limited.

Advanced liver disease is often associated with profound abnormalities in the cardiovascular system and fluid homeostasis, which is in part controlled by neurohumeral regulation. It is the intention of this review to summarize some cornerstones and recent investigations into the pathophysiology of the autonomic nervous system in patients with liver disease, predominantly cirrhosis. For purely descriptive reasons, neurohumoral elements, catecholamine metabolism, cardiovascular factors, and renal and homeostatic mechanisms are considered separately. However, the reader should be aware that each is a part of an integral framework with no singular effects or isolated functions.

II. PARASYMPATHETIC NERVOUS FUNCTION IN LIVER DISEASE

Clinical assessment of parasympathetic nervous function is difficult and has mainly been done by determination of beat-to-beat variation in heart rate[2] and measurement of the circulating level of pancreatic polypeptide,[3] both being under vagal control. In normal man, heart rate as determined from the electrocardiogram undergoes a cyclic variation governed by respiration and a parasympathetic reflex arc.[4] Pancreatic polypeptide has been localized to secretory granules in specific endocrine pancreatic cells located in the islets, acinar tissue, and duct epithelium. Vagal cholinergic stimulation and stimulation by meal are major regulators of pancreatic polypeptide secretion and thereby of the fasting plasma concentration of this peptide.[3] Beat-to-beat variation and plasma pancreatic polypeptide have been extensively studied in patients with, e.g., diabetic neuropathy,[2,4] but not in patients with liver disease.

Gastrointestinal and genital dysfunctions are relatively common in chronic liver disease. Whether these are primarily related to endocrine abnormalities or to parasympathetic neuropathy is not known. In fact, dysfunction of the parasympathetic nervous system in liver disease has never been the objective of intensive research. Degenerative changes in the vagus nerve have been described in patients with alcoholic polyneuropathy[5,6] and recovery has been seen, following prolonged abstinence.[7] It is well known that patients with advanced chronic liver disease, i.e., decompensated cirrhosis, have moderate tachycardia. It is not established whether this phenomenon is due to vagal dysfunction, as it may be seen in diabetics with autonomic neuropathy,[4] or due to enhanced sympathetic nervous activity (see later), or both. Since Lenz et al.[8] found a smaller increase in heart rate after intravenous atropine in liver patients compared to normals, they concluded that the increased activity of the sympathetic nervous system in hepatic encephalopathy is associated with a decreased parasympathetic tone.

III. SYMPATHETIC NERVOUS FUNCTION IN LIVER DISEASE

The catecholaminergic system comprises the adrenal medulla, the sympathetic nervous system (SNS) and the brain catecholamine neuron system. Norepinephrine (NE) is the neurotransmitter released from axon terminals of sympathetic postganglionic neurons which normally control cardiovascular responses during exercise and postural changes. NE and epinephrine (E) also modulate visceral functions such as metabolism and hormone secretion in the gastrointestinal tract, liver, pancreas, and genitals.

The function of SNS in man has previously been evaluated indirectly by measurements of changes in physiological variables considered to be controlled by sympathetic nerves (e.g., heart rate, blood pressure, vascular resistance). However, a major problem has been to establish whether the changes observed are really due to alterations in sympathetic nervous activity (SNA). A direct way to determine SNA is obviously to record impulses within nerve fibers.[9] This procedure has been used in anesthetized animals and in superficial sympathetic nerves to skin and muscles in conscious human subjects, but a major drawback is that this technique can not yet be applied to nerves to internal organs in man. Furthermore, enzymatic isotope-derivative techniques and high performance liquid chromatography have recently been developed, and these permit reliable measurements of NE and E concentrations in plasma.[10] This is important since NE leaks from the synaptic cleft into plasma where its concentration may reflect the neurotransmitter function and thereby the activity in SNS.

In normal supine man, circulating catecholamines are low, but the plasma concentration of NE increases with age.[11] During upright position and physical activity, procedures known to be associated with enhancement of SNA, plasma NE, and E increase substantially, reflecting increased sympathoadrenal activity.[12] Recent studies have shown that there is a close correlation between plasma NE concentrations measured in forearm venous blood and muscle sympathetic nerve activity as measured neurophysiologically.[9] This has been observed during exercise and during mental stress as well as during hypoglycemia, and both variables increase with age. The reason for this relationship is probably that muscle tissue has the greatest mass of all the tissue in the body and approximately half of NE in forearm venous plasma is derived locally from muscle tissue. The dynamics of circulating NE and E and the significance of arterial vs. venous blood samples is considered later.

A. CIRCULATING CATECHOLAMINES AND SYMPATHETIC NERVOUS ACTIVITY

There is increasing evidence that SNS plays an important role in the cardiovascular and homeostatic disarrangement seen in advanced liver disease.[13] As most of our knowledge on this topic is gained from studies of catecholamines, the kinetics of NE and E are described in detail in the following.

Circulating NE, and to some extent also E, is significantly elevated in patients with advanced liver disease with sodium and water retention, whereas in patients without ascites or edema, it is not different from controls[13-16] (Figure 1). It is now established that this increase in catecholamine concentration is not caused by diminished catabolism in the diseased liver, but is actually due to increased release from the nerve terminals.[16,17] The whole-body clearance of NE in cirrhosis is, in fact, equal to that of normal controls (approximately 1.5 1/min).[16-18] Studies with tritium-labeled NE-infusions have demonstrated that the net release is substantially increased in decompensated patients, but not in those without fluid retention.[13,16,17,19] Recently, Bernardi et al.[19a] found that even patients without

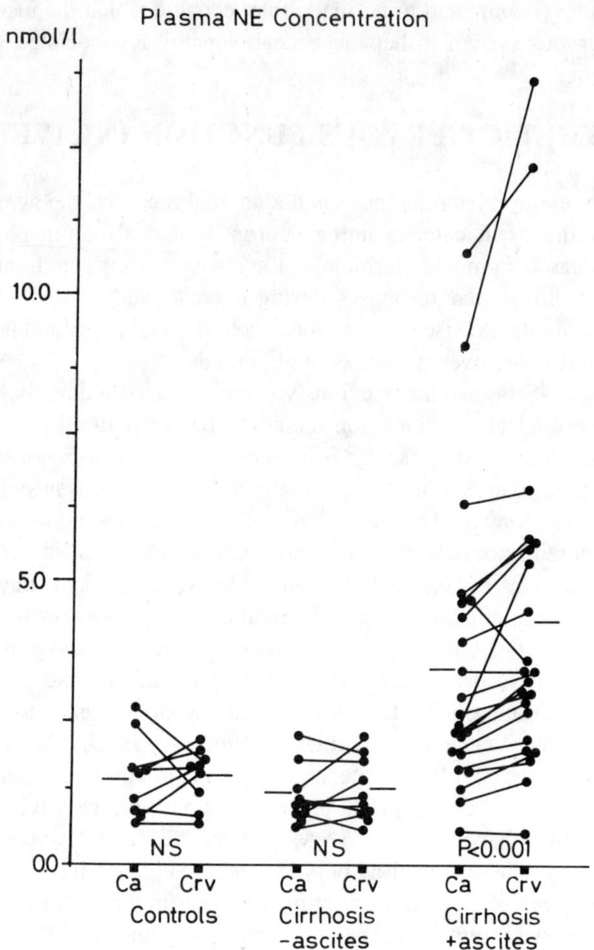

FIGURE 1.   Arterial (C_a) and renal venous (C_v) plasma concentration of endogenous norepinephrine (NE) in patients with and without fluid retention and control subjects without liver disease.

fluid retention have signs of moderately enhanced sympathetic tone as evaluated from urinary output of catecholamines. Thus, there is increasing evidence that the sympathoadrenal activity depends on the stage of the liver disease.[20,20a] In accordance with that, Hörtnagel et al. have recently reported highly increased values of both NE and E in patients with hepatic coma.[21] Whether SNA is changed in other types of chronic liver disease like hepatic fibrosis with portal venous hypertension or different types of chronic hepatitis is not known at present. However, cardiovascular and renal abnormalities exist in, e.g., hepatic failure following viral hepatitis, that may suggest sympathetic overactivity in this condition.[20] Obviously, these problems need further investigation.

B. ORGANS INVOLVED IN ENHANCED SYMPATHETIC NERVOUS ACTIVITY IN LIVER DISEASE

Preferably, SNA in individual organs should be studied by recording nerve impulses from autonomic nerve fibers supplying the organ in question or by estimating the release of NE from these organs into the veins that drain them. In order to measure the release of NE, the veno-arterial difference must be corrected for neuronal and nonneuronal reuptake, and the blood flow rate must be known. By infusion of labeled NE, it is possible to quantify these bidirectional fluxes of NE.[22-24]

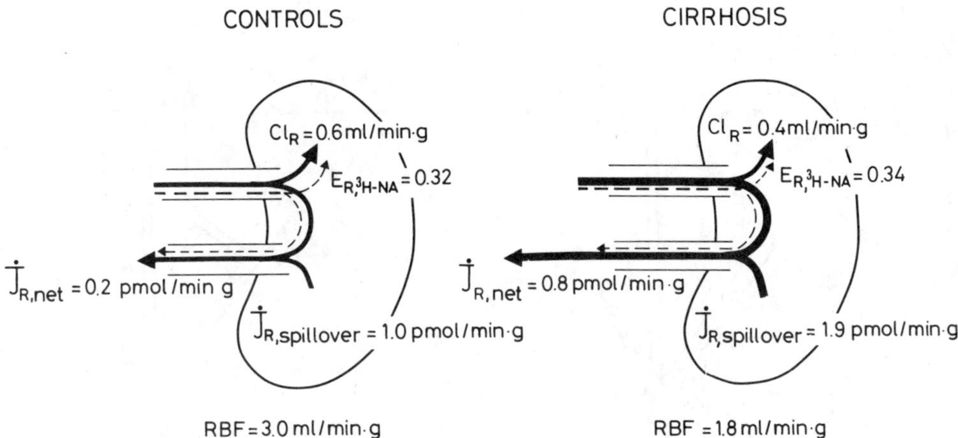

FIGURE 2.   Illustration of renal release and uptake of norepinephrine (NE) in control subjects (n = 6) and patients with moderately severe cirrhosis (n = 12). Cl_R and E_R: renal clearance and extraction ratio of labeled NE, respectively; $J_{R,net}$ and $J_{R,spillover}$: net rate and total spillover of NE from the kidney; RBF: renal blood flow.

Whether NE release and SNA are uniformly increased in patients with liver disease or the increase is limited to certain specific organs is still under debate. The increased heart rate and cardiac output in advanced liver disease[20] suggest enhanced SNA to the heart, but direct measurements are not available at present.

In the normal kidney, significant net release of NE into the systemic circulation is low or absent, since the concentration of NE is similar in arterial and renal venous plasma[25] (Figure 1). Experiments in dogs have shown that graded stimulation of the renal nerves causes increased vasoconstriction and simultaneously increased NE-release into the renal vein.[26] Thus, it seems justified to consider the size of the renal NE overflow as an index of renal sympathetic nervous tone. In patients with decompensated and recompensated cirrhosis a significant overflow of endogenous NE from the kidney has been established[16,17,25] (Figure 2). Moreover, renal blood flow has been found to be negatively correlated to the plasma NE concentration in the artery as well as in the renal vein.[17] Based on these observations, it seems reasonable to conclude that the augmented SNA in the kidney in advanced liver disease could be a main factor responsible for the observed renal vasoconstriction. The implications of these findings to homeostatic mechanisms will be considered later.

Sampling during hepatic vein catheterization in patients with raised arterial NE concentration has revealed an arterial-hepatic venous extraction of labeled NE that is greater than the extraction of endogenous NE.[27,27a] These results suggest that NE is released from sympathetic synapses within the hepato-splanchnic system (see below). No release was found in supine subjects without liver disease (Figure 3).

Sampling from different peripheral veins indicates that SNA may also be increased in skin and muscle.[28]

C. CATECHOLAMINE KINETICS

After release from postganglionic sympathetic nerve fibers, NE is removed form the synaptic cleft by different mechanisms. Spillover into plasma has been mentioned earlier. Irreversible loss is obtained by neuronal uptake as well as nonneuronal uptake. Most of NE taken up by neurons is metabolized. Only a small part is recircled through synaptic release. Metabolism includes methylation by the enzyme catechol-*o*-methyl transferase and deamination by the enzyme monamine-oxidase. The final metabolite, vanilin-mandelic-acid, is excreted through the kidney.

Since the same vascular bed may release, as well as remove NE, quantification of NE-

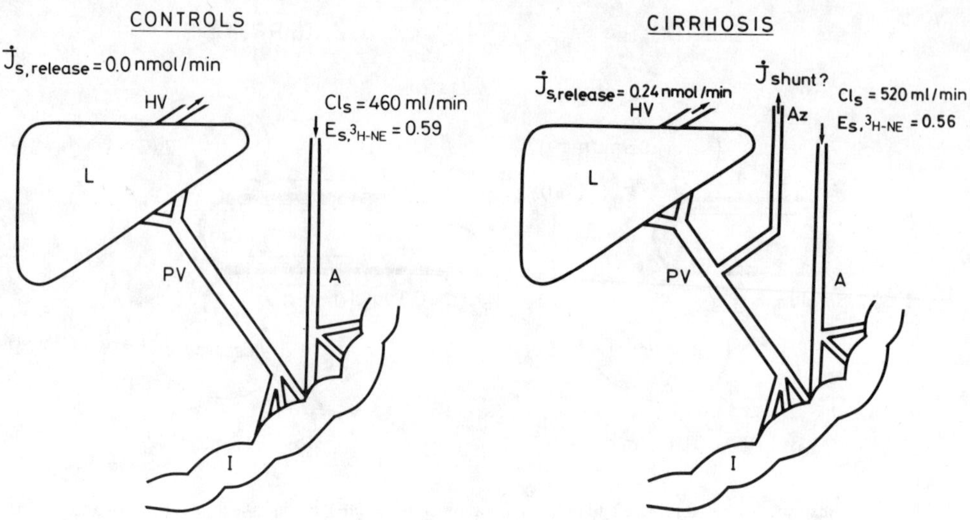

FIGURE 3.   Illustration of splanchnic release and uptake of norepinephrine (NE) in control subjects (n = 6) and patients with moderately severe cirrhosis (n = 12). Cl_S and E_S: clearance and extraction ratio of labeled NE in liver-intestine, respectively; $J_{,S,release}$ and $J_{s,shunt}$: net release of NE from liver-intestine through hepatic veins (HV) and porto-systemic collaterals (azygos vein: AZ), respectively. PV: portal vein; A: artery; L: liver; I: intestine.

kinetics in plasma demands a method such as the application of labeled NE, which is able to distinguish both fluxes. In the following, a brief description is given of plasma NE-kinetics with respect to whole-body and single organs. It is outside the scope of this review to discuss methodological problems in detail, but major and in part unsolved problems are related to the different permeability-surface area of catecholamines in the different organs, steady state problems with respect to volume of distribution of NE, and the fact that the specific activity (i.e., concentration of labeled NE relative to endogenous NE concentration) is different in plasma and in the synaptic cleft.[28a]

Infusion of tritium-labeled NE into a peripheral vein in normal subjects has revealed that the plasma turnover rate is fast with an equivalent plasma clearance of approximately 1.5 1/min.[18,27a] It is important to notice that arterial concentration of labeled NE should be used to calculate the plasma clearance because there is a considerable extraction across the forearm. Therefore, application of cubital venous plasma will reflect local, as well as systemic, mechanisms leading to erroneously high estimate of NE plasma clearance.

By multiplying the concentration of endogenous NE in arterial plasma by the plasma clearance of NE, an appearance rate of NE into plasma is obtained. It is important to notice that in advanced liver disease this appearance rate is significantly increased and positively correlated to the circulating level of NE, which may be taken as an index of NE spillover due to enhanced SNA.[22-24] However, it should be realized that, due to local degradation, the plasma appearance rate is far smaller than the rate of NE release from sympathetic postganglionic axon terminals.[27a,28a]

In individual organs, NE spillover may be determined from arterial and venous concentration of endogenous NE, and labeled NE according to the following equation.[17,24,27a]

$$\dot{J} = \text{organ plasma flow} \times C_{a,NE} \times [(C_v/C_a)_{NE} - (C_v/C_a)_{3H-NE}]$$

Table 1
Spillover Rate of Norepinephine (NE) in Kidney, Liver-Intestine and Lower Limb in Patients with Cirrhosis and Controls

	Kidney	Liver-intestine	Lower limb
	nmol/min of NE-spillover per unit (nmol/min) NE-inflow		
Cirrhosis (n = 12)	0.69[a] (0.48—1.14)	0.15 (0.0—0.38)	0.23 (0.01—0.59)
Controls (n = 6)	0.45 (0.28—0.49)	0.0[b] (−0.3—0.5)	0.49 (0.26—0.71)
p	< 0.005	< 0.025	< 0.1

Note: Figures in the table are medians; ranges are in parentheses.

[a] $p < 0.001$ compared to the lower limb and liver-intestine.
[b] $p < 0.05$ compared to kidney and lower limb.

where $\dot{J}$ denotes the release rate of NE, and $C_{a,NE}$ is the arterial concentration of endogenous NE, (C_v/C_a) is the veno-arterial ratio of endogenous and labeled NE, respectively. The extraction ratio of endogenous and labeled catecholamines can be expressed in a conventional way as arterial-venous difference divided by arterial concentration. Hence the plasma clearance of the organ is obtained as plasma flow multiplied by extraction ratio.

Kinetics of NE may be determined in man with respect to the whole body as well as individual organs, provided that organ flow can be determined and sampling from the venous outflow is obtained. Both may be performed during a diagnostic catheterization study. The spillover rate of NE per unit NE-inflow, i.e., $(C_v/C_a)_{NE} - (C_v/C_a)^3_{H-NE}$ in different locations, may indicate uniform or heterogenous distribution of SNA in different parts of the body (Table 1).

D. AFFERENT TRIGGERS OF SYMPATHETIC NERVOUS ACTIVITY

A number of stimuli may elicit increased SNA, e.g., hypoglycemia, hypovolemia (acute during gastrointestinal bleeding or more chronically as a part of the ascitic syndrome, see later) or low arterial blood pressure.[11,29,30] Recently Kostreva et al.[31] demonstrated evidence of a non-volume-dependent hepatic baroreceptor, which may elicit increased activity in renal and cardiac sympathetic fibers in animals. DiBona has suggested that a hepatic baroreceptor plays a role in human pathophysiology as well.[32] In man and animals increased sympathetic activity may be elicited by central volume depletion, and reflex loss of sympathetic activity may be seen during stretch of the atrial wall.[29] Moreover, Wallin et al. have found that the burst activity in sympathetic nerve fibers varies synchroneously with arterial blood pressure.[9] Bilateral clamping of the carotid artery, which leads to underfilling and reduced pressure in the carotid sinuses, induces reflex hypertension due to sympathetic overactivity.[33] In a similar way, low arterial blood pressure in advanced liver disease may be counteracted by enhanced SNA,[34] but apparently the increase in SNA is inadequate in overcoming the vasodilatory forces responsible for the deranged systemic and splanchnic hemodynamics (see later).

Cirrhosis is associated with several circulatory changes,[35-37] i.e., altered plasma volume, heart rate, cardiac output, and portal venous pressure, whereas arterial blood pressure and renal blood flow most often are decreased.

The mechanisms behind these hemodynamic changes including the reduced systemic vascular resistance is not yet known. The question of overfilling vs. underfilling of the central vascular bed has been disputed for a long time.[38] There is evidence in favor of either condition.[35,39,40] Thus, several studies have shown an elevation of plasma volume in cirrhosis, suggesting overfilling of the circulation. On the other hand, the low arterial blood pressure, the effect of peritoneovenous shunting and head-out water immersion (procedures that expand the central plasma volume) in bringing about a natriuresis in some patients, the activated renin-angiotensin aldosterone system, all suggest central underfilling.[41-44] Recently, a method has been developed that allows direct determination of the central and arterial blood volume. Preliminary studies by this method suggest central underfilling in cirrhosis.[45,45a] Whether this holds true in other types of advanced liver disease is unknown. Splanchnic pooling and increased capacitance of large and small veins may contain a substantial part of an enlarged total blood volume, leaving the central circulatory volume underfilled. The intrathoracic pressure may be increased in patients with cirrhosis and fluid retention, as suggested by Guazzi et al.[46] Therefore, a normal or even somewhat elevated right atrial pressure, relative to an external reference (midaxillary line), may still indicate underfilling of the central vascular bed, since the correct pressure reflecting the degree of filling and thereby the afferent sympathetic stimulus must be the transmural gradient (i.e., atrial pressure minus intrathoracic pressure).

Based on neuroendocrine alterations, reduced arterial blood volume, and low peripheral vascular resistance, a new "peripheral vasodilatation hypothesis" on renal sodium-water retention has been put forward.[46a] In advanced liver disease, the peripheral vascular resistance is reduced considerably, and the arterial blood pressure is usually lower than in normal individuals. The etiology of this hyperkinetic circulatory state is obscure, and the regions of the circulation responsible for the reduced peripheral resistance are not yet known.[47] It has been suggested that patients with liver failure have a general impairment of peripheral vasoconstriction that contributes to the arterial hypotension. Skin and muscle perfusion may be increased, but the result of studies on this topic are equivocal. Cross-circulation experiments in animals have suggested the existence of a general vasodilatator that might be produced by, or escape degradation in, the diseased liver,[48,49] but such a factor has not been yet demonstrated with certainty in patients. Hörtnagl et al.[21] have suggested that a factor with such properties could be substance P, the concentration of which is markedly increased in the plasma in patients with hepatic coma. Vasoactive intestinal polypeptide has also been suggested in this context (for survey, see References 50 and 51), but recent investigations have shown that the cirrhotic liver degrades vasoactive intestinal polypeptide almost as well as the normal liver.[51] Moreover, plasma concentration of the peptide is only moderately elevated in patients with cirrhosis, and a relation to hemodynamic changes or fluid retention has not been demonstrated.[50,51]

Direct arterial-venous shunting, which can be observed in the pulmonary, splanchnic, and peripheral circulation in advanced liver disease, has been considered of minor hemodynamic importance. However, intra- as well as extrahepatic arterial-venous shunting in the splanchnic circulation may be of greater consequence than previously estimated.[52,53] An impairment of the baroreceptor-mediated sympathetic nervous reactivity in cirrhosis has been suggested,[54] but recent studies seem to indicate that neurovascular activity is intact even in patients with very low peripheral resistance.[34]

Thus, the deranged peripheral resistance is the major unsolved problem of cardiovascular homeostasis in patients with advanced liver disease. Cardiac output and peripheral vascular resistance return to normal following successful liver transplantation.[55] Moreover, after successful implantation of a peritoneovenous shunt, Blendis et al.[43,56] have shown that the hemodynamics is partially normalized. This occurred simultaneously with normalization of circulating catecholamines, indicating that the activity in SNS returns to normal when the systemic hemodynamic abnormalities are reversed, except for the cardiac output, which was still elevated.

E. α- AND β-ADRENORECEPTORS AND SYMPATHETIC NEUROPATHY IN LIVER DISEASE

In contrast to normal subjects, α-adrenergic blockade by phentolamine in patients with decompensated cirrhosis is followed by a fall in systemic blood pressure, which indicates that sympathetic nervous tone is important for the maintenance of the blood pressure in this condition[19,57] (see Chapter 17). By tilting cirrhotic patients to 60° head-up position, Ring-Larsen et al.[34] observed a normal NE response (i.e., rapidly increasing concentrations of NE in arterial plasma). The absolute level of arterial NE was higher in these patients but the increment was normal, which indicates that baro- and volume-receptor-mediated responses were intact in the patients studied.

False or weak neurotransmitters (e.g., octopamine) in the central and peripheral nervous system have been invoked to explain hepatic encephalopathy and autonomic dysfunction in cirrhosis.[58-60] Recently, Bernardi et al.[58] reported that octopamine and β-phenylethanolamine increased in parallel with NE in patients with cirrhosis during head-up tilt. The patients did not achieve an adequate cardiovascular response, and the authors concluded that hyperproduction of weak neurotransmitters was, at least in part, responsible for the attenuation. However, postsynaptic α-adrenoceptors might already be occupied by endogenous catecholamines due to enhanced sympathetic nervous resting tone. This is in accordance with the observed blunted pressor response to exogenous NE in cirrhosis.[61] Reduced vascular reactivity to angiotensin II and NE has been described in experimental portal hypertension and cirrhosis.[62,63] However, the results on vascular reactivity by exogenous vasoconstrictive agents in man are conflicting. Thus, Lenz et al.[8] have recorded, in patients with far-advanced liver diseases, a normal increase in systolic blood pressure in response to infusion of vasoconstrictive agents, NE and angiotensin II. In fact the response was even greater than in a group of young healthy control subjects. In severely advanced liver disease, patients may have a supranormal pressor response to exogenous NE, suggesting tissue depletion of catecholamines.[64]

It has been questioned whether alcoholic sympathetic neuropathy exists. There are indications that sympathetic fibers may be damaged in patients with alcoholic neuropathy.[5,65] However, the fact that most patients with advanced alcoholic liver disease have raised levels of circulating NE does indicate a high degree of sympathetic reactivity, but that the maximal sympathetic response may be somewhat blunted is likely. However, this remains to be proven.

It should be recalled that Gerbes et al.[66] found evidence of a decreased number of β-receptors in leukocytes from patients with cirrhosis, and Ramond et al.[67] found a decreased sensitivity to isoprenaline in patients with cirrhosis. However, it is obvious that postsynaptic receptors (numbers, occupancy, ratio between α- and β-receptors, etc.), false neurotransmitters, and autonomic neuropathy in liver disease need further investigation.

IV. CIRCULATORY AND FLUID HOMEOSTASIS

Besides governing a number of essential hemodynamic functions, SNA also plays a role in the fluid homeostatis. The normal kidney is able to maintain the organism in sodium-water balance over a wide range of intake of these substances. Thus, normal subjects may excrete between 20 and 500 mmol sodium per day, and after a water load of 1 to 2 l, this volume is eliminated within a few hours. During orthostasis and volume depletion, renal blood flow (RBF) and glomerular filtration rate (GFR) decrease substantially, mainly due to enhanced sympathoadrenal and renin-angiotensin-aldosterone system activity. Stimulation of renal sympathetic nerve fibers causes not only a decrease in RBF and GFR (α-adrenoreceptor which in itself reduces urinary sodium excretion)[68] but also an increase in sodium reabsorption in the proximal parts of the nephron due to a direct effect (α-adrenoreceptor) on the proximal tubules.[68-71] Furthermore, SNA may activate the renin-angiotensin-aldosterone system[34] due to a change in the autoregulation, decreased delivery of sodium to distal parts of the nephron, and to a direct effect (β-adrenoreceptor) on the macula densa.[68,72] RBF and GRF are decreased in decompensated cirrhosis, and an inverse relationship between

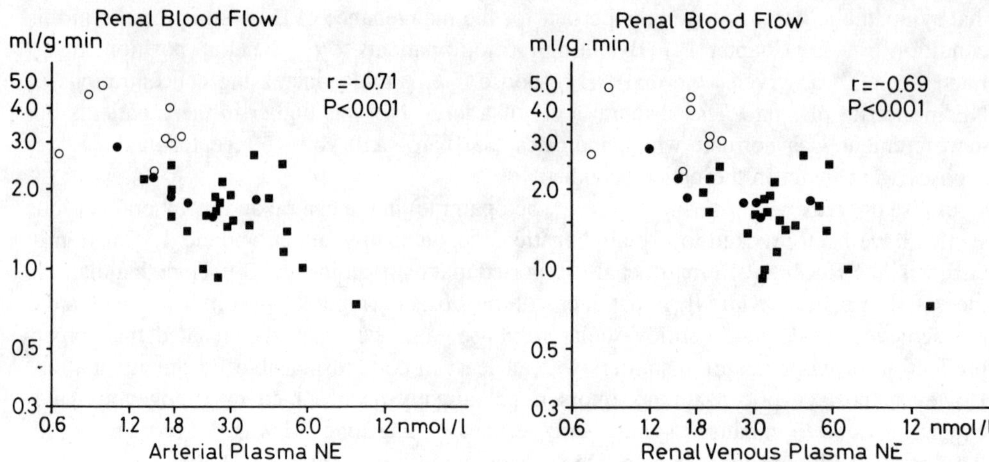

FIGURE 4.   Relationship between arterial and renal venous norepinephrine (NE) concentration and renal blood flow in controls (circles) and patients with cirrhosis (●, patients without ascites; ■, patients with ascites).

RBF and arterial and renal venous plasma concentrations of NE has been demonstrated,[17] suggesting a relationship between enhanced SNA and decreased RBF (Figure 4). The kidney in cirrhosis is not able to excrete a sodium load as quickly and as completely as a normal kidney, and in decompensated cirrhosis, the most extreme degrees of sodium retention are found. The urinary excretion of sodium may be in the order of or less than 1 mmol/d, which is the most avid sodium retention known in renal pathophysiology. Total body sodium is substantially increased, but despite this, the serum sodium concentration is low (down to 110 to 115 mmol/l) due to enhanced water retention as well. An osmotic load (mannitol) may, surprisingly, increase free water clearance in patients with decompensated cirrhosis.[72a] However, this is in accordance with the concept that the reabsorption of salt and water in the proximal tubules is substantially enhanced due to sympathetic overactivity, leaving only a small fraction of the filtrate to pass through into the distal tubules and collecting ducts. The osmotic load will increase the amount of fluid available here. Sodium molecules passing to the ascending limb of the loop of Henle and to the distal tubules are then reabsorbed in this tubular segment through an aldosterone-mediated mechanism,[73] and the urine may become hyposmotic. Moreover, varying degrees of reduced salt and water delivery to the distal tubules may explain why aldosterone antagonists (such as spironolactone), sometimes are ineffective in bringing about a natriuresis, despite highly increased levels of circulating aldosterone.

Bichet et al.[15] found a close correlation between NE and the degree of sodium and water retention following a water load in patients with decompensated cirrhosis. Moreover, these authors were able to suppress the elevated plasma NE concentration and to improve the ability to excrete water and sodium by head-out water immersion, a procedure which increases the central blood volume.[74] Recently, Blendis et al.[56] showed in six patients with massive refractive ascites and highly elevated circulating catecholamines that the plasma concentration of NE and E fell to within normal ranges 2 weeks after successful implantation of a peritoneovenous shunt. This indicates that the increased SNA in decompensated cirrhosis is a response to vascular underfilling. Bernardi et al.[58] demonstrated an inverse relationship between plasma NE concentrations and tubular rejection fraction, and urinary excretion of sodium when quantifying the changes of renal function in cirrhotic patients with ascites induced by changes in posture. In contrast to Bichet et al.,[15,75] Epstein[76] did not find plasma NE concentration changes that could be related to the increased urinary sodium excretion in patients with decompensated cirrhosis during head-out water immersion, although the plasma NE concentration was considerably increased. In contrast to this, by use of another mode of redistributing blood volume, increasing right atrial pressure without increasing total blood volume, Ring-Larsen et al.[77] found that patients with decompensated cirrhosis in the supine position had a nearly 100% better natriuretic response to a potent natriuretic drug than when in the upright position. This augmented response seemed related to a decrease in SNA, probably via a greater delivery of sodium to the part of the nephron distal to the proximal tubules, because of increased GFR and a decreased reabsorption in the proximal tubules.

The increased SNA in the "cirrhotic kidney" may be of importance for the renal sodium excretion. This is supported by animal experiments showing that stimulation of the renal nerves not only reduces RBF, but also enhances the proximal tubular sodium reabsorption independent of flow and filtration.[68,70,71] Thus, it is likely, also in man, that the increased SNA has a sodium-retaining function in reducing GFR as well as enhancing reabsorption of sodium in the proximal tubules.

Arroyo et al.[44] and Henriksen et al.[78] found a positive correlation between arterial plasma NE and renin and aldosterone concentrations. This may indicate that increased SNA leads to activation of the renin-angiotensin-aldosterone system in decompensated cirrhosis. In contrast to normal subjects, cirrhotic patients with elevated renin and aldosterone values are very sensitive to angiotensin II antagonists.[79,80] These drugs evoke significant hypotension, indicating that the blood pressure in these patients depends on the pressor effect of angiotensin II. Early studies on α-adrenoceptor blocking agents (phenotolamine) in cirrhosis suggest that arterial blood pressure also depends on α-adrenergic sympathetic tone.[57] The renal vasoconstriction in liver failure may be due to lack of a physiologic renal vasodilator, to the presence of a pathophysiological renal vascoconstrictor, or to the presence of a pathophysiologic systemic vasodilator. The latter leads to compensatory renal hypoperfusion via stimulation of central venous or arterial baroreceptors, as mentioned earlier. Renal prostaglandins (E series) are cyclized fatty acids that are synthesized in and act within the kidney as vasodilators with limited, if any, systemic effect.[81] They seem to be able to change the glomerular arteriolar resistance and thereby influence RBF and GFR. Renal prostaglandin (PG) synthesis is stimulated by renal nerve stimulation, angiotensin II, and bradykinin, and they apparently stimulate renin release, counteract vasopressin-mediated water transport, and potentiate the effect of bradykinin.[82] The role of endogenous PGE_2 in patients with decompensated cirrhosis has been demonstrated by inhibiting renal prostaglandin production.[83,84] This resulted in a reduced RBF and an approximately 50% reduction in GFR, which, however, returned to baseline value after discontinuation of drugs. Several investigators have found the urinary excretion of PGE_2 decreased in patients with renal failure following liver disease, and a deficit of endogenous PG has been implied as the cause of this kind of renal failure.[44,85]

Renal vasoconstriction in cirrhosis appears to be an integral part of the evolution of the illness. The hemodynamic changes point towards renal hypoperfusion being, at least initially, a normal physiologic response to changes in the systemic or splanchnic circulation, leading to decreased urinary sodium and water excretion. It seems possible that increased sympathoadrenal activity is a primary pathogenetic factor, but several connected systems regulating hemodynamics and sodium-water homeostasis are secondarily activated. Results of nearly all studies of these systems in liver failure indicate that they are counteracting a decreased systemic vascular resistance. The importance of some of these systems, such as SNS, vasopressin, the renin-angiotensin-aldosterone system, and endogenous renal PG for the renal hemodynamics and the renal handling of sodium and water, has been dealt with in more detail above and elsewhere in this book.

Thus, in advanced decompensated cirrhosis, the kidneys appear pathophysiologically to function like a Goldblatt kidney.[86] Experiments in dogs have shown that stimulation of the renal nerves or infusion into the renal artery of minimal doses of NE lacking any systemic effect results in a decrease of RBF. More interestingly, these experiments have revealed that the autoregulation curve in dogs is shifted to the right so that RBF is diminished at a higher perfusion pressure than without sympathetic nerve stimulation.[72,87] This situation seems similar to that observed in cirrhosis. When taking a close look at the renal perfusion pressure in advanced cirrhosis (that is, arterial pressure minus renal vein pressure) it has been demonstrated that this is very often decreased to a critical level.[20,39,86] As judged from the animal experiments this level is about 70 mmHg, a pressure which would be sufficient in normal man, but insufficient in a patient with decompensated cirrhosis and increased SNA in the kidney.

The circulatory characteristics of the cirrhotic patient dying with renal failure are those of low arterial blood pressure and an increased central venous pressure artifically kept up by infusion of various plasma expanders without any overt effect on the arterial pressure, thus, a decreased renal perfusion pressure. The importance of a normal renal perfusion pressure for filtration and sodium and water excretion has recently been shown by Lenz et al.[88] In a patient with hepatorenal syndrome, they demonstrated that keeping up the arterial blood pressure by ornipressin (8-ornithine vasopressin) GFR increased from 24 to 65 ml/min, with a subsequent increase in urinary volume and fractional sodium excretion. In this therapeutic trial the plasma NE decreased from 2.04 to 1.37 ng ml^{-1}, indicating a renal vasodilation due to a reduced sympathetic nervous activity. In its turn this is the result of a reduced stimulus to the arterial baroreceptors, since the pulmonary arterial wedged pressure was essentially unchanged during the infusion of ornipressin. The values returned to control levels after stopping ornipressin.

Similarly, Nicholls et al.[89] studied, in patients with decompensated cirrhosis, the natriuretic response to either head-out water immersion alone, expanding the central blood volume, or to intravenous infusion of NE, increasing the peripheral vascular resistance, or to a combination of the two methods. The combined maneuver resulted in the greatest increase in sodium and water excretion, probably reflecting the importance of the high-pressure as well as the low-pressure baroreceptors in the volume homeostasis in decompensated cirrhosis.

A major problem in the understanding of the circulatory changes in cirrhosis is the discordance between the vascular tone in the kidney and other parts of the circulation. Thus, the vascular resistance in the kidney is greatly increased whereas in the organism as a whole it is decreased.[20,36,37] In other clinical situations with enhanced SNA (except for mental stress), both renal and systemic vascular resistance are increased.[90] A circulatory state resembling that of decompensated cirrhosis may be observed during exercise in which situation the plasma NE concentration is high[12] and RBF decreased due to renal vascular constriction, while the overall systemic resistance is reduced due to muscular vasodilation. This superficial similarity to cirrhosis may tempt speculation that the balance between vasodilators and vasoconstrictors may be abnormal in decompensated cirrhosis.

V. CONCLUSION

In summary, the mechanisms behind the changes in renal function and water-electrolyte handling are not fully elucidated. Thus, renal sodium retention in cirrhosis may be considered a normal phenomenon, due to substantially activated volume- and pressure preserving forces or as the result of a direct pathologic influence of the diseased liver on the kidney.[38] These two extremes may operate together, simultaneously or successively, in the genesis and perpetuation of the hepatic ascites syndrome. Animal experiments have shown that the underfilling as well as the overfilling (overflow) models lead to ascites formation,[91-93] but these experiments do not conclusively solve the pathophysiologic problems in man. However, based on the present survey, the authors find that underfilling and peripheral vasodilatation

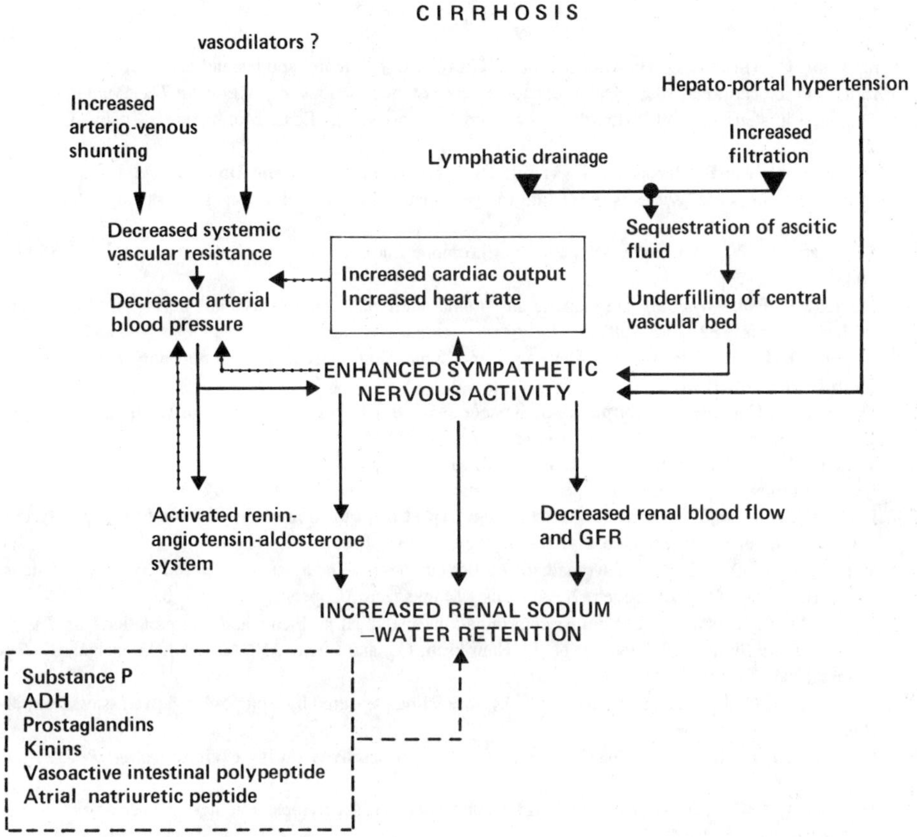

FIGURE 5. Summary of present view on the role of the sympathetic nervous system in advanced liver disease.

seem at present to fit with most available investigative data. It is the authors' conception that the sympathetic nervous system plays a vital role in the pathophysiological mechanisms involved in the hemodynamic and homeostatic changes seen in advanced liver disease (Figure 5). The pathophysiological mechanisms behind the decreased systemic hemodynamic resistance in advanced liver disease are still the major enigma. Moreover, the potential role of parasympathetic dysfunction in liver disease remains to be elucidated.

ACKNOWLEDGMENTS

This work was supported by a grant from the NOVO Foundation and Max and Anna Friedmanns Legat. The authors wish to express their gratitude to Ms. Bente Henriksen and Ms. Ruth Werner for their skillful assistance.

REFERENCES

1. **Owman, C., Hanko, J., Harebo, J., and Kåhrström, J.,** Neuropeptides and classical autonomic transmitters in the cardiovascular system: existence, coexistence, action, interaction, in *The Sympatho-Adrenal System*, Christensen, N. J., Henriksen, O., and Lassen, N. A., Eds., Munksgaard, Copenhagen, 1986, 340.
2. **Wieling, W., van Brederode, J. F. M., de Rijk, L. G., Borst, C., and Dunning, A. J.,** Reflex control of heart-rate in normal subjects in relation to age: a data base for cardiac vagal neuropathy, *Diabetologia,* 22, 163, 1982.
3. **Schwartz, T. W.,** Pancreatic polypeptide: a hormone under vagal control, *Gastroenterology,* 85, 1411, 1983.
4. **Hilsted, J.,** Pathophysiology in diabetic autonomic neuropathy: cardiovascular, hormonal, and metabolic studies, *Diabetes,* 32, 730, 1982.
5. **Novak, D. J., and Victor, M.,** The vagus and sympathetic nerves in alcoholic polyneuropathy, *Arch. Neurol.,* 30, 273, 1974.
6. **Decaux, G., Cauchie, P., Soupart, A., Kruger, M., and Delwiche, F.,** Role of vagal neuropathy in the hyponatremia of alcoholic cirrhosis, *Br. Med. J.,* 293, 1534, 1986.
7. **Tan, E. T. H., Johnson, R. H., Lambie, D. G., and Whiteside, E. A.,** Alcoholic vagal neuropathy: recovery following prolonged abstinence, *J. Neurol. Neurosurg. Psychiatr.,* 47, 1335, 1984.
8. **Lenz, K., Hörtnagl, H., and Magometschnigg, D. et al.,** Function of the autonomic nervous system in patients with hepatic encephalopathy, *Hepatology,* 5, 831, 1985.
9. **Wallin, B. G.,** Organization of sympathetic outflow in man, in *The Sympatho-Adrenal System*, Christensen, N. J., Henriksen, O., and Lassen, N. A., Eds., Munksgaard, Copenhagen, 1986, 52.
10. **Hjemdahl, P.,** Plasma catecholamine determination: analytical problems and interpretations, in *The Sympatho-Adrenal System*, Christensen, N. J., Henriksen, O., and Lassen, N. A., Eds., Munksgaard, Copenhagen, 1986, 26.
11. **Christensen, N. J.,** Plasma noradrenaline and adrenaline measured by isotope-derivative assay, *Dan. Med. Bull.* 26, 17, 1979.
12. **Christensen, N. J. and Galbo, H.,** Sympathetic nervous activity during exercise, *Annu. Rev. Physiol.,* 45, 139, 1983.
13. **Henriksen, J. H., Ring-Larsen, H., and Christensen, N. J.,** Sympathetic nervous activity in cirrhosis, *J. Hepatol.,* 1, 55, 1985.
14. **Burghardt, W., Wernze, H., and Schaffrath, I.,** Changes of circulating noradrenaline and adrenaline in hepatic cirrhosis. Relation to stage of disease, liver and renal function, *Acta Endocrinol.,* 99 (Suppl. 246), 252, 1981.
15. **Bichet, D. G., Van Putten, V. J., and Schrier, R. W.,** Potential role of increased sympathetic activity in impaired sodium and water excretion in cirrhosis, *N. Engl. J. Med.,* 307, 1552, 1982.
16. **Willet, I., Esler, M., Burke, F. et al.,** Total and renal sympathetic nervous system activity in alcoholic cirrhosis, *J. Hepatol.,* 1, 639, 1985.
17. **Henriksen, J. H., Ring-Larsen, H., and Christensen, N. J.,** Renal release and uptake of noradrenaline in cirrhosis, in *The Sympatho-Adrenal System*, Christensen, N. J., Henriksen, O., and Lassen, N. A., Eds., Munksgaard, Copenhagen, 1986, 474.
18. **Hilsted, J., Christensen, N. J., and Madsbad, S.,** Whole body clearance of norepinephrine — The significance of arterial sampling and surgical stress, *J. Clin. Invest.,* 71, 500, 1983.
19. **Moreau, R., Lee, S. S., Hadengue, A., Braillon, A., and Lebrec, D.,** Hemodynamic affects of a clonidine-induced decrease in sympathetic tone in patients with cirrhosis, *Hepatology,* 7, 149, 1987.
19a. **Bernardi, M., Trevisani, F., DePalma, R., Ligabue, A., Capani, F., Baraldini, M., and Gasbarrini, G.,** Chronobiological evaluation of sympathoadrenergic function in cirrhosis. Relationship with arterial pressure and heart rate, *Gastroenterology,* 93, 1178, 1987.
20. **Ring-Larsen, H.,** Heptatic nephropathy related to hemodynamics, *Liver,* 3, 265, 1983.
20a. **Bendtsen, F., Henriksen, J. H., Sørensen, T. I. A., and Christensen, N. J.,** Effect of oral propranolol on circulating catecholamines in cirrhosis: relationship to severity of liver disease and splanchnic haemodynamics. *J. Hepatol.* 10, 198, 1990.
21. **Hörtnagl, H., Singer, E. A., and Kenz, K. et al.,** Substance P is markedly increased in plasma of patients with hepatic coma, *Lancet,* i, 480, 1984.
22. **Christensen, N. J., Galbo, H., Gjerris, A., and Henriksen, J. H. et al.,** Whole body and regional clearance of noradrenaline and adrenaline in man, *Acta Physiol. Scand.,* 17 (Suppl. 527), 1984.
23. **Esler, M., Willet, I., Leonard, P., Hasking, G., Johns, J., Little, P., and Jennings, G.,** Plasma noradrenaline kinetics in humans, *J. Auton. Nerv. Syst.,* 11, 125, 1984.
24. **Halter, J. B., Best, J. D., and Linares, O. A.,** Measurement of catecholamine kinetics *in vivo,* in *The Sympatho-Adrenal System*, Christensen, N. J., Henriksen, O., and Lassen, N. A., Eds., Munksgaard, Copenhagen, 1986, 38.

25. **Henriksen, J. H., Ring-Larsen, H., Kanstrup, I.-L., and Christensen, N. J.,** Splanchnic and renal elimination and release of catecholamines in cirrhosis. Evidence of enhanced sympathetic nervous activity in patients with cirrhosis, *Gut,* 25, 1034, 1984.

26. **Kopp, U., Bradley, T., and Hjemdahl, P.,** Renal venous outflow and urinary excretion of norepinephrine, epinephrine and dopamine during graded renal nerve stimulation. *Am. J. Physiol.,* 244, E52, 1983.

27. **Henriksen, J. H., Ring-Larsen, H., and Christensen, N. J.,** Splanchnic uptake and release of catecholamines in alcoholic cirrhosis. Evidence of enhanced sympathetic nervous activity in the splanchnic system, *Gut,* 28, 1637, 1987.

27a. **Henriksen, J. H., Christensen, N. J. and Ring-Larsen, H.,** Continuous infusion of tracer norepinephrine may miscalculate unidirectional nerve uptake of norepinephrine in humans. *Cir. Res.* 65, 388, 1989.

28. **Henriksen, J. H., Ring-Larsen, H., and Christensen, N. J.,** Catecholamines in plasma from artery, cubital vein, and femoral vein in patients with cirrhosis. Significance of sampling site, *Scand. J. Clin. Lab. Invest.,* 46, 39, 1986.

28a. **Henriksen, J. H. and Christensen, N. J.** Plasma norepinephrine in humans: limitations in assesment of whole body norepinephrine kinetics and plasma clearance. *Am. J. Physiol.* 257, E743, 1989.

29. **Linden, R. J., Mary, D. A. S. G., and Weathreill, D.,** The nature of the atrial receptors responsible for a reflex decrease in activity in renal nerves in the dog, *J. Physiol. (London),* 300, 31, 1980.

30. **Gross, R., Hackenberg, H. M., and Hackentnal, E. et al.,** Interaction between perfusion pressure and sympathetic nerves in renin release by carotid baroreflex in conscious dogs, *J. Physiol. (London),* 313, 327, 1981.

31. **Kostreva, D. R., Castaner, A., and Kampine, J. P.,** Reflex effect of hepatic baroreceptors on renal and cardiac sympathetic nerve activity, *Am. J. Physiol.,* 238, R390, 1980.

32. **DiBona, G. F.,** Renal neural activity in hepatorenal syndrome, *Kidney Int.,* 25, 841, 1984.

33. **Pelletrier, C. L. and Shepherd, J. T.,** Relative influence of carotid baroreceptors and muscle receptors in the control of renal and hindlimb circulation, *Can. J. Physiol. Pharmacol.,* 53, 1042, 1975.

34. **Ring-Larsen, H., Hesse, B., Henriksen, J. H., and Christensen, N. J.,** Sympathetic nervous activity and renal and systemic haemodynamics in cirrhosis — Plasma norepinephrine concentration, hepatic extraction, and renal release, *Hepatology,* 2, 304, 1982.

35. **Lieberman, F. L., Denison, E. K., and Reynolds, T. B.,** The relationship of plasma volume, portal hypertension, ascites, and renal sodium retention in cirrhosis: the overflow theory of ascites formation, *Ann. N.Y. Acad. Sci.,* 170, 202, 1970.

36. **Skorecki, K. L. and Brenner, B. M.,** Body fluid homeostasis in congestive heart failure and cirrhosis with ascites, *Am. J. Med.,* 72, 323, 1982.

37. **Better, O. S, and Schrier, R. W.,** Disturbed volume homeostasis in patients with cirrhosis of the liver, *Kidney Int.,* 23, 303, 1982.

38. **Epstein, F. H.,** Underfilling versus overfilling in hepatic ascites, *N. Engl. J. Med.,* 307, 1577, 1982.

39. **Henriksen, J. H.,** Protein-kinetics and haemodynamic studies in patients with liver cirrhosis. Evidence of a lymph-imbalance theory of ascites formation, *Clin. Physiol.,* 1, 565, 1981.

40. **Wernze, H., Spech, H. J., and Müller, G.,** Studies on the activity of the renin-angiotensin-aldosterone system (RAAS) in patients with cirrhosis of the liver, *Klin. Wochenschr.,* 56, 389, 1978.

41. **Epstein, M., Puns, D. S., Schneider, N., and Levinson, R.,** Determinants of deranged sodium and water homeostasis in decompensated cirrhosis, *J. Lab. Clin. Med.,* 87, 822, 1976.

42. **Epstein, M.,** Peritoneovenous shunt in the management of ascites and the hepatorenal syndrome, *Gastroenterology,* 82, 790, 1982.

43. **Blendis, L. M.,** The use of peritoneovenous shunting in unravelling the pathogenesis of ascites in cirrhosis, *Isr. J. Med. Sci.,* 22, 78, 1986.

44. **Arroyo, V., Planas, R., and Gaya, J. et al.,** Sympathetic nervous activity, renin-angiotensin system and renal excretion of prostaglandin E_2 in cirrhosis. Relation to functional renal failure and sodium and water excretion, *Eur. J. Clin. Invest.,* 13, 271, 1983.

45. **Henriksen, J. H., Schütten, H. J., Bendtsen, F., and Warberg, J.,** Circulating atrial natriuretic peptide (ANP) and central blood volume (CBV) in cirrhosis, *Liver,* 6, 361, 1986.

45a. **Henriksen, J. H., Bendtsen F., Sørensen, T. I. A., Stadeaqer, C., and Ring-Larsen, H.,** Reduced central blood volume in cirrhosis. *Gastroenterology,* 97, 1506, 1989.

46. **Guazzi, M., Polese, A., and Matrini, F. et al.,** Negative influence of ascites on the cardiac function of cirrhotic patients, *Am. J. Med.,* 59, 165, 1975.

46a. **Schrier, R. W., Arroyo, V., Bernardi, M., Epstein, M., Henriksen, J. H., and Rodés, J.** Peripheral arterial vasodilatation hypothesis: a proposal for the initiation of renal sodium and water retention in cirrhosis, *Hepatology,* 8, 1151, 1988.

47. **Ring-Larsen, H. and Henriksen, J. H.,** Pathogenesis of ascites formation and hepatorenal syndrome: humoral and hemodynamic factors, *Sem. Liv. Dis.,* 6, 341, 1986.

48. **Shorr, E.,** Hepatorenal Vasotropic Factors, Experimental Cirrhosis, Liver Injury, Trans. 6 Conference, May 1 to 2, 1947, New York, Josiah Macy Foundation, 1947, 33.

49. **Korthuis, R. J., Benoit, J. N., Kvietys, P. R., Townsley, M. I., Taylor, A. E., and Granger, D. N.,** Humoral factors may mediate increased rat hindquarter blood flow in portal hypertension, *Am. J. Physiol.,* 249, H827, 1985.

50. **Henriksen, J. H., Staun-Olsen, P., Fahrenkrug, J., and Ring-Larsen, H.,** Vasoactive intestinal polypeptide in cirrhosis: arteriovenous extraction in different vascular beds, *Scand. J. Gastroenterol.,* 15, 787, 1980.

51. **Henriksen, J. H., Staun-Olsen, P., Mogensen, N. B., and Fahrenkrug, J.,** Circulating endogeneous vasoactive intestinal polypeptide (VIP) in patients with uremia and liver cirrhosis, *Eur. J. Clin. Invest.,* 16, 211, 1986.

52. **Huet, P.-M., Pomier-Layaragues, G., Villeneuve, J.-P., Varin, F., and Viallet, A.,** Intrahepatic circulation in liver disease, *Sem. Liv. Dis.,* 6, 277, 1986.

53. **Blei, A. T.,** Pharmacokinetic-hemodynamics interactions in cirrhosis, *Sem. Liv. Dis.,* 6, 299, 1986.

54. **Lunzer, M., Newman, S.-P., and Sherlock, S.,** Skeletal muscle blood flow and neurovascular reactivity in liver disease, *Gut,* 14, 354, 1973.

55. **Vera, S. R., Williams, J. W., Peters, T. G., and Britt, L. G.,** Hemodynamic changes after liver transplantation, *Hepatology,* 5, 1024, 1985.

56. **Blendis, L. M., Sole, M. J., Campbell, P., Lossing, A. G., Greig, P. D., Taylor, B. R., and Langer, B.,** The effect of peritoneovenous shunting on catecholamine metabolism in patients with hepatic ascites, *Hepatology,* 7, 143, 1987.

57. **Epstein, M., Berk, D. P., and Hollenberg, N. K. et al.,** Renal failure in the patient with cirrhosis — The role of active vasoconstriction, *Am. J. Med.,* 49, 175, 1970.

58. **Bernardi, M., Trevisani, F., and Landini, C. et al.,** Plasma norepinephrine, weak neurotransmitters and renin activity during active tilting in liver cirrhosis — Relationship with cardiovascular homeostasis and renal function, *Hepatology,* 3, 56, 1983.

59. **Cuilleret, G., Pomier-Laryargues, G., and Pons, F. et al.,** Changes in brain catecholamine levels in human cirrhotic hepatic encephalopathy, *Gut,* 21, 565, 1980.

60. **Gentilini, P., Sicuteri, F., and Laffi, G. et al.,** The renin system and other vasoactive substances in chronic liver disease, *Adv. Exp. Med. Biol.,* 156B, 1161, 1983.

61. **Ames, R. P., Borkowski, A. J., Siciuski, A. M., and Laragh, J. H.,** Prolonged infusions of angiotensin II and norepinephrine and blood pressure, electrolyte balance, and aldosterone and cortisol secretion in normal man and in cirrhosis with ascites, *J. Clin. Invest.,* 44, 1171, 1965.

62. **Murray, B. M. and Paller, M. S.,** Decreased pressor reactivity to angiotensin II in cirrhotic rats. Evidence for a post-receptor defect in angiotensin action, *Circ. Res.,* 57, 424, 1985.

63. **Bomzon, A. and Blendis, L. M.,** Vascular reactivity in experimental portal hypertension, *Am. J. Physiol.,* 252, G158, 1987.

64. **Mashford, M. L., Makow, W. A., and Chalmers, T. C.,** Studies of the cardiovascular system in the hypotension of liver failure, *N. Engl. J. Med.,* 267, 1071, 1962.

65. **Eisenhofer, G., Whiteside, E. A., and Johnson, R. H.,** Plasma catecholamine responses to change of posture in alcoholics during withdrawal and after continued abstinence from alcohol, *Clin. Sci.,* 68, 71, 1985.

66. **Gerbes, A. L., Jüngst, D., Remine, J., Sauerbruch, T., Paum-Gartner, B.,** Evidence for downregulation of beta-2-adrenoceptors in cirrhotic patients with severe ascites, *Lancet,* i, 1409, 1986.

67. **Ramond, M.-J., Comoy, E., and Lebrec, D.,** Alterations in isoprenaline sensitivity in patients with cirrhosis: evidence of abnormality of the sympathetic nervous activity. *Br. J. Pharmacol.,* 21, 191, 1986.

68. **DiBona, G. F.,** The functions of the renal nerves, *Rev. Physiol. Biochem. Pharmacol.,* 94, 75, 1982.

69. **DiBona, G. F.,** Neurogenic regulations of renal tubular sodium reabsorption, *Am. J. Physiol.,* 233, F-73, 1977.

70. **Proznits, E. H. and DiBona, G. F.,** Effect of decreased renal sympathetic nerve activity of renal tubular sodium reabsorption, *Am. J. Physiol.,* 235, F551, 1978.

71. **Bello-Ruess, E.,** Effect of catecholamines in fluid reabsorption by the isolated proximal convoluted tubule, *Am. J. Physiol.,* 238, F-347, 1980.

72. **Langaard, Ø., Holdaas, H., Eide, I., and Kiiel, F.,** Conditions for humoral α-adrenoceptor stimulation of renin release in anesthetized dogs, *Scand. J. Clin. Lab. Invest.,* 3, 265, 1983.

72a. **Scheld, H. P. and Bartter, F. C.,** An explanation for and experimental correction of the abnormal water diuresis in cirrhosis, *J. Clin. Invest.,* 39, 248, 1969.

73. **Wilkinson, S. P. and Williams, R.,** Renin-angiotensin-aldosterone system in cirrhosis, *Gut,* 21, 545, 1980.

74. **Bichet, D., Groves, B., and Schrier, R. W.,** Mechanisms of improvement of water and sodium excretion by enhancement of central hemodynamics in decompensated cirrhosis, *Clin. Res.,* 31, 75A, 1983.

75. **Bichet, D. G., Groves, B. M., and Schrier, R. W.,** Mechanisms of improvement of water and sodium excretion by immersion in decompensated cirrhotic patients, *Kidney Int.,* 24, 788, 1983.

76. **Epstein, M.,** *N. Engl. J. Med.,* 308, 1030, 1983, (letter).

77. **Ring-Larsen, H., Henriksen, J. H., and Wilken, C. et al.,** Diuretic treatment in decompensated cirrhosis and congestive heart failure: effect of posture, *Br. Med. J.,* 292, 1351, 1986.
78. **Henriksen, J. H., Ring-Larsen, H., and Christensen, N. J.,** Plasma noradrenaline in patients with liver cirrhosis in relation of ascites and treatment, *Clin. Physiol.,* 1 (Suppl. 1), 66, 1981.
79. **Schroeder, E. T., Anderson, G. H., and Goldmann, S. H. et al.,** Effect of blockade of angiotensin II on blood pressure, renin and aldosterone in cirrhosis, *Kidney Int.,* 9, 511, 1976.
80. **Shepherd, A. N., Neligan, P., and Hayer, P. C.,** Captopril and resistant ascites, *Lancet,* i, 139, 1983.
81. **Morrison, A. R.,** Biochemistry and pharmacology of renal arachidonic acid metabolism, *Am. J. Med.,* 780 (Suppl. 1A), 3, 1986.
82. Editorial, Prostaglandins in the kidney, *Lancet,* 2, 343, 1981.
83. **Boyer, T. D., Zia, P., and Reynolds, T. B.,** Effects of indomethacin and prostaglandin A on renal function and plasma renin activity in alcoholic liver disease, *Gastroenterology,* 77, 215, 1979.
84. **Planas, R., Arroyo, V., and Timola et al.,** Acetacyclic acid suppresses the renal haemodynamic effect and reduces the diuretic action of furosemide in cirrhosis with ascites, *Gastroenterology,* 84, 247, 1983.
85. **Zipser, R. D., Radvan, G. M., and Kronborg, I. J. et al.,** Urinary thromboxane E_2 and prostaglandin E_2 in the hepatorenal syndrome: evidence for increased vasoconstrictor and decreased vasodilator factors, *Gastroenterology,* 84, 697, 1983.
86. **Lassen, N. A., Ring-Larsen, H., and Henriksen, J. H.,** Is the cirrhotic kidney a bilateral Goldblatt kidney as modified by salt depletion and increased sympathetic tone?, in *The Sympatoadrenal System,* Christensen, N. J., Henriksen, O., and Lassen, N. A., Eds., Munksgaard, Copenhagen, 1986, 490.
87. **Finke, R., Gross, R., and Hackenthal, E. et al.,** Threshold pressure for the pressure-dependent renin release in the autoregulating kidney of conscious dogs, *Pfluegers Arch.,* 399, 102, 1983.
88. **Lenz, K., Druml, W., and Kleinberg, G. et al.,** Enhancement of renal function with ornipressin in a patient with decompensated cirrhosis, *Gut,* 26, 1385, 1985.
89. **Nicholls, K. M., Shapiro, M. D., and Kluge, R. et al.,** Sodium excretion in advanced cirrhosis: effect of expansion of central blood volume and suppression of plasma aldosterone, *Hepatology,* 6, 235, 1986.
90. **Christensen, N. J., Henriksen, O., and Lassen, N. A.,** *The Sympathetho-Adrenal System,* Munksgaard, Copenhagen, 1986.
91. **Ball, W. C., Davis, J. D., and Goodkind, M. J.,** Ascites formation without sodium intake in dogs with thoracic inferior vena cava constriction and in dogs with right-sided congestive heart failure, *Am. J. Physiol.,* 188, 578, 1957.
92. **Watkins, L., Burton, J. A., and Habert, et al.,** The renin-angiotensin-aldosterone system in congestive failure in conscious dogs, *J. Clin. Invest.,* 57, 1606, 1976.
93. **Levy, M.,** Urinary sodium retention in chronic liver disease: a summary, *Isr. J. Med. Sci.,* 22, 67, 1986.

Chapter 5

THE HEART IN LIVER DISEASE

Samuel S. Lee and Arieh Bomzon

TABLE OF CONTENTS

I. INTRODUCTION

Clinical observations extending over the past century have linked alterations in heart function with the existence of liver disease. Within the last four decades, development of sophisticated techniques has allowed accurate description of the mechanical, electrophysiological and biochemical cardiac changes. In addition, animal experimental studies have led to some insights into pathogenic mechanisms of these changes. This chapter reviews these phenomena of altered cardiac function in the presence of acute and chronic liver disease.

II. THE HEART IN ACUTE LIVER DISEASE

A. ACUTE HEPATITIS

The heart is generally not directly affected in typical cases of acute viral hepatitis.[1] However, in severe or fulminant viral hepatitis, cardiovascular derangement has been well documented and takes three forms. The first is the appearance of an hyperkinetic circulation manifested by increased heart rate and cardiac output associated with decreased peripheral vascular resistance and arterial hypotension.[2,3] The pathogenesis of this syndrome is unclear and surprisingly little experimental study has been made of this phenomenon in acute hepatitis. For instance, in contrast to the situation in chronic liver disease, blood volume in acute hepatitis has not been examined. Given the critical multi-organ problems such as cerebral edema, acute renal failure, coagulopathy, acidosis, and electrolyte disorders that complicate fulminant hepatitis, perhaps it is understandable that the appearance of circulatory hyperkineticism is assumed to be a natural consequence of these phenomena.

The second and more clinically threatening cardiac complication is the onset of arrhythmias. Several reports have documented a variety of arrhythmias including ventricular ectopic beats, ventricular tachycardia, second- and third-degree AV blocks, sinus bradycardia, and cardiac asystole.[4-9] The high incidence of arrhythmias thus necessitates continuous electrocardiographic monitoring of every patient with fulminant hepatitis. All forms of fulminant hepatitis, whether caused by hepatitis viruses A, B, non-A, non-B, or drugs such as acetaminophen or halothane, appear to be associated with arrhythmias.[8-10] In addition, more classically cardiopathic viruses such as Coxsackie B can rarely cause concomitant icteric hepatitis,[11] but not fulminant hepatitis.

A third form of cardiac involvement is myocarditis. Pathologic findings in the heart include scattered petechial hemorrhages, inflammatory lymphocytic infiltrates, fatty degeneration, small pericardial effusions, dilated flabby ventricles, and edematous subendocardial connective tissue.[4-9] This myocarditis has generally been ascribed to either direct viral involvement or drug (acetaminophen) effect. Hepatotoxic doses of acetaminophen (paracetamol) in particular, seem to have a propensity for causing myocarditis, presumably due to direct cardiac toxicity.[9,10] The hemorrhages are probably precipitated or aggravated by the typically severe coagulation defect.

It would be logical to ascribe the arrhythmias to the myocarditis, but this is not supported by the retrospective studies that examined this issue: there seems to be no relation between the pathological changes of myocarditis and the existence of arrhythmias.[8,9] However, against the background of cerebral edema, acidosis, hypoxemia, and electrolyte imbalances, all known arrhythmogenic factors, the high incidence of arrhythmias is not surprising. Moreover, old and recent studies have suggested that bile salts, bilirubin, or some other component of icteric serum may exert toxic or irritant effects on cardiac tissue, and in particular may be important in inducing sinus bradycardia and conduction defects.[12-16]

The presence of myocarditis does not lead to acute ventricular failure. Although pulmonary vascular congestion and frank pulmonary edema are well-known complications of

TABLE 1

Summary of the Clinical Data on Jaundiced Patients Pertaining to the Plasma Total Bilirubin and Bile Acids together with the Heart Rate and Mean Arterial Blood Pressure

First author and year	Bilirubin (μmol/l)	Bile acids (μmol/l)	Heart rate (beats/min)	Mean arterial blood pressure (mmHg)	Ref.
Saito, 1981	280.5 ± 35.7	Not stated	71 ± 12	101 ± 2	22
	270.3 ± 49.3	Not stated	87 ± 14[b]	92 ± 3[a]	
Song, 1981	262.2 ± 7.1	251.1 ± 28.1	74.1 ± 1.7	Not stated	23
Lumlertgol, 1987	498.1 ± 56.1	Not stated	84.1 ± 5.8	98.1 ± 7.7	24

[a] $p < 0.02$.

[b] $p < 0.01$ and refers to the significance of the difference from the author's control group. Two values are presented for Saito, who described two groups of patients.

fulminant hepatic failure, hemodynamic studies from the King's College liver unit have demonstrated that pulmonary capillary wedge pressure is normal in these patients.[17] There was an association with concurrent cerebral edema in some of these patients, suggesting either a neurogenic etiology of pulmonary edema or a common pathogenesis, perhaps a multisystem "capillary leak" syndrome.

B. CHOLESTASIS

It is still widely accepted that cholestasis be included in the differential diagnosis for bradycardia.[18] This phenomenon consists of two aspects: an absolute bradycardia, i.e., a resting heart rate less than 50 beats/min and a "relative" bradycardia, i.e., an inadequate tachycardiac response following sympathetic stimulation. One of the earliest descriptions of absolute bradycardia in cholestasis was made by Meakin in 1932 where he noted that it was a common clinical feature in jaundiced patients.[19] In 1956, Zollinger and Williams proposed that patients with cholestasis have a "relative" bradycardia, i.e., an impaired tachycardiac response following sympathetic stimulation of the heart.[20]

The etiological factors responsible for these two phenomena are unknown. However, the plasma accumulation of bile acids has long been considered to be the causative humoral factors since their concentration can rise a thousand-fold from 1 to 2 $\mu M/l$ to 1 to 2 mM/l. Many of the experiments performed in the 19th century on the effect of bile and bile acids were reviewed by Meakin.[19] Since this report, only a few clinical studies on the effects of cholestasis and cholemia on cardiovascular function have been published. The paucity of reports probably prompted Heaton in 1972 to note that "the bradycardia of obstructive jaundice attributable to bile acids does not seem to have been investigated by modern methods".[21]

From these introductory comments, it is obvious that three questions need answering:

1. What is the basis of the absolute bradycardia?
2. What is the basis of the relative bradycardia?
3. Are bile acids the etiological factors responsible for the cardiac dysfunction?

1. Absolute Bradycardia in Cholestasis

Contrary to older studies, the modern literature does not provide evidence for the existence of an absolute bradycardia in cholestasis, irrespective of the degree of hyperbilirubinemia. Table 1 summarizes data obtained from jaundiced patients by three groups of investigators.[22-24] None of these investigators found the existence of an absolute bradycardia.

In fact, in some of the patients it would appear that the heart rate was elevated. Saito[22] found in jaundiced patients with a concomitant hyperkinetic circulation that the heart rate was significantly elevated above that observed in a group of age-matched controls.

Similarly, the existence of absolute bradycardia in jaundiced experimental animals remains to be established. Tables 2 and 3 summarize data obtained from jaundiced bile duct-ligated dogs and rats, respectively.[25-40] Four factors complicate the interpretation of this data: (1) the influence of anesthesia, especially sodium phenobarbitone; (2) the varying duration of bile duct ligation; (3) the depth of jaundice; and (4) the nondetermination of plasma bile acid concentration. In the dog studies (Table 2), phenobarbitone anesthesia almost doubled the heart rate in control and jaundiced animals. Moreover, the magnitude of hyperbilirubinemia in these animals is only about half of that observed in the human studies. This is related to the duration of the ligation and whether the bile duct was only ligated or ligated and sectioned.[41] The exception is the study of Green et al.[29] where the plasma total bilirubin was as high as 568 μmol/l in conscious dogs with choleductocaval anastomosis.

In jaundiced rats, the existence of bradycardia is also unsettled (Table 3). Two of four studies in conscious icteric rats demonstrated slower heart rates than control rats. Heart rates of anesthetized jaundiced rats in all five studies were not different from anesthetized control groups.

Last, it should be noted that the heart rate appears to be a labile variable since even values, which are considered significantly different from the control, often lie within the normal range. Two examples of this point can be found in the data presented in Tables 1 and 3. Saito[22] found that his jaundiced patients had tachycardia, but the absolute values are considered to lie within the normal clinical range (Table 1). Joubert[32] found that his jaundiced rats had bradycardia in the first 4 days postoperatively. Yet, the reported values for both tachycardia and bradycardia lie within the range that other investigators consider to be normal (Table 3).

2. Relative Bradycardia in Cholestasis

Cholestasis is invariably associated with a decrease in the total peripheral resistance which is a stimulus for reflex tachycardia. The absence of significant changes in heart rate in cholestatic patients and animals may, in fact, be a reflection of the inability of the heart to respond to sympathetic stimulation. In other words, a "relative" bradycardia exists in cholestasis. Lumlertgol et al.[24] evaluated the positive inotropic and chronotropic response of their patients to the selective β_1- adrenoceptor agonist dobutamine, using cardioscintigraphy. Although the changes in blood pressure and heart rate were comparable in the control and jaundiced patients, the rate of increase of the left ventricular ejection fraction to the agonist was diminished in the jaundiced patient.

Although their study still requires clinical confirmation, studies in conscious and anesthetized jaundiced animals indicate the existence of altered cardiac responsiveness to β-adrenergic stimulation (Tables 2 and 3). However, examination of the *in vivo* and *in vitro* data suggests that the failure to respond to β-adrenergic agonists is species-dependent. Bomzon et al.[30] showed an attenuated chronotropic response to the nonselective β-adrenoceptor agonist isoproterenol, in conscious bile duct-ligated dogs. This has also been shown *in vitro*[42] (Figure 1). On the other hand, if the same studies are done in conscious bile duct-ligated rats or isolated cardiac tissue from such animals, normal or intact responses are found[37] (Figure 2).

Ludatscher and her colleagues[41] showed that the myocardium of bile duct-ligated dogs is histologically normal. Since these same dogs have blunted responses to β-adrenoceptor agonists, this suggests that the hyporesponsiveness to β-stimulation may be due to altered receptor function. In contrast, in the jaundiced rat, whose heart responds normally to β-adrenergic agonists, it has been reported that there are pathological intracellular changes within the cardiac myocytes.[33]

TABLE 2

A Summary of the Data Pertaining to Heart Rates, Mean Arterial Blood Pressure (MABP), Plasma Total Bilirubin Concentrations and Responsiveness to Pressor Agents in Jaundiced Dogs. Plasma Bile Acids Were Not Determined in Any of These Studies

First author and year	Duration of ligation (weeks)	Heart rate (beats/min)	MABP (mmHg)	Bilirubin (μmol/l)	Comments	Ref.
Finberg, 1981	1 and 3	Not stated	104 ± 5.8[a] 97.6 ± 5.7[a]	207.4 ± 17	Conscious; intact tachycardic response to isoproterenol and bradycardic responses to pressor agents	25
Bosch, 1983	8	168 ± 4	110 ± 4[a]	105.4 ± 22.1	Phenobarbitone anesthetized	26
Willems, 1986	6—12	$163 \pm 9+$	$105 \pm 5+$	Not stated	Phenobarbitone anesthetized	27
Bomzon, 1986	1 and 3	Not stated	107.2 ± 3.0	144.5 ± 42.5	Conscious; blunted response to norepinephrine has a cardiac origin	28
Green, 1986	CDCA 2	Not stated	103 ± 11	567.8 ± 18.2	Impaired left ventricular function; intact response to ouabain	29
Bomzon, 1990	2—3	98 ± 11	105.6 ± 3.7	Not known	Conscious; blunted chronotropic response to isoproterenol	30
	2—3	150 ± 28	101.6 ± 3.7	Not known	Phenobarbitone anesthetized; blunted chronotropic response to isoproterenol	
Bomzon, 1988	12—14	94 ± 10	117.5 ± 3.7	Not known	Conscious; intact chronotropic response to isoproterenol	31

[a] $p < 0.05$ and refers to significance from the control group of the investigators; $+$ values estimated from figures within the text since absolute values were not stated; CDCA = choleductocaval dogs.

TABLE 3

A Summary of the Data Pertaining to Heart Rates, Mean Arterial Blood Pressure (MABP), Plasma Total Bilirubin Concentrations and Responsiveness to Isoproterenol in Jaundiced Rats

First author and year	Duration of ligation (d)	Heart rate (beats/min)	MABP (mmHg)	Bilirubin (μmol/l)	Comments	Ref.
Joubert, 1978	5—8	348 ± 6[a]	Not stated	Not stated	Conscious; bradycardia preceded by 4 days tachy-cardia (1—4 days) postoperatively	32
Tajuddin, 1980	5 and 10	Not stated	Not stated	97 ± 9	Bradycardia reported	33
Finberg, 1982	7	Not stated	99.1 ± 4.8	63.6 ± 11.2	Urethane anesthetized	34
Lee, 1986	28	339 ± 17[a]	100 ± 3[a]	Not stated	Conscious	35
	28	396 ± 17	99 ± 6	Not stated	Pentobarbital anesthetized	
Heidenreich, 1987	6	Not stated	110.3 ± 1.8	169.1 ± 17.9	Conscious	36
Bomzon, 1988	3	388 ± 31	106 ± 6	161.5 ± 50	Conscious; intact chronotropic response to isopro-terenol; serum bile acids 3.79 ± 0.81 μmol/l	37
Jacob. 1988	3	301 ± 26	139.8 ± 11.9	Not known	Ketamine anesthetized	38
	35	366 ± 16	122 ± 14	Not known	Ketamine anesthetized	
Sikuler, 1988	21	379 ± 17	107 ± 6[a]	Not stated	Ketamine and ether anesthetized	39
Lee, 1990	28	354 ± 17	100 ± 7[a]	Not stated	Conscious; blunted positive chronotropic response to isoproterenol	40

[a] $p < 0.05$ and refers to significance from the control group of the investigator.

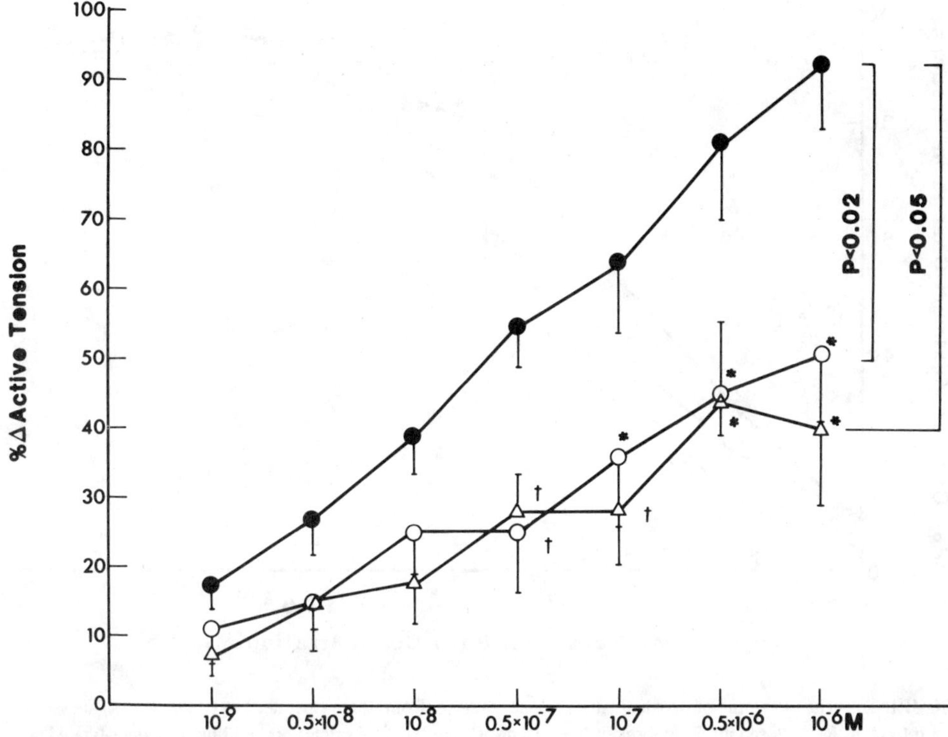

FIGURE 1.   The effect of different doses of isoproterenol on the change in active tension of isolated ventricular muscle strips from normal and jaundiced dogs. Key: closed circle, sham-operated (N = 9); open circle, chronic bile duct-ligated (N = 5); open triangle, choleductocaval-anastomosed dogs (N = 5). P value for the ANOVA test is shown on right hand side of figure. (Reprinted by permission from *Clin. Sci.*, Vol. 69, pp. 647—653, copyright © 1985, The Biochemical Society, London.)

On the basis of this evidence, it would appear that the bile duct-ligated dog is the most appropriate model in which to study cardiac function in cholestasis. However, it should be noted that as the duration of the cholestasis lengthens, the situation appears to reverse itself inasmuch as normal responses to isoproterenol become apparent in the dog[31], whereas blunted responses to the same agonist occur in the rat.[40] In these circumstances, the animal is a model of cirrhosis with portal hypertension and not cholestasis per se.[42]

3. Bile Acids and the Pathogenesis of Cardiac Dysfunction

Experiments to identify the etiological humoral factors responsible for cardiac dysfunction in cholestasis began over 100 years ago. Early investigators showed that the injection of bile and bile acids caused bradycardia with a concomitant fall in blood pressure. By the 1930s, it had become widely accepted that bile acids accounted for the bradycardia of obstructive jaundice.[19]

For obvious ethical reasons, there are almost no clinical studies on the effects of bile acids on cardiac function. However, in 1928, Dumitresco-Mante reported that the injection of bile acids into human volunteers induced a bradycardia.[43] More recently, the National Cooperative Gallstone Study Group in the U.S. published their findings on the use of chenodeoxycholic acid for gallstone dissolution.[44] In this study involving 916 patients who took the bile acid for as long as 2 years, they observed bradycardia after 24 months of treatment. The investigators considered these changes to be of "no clinical significance" and commented that the findings were "compatible with the traditional concept that bile acids cause bradycardia associated with jaundice".

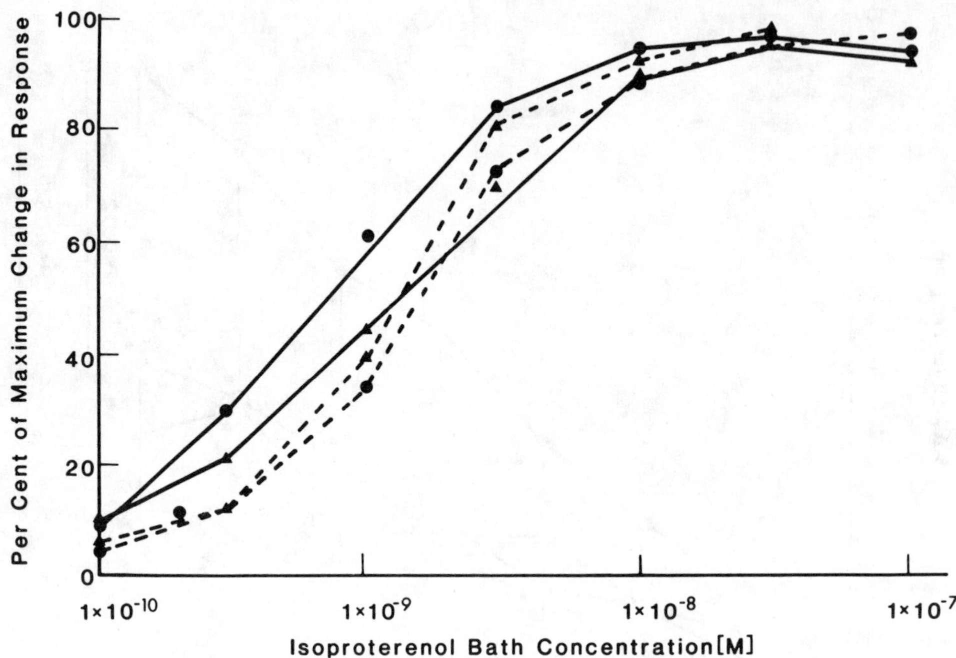

FIGURE 2.   The response of isolated atrial tissue excised from sham-operated and bile duct-ligated rats to isoproterenol. Key: closed circle, unbroken line, sham-operated; closed circle, broken line, bile duct-ligated spontaneous right atrium (chronotropic) responses; closed triangle, unbroken line, sham-operated; closed triangle, broken line, bile duct-ligated electrically driven left atrium (inotropic) responses. The EC_{50} for the sham-operated (N = 8) and bile duct-ligated (N = 9) dose response curves were 0.7 nmol and 1.25 nmol, respectively.[174]

The results of all the experiments performed in laboratory animals indicate that bile acids have a negative inotropic or chronotropic effect on the heart at concentrations that are within the pathophysiological range.[42,45] Using anesthetized rats, Joubert[32] demonstrated that the intravenous administration of cholic acid elicited a dose-dependent negative chronotropic effect. Bogin et al.[46] and Enriquez de Salamanca et al.[47] showed a negative chronotropic effect of bile acids on isolated rat cardiac myocytes and in the isolated perfused heart, respectively. This latter effect of the bile acids can be observed at concentrations as low as 100 nM/l.[16]

The mechanism whereby bile acids exert their effects on the heart is unresolved but three hypotheses have been proposed: (1) mechanical interference by forming a monolayer on the cell membrane surface,[32] (2) interfering with the ability of the membrane to conduct action potentials by reducing the slow inward current of calcium,[16] (3) acting as a muscarinic antagonist since their effects can be reversed by atropine or potentiated by physostigmine.[32,47,48]

Despite the evidence favoring the hypothesis that bile salts could be the humoral causative factors, it is still premature to accept this theory in its entirety. As noted previously, the majority of investigators did not measure plasma bile acid concentrations (Tables 1 through 3). Second, it should be noted that Song and colleagues[23] were unable to show a correlation between bile acid concentrations and sinus bradycardia because the latter was not observed. Third, most of the animal studies were undertaken in normal rats and this data may not correlate with the findings observed in jaundiced rats.

Nevertheless, in summarizing the cardiovascular effects of bile acids, the evidence suggests that bile acids probably are the etiological factors responsible for cardiac dysfunction in cholestasis. However, the exact mechanism of action of bile acids on cardiac function needs to be elucidated.

III. THE HEART IN CHRONIC LIVER DISEASE

A. HYPERKINETIC CIRCULATION

The circulation becomes hyperkinetic in patients with cirrhosis. As mentioned previously, this consists of increased cardiac output associated with decreased peripheral vascular resistance and a tendency toward arterial hypotension. In addition, circulation times are shortened.[49,50] In 1953, using a dye-dilution technique, Kowalski and Abelmann showed that the cardiac output was increased in patients with cirrhosis as compared with controls.[49] Subsequently numerous studies, using various methods, confirmed these findings.[50-59] The augmented output is due to increases in both stroke volume and heart rate in most patients and solely to increased heart rate in a minority.[49-59] However, the increased cardiac output is not a uniform feature of cirrhosis; in different series about 30 to 70% of patients have elevated values while the rest are within normal ranges.[49-59] Nevertheless the mean of any group of cirrhotic patients is almost invariably higher than an age-matched control group. The lack of uniformity in elevations of cardiac output may be due to differing study populations. It is now clear that the degree of circulatory hyperkinesis correlates with advancing stages of liver insufficiency, i.e., early stages of chronic liver disease are associated with normal or modest elevations of cardiac output, while late stages have marked hyperkinesis.[60-63] It is likely that the circulatory abnormalities in chronic liver disease lie on a spectrum from normalcy to severe hyperkinesis. Careful longitudinal studies documenting the hemodynamic changes in patients with precirrhosis, as their liver disease progresses, are needed.

The pathogenesis of the increased cardiac output has been the subject of much speculation and study. In this regard, animal experimentation has been helpful, since to date, every animal model of cirrhosis develops a hyperkinetic circulation.[35,64-66] Moreover, even animals with prehepatic portal hypertension and normal liver develop a hyperkinetic circulation. Partial ligation of the infrahepatic portal vein in the rat[66,67] and rabbit[68] with consequent portal vein stenosis results in portal hypertension, extensive portosystemic collateral formation, and hyperkinetic circulation with increased cardiac output. The livers of these animals remain functionally and histologically normal. This situation mirrors human prehepatic portal vein thrombosis wherein hyperkinetic circulation has been demonstrated in the presence of normal livers.[69]

It therefore follows that the prerequisite for the development of circulatory hyperkineticism is not liver disease but rather portal hypertension, or at least some phenomenon associated with portal hypertension. Indeed, Braillon and colleagues recently suggested that the development of portosystemic collaterals and not portal hypertnesion per se leads to the increase in cardiac output.[70] They based this conclusion on a significant correlation between cardiac output and portal tributary blood flow in both portal-stenosed rats and rats with surgical portocaval shunts. Control rats lacked this correlation. The portocaval shunted-rats, with 100% portosystemic shunt and normal portal pressure, had the highest cardiac outputs. The portal-stenosed rats, with 60 to 90% shunts and portal hypertension had lesser elevations of cardiac output, although still greater than controls. While these data are compatible with the authors' hypothesis, they are not conclusive and a more prudent interpretation would be that in these models, changes in cardiac output are linked to a splanchnic circulatory factor.

According to one line of reasoning, this splanchnic circulatory factor could be splanchnic venous pooling. Portal hypertension and a large portosystemic collateral bed would induce changes in the splanchnic venous capacitance such that blood could pool in this reservoir. This would decrease the so-called "effective circulating volume" and set off a compensatory cascade of renal sodium retention, expansion of the plasma volume, and sympathetic nervous activation. The hyperkinetic circulation would then result from the augmented plasma volume and sympathetic overactivity. The difficulty in trying to verify this hypothesis is that, at present, no methods yet exist to quantify either splanchnic venous capacitance or "effective circulating volume".

A portocaval shunt may be thought of as a surgical exaggeration of naturally occurring portosystemic collaterals. A number of investigations have examined the hemodynamic consequences of performing a portocaval shunt. The shunt would have two major effects: (1) allow vasoactive substances in the portal circulation to bypass the liver and directly access the heart, and (2) allow the mesenteric blood to short circuit the liver resistor and increase cardiac preload. This would occur since some splanchnic venous blood, at normal portal venous pressures would remain pooled in the splanchnic compartment, instead is displaced to the central compartment. Both the preceding effects could be total or partial depending on the type of shunt; the end-to-side shunt produces 100% shunting while the side-to-side shunt probably induces very high-grade shunting, at least initially. Long-term (months to years) outcomes of side-to-side shunts have been shown to be reversal of flow direction, with hepatofugal portal flow, in two thirds of cirrhotic patients.[71]

In patients with cirrhosis, the creation of a portocaval shunt further elevates the already increased cardiac output.[72-74] This elevation persists even several years after surgery if the shunt remains patent.[75] Most animal shunt experiments have been done in normal animals and in these cases, the procedure augments cardiac output in dogs[76,77] and rats.[70,78] Most attention has been focused on the first aforementioned mechanism as the cause of the hyperkinetic circulation after shunt surgery. Credit for this hypothesis of the humoral vasoactive substances, in the pathogenesis of cirrhotic circulatory disturbances, is usually attributed to Shorr and colleagues, based on studies done four decades ago.[79] However, it should be noted that their hypothesized "vasodepressor" and "vasoexcitatory" material resulted from experiments in an anesthetized dog model of hemorrhagic shock. This condition is not relevant to the hyperkinetic state seen in cirrhosis.

In more recent times, glucagon has been suggested as the mediator of the hyperkinetic circulation since it is known to be a vasodilator and positive ionotrope, is produced by the gut, and is inactivated by the liver.[80] However serum glucagon levels do not correlate with the increased cardiac output in portal-stenotic rats with high-grade portosystemic collateral formation,[81] nor in rats with surgical portocaval shunts.[78] Physiologic doses of glucagon do not affect cardiac output in normal dogs[82] or rats.[83] Finally, in humans with cirrhosis and naturally occurring portosystemic collaterals, modestly supraphysiological doses of glucagon do not affect cardiac output or peripheral vascular resistance.[84] It thus appears that glucagon is not involved.

Martini and colleagues[85] investigated the hypothesis that histamine could be the vasodilator material. Infusion of this substance into cirrhotic patients induced circulatory hyperkinesis and decreased the peripheral arteriovenous oxygen gradient. However, the histamine doses used were pharmacologic, thus complicating interpretation of these results.

Although the second hemodynamic effect of portocaval shunt, that of bypassing the liver resistor and increasing preload, has not been extensively investigated, Mooney and colleagues conducted a dog study pertinent to this issue.[86] They found that constructing an arteriovenous shunt in the mesenteric vascular bed, and thus interposing the liver in the venous side of the circuit, prevented the expected increase in cardiac output. This contrasts with construction of nonsplanchnic arteriovenous shunts, which cause increased cardiac output and decreased peripheral vascular resistance.[86,87]

Hemodynamic effects of portocaval shunts have also been studied in cirrhotic animals.[88-91] Levy and colleagues have conducted some interesting studies with end-to-side and side-to-side protocaval shunts in dogs made cirrhotic by bile duct ligation. Surprisingly, the dogs with end-to-side shunts developed the typical hyperkinetic circulation with sodium retention and increases in plasma volume and cardiac output,[88] while the side-to-side shunted dogs did not retain sodium, remained euvolemic and did not develop circulatory hyperkineticism.[89] These authors suggested that their findings support the hypothesis that the hyperkinetic circulation is caused by expansion of the plasma volume. An intriguing question left unanswered by the study is why the side-to-side group did not retain sodium and reamined euvolemic. It should be noted that species differences may be important here, as cirrhotic humans with both end-to-side and side-to-side portocaval shunts have expanded plasma volume.[92]

The phenomenon of blood volume augmentation in cirrhosis was first documented by Perera in 1946.[93] Numerous subsequent studies confirmed the finding.[52,53,92,94,95] The total red cell mass remains normal or is somewhat low, and plasma volume is increased so hemodilutional anemia results. The combination of hemodilution and volume expansion was hypothesized to augment cardiac output, but experimental evidence does not support this idea, because most studies find no correlation between degree of hemodilution or plasma volume and cardiac output.[53,57,59,95]

Given the clinical evidence of peripheral arteriovenous anomalies such as vascular, spider nevi, telangiectasia, and finger clubbing, some investigators have proposed the presence of arteriovenous shunts as an explanation for the increased cardiac output. Pathologic and hemodynamic studies confirm the presence of small arteriovenous connections in the skin and subcutaneous tissue.[96-99] Whether these small arteriovenous shunts are significant enough to raise the cardiac output or even cutaneous blood flow, is not clear. Early plethysmographic studies found forearm blood flow to be increased in patients with cirrhosis,[58,96,100] but more recent studies using plethysmography and xenon clearance have failed to demonstrate baseline differences between cirrhotics and controls.[101-103]

Hypoxia can occur in patients with cirrhosis and also has been hypothesized to be a contributory factor in the development of circulatory hyperkinesis.[53,57,104,105] (See also Chapter 11.) According to this line of reasoning, with the progression of liver disease, a state of relative tissue hypoxia starts manifesting itself. This is suggested by the following evidence: (1) Arterial oxygen tension is frankly low in many cirrhotic patients.[53,57,63,104-106] (2) Altered hepatic and total-body redox states can be demonstrated.[63,105,107,108] (3) In severe liver disease, serum lactate levels are elevated.[63,105,108] (4) A subtle sign of tissue hypoxia in patients with the adult respiratory distress syndrome (ARDS) is oxygen supply-demand dependency.[109] That is, oxygen uptake is directly linked to oxygen transport at all levels of oxygen transport. In other words, the body utilizes all available oxygen transported to the tissues. This same supply-demand dependency has been demonstrated for patients with liver failure from fulminant hepatitis[110] and cirrhosis.[110] The link between increasing circulatory hyperkinesis and degree of liver failure may lie in the observation that the latter also tends to be correlated to the degree of tissue hypoxia.[60-63] The underlying cause of this latent tissue hypoxia may be either impaired oxidative metabolism at the mitochondrial level,[112] or microcirculatory shunting caused by imbalances in vasoconstrictive and vasodilator actions, such as the α- and β-adrenoceptor effects of catecholamines.[113] The increase in cardiac output (and thus oxygen delivery) would be a homeostatic response to the latent tissue hypoxia.

B. CARDIOMYOPATHY

Despite the fact that cardiac output is generally increased in patients with cirrhosis, an uncertain but probably significant percentage of cirrhotic patients appear to have overt or latent signs of cardiomyopathy. In a few patients, this takes the form of a typical high-output heart failure of which beriberi cardiomyopathy is the classical example. In view of the tendency of cirrhotic patients, particularly alcoholics, to be malnourished, a small percentage undoubtedly suffer from thiamine deficiency as a primary or aggravating cause of heart failure. However, the great majority of cirrhotic patients with cardiac failure do not respond to thiamine supplementation.[114,115]

Studies of cardiac function in chronic liver disease are enormously complicated by the heterogeneous patient population. In western countries, alcohol is the commonest cause of cirrhosis and, of course, a well-shown cardiotoxin. Nonalcoholic causes such as postnecrotic viral hepatitis and autoimmune chronic hepatitis account for a significant percentage of cirrhosis in the West and the majority of cirrhosis in the rest of the world. Thus separating the possible cardiac dysfunction associated with chronic liver disease and that due to the effects of alcohol is not a simple task. In interpreting the following investigations, one should carefully note the type of patient population being studied. A large number of studies have delineated the pattern of myocardial dysfunction in alcoholics.[116-125] It appears that alcoholic cardiomyopathy represents a spectrum of disease starting with a pattern of high resting output and subtle evidence of decompensation with stress, to asymptomatic but with resting subtle evidence of insufficiency, to the end-stage symptomatic low-output failure.

In patients in the middle portion of the spectrum, the role of peripheral vasodilatation and decreased systemic vascular resistance should be considered. This afterload reduction may mask latent ventricular failure, which only becomes manifest under conditions that physiologically or pharmacologically stress myocardial function. Several experimental studies support this concept. Gould and colleagues performed cardiac catheterizations in patients with chronic alcoholic liver disease and found resting cardiac outputs to be increased with normal left ventricular filling pressures.[116] However on exercise, all patients increased left ventricular end-diastolic and pulmonary artery pressures while stroke index fell or remained the same; this pattern represents a clearly abnormal ventricular response. Limas and colleagues studied patients with alcoholic cirrhosis and no clinical evidence of heart disease.[121] They found, as expected, in the resting state, high cardiac output, low peripheral vascular resistance (mean 825 dyn/s·cm^{-5}) and normal pulmonary capillary wedge pressure (10 mmHg). Infusion of angiotensin in doses sufficient to increase diastolic pressure 20 mmHg and "normalize" the peripheral vascular resistance to 1140 dyn/s · cm^{-5}, caused the pulmonary wedge pressure to rise strikingly to 19 mmHg while cardiac output remained unchanged. This suggested that the low peripheral resistance exerted a beneficial protective on LV function and normalization of this afterload unmasked acute left ventricular decompensation. Kelbaek et al. studied asymptomatic patients with alcoholic cirrhosis.[124] In the resting state, echocardiographic systolic time intervals and radionuclide ventricular ejection fractions were not different from age-matched controls. On submaximal exercise, LV ejection fraction increased only 6% in cirrhotics versus 14% in controls, a significant difference. In a group of mixed alcoholic and nonalcoholic cirrhotic patients, even eating a liquid meal induced small but significant decreases in cardiac output and increased systemic vascular resistance.[126] Finally, despite the resting tachycardia, cirrhotic patients exhibited blunted chronotropic responses to the β-adrenoceptor agonist, isoproterenol.[127]

In view of the ubiquity of alcohol and the prevalence of chronic alcohol abuse, one might expect that cirrhosis and overt alcoholic cardiomyopathy would frequently coexist in the same patient. However, studies support the clinical impression that the combination of the two conditions is relatively rare.[59,115] This may reflect, in part, the veracity of the cardiologists' contention that hepatologists cannot hear murmurs or gallop rhythms and the hepatologists' suspicion that cardiologists abort their interest and examination at the level of the diaphragms. Another factor accounting for the rarity of concurrence of these two disorders may be Berkson's bias. Berkson's statistical analyses suggested that any two lethal diseases will demonstrate a negative association at autopsy.[128,129] Subsequent testing of his hypothesis has confirmed this negative association for diseases such as cirrhosis and hepatic metastases and brain tumor and myocardial infarction.[129-131]

Finally, as mentioned previously, the peripheral vasodilatation and low afterload of advanced liver disease seem to not only mask subclinical heart failure but may even exert a protective effect on the development of overt ventricular failure. This is logical, since afterload reduction is now the mainstay of drug treatment in chronic congestive cardiomyopathy not associated with liver disease.[115]

Most patients with nonalcoholic cirrhosis have normal resting ventricular function as assessed by different invasive or noninvasive techniques. Echocardiographic systolic time intervals and radionuclide ejection fractions in these patients are generally normal.[132,133] Occasional patients in these studies had accentuated indices of systolic function, consistent with a marked hyperkinetic circulation. Although low-output congestive cardiomyopathy, like that seen in alcoholics, has not been described in patients with nonalcoholic cirrhosis, there is a suspicion that the hyperkinetic hearts of the latter group might react abnormally, if sufficiently stressed. However, no human studies have systematically examined this notion.

In this regard, animal experiments are interesting. Volume infusion in rats with carbon tetrachloride-induced cirrhosis resulted in acute ventricular failure with a 50% decrease in cardiac output.[134] Rats with portal vein stenosis[135] as well as biliary cirrhosis[40, 136] also display impaired chronotropic responses to isoproterenol. These experiments support the concept that chronic liver disease per se, and not just alcohol, is associated with ventricular dysfunction, since laboratory animals would have difficulty acquiring alcohol.

Pathological heart changes in patients with cirrhosis have been described in several autopsy series.[137-140] Lunseth et al. documented a subgroup of 12 of 108 autopsied patients in whom idiopathic ventricular hypertrophy and dilatation were found in the absence of hypertension, ischemia, or valvular disease.[137] Myocardial fibrosis, usually of delicate and diffuse pattern, mild subendocardial edema, and nuclear and cytoplasmic vacuolation are seen.[137,139,140] Cardiac hypertrophy was also noted in other series and ascribed to the hyperkinetic circulation.[138-140] As will be discussed later, significant coronary arteriosclerosis and evidence of ischemic heart disease appeared to be rare (see Section C).

The biochemical pathogenesis of cirrhotic cardiomyopathy remains obscure. Severe ventricular failure seems to be limited to those with alcoholic liver disease and alcohol may have a number of toxic effects at the mitochondrial and membrane biochemical level.[141-143] In addition, patients with cirrhosis of any etiology have high serum catecholamine levels[144] and these substances have been shown to cause cardiomyopathy.[115,145]

Cardiac myocyte membrane changes in chronic liver disease have not been studied in humans. β-Adrenoceptors on human lymphocytes generally mirror the status of cardiac β-receptors, and Gerbes et al. have shown that decompensated cirrhosis is associated with decreased β-adrenoceptor density, as compared to controls.[146] In rats with biliary cirrhosis, ventricular β_1- adrenoceptor density was significantly decreased compared to controls.[40] These receptor studies may explain the cardiac adrenergic hyporesponsiveness of the cirrhotic patient. Further work at the receptor level should prove rewarding in helping delineate the cardiovascular phenomena.

Finally, based on the foregoing discussion, what treatment recommendations can be made for patients with cardiac decompensation? In alcoholics, abstinence may be expected to improve or at least slow the rate of deterioration of hepatic as well as cardiac function.[114,115,147,148] Prolonged bed rest was helpful in one study of alcoholic cardiomyopathy, although this may have been due to the effects of abstinence.[149] As far as active treatment in all types of cirrhotic patients is concerned, those with normal cardiac function at rest should not need drug therapy. Those with more overt cardiomyopathy should have careful drug therapy to decrease cardiac loading conditions.[115] One study showed that cardiac glycosides were completely ineffective in improving ventricular contractility, so these drugs cannot be recommended.[121]

C. ASCITES

The pathogenesis of ascites is not discussed here, but rather its effects on cardiac function. Severe ascites is thought to impede preload chiefly by hydrostatic pressure on the diaphragm, causing increased intrathoracic and intrapleural pressure with consequent reduction of cardiac transmural filling pressure.[114,150,151] An early study by Kowalski and colleagues failed to demonstrate significant cardiac dynamic changes with paracentesis.[152] Knauer and Lowe reported a biphasic response, with increases in cardiac output after removal of small amounts of ascitic fluid (100 to 250 ml) and progressive decreases with paracentesis volumes greater than one litre.[150] They ascribed the decreases to fluid shift from intravascular to extravascular compartments. On the other hand, Guazzi and colleagues found that removal of ascitic volumes up to 7 liters resulted in progressive increases in stroke volume and cardiac output, although the hemodynamic changes tended to plateau at 3 to 4 liters of removed fluid.[151] The authors did not state how they selected their study patients. This is unfortunate since they seem to have chosen a group of patients with moderately or severely advanced cirrhosis but atypical hemodynamic characteristics: baseline mean arterial pressure, cardiac output, and total peripheral resistance were all normal.

Another way to mobilize large volumes of ascitic fluid in a more physiologic fashion directly into the intravascular compartment, is by inserting a peritoneovenous shunt. Blendis and colleagues have examined the short-and long-term hemodynamic effects of these shunts.[153-154] In their patients with cirrhosis mostly of alcoholic origin, the short-term cardiac response was normal, with significant increases in cardiac output and stroke volume with no change in pulmonary capillary wedge pressure. By the 10th postoperative day, cardiac output had returned to preoperative levels. When remeasured several months later, cardiac output had not significantly changed. These results suggest that the cardiac response to these shunts is generally normal.

D. ISCHEMIC HEART DISEASE

Several autopsy reviews starting in the 1950s confirmed the widely held clinical impression that coronary atherosclerosis was infrequent in patients with cirrhosis, particularly alcoholic cirrhosis.[155-158] The first review to address this issue, conducted in 782 autopsied cases of cirrhosis by Hall et al., found an apparently decreased prevalence of coronary atherosclerosis. However, this study was flawed by lack of a proper control group, since they used controls from other centers' studies.[155] Subsequent studies using control noncirrhotic autopsied cases from their own center's material, confirmed the significantly lower prevalence of both fatal myocardial infarctions[157] and significant coronary artery disease.[156,158] The differences between cirrhotic and noncirrhotic subjects are striking. For example, in the myocardial infarction study, only 3.3% of cirrhotic patients died of myocardial infarcts, while the corresponding mortality in noncirrhotic patients was 11.4%.[157] To a certain extent, these results are likely a reflection of the aforementioned Berkson's bias. However, (1) the differences are highly significant, (2) other epidemiological data support the negative association, (3) coronary angiography in chronic alcoholics is almost always normal,[128] and (4) the clinical impression of the negative association of two disorders is so universal. Thus, the paucity of coronary ischemic events in patients with cirrhosis appears to be a real phenomenon.

The other epidemiologic data referred to are several large cohort analyses of drinking patterns and cardiovascular mortality and morbidity.[161-163] These suggest that moderate alcohol intake (2 to 3 drinks daily) is associated with a significantly decreased risk of cardiac ischemic events. The reasons for this are not obvious, but may be related to alcohol effects on serum lipid levels or enhanced fibrinolytic activity.

The effects of acute and chronic alcohol ingestion on serum lipids and ultimately, atherogenesis, are complex and far from fully elucidated. Moderate ethanol ingestion appears to increase serum levels of HDL-cholesterol, a type of cholesterol which may help transport other lipids out of vessels and thus hinder atherogenesis.[163] In addition, since the liver is the central regulator of lipid synthesis and metabolism, chronic liver disease per se will also critically affect the lipid profile, and thus atherogenesis. An example of this phenomenon is found in patients with primary biliary cirrhosis; in the early stages of disease, VLDL levels are normal and HDL levels are high while in the advanced stages, VLDL levels increase and HDL becomes low. The elevated HDL levels until very late in the disease course have been offered as the explanation for the rarity of vascular arteriosclerotic events in patients with primary biliary cirrhosis.[164]

Although it is now clear that alcohol abuse tends to elevate arterial blood pressure and interfere with treatment of established hypertension,[165] paradoxically, with the onset of alcoholic cirrhosis, arterial pressure normalizes and may even decline to hypotensive levels.[155,166-168] This hypotensive pattern of advanced cirrhosis is seen with both alcoholic and nonalcoholic causes. The hypotension thus removes an important risk factor for coronary atherosclerosis.

Some of these unclear issues could be clarified by a long-term prospective study of a large cohort of patients with alcoholic and nonalcoholic liver disease in mild stages, with careful monitoring of blood pressure, lipid patterns, smoking and other risk factors.

E. PERICARDIAL DISEASE

Although constrictive pericarditis is well known as a cause of cardiac cirrhosis, the converse, cirrhosis causing pericardial disease is almost unreported in the literature. Aside from isolated case reports of spontaneous hemopericardium with fatal tamponade[169] and small silent pericardial effusions in cirrhosis,[170] the only formal study was recently conducted by Shah and Variyam.[171] Of 27 alcoholic cirrhotic patients, 63% had clinically silent pericardial effusions detected by echocardiography. These were all in conjunction with gross ascites. Abnormal systolic motions of the mitral valve or interventricular septum were seen in eight patients, but these disappeared with resolution of the ascites. Since pericardial effusions are commonly seen in other edematous states such as nephrotic syndrome, it appears that cirrhosis with ascites can also be added to this list. These effusions do not seem to be clinically significant.

F. BACTERIAL ENDOCARDITIS

Since the liver plays a critical role as the bacterial "filter" of the portal circulation, severe liver disease might be expected to lead to greater frequency of bacteremia and complications thereof. Indeed, the polyclonal gammopathy typical of chronic liver disease is usually ascribed to immune system processing of bacterial antigen that has "spilled over" into the peripheral circulation by either portosystemic collaterals or inadequate removal by the diseased liver or both.[172] Again, aside from an isolated case report,[173] there is only one formal study of this problem. Snyder and colleagues found an autopsy frequency of endocarditis to be 1.8% in cirrhotics versus 0.9% in controls.[131] Although the formal p value for this difference is 0.06, in view of Berkson's bias, this probably represents a significant difference. In reviewing 41,151 hospital admissions, the incidence of endocarditis was 0.34% in cirrhotics versus 0.1% in noncirrhotics ($p < 0.001$). These data suggest that the cirrhotic patient is at increased risk for infective endocarditis, particularly with enteric organisms.

IV. SUMMARY

Cardiac abnormalities are found in fulminant hepatitis, subacute biliary obstruction, and established cirrhosis. In fulminant hepatitis, the circulation is hyperkinetic, arrhythmias are frequent, and pathologic myocarditis is generally subclinical. Despite the not uncommon occurrence of pulmonary edema, this is of noncardiogenic origin, and ventricular failure is rare.

Acute and subacute cholestasis is associated with normal or hyperkinetic circulation but impaired cardiovascular homeostatic responses. Although the notion is entrenched in the literature, it is still not clear whether deep jaundice can cause bradycardia. However, both peripheral vascular responses and myocardial function have been shown to be depressed in animal models and a few clinical observations. The toxic factors and mechanism responsible have not yet been elucidated but much attention has been focused on the cardiodepressant effects of bile salts.

Cirrhosis is associated with circulatory hyperkinesis. As well, there is evidence of latent or overt cardiomyopathy in some patients. The etiology of the hyperkinesis is still unclear, although numerous theories have been proposed. Hepatocellular insufficiency is not essential for its development, but advancing liver dysfunction is associated with increasing circulatory hyperkinesis.

The majority of cirrhotic patients appear to have normal ventricular function but a significant minority, especially among alcoholics, appear to have latent subclinical cardiomyopathy that only becomes manifest under stress. End-stage low-output congestive cardiomyopathy has to date only been described in those with alcoholic-origin cirrhosis. Ascites is associated with some embarrassment of cardiac function, even though the majority of patients still maintain a hyperkinetic circulation. Partial relief of ascites by paracentesis or peritoneovenous shunting results in at least temporary increase in cardiac output. Small clinically silent pericardial effusions are seen in ascitic patients, but formal study of pericardial function in cirrhotics has not yet been done. Cirrhotic patients appear to be at increased risk for bacterial endocarditis and decreased risk for coronary arteriosclerosis.

ACKNOWLEDGMENTS

We thank Dr. John V. Tyberg for thoughtfully reviewing the manuscript and Diane Buzan for typing the manuscript.

REFERENCES

1. **Koff, R. S., and Galambos, J.,** Viral hepatitis, in *Diseases of the Liver,* 5th ed., Schiff, L. and Schiff, E. R., Eds., J. B. Lippincott, Philadelphia, 1982, 461.
2. **Ritt, D., Whelan, G., Werner, D., Eigenbrodt, E., Schenker, S., and Combes, B.,** Acute hepatic necrosis with stupor and coma. An analysis of 31 patients, *Medicine (Baltimore)* 48, 151, 1979.
3. **Rueff, B. and Benhamou, J.-P.,** Acute hepatic necrosis and fulminant hepatic failure, *Gut,* 14, 805, 1973.
4. **Hoagland, C. L. and Shank, R. E.,** Infectious hepatitis: a review of 200 cases, *J. Am. Med. Assoc.,* 130, 615, 1946.
5. **Dehn, H., Feil, H., and Rinderknecht, R.,** Electrocardiographic changes in cases of infectious hepatitis, *Am. Heart J.,* 31, 183, 1946.
6. **Adler, E. and Lyon, E.,** Cardiac disorders associated with infectious hepatitis, *Cardiologia,* 11, 111, 1947.
7. **Saphir, O., Amromin, G. D., and Yokoo, H.,** Myocarditis in viral (epidemic) hepatitis, *Am. J. Med. Sci.,* 231, 168, 1956.
8. **Bell, H.,** Cardiac manifestations of viral hepatitis, *J. Am. Med. Assoc.,* 218, 387, 1971.
9. **Weston, M. J., Talbot, I. C., Howorth, P. J. N., Mant, A. K., Capildeo, R., and Williams, R.,** Frequency of arrhythmias and other cardiac abnormalities in fulminant hepatic failure. *Br. Heart J.,* 38, 1179, 1976.
10. **Pimstone, B. L. and Uys, C. J.,** Liver necrosis and myocardiopathy following paracetamol overdosage, *S. Afr. Med. J.,* 42, 259, 1968.
11. **Sun, N. C. and Smith, V. M.,** Hepatitis associated with myocarditis, *New Engl. J. Med.,* 274, 190, 1966.
12. **Meltzer, S. J. and Salant, W.,** Studies on the toxicity of bile: the effects of intravenous injections of bile upon the blood pressure, *J. Exp. Med.,* 7, 280, 1905.
13. **Emerson, W. C.,** The toxic constituent of the bile, *J. Lab. Clin. Med.,* 14, 635, 1929.
14. **Zetterstrom, R. and Ernster, L.,** Bilirubin, an uncoupler of oxidative phosphorylation in isolated mitochondria, *Nature,* 178, 1335, 1956.
15. **Bomzon, A., Finberg, J. P. M., Tovbin, D., Naidu, S. G., and Better, O. S.,** Bile salts, hypotension and obstructive jaundice, *Clin. Sci.,* 67, 117, 1984.

16. **Binah, O., Rubinstein, I., Bomzon, A., and Better, O. S.,** Effects of bile acids on ventricular muscle contraction and electrophysiological properties: studies in rat papillary muscle and isolated ventricular myocytes, *Arch. Pharmacol.,* 335, 160, 1987.

17. **Trewby, P. N., Warren, R., Contini, S., Crosbie, W. A., Wilkinson, S. P., Laws, J. W., and Williams, R.,** Incidence and pathophysiology of pulmonary edema in fulminant hepatic failure, *Gastroenterology,* 74, 859, 1978.

18. **Sherlock, S.,** *Diseases of the Liver and Bililary System,* 5th ed., Blackwell Scientific, Oxford, 1975.

19. **Meakin, J. C.,** Jaundice and blood pressure, *Med. Clin. N. Am.,* 16, 715, 1932.

20. **Zollinger, R. M. and Williams, R. D.,** Surgical aspects of jaundice, *Surgery,* 39, 1016, 1956.

21. **Heaton, K. W.,** *Bile Acids in Health and Disease,* Churchill Livingstone, London, 1972.

22. **Saito, H.,** Clinical and experimental studies on the hyperdynamic states in obstructive jaundice, *J. Jpn. Surg. Soc.,* 82, 483, 1981.

23. **Song, E.,Segal, I., Hodkinson, J., and Kew, M. C.,** Sinus bradycardia in obstructive jaundice: correlation with total serum bile acid concentrations, *S. Afr. Med. J.,* 64, 548, 1983.

24. **Lumlertgol, D., Boonyaprapa, S., Bunnacheck, D., Thanachaikun, N., Praisontarangkul, O. A., Phornphutkul, K., and Keoplung, M.,** The jaundiced heart: evidence for blunted response to positive inotropic stimulation, personal communication, 1987.

25. **Finberg, J. P. M., Syrop, H. A., and Better, O. S.,** Blunted pressor response to angiotensin and sympathetic amines in bile duct-ligated dogs, *Clin. Sci.,* 61, 535, 1981.

26. **Bosch, J., Enriquez, R., Groszmann, R. J., and Storer, E. H.,** Chronic bile duct ligation in the dog: hemodynamic characterization of a portal hypertensive model, *Hepatology,* 3, 1002, 1983.

27. **Willems, B., Villeneuve, J. P., and Huet, P. M.,** Effect of propranolol on hepatic and systemic hemodynamics in chronic bile duct ligation, *Hepatology,* 6, 92, 1986.

28. **Bomzon, A., Rosenberg, M., Gali, D., Binah, O., Mordechowtiz, D., Better, O. S., Greig, P. D., and Blendis, L. M.,** Systemic hypotension and decrease pressor response in dog with chronic bile duct ligation (CBDL), *Hepatology,* 6, 595, 1986.

29. **Green, J., Beyar, R., Sideman, S., Mordechovitz, D., and Better, O. S.,** The "jaundiced" heart": a possible explanation for positive shock in obstructive jaundice, *Surgery,* 100, 14, 1986.

30. **Bomzon, A., Monies-Chass, I., Kamenetz, L., and Blendis, L. M.,** Anesthesia and pressor responsiveness in chronic bile duct-ligated (CBDL) dogs, *Hepatology,* 11, 551, 1990.

31. **Bomzon, A., Binah, O., and Blendis, L. M.,** Temporal changes in pressor and contractile responsiveness in the conscious chronic bile duct ligated (CBDL) dog, *Hepatology,* 8 (Abstr.), 1393, 1988.

32. **Joubert, P.,** An *in vivo* investigation of the negative chronotropic effect of cholic acid in the rat, *Clin. Exp. Physiol. Pharmacol.,* 5, 9, 1978.

33. **Tajuddin, M., Tariq, M., Bilgrami, N. I., and Kumar, S.,** Biochemical and pathological changes in the heart following bile duct ligation, in *Advances in Myocardiology,* Vol. 2, Tajuddin, M., Bhatia, B., Siddiqui, H. H., and Rona, G., Eds., University Park Press, Baltimore, 1980, 209.

34. **Finberg, J. P. M., Sideman, R., and Better, O. S.,** Cardiovascular responsiveness to vasoactive agents in rats with obstructive jaundice, *Clin. Exp. Physiol. Pharmacol.,* 9, 639, 1982.

35. **Lee, S. S., Girod, C., Braillon, A., Hadengue, A., and Lebrec, D.,** Hemodynamic characterization of chronic bile duct-ligated rats: effect of pentobarbital sodium, *Am. J. Physiol.,* 251, G176, 1986.

36. **Heidenreich, S., Brinkema, E., Martin, A., Dusing, R., Kipnowski, J., and Kramer, H. J.,** The kidney and cardiovascular system in obstructive jaundice: functional and metabolic studies in conscious rats, *Clin. Sci.,* 73, 593, 1987.

37. **Bomzon, A., Weinbroum, A., and Kamenetz, L.,** Systematic hypotension and pressor responsiveness in cholestasis: a study in conscious 3-day bile duct ligated rats, *J. Hepatol.,* in press.

38. **Jacob, G., Bishara, B., Bomzon, A.,** unpublished results, 1988.

39. **Sikuler, E.,** personal communication, 1988.

40. **Lee, S. S., Marty, J., Mantz, J., Samain, E., Braillon, A., and Lebrec, D.,** Desensitization of myocardial beta-adrenergic receptors in cirrhotic rats, *Hepatology,* in press.

41. **Ludatscher, R. M., Binah, O., Bomzon, A., Better, O. S., and Lightig, C. M.,** Ultrastructure of the myocardium in dogs with induced jaundice, *Acta Anat.,* 130, 242, 1987.

42. **Better, O. S. and Bomzon, A.,** The effects of cholemia on the renal and cardiovascular systems, in *The Kidney in Liver Disease,* 3rd ed., Epstein, M., Ed., Williams & Wilkins, Baltimore, 1988, 508.

43. **Dumitresco-Mante, H. D.,** Action des injections intraveineuses de sels biliaires sur le rhythme de pouls normal chez l'homme, *C. R. Séances Soc. Biol. Paris,* 99, 913, 1928.

44. **Schoenfield, L. J., Lachin, J. M., and the National Cooperative Gallstone Study Group,** Chenodiol (Chenodeoxycholic acid) for the dissolution of gallstones: the national cooperative study, *Ann. Int. Med.,* 95, 257, 1981.

45. **Binah, O., Bomzon, A., Blendis, L. M., Mordohovich, D., and Better, O. S.,** Obstructive jaundice blunts myocardial contractile response to isoprenaline in the dog: a clue to the susceptibility of jaundiced patients to shock? *Clin. Sci.,* 69, 647, 1985.

46. **Bogin, E., Better, O. S., and Harari, I.,** The effect of jaundiced sera and bile salts on cultured beating rat heart cells, *Experientia,* 39, 1307, 1983.

47. **Enriquez de Salamanca, R., Toni, P., Montes, M. J., Sanz, L., and Gilsanz, V.,** Negative chronotropic effect of cholic acid on isolated rat heart, *Med. Chir. Dig.,* 14, 585, 1985.

48. **Dave, M., Prabhu, S., Arora, S., and Sanyal, R. K.,** Some cardiovascular actions of sodium taurocholate, *Indian Physiol. Pharmacol.,* 18, 93, 1974.

49. **Kowalski, H. J., and Abelmann, W. H.,** The cardiac output at rest in Laennec's cirrhosis, *J. Clin. Invest.,* 32, 1025, 1953.

50. **Cohn, J. D., Greenspan, M., Goldstein, C. R., Godwin, A. L., Siegel, J. H., and Del Guercio, R. L. M.,** Arteriovenous shunting in high cardiac output shock syndromes, *Surg. Gynecol. Obstet.,* 1217, 282, 1968.

51. **Martini, G. A. and Hagemann, J. E.,** Über Fingernagelveranderungen bei Leberzirrhose als Folge veranderter peripheren Durchblutung, *Klin. Wochenschr.,* 34, 25, 1956.

52. **Claypool, J. G., Delp, M., and Lin, T. K.,** Hemodynamic studies in patients with Laennec's cirrhosis, *Am. J. Med. Sci.,* 244, 48, 1957.

53. **Murray, J. F., Dawson, A. M., and Sherlock S.,** Circulatory changes in chronic liver disease, *Am. J. Med.,* 24, 358, 1958.

54. **Mashford, M. L., Mahon, W. A., and Chalmers, T. C.,** Studies of the cardiovascular system in the hypotension of liver failure, *N. Engl. J. Med.,* 267, 1071, 1962.

55. **Schwab, M., Schroder, R., Dissmann, Tu. W., Heimberg, P., Huttemann, U., and Schuren, K.-P.,** Venose beimischung and Lungendreislauf bei Leberzirrhose, *Klin. Wochenschr.,* 41, 469, 1963.

56. **Williams, J. H. and Abelmann, W. H.,** Portopulmonary shunts in patients with portal hypertension, *J. Lab. Clin. Med.,* 62, 715, 1963.

57. **Bayley, T. J., Segel, N., and Bishop, J. M.,** The circulatory changes in patients with cirrhosis of the liver at rest and during exercise, *Clin. Sci.,* 26, 227, 1964.

58. **Kontos, H. A., Shapiro, W., Mauck, H. P., and Patterson, J. L.,** General and regional circulatory alterations in cirrhosis of the liver, *Am. J. Med.,* 37, 526, 1964.

59. **Massumi, R. A., Rios, J. C., and Ticktin, H. E.,** Hemodynamic abnormalities and venous admixture in portal cirrhosis, *Am. J. Med., Sci.,* 250, 275, 1965.

60. **Siegel, J. H., Goldwyn, R. M., Farrell, J., Gallin, P., and Friedman, P.,** Hyperdynamic states and the physiologic determinants of survival, *Arch. Surg.,* 108, 283, 1974.

61. **Dicarlo, V., Staudacher, C., Chiesa, R., Andreoni, B., Cristallo, M., and Ronchetti, E.,** The role of cardiovascular hemodynamics and liver histology in evaluating bleeding cirrhotic patients, *Ann. Surg.,* 2, 218, 1979.

62. **Valla, D., Poynard, T., Bercoff, E., Bataille, C., Coldfarb, G., and Lebrec, D.,** Le syndrome d'hypercinésie circulatoire systémique chez les malades atteints de cirrhose. Relations avec l'insuffisance hépatocellulaire et l'hypertension portale, *Gastroenterol. Clin. Biol.,* 8, 321, 1984.

63. **Moreau, R., Lee, S. S., Soupison, T., Roche-Sicot, J., and Sicot, C.,** Abnormal tissue oxygenation in patients with cirrhosis and liver failure, *J. Hepatol.,* 4, 98, 1988.

64. **Vorobioff, J., Bredfeldt, J. E., and Groszmann, R. J.,** Increased blood flow through the portal system in cirrhotic rats, *Gastroenterology,* 87, 1120, 1984.

65. **Bosch, J., Enriquez, J., Groszmann, R. J., and Storer, E. H.,** Chronic bile duct ligation in the dog: hemodynamic characterization of a portal hypertensive model, *Hepatology,* 3, 1002, 1983.

66. **Groszmann, R. J., Vorobioff, J., and Riley, E.,** Measurement of splanchnic hemodynamics in portal hypertensive rats: application of gamma-labeled microspheres, *Am. J. Physiol.,* 242, G156, 1982.

67. **Lee, S. S., Girod, C., Valla, D., Geoffroy, P., and Lebrec, D.,** Effects of pentobarbital sodium anesthesia on the splanchnic hemodynamics of normal and portal-hypertensive rats, *Am. J. Physiol.,* 249, G528, 1985.

68. **Jensen, L. S., Krarup, N., Larsen, J. A., Juhl, C., Nielsen, T. H., and Dybdahl,** Chronic portal venous hypertension, *Scand. J. Gastroenterol.,* 22, 463, 1987.

69. **Lebrec, D., Bataille, C., Bercoff, E., and Valla, D.,** Hemodynamic changes in patients with portal venous obstruction, *Hepatology,* 3, 550, 1983.

70. **Braillon, A., Lee, S. S., Girod, C., Peignoux-Martinot, M., Valla, D., and Lebrec, D.,** Role of portasystemic shunts in the hyperkinetic circulation of the portal hypertensive rat, *J. Lab. Clin. Med.,* 108, 543, 1986.

71. **Reynolds, T. B.,** Hepatic circulatory changes after shunt surgery, *Ann. N.Y. Acad. Sci.,* 170, 379, 1970.

72. **Even, P., Nicollo, F., Benhamou, J.-P., and Fauvert, R.,** Le débit cardiaque au cours des maladies du foie. Effets de l'anastomose porto-cave et des diurétiques, *Rev. Int. Hepatol.,* 16, 955, 1966.

73. **Levi, J. U., Zeppa, R., and Hutson, D. G.,** Early hemodynamic effects of the distal spenorectal shunt, *Surg. Forum,* 27, 370, 1976.

74. **Reichle, F. A. and Owen, O. E.,** Hemodynamic patterns in human hepatic cirrhosis, Ann. Surg, 190, 523, 1979.

75. **Sherlock, S.,** Portal hypertension, in *The Liver,* Read, A. E., Ed., Butterworths, London, 1967, 261.

76. **Gurll, N. J., Reynolds, D. G., Coon, D., and Shirazi, S. S.,** Acute and chronic splanchnic blood flow responses to portacaval shunt in the normal dog, *Gastroenterology,* 78, 1432, 1980.
77. **Shatney, C. H., Harmon, J. W., and Rich, N. M.,** Effects of portasystemic shunting on visceral and portal blood flow in the dog, *Gastroenterology,* 83, 1170, 1982.
78. **Kravetz, D., Arderiu, M., Bosch, J., Fuster, J., Visa, J., Casamitjana, R., and Rodès, J.,** Hyperglucagonemia and hyperkinetic circulation after portocaval shunt in the rat, *Am. J. Physiol.,* 252, G257, 1987.
79. **Shorr, E., Zweifach, B. W., Furchgott, R. F., and Baez, S.,** Hepatorenal factors in circulatory homeostasis, *Circulation,* 3, 42, 1951.
80. **Benoit, J. N., Barrowman, J. A., Harper, S. L., Kvietys, P. R., and Granger, D. N.,** Role of humoral factors in the intestinal hyperemia associated with chronic portal hypertension, *Am. J. Physiol.,* 247, G486, 1984.
81. **Sikuler, E. and Groszmann, R. J.,** Hemodynamic studies in long- and short-term portal hypertensive rats: the relation to systemic glucagon levels, *Hepatology,* 6, 414, 1986.
82. **Premen, A. J., Hall, J. E., and Smith, M. J.,** Postprandial regulation of renal hemodynamics: role of pancreatic glucagon, *Am. J. Physiol.,* 248, F656, 1985.
83. **Cerini, R., Koshy, A., Hadengue, A., Lee, S. S., Garnier, P., Lebrec, D.,** Effects of glucagon on systemic and splanchnic hemodynamics in rats with biliary cirrhosis, *J. Hepatol.,* 4, (Abstr.), S19, 1988.
84. **Lee, S. S., Moreau, R., Hadengue, A., Cerini, R., Koshy, A., and Lebrec, D.,** Glucagon selectively increases splanchnic blood flow in patients with well-compensated cirrhosis, *Hepatology,* 8, 1501, 1988.
85. **Martini, G. A., Arndt, H., Baltzer, G., Buchta, I., Hardewig, A., Marsch, W., and Schmidt, H. A.,** Pulmonary circulation in portal hypertension, *Ann. N.Y. Acad. Sci.,* 170, 280, 1970.
86. **Mooney, C. S., Honaker, A., and Griffen, W. O.,** Influence of the liver on arteriovenous fistulas, *Arch. Surg.,* 100, 154, 1979.
87. **Warren, J. V., Nickerson, J. L., and Elkine, D.,** The cardiac output in patients with arteriovenous fistulas, *J. Clin. Invest.,* 30, 210, 1951.
88. **Unikowsky, B., Wexler, M. J., and Levy, M.,** Dogs with experimental cirrhosis of the liver but without intrahepatic hypertension do not retain sodium or form ascites, *J. Clin. Invest.,* 72, 1594, 1983.
89. **Levy, M., Maher, E., Wexler, M. J.,** Euvolemic cirrhotic dogs in sodium balance maintain normal systemic hemodynamics, *Can. J. Physiol. Pharmacol.,* 66, 80, 1988.
90. **Jenkins, S. A., Baxter, J. N., Waxman, K., and Whang, J., et al.,** Effects of total and selective portasystemic shunting on hepatic haemodynamics and some aspects of liver function in the cirrhotic rat, *Clin. Exp. Pharmacol. Physiol.,* 9, 671, 1986.
91. **Jenkins, S. A., Devitt, P., Day, D. W., Baxter, J. N., and Shields, R.,** Effects of somatostatin on hepatic haemodynamics in the cirrhotic rat, *Digestion,* 33, 126, 1986.
92. **Lieberman, F. L. and Reynolds, T. B.,** Plasma volume in cirrhosis of the liver: its relation to portal hypertension, ascites and renal failure, *J. Clin. Invest.,* 46, 1297, 1967.
93. **Perera, G. A.,** The plasma volume in Laennec's cirrhosis of the liver, *Ann. Int. Med.,* 24, 643, 1946.
94. **Eisenberg, S.,** Blood volume in patients with Laennec's cirrhosis of the liver as determined by radioactive chromium-tagged red cells, *Am. J. Med.,* 20, 189, 1956.
95. **Bosch, J., Arroyo, V., Betriu, A., Mas, A., Carrilho, F., Rivera, A., Navarro, F., and Rodes, J.,** Hepatic hemodynamics and the renin-angiotensin-aldosterone system in cirrhosis, *Gastroenterology,* 78, 92, 1980.
96. **Clark, E. R.,** A-V anastomosis, *Physiol. Rev.,* 18, 229, 1938.
97. **Bean, W. B.,** *Vascular Spiders and Related Lesions of the Skin,* Charles C Thomas, Springfield, IL, 1958.
98. **Fisher, C. J., Eich, R., and Faloon, W. W.,** Arteriovenous shunting in palmar erythema: the effect upon blood ammonia determination, *J. Lab. Clin. Med.,* 51, 118, 1958.
99. **Dal Palu, C., Donnaggio, G., Dal Zotto, I., and Pessina, A. C.,** Arterio-venous shunts in cirrhotic patients studied with human serum albumin macroaggregates tagged with I^{131}, *Sand. J. Gastroenterol.,* 3, 425, 1968.
100. **Abramson, D. I. and Lichtman, S. S.,** Influences of ergotamine tartrate upon peripheral blood flow in subjects with liver disease, *Proc. Soc. Biol. Ed.,* 37, 262, 1937.
101. **Lunzer, M., Newman, S., and Sherlock, S.,** Skeletal muscle blood flow and neurovascular reactivity in liver disease, *Gut,* 14, 354, 1973.
102. **Lunzer, M., Manghani, K., Newman, S., Sherlock, S., Bernard, A., and Ginsberg, J.,** Impaired cardiovascular responsiveness in liver disease, *Lancet,* ii, 382, 1975.
103. **Jiron, M. I., Lee, S. S., Cerini, R., Pugliese, D., Hadengue, A., and Lebrec, D.,** Effects of nitroglycerin on forearm haemodynamics in patients with cirrhosis, *Clin. Sci.,* 74, 433, 1988.
104. **Williams, R. H. and Bissell, G. W.,** Thiamine metabolism with particular reference to the role of the liver and kidneys, *Arch. Int. Med.,* 73, 203, 1944.
105. **Amatuzio, D. S. and Nesbitt, S. A.,** A study of pyruvic acid in blood and spinal fluid of patients with liver disease with and without hepatic coma, *J. Clin. Invest.,* 29, 1486, 1950.

106. **Georg, J., Mellemgaard, K., Tygstrup, N., and Winkler, K.,** Venoarterial shunts in cirrhosis of the liver, *Lancet,* 1, 852, 1960.

107. **Lieber, C. S.,** Alcohol and the liver: 1984 update, *Hepatology,* 4, 1243, 1984.

108. **Bihari, D. F., Gimson, A. E. S., and Williams, R.,** Disturbances in cardiovascular and pulmonary function in fulminant hepatic failure, *Clin. Crit. Care Med.,* 9, 47, 1986.

109. **Cain, S. M.,** Peripheral oxygen uptake and delivery in health and disease, *Clin. Chest Med.,* 4, 139, 1983.

110. **Gimson, A., Bihari, D., Wilson, C., and Williams, R.,** Delivery dependent oxygen consumption in acute liver failure, *Clin. Sci.,* 66, (Abstr.), 12, 1984.

111. **Moreau, R., Lee, S. S., Hadengue, A., Ozier, Y. Sicot, C., and Lebrec, D.,** Relation between oxygen transport and consumption during vasoactive drug administration in patients with cirrhosis, *Hepatology,* 9, 427, 1989.

112. **Arai, M., Leo, M. A., Nakano, M., Gordon, E. R., Lieber, C. S.,** Biochemical and morphological alterations of baboon hepatic mitochondria after chronic ethanol administration, *Hepatology,* 4, 165, 1984.

113. **Berk, J., Hagen, J., Mary, G., Koo, R.,** The treatment of shock with β-adrenergic blockade, *Arch. Surg.,* 104, 46, 1972.

114. **Rapaport, E.,** Cardiopulmonary complications of liver disease, in *Hepatology: A Textbook of Liver Disease,* Zakim, D., and Boyer, T. D., Eds., W. B. Saunders, Philadelphia, 1982, 529.

115. **Wynne, J. and Braunwald, E.,** The cardiomyopathies and myocarditis, in *Heart Disease,* Braunwald, E., Ed., W. B. Saunders, Philadelphia, 1988, 1410.

116. **Gould, L., Shariff, M., Zahir, M., and Lieto, M.,** Cardiac hemodynamics in alcoholic patients with chronic liver disease and a presystolic gallop, *J. Clin. Invest.,* 48, 860, 1969.

117. **Regan, T. J., Levinson, G. E., Oldewurtel, H. A., Frank, M. J., Weisse, A. B., and Moschos, C. B.,** Ventricular function in noncardiacs with alcoholic fatty liver: role of ethanol in the production of cardiomyopathy, *J. Clin. Invest.,* 48, 397, 1969.

118. **Kolde, T., Machida, K., Nakanishi, A., Ozeki, K., Mashima, S., and Kono, H.,** Cardiac abnormalities in chronic alcoholism, *Jpn. Heart J.,* 13, 418, 1972.

119. **Spodick, D. H., Pigott, V. M., and Chirife, R.,** Preclinical cardiac malfunction in chronic alchoholism, *N. Engl. J. Med.,* 287, 677, 1972.

120. **Demakis, J. G., Proskey, A., Rahimtoola, S. H., Jamil, M., Sutton, G. C., Rosen, K. M., Gunnar, R. M., and Tobin, J. R., Jr.,** The natural course of alcoholic cardiomyopathy, *Ann. Intern. Med.,* 80, 293, 1974.

121. **Limas, C. J., Guiha, N. H., Lekagui, O., and Cohn, J. N.,** Impaired left ventricular function in alcoholic cirrhosis with ascites, *Circulation,* 49, 755, 1974.

122. **Askanas, A., Udoshi, M., and Sadjadi, S. A.,** The heart in chronic alcoholism. A noninvasive study, *Am. Heart J.,* 99, 9, 1980.

123. **Kino, M., Imamitchi, H., Morigutchi, M., Kawamura, K., and Takatsu, T.,** Cardiovascular status in asymptomatic alcoholics, with reference to the level of ethanol consumption, *Br. Heart J.,* 46, 545, 1981.

124. **Kelbaek, H., Erikson, J., Brynjolf, I., Raboel, A., Lund, J. O., Munck, O., Bonnevie, O., and Godtfredsen, J.,** Cardiac performance in patients with asymptomatic alcoholic cirrhosis of the liver, *Am. J. Cardiol.,* 54, 852, 1984.

125. **Ahmed, S. S., Howard, M., ten Hove, W., Leevy, C. M., and Regan, T. J.,** Cardiac function in alcoholics with cirrhosis: absence of overt cardiomyopathy — myth or fact?, *J. Am. Coll. Cardiol.,* 3, 696, 1984.

126. **Lee, S. S., Hadengue, A., Moreau, R., Sayegh, R., Hillon, P., and Lebrec, D.,** Postprandial hemodynamic responses in patients with cirrhosis, *Hepatology,* 8, 647, 1988.

127. **Ramond, M. J., Comoy, E., and Lebrec, D.,** Alterations in isoprenaline sensitivity in patients with cirrhosis: evidence of abnormality of the sympathetic nervous activity. *Br. J. Clin. Pharmacol.,* 21, 191, 1986.

128. **Berkson, J.,** Limitations of the application of four-fold table analysis to hospital data, *Biomed. Bull.,* 2, 47, 1947.

129. **Mainland, D.,** The risk of fallacious conclusions from autopsy data on the incidence of disease with applications to heart disease, *Am. Heart J.,* 45, 644, 1953.

130. **Gall, E. A.,** Primary and metastatic carcinoma of the liver. Relationship to hepatic cirrhosis, *Arch. Pathol.,* 70, 226, 1960.

131. **Synder, N., Atterbury, C. E., Pinto-Correia, J., and Conn, H. O.,** Increased concurrence of cirrhosis and bacterial endocarditis, *Gastroenterology,* 73, 1107, 1977.

132. **Lewis, B. S., Tur-Kaspa, R., Lewis, N., Gotsman, M. S., and Eliakim, M.,** Left ventricular function in liver cirrhosis: an echocardiographic study, *Isr. J. Med. Sci.,* 16, 489, 1980.

133. **Morace, G., Malfanti, P. L., Porciani, M. C., Barletta, G. A., Bellandi, F., Bisi, G., Pedenovi, P., and Simondi, P.,** La funzione cardiaca nella cirrosi epatica, *Cardiologia,* 28, 523, 1983.

134. **Fernandez-Munoz, D., Caramelo, C., Santos, J. C., Blanchart, A., Hernando, L., and Lopez-Novoa, J.,** Systemic and splanchnic hemodynamic disturbances in conscious rats with experimental liver cirrhosis without ascites, *Am. J. Physiol.,* 249, G316, 1985.

135. **Lee, S. S., Braillon, A., Girod, C., Geoffroy, P., and Lebrec, D.,** Haemodynamic rebound phenomena after abrupt cessation of propranolol therapy in portal hypertensive rats, *J. Hepatol.,* 3, 38, 1986.

136. **Geoffroy, P., Lhoste, F., Girod, C., Valla, D., and Lebrec, C.,** Impairment of chronotropic response to the beta agonist isoproterenol in rats with portal hypertension due to portal vein stenosis or bile-duct ligation, *J. Hepatol.,* 1, (Abstr.), S59, 1985.

137. **Lunseth, J. H., Olmstead, E. G., Forks, G., and Abbound, F.,** A study of heart disease in 180 hospitalized patients dying with portal cirrhosis, *A.M.A. Arch. Intern. Med.,* 102, 405, 1958.

138. **Cohn, M. D.,** The relationship of cardiac hypertrophy to cirrhosis of the liver, *Surgery,* 46, 887, 1959.

139. **Inagaki, Y. and Terao, K.,** Some problems upon the interrelationship between Wuhrmann's myocardiosis and Hegglin's syndrome with the special reference to their clinical and pathological diagnosis, *Jpn. Circ. J.,* 28, 156, 1964.

140. **Shozawa, T. and Otsu, Shoichi.,** Pathology of the myocardium in cases of chronic liver disease, especially of liver cirrhosis, *Jpn. Circ. J.,* 28, 163, 1964.

141. **Rubin, E.,** Alcoholic myopathy in heart and skeletal muscle, *N. Engl. J. Med.,* 301, 28, 1979.

142. **Lange, L. G. and Sobel, B. E.,** Impaired cardiac mitochondrial function induced by specific metabolites of ethanol, *J. Am. Coll. Cardiol.,* 1, 667, 1983.

143. **Tsiplenkova, V. G., Vikher, A. M., and Cherpachenko, N. M.,** Ultrastructural and histochemical observations in human and experimental alcoholic cardiomyopathy, *J. Am. Coll. Cardiol.,* 8, 22, 1986.

144. **Henriksen, J. H. Ring-Larsen, H., and Christensen, N. J.,** Sympathetic nervous activity in cirrhosis. A survey of plasma catecholamine studies, *J. Hepatol.,* 1, 55, 1985.

145. **Szakacs, J. E. and Mehlman, B.,** Pathologic changes induced by 1-norepinephrine, *Am. J. Cardiol.,* 5, 619, 1960.

146. **Gerbes, A. L., Remien, J., Jungst, D., Sauerbruch, T., and Paumgarter, G.,** Evidence for down-regulation of beta-2-adrenoceptors in cirrhotic patients with severe ascites, *Lancet,* 1, 1409, 1986.

147. **Baudet, M., Rigaund, M., and Rocha, P., et al.,** Reversibility of alcoholic cardiomyopathy with abstention from alcohol, *Cardiology,* 64, 317, 1979.

148. **Schwartz, L., Sample, K. A., and Wigle, E. D.,** Severe alcoholic cardiomyopathy reversed with abstention from alcohol, *Am. J. Cardiol.,* 36, 963, 1975.

149. **McDonald, C. D., Burch, G. E., and Walsh, J. J.,** Alcoholic cardiomyopathy managed with prolonged bed rest, *Ann. Intern. Med.,* 74, 681, 1971.

150. **Knauer, M. C. and Lowe, H. M.,** Hemodynamics in the cirrhotic patient during paracentesis, *N. Engl. J. Med.,* 276, 492, 1967.

151. **Guazzi, M., Polese, A., Magrini, F., Fiorentini, C., and Olivari, M.,** Negative influences of ascites on the cardiac function of cirrhotic patients, *Am. J. Med.,* 59, 165, 1975.

152. **Kowalski, H. J., Abelmann, W. H., and McNeely, W. F.,** Cardiac output in patients with cirrhosis of liver and tense ascites with observations on effect of paracentesis, *J. Clin. Invest.,* 33, 768, 1954.

153. **Blendis, L. M., Greig, P. D., Langer, B., Baigrie, R. S., Ruse, J., and Taylor, B. R.,** The renal and hemodynamic effects of the peritoneovenous shunt for intractable hepatic ascites, *Gastroenterology,* 77, 250, 1979.

154. **Greig, P. D., Blendis, L. M., Langer, B., Taylor, B. R., and Colapinto, R. F.,** Renal and hemodynamic effects of the peritoneovenous shunt: II. Long-term effects, *Gastroenterology,* 80, 119, 1981.

155. **Hall, E. M., Olsen, A. Y., and Davis, F. E.,** Portal cirrhosis, *Am. J. Pathol.,* 29, 993, 1953.

156. **Creed, D. L., Baird, W. F., and Fisher, E. R.,** The severity of aortic arteriosclerosis in certain diseases, *Am. J. Med. Sci.,* 230, 385, 1955.

157. **Grant, W. C., Wasserman, F., Rodensky, P. L., and Thompson, R. V.,** The incidence of myocardial infarction in portal cirrhosis, *Ann. Int. Med.,* 51, 774, 1959.

158. **Platt, D., Kie, F. E., and Luboeinski, H. P.,** Effect of age on the negative syntropy between malignant tumors, liver cirrhosis and arteriosclerotic structural changes in the aortic wall, the coronary and cerebral arteries, *Klin. Wochenschr.,* 51, 176, 1973.

159. **Alderman, E. L. and Coltart, D. J.,** Alcohol and the heart, *Br. Med. Bull.,* 38, 77, 1982.

160. **Klatsky, A. L., Friedman, G. D., Siegelabu, A. B.,** Alchoholic consumption before myocardial infarction: results from the Kaiser-Permanente epidemiologic study of myocardial infarction, *Ann. Intern. Med.,* 81, 292, 1974.

161. **Yano, K., Rhoads, G. G., and Kagan, A.,** Coffee, alcohol and risk of coronary heart disease among Japenese men living in Hawaii, *N. Engl. J. Med.,* 297, 405, 1977.

162. **Kozararevic, D. J., McGee, D., Vojvodic, N., Racic, Z., Dawber, T., and Gordon, T.,** Frequency of alcohol consumption and morbidity and mortality: Yugoslavia cardiovascular disease study, *Lancet,* 1, 613, 1980.

163. **Ginberg, H., Olefsky, J., and Farquhar, J. W. et al.,** Moderate ethanol ingestion and plasma triglyceride levels: a study in normal and hypertriglyceridemic persons, *Ann. Intern. Med.,* 80, 143, 1974.

164. **Jahn, C. E., Schaefer, E. J., Tam, L. A., Hoofnagle, J. H., Lindgren, F. T., Albers, J. J., Jones, E. A., and Brewer, H.,** Lipoprotein abnormalities in primary biliary cirrhosis: association with hepatic lipase inhibition as well as altered cholesterol esterification, *Gastroenterology,* 89, 1266, 1985.

165. **Klatsky, A. L., Friedman, G. D., Siegelaub, A. B., and Gerard, M. J.,** Alcohol consumption and blood pressure, *N. Engl. J. Med.,* 296, 1194, 1977.
166. **Bouchut, L., Froment, R., and Grasset, E.,** État du système cardiovasculaire dans la cirrhose éthylique du foie d'après 160 observations avec vérification anatomique, *Lyon Med.,* 160, 3, 1947.
167. **Spatt, S. D. and Rosenblatt, P.,** The incidence of hypertension in portal cirrhosis: a study of 80 necropsied cases of portal cirrhosis, *Ann. Int. Med.,* 31, 479, 1949.
168. **Loyke, H. F.,** The relationship of cirrhosis of the liver to hypertension: a study of 504 cases of cirrhosis of the liver, *Am. J. Med. Sci.,* 230, 627, 1955.
169. **Kopferschmitt, J., Doffoel, M., Schneider, R., and Bockel, R.,** Fatal spontaneous hemopericardium in cirrhotic, *Nouv. Presse Med.,* 8, 366, 1979, letter.
170. **Fischer, D. M., Casanova, R., and Aldi, M.,** High-output heart failure in hepatic cirrhosis, *G. Ital. Cardiol.,* 11, 1520, 1981.
171. **Shah, A. and Variyam, E.,** Pericardial effusion and left ventricular associated with ascites secondary to hepatic cirrhosis, *Arch. Int. Med.,* 148, 585, 1988.
172. **Triger, D. R. and Wright, R.,** Hypergammaglobulinemia in liver disease, *Lancet,* 1, 1494, 1973.
173. **Pederson, C., Josephsen, P., Hegholm, A., and Josephsen, I. L.,** *Yersinia enterocolitica* endocarditis, *Ugeskr. Laeg.,* Jul., 8, 147, 1985.

Chapter 6

THE PULMONARY CIRCULATION IN LIVER DISEASE

M. D. Voigt, E. D. Bateman, S. J. Louw, and R. E. Kirsch

TABLE OF CONTENTS

I. INTRODUCTION

A wide spectrum of pulmonary abnormalities have been reported in patients with liver disease. These are listed, with references, in Table 1. This chapter will focus on the pulmonary circulation in patients with cirrhosis and portal hypertension. The prevalence, pathogenesis, pathophysiology, clinical manifestations, and current management of pulmonary hypertension and pulmonary arterial oxygen desaturation will be discussed. No attempt will be made to cover the several disorders of lung function seen in different forms of liver disease except as they relate to changes in the pulmonary vasculature.

II. PULMONARY HYPERTENSION

A. PREVALENCE

While there is broad agreement that the prevalence of pulmonary hypertension is increased in patients with cirrhosis and portal hypertension,[1-11] its incidence has not been established. This is due, in part, to a lack of adequately controlled studies, but also to the relative insensitivity of clinical signs and routine pathological criteria and the invasiveness of methods previously employed for determining pulmonary arterial pressure (PAP). Although the former remains a problem, the availability of noninvasive methods, such as Doppler ultrasonography, for measuring PAP have enhanced the investigator's ability to study the relationship between cirrhosis and the pulmonary vascular response.[12]

The reported prevalence of pulmonary hypertension is shown in Table 2. The differing prevalences appear to depend upon the sensitivity of the diagnostic methods employed. In the largest of these series, involving 2459 patients with biopsy-proven hepatic cirrhosis and 1241 subjects in whom cirrhosis was confirmed at autopsy, McDonnell et al. found a clinical diagnosis of pulmonary hypertension in 0.61% and autopsy evidence of pulmonary hypertension in 0.73%. These figures are higher than the prevalence of 0.13% in their control group of 17,901 autopsies performed on unselected patients older than 1 year of age ($p < .001$).[10]

Lai et al. found clinical evidence of pulmonary hypertension in 2.1% of 728 prospectively evaluated patients with recurrent pyogenic cholangitis admitted to the Queen Mary Hospital, Hong Kong.[11] In a subgroup of patients with frequent exacerbations of cholangitis over 8 years or more, the prevalence was 7.6%. All patients with pulmonary hypertension had scarred livers, and portal-hepatic venous shunts were demonstrated within these scars.

O'Brien et al. used pulmonary function and exercise studies to test for pulmonary vascular disease in 11 patients with cirrhosis and portal hypertension and in 10 patients with extrahepatic portal hypertension and normal livers.[13] Evidence of pulmonary hypertension was found in roughly 30% in each group.

In the only other major prevalence study from results of routine autopsy reports, Ruttner et al. found 765 cases of cirrhosis in a series of 11,998 autopsies in patients older than 20 years.[8] Only two of the 765 cases with cirrhosis had unexplained cor pulmonale and plexogenic pulmonary hypertension, a prevalence in cirrhosis of 0.26% and an overall prevalence of 0.016%. Accurate autopsy diagnosis of pulmonary hypertension is difficult in all but the most severe forms of this condition. Morphometric analysis is essential and involves the assessment of increases in musculature of small pulmonary arteries and of the muscularization of small, usually nonmuscular, pulmonary arterioles. Using such methods, Matsubara et al. studied 21 cases, randomly selected from a group of 94 adults, with autopsy evidence of severe liver disease.[5] The mean wall thickness of pulmonary vessels in cirrhotic patients was found to be significantly higher than that in 19 control patients (21.2 ± 10.4 μm 15.3 ± 7.5 μm, respectively). The ratio of wall thickness to vessel radius was 0.21 ± 0.09 in the cirrhotic group and 0.13 ± 0.07 in the controls ($p<.005$). Features of pulmonary

TABLE 1
Diseases Affecting both Liver and Lung

Diseases secondarily affecting liver and/or lung

Disease	Liver	Lung
Alpha-1 protease inhibitor deficiency	Neonatal hepatitis-cholestasis;[177,179] cirrhosis;[175-178] hepatocellular carcinoma[177,179]	Panasinar emphysema Bronchiectasis
Sarcoidosis and other granulomatous diseases	Granulomas;[180-182] cholestasis;[180] portal hypertension[181,182]	Granulomas; interstitial disease, adenopathy, pleural effusions, and angiocentric granulomatosis
Schistosomiasis	Periportal fibrosis; portal hypertension	Pulmonary arteritis;[189] pulmonary hypertension[190]

Entities associated with specific liver conditions

Acute liver disease	
Fulminant hepatic failure	Non-cardiogenic pulmonary edema[34]
Injection sclerotherapy	Acute respiratory failure[162]
Chronic liver disease	
Primary biliary cirrhosis	Lymphocytic interstitial pneumonitis; chronic airflow obstruction; reduced diffusing capacity[182-184]
Chronic active hepatitis	Interstitial pneumonitis[185,186] and pleural effusions[127]
Sclerosing cholangitis	Bronchiectasis and chronic bronchitis[187,188]
Hepatocellular carcinoma	Pulmonary hypertension[191,192]

TABLE 2
Prevalence Rates of Portapulmonary Hypertension

Study	Cases	Prevalence (%)	Comments	Ref.
Bayley et al.	15	87	Nonrandomized; historical controls; normal values not given; absolute values of pulmonary vascular resistance not raised; no clinical case of pulmonary hypertension	1
Senior et al.	11	54	Probably selected cases; pressures measured by catheterization	9
O'Brien et al.	21	35	Pulmonary vascular disease inferred from exercise response; pressure not measured; previous sclerotherapy in 4 patients	13
Matsubara et al.	94	31	Prevalence determined by qualitative pathology Subjective and unblinded; retrospective	5
Lai et al.	728	2.1—7.6	Patients had recurrent pyogenic cholangitis; pathogenesis of pulmonary hypertension may be different; no catheterization data.	11
McDonnel et al.	17,901	.73	Pathological; retrospective	10
	1,241	.61	Clinical; retrospective	10
Ruttner et al.	765	.26	Retrospective; only gross pathological changes sought (Gr 4 and above); insensitive method for detecting right ventricular hypertrophy	8
Lebrec et al.	2000	0.25	No pressure data; retrospective	2
Senior et al. (retrospective)	70	0	Pulmonary pressures not measured	9
Rodriguez-Roisin et al.	15	0	Compensated cirrhosis; low pulmonary artery pressure on catheterization	14
Naeije et al.	24	0	Low pulmonary pressures; loss of pulmonary vascular reflexes; possibly selected cases	15

hypertension were found in roughly 30% of their 94 patients, but it is worth noting that the criteria for hypertension were more sensitive than those generally applied.[5] Nevertheless, these results suggest that a degree of subclinical pulmonary hypertension might be present in a high proportion of patients with chronic liver disease.

Pulmonary artery catheterization studies of patients with cirrhosis have yielded inconsistent results. Bayley et al. found mean pulmonary arterial pressures of greater than 20 mmHg in 13 of 15 patients with cirrhosis.[1] The mean PAPs in the cirrhotic group (24.4 ± 3.7) differed significantly from those of 77 normal subjects (17.9 ± 3.2). The use of historical controls and lack of information regarding the selection of the cirrhotic patients limit the interpretation of this data. Despite these reservations, 87% of their subjects had pulmonary hypertension.

Of 11 cirrhotic patients prospectively studied by Senior et al. 54% had marked pulmonary hypertension.[9] Conversely, 15 patients with well compensated cirrhosis studied by Rodriguez-Roisin et al. had a mean pulmonary artery pressure below normal (6.3 ± 0.6 mmHg). Normal control values were not given.[14] Mean pulmonary arterial pressures were 11.9 ± 0.8, in 24 patients with alcoholic cirrhosis studied by Naeije et al.,[15] and 15 ± in 10 studied by Daoud et al.[16] Only 2 of 18 patients with alcoholic cirrhosis prospectively studied by Massumi et al. had PAPs greater than 20 mmHg.[17] These discrepant results may reflect differences in patient selection,[18] the type or duration of liver disease, or other factors such as the size of the portal-systemic shunt.

B. PATHOGENESIS

There is increasing evidence that the pulmonary hypertension associated with liver disease is due to portal systemic shunting (portapulmonary hypertension) and not to hepatocellular dysfunction. This is based on descriptions of pulmonary hypertension in patients with portal vein thrombosis without liver disease, patients with surgically created portal-systemic shunts, and on experimental studies in dogs and rats.

The first description of portapulmonary hypertension was that of a 53-year-old woman with portal vein thrombosis, a large spontaneous portal-systemic shunt, and normal liver histology.[4] Subsequently, there have been several reports of pulmonary hypertension complicating portal hypertension in the absence of liver disease.[2,3,7,19-22] Lebrec et al.[2] and Yutani et al.[23] also described 3 patients with pulmonary hypertension who had minimal liver dysfunction, due to nodular regenerative hyperplasia.

Lebrec et al. suggested that surgical portal-systemic shunting increases the risk of portalpulmonary hypertension.[2] His impression was based on cases in the literature and his own finding that 6 of 9 patients who had undergone surgical portal-systemic shunting had developed pulmonary hypertension. Senior et al. measured PAPs in 11 patients who had survived for 2 years or more after surgical portal systemic shunts.[9] Six (54%) had pulmonary hypertension with mean PAPs ranging from 26 to 51 mmHg (mean 44.3 ± 1.7 mmHg). Clinical features of pulmonary hypertension were present in only the four most severely affected patients. Although there are no controlled data, the figure for the incidence of pulmonary hypertension after surgical shunts is not higher than the prevalence found by Bayley et al. in their group of unoperated cirrhotic patients.[1]

The first experimental study suggesting an association between portal systemic shunting and pulmonary hypertension was that of Cohn, who found that dogs developed cardiac hypertrophy after surgical shunting of portal blood into the left side of the circulation.[24] Some years later, Lunseth demonstrated cardiac hypertrophy in rats with carbon tetrachloride-induced cirrhosis.[25] We have recently shown that pulmonary hypertension develops in rats with surgically created portacaval shunts and normal liver histology.[26]

A variable and often considerable delay exists between the onset of portal hypertension and the development of pulmonary hypertension (Table 2). This is not surprising, since pulmonary hypertension is known to have a long silent period. The influence of the size of the portal-systemic shunt on the development of pulmonary hypertension is not known. The likelihood of hypertension resulting may not relate to the degree of shunting. Cohen et al. described a patient with portal vein thrombosis and pulmonary hypertension whose portal shunt at autopsy was not apparent.[21] However, the rate and volume of blood flow through the shunt during life was not known, and the patient had received sclerotherapy prior to his death, which may have obliterated portal-systemic channels, thus masking the size of the shunt that had been present while he developed pulmonary hypertension.

The mechanism whereby liver disease and/or spontaneous or surgical portal-systemic shunting causes pulmonary hypertension is unknown. Theoretical explanations include increased blood volume and cardiac output, autoimmunity, bacterial and dietary products bypassing the liver, and *in situ* thrombosis or thromboembolism.

1. Increased Cardiac Output and Circulating Blood Volume

In congenital cardiac shunting, the prolonged elevation of cardiac output is thought to cause pulmonary endothelial damage which ultimately leads to the development of pulmonary hypertension.[27] A similar mechanism may account for pulmonary hypertension in liver disease, the increased flow being secondary to an increased circulating blood volume. Bayley et al. measured cardiac output in 15 cirrhotic patients, 14 of whom had mean pulmonary artery pressures above 20 mmHg and 7 pressures of 25 mmHg or more.[1] Resting cardiac output was significantly increased (5.13 ± 1.44 vs 4.04 ± 0.64 l/min/m^2, $p < .001$), while pulmonary vascular resistance was similar to that of controls. However, in many, if not most patients with liver disease, pulmonary artery pressures remain normal in spite of increased flow.[17] Massumi et al. found that 17 of 18 patients with cirrhosis and raised cardiac output (5.25 ± 1.63 l/min/m^2) had normal pulmonary arterial pressures.[17] Similarly, in a study by Rodriguez-Roisin et al. in 15 consecutive male patients with cirrhosis, admitted for treatment of variceal bleeding, mean pulmonary artery pressure and pulmonary vascular resistance were decreased in spite of the presence of a mild hyperkinetic circulatory state with increased cardiac output, reduced mean arterial pressure, and systemic vascular resistance.[14] These findings argue against a direct relationship between cardiac output and pulmonary hypertension.

2. Autoimmunity

The known association between several autoimmune diseases and pulmonary hypertension and the association of hepatitis B with immunological phenomena and with polyarteritis nodosa have led to the suggestion that autoimmune mechanisms may be involved in the pulmonary hypertension of liver disease.[6,28] While it is possible that patients with autoimmune chronic active hepatitis, systemic lupus erythematosus, or polyarteritis nodosa have pulmonary hypertension as part of their autoimmune disease, there is no evidence to suggest that autoimmunity plays any role in the majority of patients with pulmonary hypertension secondary to liver disease.

3. Bacterial and Dietary Products Bypassing the Liver

Antibodies to bacterial and dietary products are found in patients with chronic liver disease.[29,30] Endotoxin has been demonstrated in the systemic circulation of patients with fulminant hepatic failure and in patients with cirrhosis.[31-36] Bacterial toxins, including endotoxin, have been shown to cause acute lung injury and chronic pulmonary hypertension in numerous animal models.[37-43] Many of the pulmonary features of liver disease such as ventilation perfusion imbalance, loss of hypoxic pulmonary vasoconstriction, hypoxia, platelet consumption, intravascular coagulation, and pulmonary hypertension have been described in animals subjected to systemic endotoxemia. Endotoxins are normally cleared by both

Kupffer cells and hepatocytes, but in portal systemic shunting, these substances reach the pulmonary circulation[44] and may play a role in the pathogenesis of portapulmonary hypertension.

4. *In Situ* Thrombosis or Thromboemboli

Many authors have argued that the pulmonary hypertension associated with liver disease is due to emboli arising from the portal circulation.[3,4,7,11,21] This view is based on the demonstration of thrombi in pulmonary vessels. For example, thrombi were found in small pulmonary vessels of all six cases described by Naeye,[7] in 8 of 12 patients described by Edwards et al.,[19] and in several smaller series and case reports.[4,9,45] While there is little doubt that such thrombi exist, their site of origin is usually not manifest. Naeye was able to demonstrate a potential source for emboli in only three of his six patients[7] and Edwards et al. in 2 of their 12 cases.[19] Only 4.3% of the 94 patients studied by Matsubara et al. had thrombi in both portal and pulmonary vessels.[5] Edwards et al. speculated that the thrombi arise in pulmonary arteries in situ as a result of stasis, local endothelial injury, or a generalized hypercoagulable state.[19] In keeping with this hypothesis, elevated intravascular pressure or flow in patients with right to left shunts due to congenital cardiac disease has been found to disrupt normal endothelium[27] This damage may change the environment of the vascular bed from anti-coagulant to pro-coagulant.[45,46]

We have previously shown that patients with cirrhosis and portal hypertension and patients with extrahepatic portal hypertension have increased concentrations of fibrinogen and fibrin degradation products in their plasma, strongly suggesting active coagulation and lysis.[47] These changes also occur in rats after surgical portacaval shunts[48] and have been found in primary pulmonary hypertension.[49,50]

It is thus probable that in situ fibrin deposition and thrombus formation, rather than thromboembolism, play a role in the development of pulmonary hypertension associated with liver disease.

C. PATHOLOGY

Descriptions of the pathology of pulmonary hypertension in man are limited to features of severe disease, but animal models have been used to characterize changes that occur during the early stages of this condition. The earliest recognized changes of the tunica media are muscularization of smaller pulmonary arteries and medial hypertrophy.[51] These are found in virtually all models, whether induced by surgical left to right shunts,[52] crotolaria,[53-56] *Senechio jacobaea*,[57] hypoxia,[58-60] hyperoxia,[61] or infusions of *Escherichia coli* endotoxin.[37-43,62] These changes may develop rapidly; in hypoxic rats, subendothelial blebs and edema are present at 1 h, increased subendothelial fibroblasts at 24 h, and smooth muscle cells at 2 days.[63] Hislop and Reid found neomuscularization and medial thickening of small arteries after only 3 days,[60] changes similar to those that occur in humans with liver disease.[5]

The commonly observed intimal lesions are proliferation followed by fibrosis. These are seen as whorls of cellular or fibrous tissue which may occlude the vessel lumen.[64] In more advances cases, there is disruption of the media and focal aneurysmal dilatation of small vessels. Some of these microaneurysms contain complex proliferative tufts of intimal cells and capillary channels known as plexiform lesions.[64] Plexiform lesions are nonspecific and occur in primary pulmonary hypertension and pulmonary hypertension secondary to chronic liver disease, congenital heart disease, and chronic hypoxia.[65,66] Angiomatoid lesions, consisting of clusters of dilated and tortuous vascular channels, may occur distal to plexiform lesions. In severe cases necrotizing pulmonary arteritis may be found. Finally, long-standing pulmonary hypertension may lead to right ventricular hypertrophy and dilatation.

D. CLINICAL FEATURES OF PORTAPULMONARY HYPERTENSION

The symptoms and signs of the patients with portapulmonary hypertension reported in

TABLE 3
Clinical Features of Portal-Pulmonary Hypertension

Number of cases reported	97
Clinical information	42
Age at presentation	41.7 years (median 40, range 5—76)
Male to female ratio	1:1
Interval between diagnosis of liver disease and diagnosis of pulmonary hypertension	8.7 (SD 6.1); range 0—27 years
Survival interval after diagnosis of pulmonary hypertension	1.43 years (SD 1.5; range 0 to 7 years) (23% alive at time of reporting)
Type of liver disease	Percentage
Alcoholic cirrhosis	36
Crypogenic cirrhosis	16
Portal vein thrombosis	9
Hepatitis-associated cirrhosis	6.9
Autoimmune chronic active hepatitis	6.9
Miscellaneous	25.2
Cases with surgical portal-systemic shunt	39
Interval between shunt and development of pulmonary hypertension	7.81 (SD 4.9 years)
Presenting symptom(s)	
Exertional dyspnea	67
Precordial chest pain	19
Effort syncope	19
Right heart failure	16.7
Hemoptysis	7
Palpitations	5
Sudden death	5
Incidental finding	7
Clinical features	
Exertional dyspnea	67
Right heart failure	38
Precordial chest pain	21
Effort syncope	19
Hemoptysis	12
Sudden death	12
Palpitations	5
Accentuated pulmonic second sound (P2)	48
Pulmonary ejection systolic murmer	33
Raised jugular venous pressure	29
Right ventricular lift	14
Tricuspid regurgitation	13
4th Heart sound	12
Chest X-ray	
Cardiomegaly	59.6
Prominent pulmonary artery	47
Electrocardiogram	
Right ventricular hypertrophy	60
Right axis deviation	54
Right bundle branch block	16

From References 2 to 11, 13, 19, 21 to 26, 28, 45, and 165 to 172.

the English literature are summarized in Table 3. They are essentially the same as those seen in primary pulmonary hypertension.

1. Diagnosis

When pulmonary hypertension is identified in patients with liver disease, a variety of alternative causes of pulmonary hypertension must be considered and excluded before the raised pulmonary arterial pressure can be attributed to liver disease. These include valvular heart disease (e.g., silent mitral stenosis), pulmonary veno-occlusive disease, interstitial lung disease (including cryptogenic fibrosing alveolitis), and recurrent pulmonary thromboembolism. A combination of tests, such as detailed lung function testing, venography of the lower limbs and iliac veins, six-view perfusion lung scan or ventilation-perfusion lung scan, and noninvasive cardiac examinations such as echo-cardiography, are useful means of excluding nonhepatic causes of pulmonary hypertension. Segmental or larger perfusion defects are found in most patients with thromboembolic pulmonary hypertension, while ventilation scans are normal.[67,68] In "primary" forms of pulmonary hypertension, lung scans are either normal or show multiple bilateral subsegmental patches of decreased perfusion. In a study by Chapman et al.,[69] all patients with thromboembolic pulmonary hypertension (confirmed by pulmonary angiography) had scans indicating a high probability of pulmonary embolism, whereas patients with primary pulmonary hypertension had normal scans or minor features indicative of a low probability of pulmonary embolism. The importance of recognizing patients with thromboembolic pulmonary hypertension lies in their improved survival on long-term anticoagulant therapy.[69,70]

2. Management of Pulmonary Hypertension

Treatment options for patients with liver-associated pulmonary hypertension are limited, because the disease is usually far advanced and vascular abnormalities are irreversible at the time of detection. In general, the treatment of pulmonary hypertension has been along similar lines to that of primary pulmonary hypertension and pulmonary hypertension associated with such conditions as systemic lupus erythematosus and systemic sclerosis. Since vasoconstriction may be an important feature in the early stages of pathogenesis, vasodilator agents offer the hope of reversing vasoconstriction before irreversible changes such as medial hypertrophy of the muscular arteries and muscularization of arterioles develop. Relatively few studies provide convincing evidence that the use of conventional vasodilator drugs provide short term benefit,[71-76] and fewer still claim a lasting effect.[75-81] Drugs previously evaluated include antihypertensive agents such as hydralazine,[69,77-79,82,83] diazoxide, nitrates[76] (isosorbide dinitrate and amyl nitrate),[69] calcium channel blockers including nifedipine,[71,72] diltiazem,[85] prazosin,[66] isoprenaline,[75,84] phenylephrine, labetolol, and captopril.[73,86] Atenolol has been used successfully in a patient with portapulmonary hypertension and raised cardiac output.[20] Although a transient reduction in pulmonary vascular resistance has been achieved with all of the above in occasional patients, these benefits are overshadowed by unacceptable tachycardia and peripheral vasodilation which, occasionally, may be life threatening.[73,87] Because of the potential hazards arising during the assessment of the efficacy of these drugs,[73,82] it is recommended that the agents should be given by mouth (and not intravenously), and that patients should be observed in an intensive care unit where appropriate hemodynamic monitoring and resuscitation can be performed. Hemodynamic monitoring by Swan Ganz catheter and cardiac output studies are preferred at the initial evaluation, but subsequent monitoring of the effects of treatment may be done by Doppler ultrasonography.

Epoprostenol (prostacyclin, PGI_2) administered as a continuous intravenous infusion has been shown to be a powerful pulmonary vasodilator and is being used with success, as a temporary measure, to lower pulmonary vascular resistance in patients awaiting heart lung transplantation.[88] It has a relatively small effect on systemic vascular resistance and tolerance does not appear to develop. The drug acts rapidly and has a short half-life, thus permitting its accurate titration according to the patient's needs. The effectiveness of this agent suggests that chronic vasodilation of vessels can be achieved even in patients with severe disease and raises the hope that a suitable oral agent may be found. However, current long term pulmonary vasodilatory agents are ineffective in the majority of patients, thus the definitive treatment option appears to be heart-lung or heart-lung-liver transplantation. It is not known whether the pulmonary vascular abnormalities will regress after liver transplantation alone, or whether they will recur if heart lung transplantation alone is performed.

Prevention might in the future depend on early identification of patients at risk and by attempting to eliminate or neutralize the causative mechanisms. Prognosis is poor in patients once they have clinically detectable pulmonary hypertension, with a mean survival time of 1.43 years.

III. HYPOXEMIA IN CHRONIC LIVER DISEASE

Hypoxemia occurring in association with liver disease may be the consequence of specific pathologic entities that affect both liver and lung or due to pulmonary functional-anatomical changes that occur in relation to any form of severe chronic liver disease. Some diseases in the former category are listed in Table 1 and will not be considered in this review.

Arterial oxyhemoglobin desaturation in patients with chronic liver disease is widely recognized,[89,119] but imperfectly understood. Keys and Snell reported a prevalence of hypoxemia of 80% in 61 unselected patients with chronic liver disease,[90,91] but in more recent studies, arterial oxygen saturation of less than 90% was found in only 16% of 57 patients with chronic liver disease[92] and in 41% of 25 patients with alcoholic cirrhosis.[17] In the latter study, 76% of the entire group failed to attain a PaO_2 of greater than 500 mmHg on breathing 100% oxygen for 15 min, indicating disordered gas exchange despite normal baseline values. In another study of pulmonary function and blood gases in 105 patients with cirrhosis, selected on the basis that there were no clinical features of cardiopulmonary disease, 30% had an arterial PaO_2 of less than 80 mmHg.[93]

A. CLINICAL FEATURES OF HYPOXEMIA IN LIVER DISEASE

Most patients with mild hypoxemia have few cardiorespiratory symptoms. Patients with severe hypoxemia appear to form a separate subgroup and often have severe dyspnea and reduced effort tolerance. Debilitating symptoms are present in up to 5% of the patients with cirrhosis.[94-96] These patients often have platypnea (dyspnea worsening on assuming the upright position)[96] and exercise-aggravated hypoxemia.[94]

All forms of cirrhosis may be associated with hypoxemia[97] and clinical features of pulmonary vascular abnormalities occasionally precede signs of liver disease.[7,98] Affected patients are cyanosed, clubbed, have marked palmar erythema, plethoric facies, and usually,[95,99] but not invariably,[98] have numerous spider nevi and dilated facial vessels. The pulse is bounding, the precordium hyperdynamic, and flow murmurs are often present. The degree of hypoxemia does not appear to correlate with the severity of the liver disease, the presence of ascites or edema, splenomegaly, or portal hypertension,[98,100-102,104] and occasionally occurs in patients with extrahepatic portal vein thrombosis.[114] Results of lung function tests correlate roughly with severity of hypoxemia. Up to 20% of patients with chronic liver disease have a reduced diffusing capacity for carbon monoxide.[104,105] Patients with mild hypoxemia may have evidence of altered mechanics,[93,106] restrictive defects,[106] increased closing volumes,[93,108] and/or mild airflow obstruction.[93,106] PaO_2 drops significantly, in some cases by up to 19 mmHg,[95] in the majority of patients with severe hypoxemia, when they stand up.[95,97] The chest X-rays show basal mottling in approximately 6% of unselected patients with cirrhosis.[104] This is thought to be due to abnormal pulmonary vessels, but mottling is not invariable, even in the most severe cases.[97] Patients with mottled chest X-rays are more often clubbed, tend to have lower diffusing capacities, lower PaO_2 and higher cardiac outputs than patients without basal mottling.[104] Lung perfusion scans are abnormal in the majority of cases, with diffuse or patchy reduction in isotope uptake by the pulmonary vasculature.[101] Catheterization studies show a hyperdynamic circulation with normal or reduced pulmonary and systemic pressures.[14,95] Angiography is often normal, or may have a spongy appearance during the capillary phase,[95,101,109,110] suggestive of diffuse small-vessel abnormalities. Large arteriovenous malformations are not a feature of this condition. Angiographic abnormalities are often asymmetrical, and may involve the upper lung zones.[97]

B. PATHOPHYSIOLOGY OF HYPOXEMIA

Several mechanisms have been proposed to explain the hypoxia associated with cirrhosis. These include (1) changes in the affinity of hemoglobin for oxygen; (2) ventilation-perfusion mismatch; and (3) intrapulmonary shunts and pulmonary perfusion-diffusion abnormalities.

1. Altered Hemoglobin Affinity for Oxygen

Early attempts to explain arterial desatuation in cirrhosis suggested that a shift in the Hb-O_2 dissociation curve to the right, with resultant decreased affinity of blood for oxygen, might be responsible for this abnormality.[91] Although this phenomenon has been observed in some cirrhotic patients,[91,111-116] it is not invariable and is insufficient to account for significant hypoxemia.[111-116] In a study by Balzer et al. no shift to the right (expressed as oxygen tension at 50% saturation (p50)), was found in cirrhotic patients; 14 controls had a mean p50 of 22.4 $\pm$ 2.8 mmHg compared with 21.8 $\pm$ 2.2 in the 30 patients with cirrhosis.[115] The cirrhotic patients did, however, have significantly higher 2,3-diphosphoglycerate (DPG) levels than controls (21.5 $\pm$ 6.4 vs 14.9 $\pm$ 4.3 μmol/10^{11} cells)[115] a metabolic event which usually shifts the Hb-O_2 dissociation curve to the right. It is worth noting that chronic hypoxia also results in elevated levels of 2,3-DPG and the observed elevation of 2,3-DPG might thus be an effect of hypoxemia rather than its cause. Direct measurements of hemoglobin-oxygen affinity in cirrhotic subjects have shown negligible differences between measured and predicted values at a variety of oxygen tensions.[111-114] These studies provide powerful evidence that alterations of the Hb-O_2 dissocation curve are not responsible to any significant extent for the hypoxemia of cirrhosis.

2. Ventilation-Perfusion Abnormalities

Imperfect matching of ventilation and perfusion within different regions of the lung accounts for the hypoxia found in most form of lung disease. V/Q inequality may also be the dominant cause of hypoxia in patients with cirrhosis. (See References 14—16, 92, 93, 97, 106—108, and 114—117.)

Several physiological sequelae of liver disease provide the basis for $\dot{V}/\dot{Q}$ inequality. These include (a) alteration in regional ventilation; (b) impairment of hypoxic pulmonary vasoconstrictor responses; and (c) altered pulmonary hemodynamics.

a. Alterations in Regional Ventilation

Changes in regional ventilation are easily recognized in subjects with ascites and pleural effusion, but similar changes are also found in patients without these obvious mechanical abnormalities. Ascites and/or pleural effusions[118-127] affect pulmonary mechanics by raising the diaphragm and compressing the lung bases. There is frequently associated interstitial pulmonary edema which has further restrictive effects on pulmonary mechanics.[106,128] Yao et al. demonstrated significant restrictive changes, with reduced total lung capacity, decreased residual volume, decreased functional residual capacity, and a reduced ratio of residual to total lung capacity, in 21 patients with cirrhosis, 13 of whom had mild and 8 severe ascites. Mild airflow limitation may also be present in such patients, but the restrictive defects dominate.[106]

Airflow limitation and gas trapping in the lung bases also occurs in the absence of pleural effusion or ascites.[93,108] Furukuwa et al. were unable to find any evidence of restrictive pulmonary defects in 105 cirrhotics without ascites, but showed reductions in PEF25 (peak expiratory flow rates at 25% of vital capacity) suggesting small airway obstruction in most of these patients.[93]

Increased closing volumes (CV) have also been found in cirrhotic patients in the absence of cardiopulmonary disease, ascites or pleural effusions.[93,107,108] Ruff et al. demonstrated closing volumes above functional residual capacity (FRC) in 9 out of 11 patients, one of whom was an 11-year-old girl.[108] This increase was similar in smokers and nonsmokers, suggesting that smoking was not responsible for the alterations. Regional ventilation and perfusion studies in the 5 most severely hypoxemic patients (mean PaO_2 56.2 mmHg), confirmed a $\dot{V}/\dot{Q}$ ratio of below 0.5 at the lung bases, suggesting that gas trapping occurred predominantly in these regions. The severity of hypoxemia did not appear to correlate with the severity of the liver disease. The authors suggest that in cirrhosis, gas trapping in the lower zones, both at residual volume and at functional residual capacity, results from premature airway closure, and produces very low regional $\dot{V}/\dot{Q}$ ratios, thereby contributing significantly to hypoxemia. They speculate that airway closure may be due to inapparent interstitial pulmonary edema, or to compression of small airways by dilated blood vessels in these well perfused basal segments. None of the patients studied by Ruff et al. had ascites.

Furukuwa et al.[93] studied 105 cirrhotic patients and compared these to 100 male and 100 female controls. All of their cirrhotic patients had varices and 30% had hypoxemia. Closing volume to residual volume ratios were significantly increased in both male and female cirrhotic patients. The value for functional residual capacity minus closing capacity (FRC − CC) was significantly reduced in the cirrhotic group (190 ± 320 vs. 720 ± 410 ml in males; 170 ± 320 vs. 650 ± 390 ml in females). Furthermore, cirrhotic patients with hypoxemia had significantly higher CV/VC ratios (33.1 ± 7.5% vs. 29.5 ± 7.2, $p < 0.05$) and FRC − CC values (-90 ± 262 vs. 317 ± 363, $p < .001$) than normoxemic patients with cirrhosis. The negative values for FRC − CC in hypoxemic cirrhotics confirm that airway closure occurs prematurely in the lung bases under conditions of resting ventilation. Ventilation perfusion mismatching in these zones may lead to hypoxemia. This opinion is supported to some extent by the finding of a positive correlation between the FRC − CC values and PaO_2 (r = 0.62).[93]

b. Impairment of Hypoxic Vasoconstrictor Response and Altered Pulmonary Hemodynamics

In addition to the changes in regional ventilation described above, ventilation/perfusion mismatching in cirrhosis may be caused by alterations in pulmonary vascular reflexes. This has been examined by Rodriguez-Roisin et al.[14] using the multiple inert gas elimination technique coupled with hemodynamic measurements during hypoxic and hyperoxic conditions. Patients with cirrhosis were divided into two groups according to the presence or absence of multiple spider nevi. The study provides one of the most useful descriptions of the altered physiological changes in cirrhotics as a group. Clear-cut differences between those with cutaneous spider nevi and those without were shown. All 15 patients studied had well-compensated cirrhosis with no evidence of fluid retention, ascites or cardiopulmonary disease, but under basal conditions they had a mild to moderate hyperkinetic circulatory state, reduced systemic and pulmonary vascular resistance, and mild hypocapnia. Only two subjects were slightly hypoxemic (75.9 and 78.8 mmHg), the other 13 having PaO_2 values greater than 80 mmHg. There was little evidence of shunting (range 0 to 7.8%) breathing room air, but the percentage of the total perfusion ($\dot{Q}_t$) to poorly ventilated areas was mildly increased (mean 5%; range 0 to 20%). These data suggest that, at least in well-compensated cirrhosis, anatomical shunts, as described by Rydell et al.,[129] Calabresi et al.,[130] and others,[131-137] are uncommon and functionally insignificant. To examine whether the excess perfusion to low $\dot{V}/\dot{Q}$ areas was primarily due to a ventilation or perfusion abnormality, the $\dot{V}/\dot{Q}$ ratio at mean of blood flow distribution ($\bar{Q}$) and ventilatory ($\bar{V}$) distribution was determined. The $\dot{V}/\dot{Q}$ ratio was slightly less than normal at the mean of the blood flow distribution (range, 0.36 to 1.3), but was normal at the mean of ventilatory distribution. In addition, the dispersion of blood flow distribution to areas of varying V/Q ratio (log SD Q), was wider than normal. No correlation was found between expiratory rate at 75% of vital capacity (V_{75}) and either PaO_2, or the dispersion of blood flow distribution (logSD Q). Taken together, these findings strongly suggest that the V/Q disturbance found in these patients is due primarily to maldistribution of blood flow, to areas of low ventilation, and is not due primarily to a ventilatory disturbance.

Since hypoxic pulmonary vasoconstriction (HPV) is responsible for the normal reduction of blood flow to poorly ventilated areas, Rodriguez-Roisin et al. next examined pulmonary vascular reactivity.[14] This was achieved by measuring V/Q ratios and pulmonary artery pressure responses to breathing 11 and 98% oxygen. Normal control data were not given since patients acted as their own controls. There was a significant increase in mean PAP in response to breathing a mixture containing 11% oxygen, when compared to pressures measured while the patient was breathing room air (21% oxygen). Mean PAP rose from 6.3 ± 0.6 to 9.4 ± 0.8 mmHg, indicating that HPV does occur in these patients. However, when stressed with the 11% O_2 mixture, pulmonary vascular resistance rose by only 26.7 ± 4% in cirrhotic patients who were hypoxemic under basal conditions, as compared to 93.1 ± 10.8% in nonhypoxemic cirrhotic patients, indicating that the hypoxemic patients had relatively incomplete vascular responses to alveolar hypoxia. In addition, the normal improvement of V/Q distribution during hypoxic stress (on 11% O_2 mixture) was not seen in the hypoxemic cirrhotic patients. With hyperoxia (breathing a 98% O_2 mixture), small but significant shunts developed where previously absent, and where previously present, these increased, and the index of dispersion of blood flow distribution increased. These findings suggest that the blunted pulmonary vascular reactivity in cirrhotic patients is responsible for the V/Q mismatch observed. The data also suggest that ventilatory abnormalities do not contribute significantly to this mismatch. Significant pulmonary arteriovenous shunting, the presence of a diffusion barrier and altered Hb-O_2 affinity were all excluded as causes of hypoxemia in the patients studied, adding further weight to the authors' claim that the V/Q abnormality was responsible for the hypoxemia. The postulated mechanism for the V/Q abnormality is due to precapillary vasodilation. When patients with cutaneous spider nevi were compared to those without, the former had evidence of more systemic and pulmonary vasodilation, less hypoxic pulmonary vasoconstriction, and more V/Q mismatch. On breathing 98% oxygen, those with spider nevi had lower systemic and pulmonary vascular resistances, their V/Q relationships deteriorated, and shunt fractions increased. The authors suggest that the presence of spider nevi might be considered a valuable clinical marker of extrahepatic involvement and possible hemodynamic derangement.

The patients studied by Rodriguez-Roisin et al. had relatively mild liver disease, and were studied soon after clinical recovery from acute variceal bleeding. Thus it might not be appropriate to extrapolate their findings to all hypoxemic cirrhotic patients. The absence of a control group consisting of normal subjects is unfortunate since this limits the interpretation of data from the nonhypoxemic cirrhotic patients, and it is unclear whether their pulmonary vascular responses are entirely normal. It is possible that more severe hypoxemia may result from the progression of these pulmonary vascular abnormalities or from other factors such as the development of anatomical shunts. It is also unclear whether the effects on the pulmonary vascular bed are dependent on the duration or severity of the liver disease.

The extent of the difference in hypoxic pulmonary vasoconstriction between volunteers with normal livers and patients with severe alcoholic cirrhosis and hypoxemia, was established in a study by Daoud et al.[16] These cirrhotic patients had more severe hypoxemia than those studied by Rodriguez-Roisin et al.[14] and all had increased cardiac output and decreased pulmonary vascular resistance. In the cirrhotic group, the mean pulmonary artery pressure minus pulmonary capillary wedge pressure rose by only 11.8% in response to hypoxia compared to 158% in the 18 control patients. The control group included patients with many features also seen in liver disease, such as anemia, high cardiac output, and alkalosis, suggesting that these factors are not responsible for the lack of hypoxic pulmonary vasoconstriction seen in cirrhotic patients.

Not all reports agree with the findings in the above studies. Naeije et al.[15] found normal responses to hypoxia in 24 patients with liver disease. These patients, however, were alcoholics, the nature of their liver disease was poorly defined, and it is not clear whether all had cirrhosis. Twenty-two had abnormal liver scans, 14 had biopsy proven cirrhosis, and 18 had varices. Thirty percent had a minimal response to alveolar hypoxia (breathing a 12.5% O_2 mixture), but in the group as a whole, the pulmonary vascular resistance increased by 50%. There was no control group. Thus, although the authors demonstrated a response to hypoxia in 70% of their patients, the lack of a control group precludes any comment on whether this response was normal.

In summary, there is increasing evidence that pulmonary vascular responses are abnormal, even at an early stage of liver disease, and that this may play a major role in producing $\dot{V}/\dot{Q}$ mismatch, and hence the hypoxemia commonly seen in cirrhosis. Much of the venous admixture formerly ascribed to anatomical shunts (see below), is probably due to the $\dot{V}/\dot{Q}$ mismatch, as shunts are not always demonstrated in patients with severe hypoxemia.[92]

C. INTRAPULMONARY SHUNTS AND PULMONARY "PERFUSION-DIFFUSION" ABNORMALITIES

Intrapulmonary shunting has been proposed as a cause of arterial hypoxemia in patients with cirrhosis. Different mechanisms may give rise to intrapulmonary shunting, including nonventilation of perfused gas exchange units, direct vascular communication between pulmonary artery and vein,[137] and poor contact of blood with alveolar gas because of abnormal capillaries (perfusion-diffusion defect).[94] The nature of the shunts in patients with liver disease remains controversial, because most studies have failed to distinguish between these types of defect.[94,95,98,102-104,113-117,138-143]

1. Anatomy of Intrapulmonary Shunts

Pre-capillary arteriovenous fistulas[95,109,110,129,132-134,144] and capillary and pre-capillary vasodilation[97,99,112,131] are the predominant lesions found in hypoxic patients with cirrhosis. In 1956 Rydell and Hoffbauer[129] first described the association of arteriovenous fistulas and liver disease, in a patient with juvenile cirrhosis. A plastic cast of the pulmonary vessels revealed direct pulmonary arteriovenous communications of the large vessels near the hilum, throughout the more peripheral pulmonary vascular bed and subpleurally. These channels had a diameter of up to 1 mm. Berthelot et al.[131] showed marked arterial dilatation of small pulmonary arteries in the lungs of 13 cirrhotic patients, but not in 7 controls. Marked pre-capillary vasodilatation, similar in structure to cutaneous spider nevi, was seen in six patients. Peripheral arteriovenous shunts were only apparent in 1 case. Karlish et al.[132] described similar changes in a 31-year-old patient with cirrhosis associated with cyanosis and clubbing. Apart from arterial dilatation, numerous arteriovenous communications were noted on the infra-hilar and diaphragmatic pleural surfaces.

2. Physiology of Intrapulmonary Shunts

The amount of blood passing through abnormal intrapulmonary vascular channels has been estimated by measuring the proportion of 20 to 50 μm technetium-99-labeled albumin macroaggregates (MAA) which escape trapping in the pulmonary circulation.[95,98,141-143,145,146] Up to 70% of MAA may pass through the pulmonary circulation in cirrhotic patients with severe hypoxemia, compared to 3 to 8% in controls.[142] Characteristically, such patients have abnormal diffusing capacities for carbon monoxide, but have normal spirometry and lung mechanics and the closing volumes may also be normal. Cardiac output is increased, pulmonary arterial pressures are normal, and PaO_2 falls significantly in the upright position (orthodeoxia) and on exercise. Schomerus et al. suggested that abnormal pulmonary capillary vasodilation may decrease diffusing capacity by increasing the distance gas has to diffuse to reach erythrocytes at the center of the column of blood.[140] The increased cardiac output[138,147] causes an apparent aggravation of diffusion defect by reducing the capillary transit time, which results in insufficient exposure time of the capillary blood to the alveolus to become fully oxygenated, an effect that worsens on exercise.[94] The resulting abnormality has been called a diffusion/perfusion defect (alveolar capillary oxygen dysequilibrium) by Davis.[99]

D. PORTAPULMONARY SHUNTS

Several groups have examined the possible role of portapulmonary shunts as a cause of the hypoxemia associated with cirrhosis.[130,148-150] Calabresi and Abelmann[130] performed autopsy studies on 10 patients with severe, decompensated cirrhosis, 6 patients with heart failure, and 4 patients without cardiorespiratory disease. Portapulmonary venous anastomoses were demonstrated in two of the cirrhotic group. Unfortunately, data on blood flow and blood gases were not available. Shaldon et al.,[100] using radioactive krypton (^{85}Kr) in solution, injected intrasplenically and intravenously (antecubital vein), calculated the proportions of blood flowing through portapulmonary shunts in 12 patients with cirrhosis, four of whom had reduced SaO_2. Significant shunting was present in only one of the 12, and no correlation was found between oxygen desaturation and the proportion of shunted blood. Similar results were obtained by Williams and Abelmann,[148] who used indicator dilution techniques in 5 patients with cirrhosis and found portapulmonary shunting in one. The authors calculated that 27% of portal blood flow, equivalent to 6.8% of the cardiac output, passed through this shunt. Nakamura et al.,[149] using ^{85}Kr, found significant portapulmonary venous shunting in 2 of 12 patients with cirrhosis, the maximum shunt being 14.4% of portal blood flow. Once again there was no correlation between the size of the shunt and the degree of desaturation. Mellemgaard et al.[103] demonstrated portapulmonary shunts in 6 of 19 patients with cirrhosis, by means of an insoluble inert gas elimination technique. However, quantitative analyses revealed that these shunts were of an insignificant size. Similar results were obtained by Fritts et al.[151] following duodenal instillation of ^{85}Kr.

It therefore appears that portapulmonary venous anastomoses are found in a small proportion of patients with cirrhosis and are generally not large enough to account for the hypoxia of liver disease. Furthermore, none of the reported studies have shown a correlation between portapulmonary shunts and the presence or degree of hypoxia.

E. TREATMENT OF HYPOXEMIA OF LIVER DISEASE

Detailed investigations should be undertaken in all hypoxemic patients, to delineate potentially reversible defects, and because the finding of intrapulmonary shunting has major implications for therapy. Intrapulmonary vascular abnormalities may be confirmed by ^{131}I-MAA pulmonary perfusion scanning and measuring peripheral dispersion of the labeled particles,[95,142] or by two-dimensional echocardiography, following intravenous injection of echo-dense contrast media, such as saline or indocyanine green.[152,153]

Management of severe hypoxemia is difficult. High flow rates of supplemental oxygen may improve patients symptomatically,[95,137] but there is no evidence that it affects the prognosis. Almitrine bismesylate, which alters $\dot{V}/\dot{Q}$ relationships in obstructive airways disease, was given to five patients with severe hypoxemia; one patient improved symptomatically on high doses of the drug and showed an improvement in PaO_2, one patient got worse, and in three there was no effect.[97] Severe hypoxemia may or may not be considered an absolute contraindication to liver transplantation,[154] because this does not appear to reverse the intrapulmonary shunting in patients with severe capillary abnormalities.[155,156] Transplantation in hypoxemic patients may be dangerous, since air embolism from the surgical venous beds may reach the cerebral circulation, leading to stroke.[157] However, transplantation has been shown to improve ventilatory control and alveolar-oxygen difference in 16 patients who did not have severe hypoxemia,[158] indicating that some of the pulmonary vascular effects of liver disease are potentially reversible with liver transplantation.

IV. THE PULMONARY VASCULAR EFFECTS OF SCLEROTHERAPY

The acute and long-term effects of sclerotherapy on the pulmonary vasculature are poorly documented. Radiological studies have shown that pulmonary changes occur within 48 h after sclerotherapy of esophageal varices. Subsegmental atelectasis, dilation of peripheral vessels, and irregular nodular densities have been demonstrated using computed tomography, in patients injected with ethanolamine oleate.[159] Various irregular nodular and linear densities, segmental and subsegmental atalectasis, and pleural effusions have been described on routine chest X-rays of patients receiving sodium morrhuate.[160]

In a prospective study of 11 patients undergoing esophageal injection sclerotherapy, less than 20% of injected sodium morrhuate reached the pulmonary circulation, and no changes in diffusing capacity were documented, suggesting that sclerotherapy does not have a significant effect on the lungs.[161] Monroe el al., however, reported that 2 of 30 patients developed acute respiratory failure within 36 h of receiving sodium morrhuate esophageal injection therapy. In order to assess whether the sclerosant could have caused this acute noncardiogenic pulmonary edema, the authors studied the pulmonary effects of intravenously injected sodium morrhuate in sheep. Transient pulmonary hypertension and increased flow of protein-poor lymphatic fluid from the lungs occurred, suggesting that the sclerosant may have caused the pulmonary edema.[162] This is a rare complication of sclerotherapy, and other factors, such as aspiration, may play a role. Cacciola et al.[163] have shown that sclerosants may cause contact activation of blood coagulation, which Musso et al.[164] postulate may lead indirectly to pulmonary vascular damage. There is currently no information available on the long-term effects of esophageal injection sclerotherapy on pulmonary function or the pulmonary vasculature.

V. CONCLUSION

In this review of the pulmonary circulation in chronic liver disease, we have cited the principal studies performed to date. These have shown that pulmonary hypertension and hypoxemia are not infrequently seen in patients with cirrhosis. As indicated, there is increasing evidence in both animals and man that portapulmonary hypertension is related to portal systemic shunting rather than to intrinsic liver disease. In contrast, hypoxemia does appear to be related to intrinsic liver disease. The two entities seldom occur together, and the pulmonary vascular resistance of patients with hypoxemia tends to be low. Intrinsic hepatocyte dysfunction appears to be a prerequisite for the development of the hypoxemia, while the role of portal hypertension may be permissive. No serial studies have been done, but the changes leading to hypoxia appear to occur early in the course of the liver disease. It is unclear whether the hypoxemia correlates with the severity of the liver disease or its duration. The hypoxemia associated with liver disease has a poorly understood natural history, obscure etiology, and complex pathophysiology, involving disturbances in ventilation-perfusion and diffusion-perfusion relationships, and is difficult to treat.

REFERENCES

1. **Bayley, T. J., Segel, N., and Bishop, J. M.,** The circulatory changes in patients with cirrhosis at rest and during exercise, *Clin. Sci.,* 26, 227, 1964.
2. **Lebrec, D., Capron, J.-P., Dhumeaux, D., and Benhamou, J.-P.,** Pulmonary hypertension complicating portal hypertension, *Am. Rev., Respir. Dis.,* 120, 849, 1979.
3. **Levine, O. R., Harris, R. C., Blanc, W. A., and Mellins, R. B.,** Progressive pulmonary hypertension children with portal hypertension *J. Ped.,* 83, 964, 1973.
4. **Mantz, F. A. and Craige, E.,** Portal axis thrombosis with spontaneous portacaval shunt and resultant cor pulmonale, *AMA Arch. Pathol.,* 52, 91, 1951.
5. **Matsubara, O., Nakamura, T., Uehara, T., and Kasuga, T.,** Histometrical investigation of the pulmonary artery in severe liver disease, *J. Pathol.,* 143, 31, 1984.
6. **Morrison, E. B., Gaffney, F. A., Eigenbrodt, E. H., Reynolds, R. C., and Buja, L. M.,** Severe pulmonary hypertension associated with macronodular (postnecrotic) cirrhosis and autoimmune phenomena, *Am. J. Med.,* 69, 513, 1980.
7. **Naeye, R. L.,** Primary pulmonary hypertension with coexisting portal hypertension. A retrospective study of six cases, *Circulation,* 22, 376, 1960.
8. **Ruttner, J. R., Bartschi, J.-P., Niedermann, R., and Schneider, J.,** Plexogenic pulmonary arteriopathy and liver cirrhosis, *Thorax,* 35, 133, 1980.
9. **Senior, R. M., Britton, R. C., Turino, G. M., Wood, J. A., Langer, G. A., and Fishman, A. P.,** Pulmonary hypertension associated with cirrhosis of the liver and with portacaval shunts, *Circulation,* 37, 88, 1968.
10. **McDonnell, P. J., Toye, P. A., and Hutchins, G. M.,** Primary pulmonary hypertension and cirrhosis: are the related?, *Am. Rev. Respir. Dis.,* 127, 437, 1983.
11. **Lai, K. S., McFadzean, A. J. S., and Yeung, R.,** Microembolic pulmonary hypertension in pyogenic cholangitis, *Br. Med. J.,* 1, 22, 1968.
12. **Currie, P. J., Seward, J. B., Chan, K. L., Fyfe, D. A., Hagler, D. J., Mair, D. D., Reeder, G. S., Nashimura, R. A., and Tajik, A. J.,** Continuous wave Doppler determination of right venticular pressure: a simultaneous Doppler-catheterization study in 127 patients, *J. Am. Coll. Cardiol.,* 6, 750, 1985.
13. **O'Brien, J. A., Morrison, S. C., Raine, R. I., Benatar, S. R., and Kirsch, R. E.,** The role of portal hypertension in the pathogenesis of pulmonary abnormalities associated with chronic liver disease, submitted.
14. **Rodriguez-Roisin, R., Roca, J., Agusti, A. G. N., Mastai, R., Wagner, P. D., and Bosch, J.,** Gas exchange and pulmonary vascular reactivity in patients with liver cirrhosis, *Am. Rev. Respir. Dis.,* 135, 1085, 1987.
15. **Naeije, R., Hallemans, R., Mols, P., and Melot, C.,** Hypoxic pulmonary vasoconstriction in liver cirrhosis, *Chest,* 80, 570, 1981.
16. **Daoud, F. S., Reeves, J. T., and Schaefer, J. W.,** Failure of hypoxic pulmonary vasoconstriction in patients with liver cirrhosis, *J. Clin. Invest.,* 51, 1076, 1972.
17. **Massumi, R. A., Rios, J. C., and Ticktin, H. E.,** Hemodynamic abnormalities and venous admixture in portal cirrhosis, *Am. J. Med., Sci.,* 250, 275, 1965.
18. **Schaefer, J. W. and Reeves, J. T.,** The lung and the liver (editorial), *Chest,* 80(5), 526, 1981.
19. **Edwards, B. S., Weir, E. K., Edwards, W. D., Ludwig, J., Dykoski, R. K., and Edwards, J. E.,** Coexistent pulmonary and portal hypertension: morphological and clinical features, *J. Am. Coll. Cardiol.,* 10, 1233, 1987.
20. **Boot, H., Visser, F. C., Thijs, J. C., and Meuwissen, S. G. M.,** Pulmonary hypertension complicating portal hypertension. A case report with suggestions for a different therapeutic approach, *Eur. Heart J.,* 8, 656, 1987.
21. **Cohen, M. D., Rubin, L. J., Taylor, W. E., and Cuthbert, J. A.,** Primary pulmonary hypertension: an unusual case associated with extrahepatic portal hypertension, *Hepatology,* 3, 588, 1983.
22. **Sallam, E. and Watson, W. C.,** Pulmonary hypertension due to micro-thromboembolism for splenic and portal veins after portal anastomosis, *Br. Heart J.,* 32, 269, 1970.
23. **Yutani, C., Imakita, M., Ishibashi-ueda, H. et al.,** Nodular regenerative hyperplasia of the liver associated with primary pulmonary hypertension, *Hum. Pathol.,* 19, 726, 1988.
24. **Cohn, R.,** The relationship of cardiac hypertrophy to cirrhosis of the liver, *Surgery,* 46(5), 887, 1959.
25. **Lunseth, J. H.,** Cardiac hypertrophy in rats, *Arch Pathol.,* 79, 644, 1965.
26. **Voigt, M. C., Bateman, E. D., Adams, L. P., Engelbrecht, G., and Kirsch, R. E.,** Pulmonary hypertension in porta-caval shunted rats (Abstr.), *Hepatology,* 8, 1391, 1988.
27. **Rabinovitch, M., Bothwell, T., Hayakawa, B. N., Williams, W. G., Trusler, G. A., Rowe, R. D., Olley, P. M., and Cutz, E.,** Pulmonary artery endothelial abnormalities, in patients with congenital heart defects and pulmonary hypertension, *Lab. Invest.,* 55(6), 632, 1986.

28. **Mukada, T., Itsaka, K., Miyazaki, S., Hirikawa, H., Kashiwagura, J., Sasaki, Y., Andoh, S., Shinzawa, A., and Sendoh, F.,** Pulmonary hypertension with liver cirrhosis and hepatitis-B antigenemia, *Tohoku J. Exp. Med.,* 139, 83, 1983.
29. **Triger, D. R., Alp, M. H., and Wright, R.,** Bacterial and dietary antibodies in liver disease, *Lancet,* i, 60, 1972.
30. **Bjorneboe, M., Prytz, H., and Orskov, F.,** Antibodies to intestinal microbes in serum of patients with cirrhosis of the liver, *Lancet,* i, 58, 1972.
31. **Liehr, H., Grun, M., and Brunswig, D.,** Endotoxaemia in acute hepatic failure, *Acta Hepata-Gastroenterol.,* 23, 235, 1976.
32. **Wardle, E. N.,** Fibrinogen in liver disease, *Arch. Surg.,* 109, 741, 1974.
33. **Wilkinson, S. P., Arroyo, V., Gazzard, B. G., Moodie, H., and Williams, R.,** Relation of renal impairment and haemorrhagic diathesis to endotoxaemia in fulminant hepatic failure, *Lancet,* 1, 522, 1974.
34. **Trewby, P. N., Waren, R., Contini, S., Crosbie, W. A., Wilkinson, S. P., Laws, J. W., and Williams, R.,** Incidence and pathophysiology of pulmonary edema in fulminant hepatic failure, *Gastroenterology,* 74(5), 859, 1978.
35. **Prytz, H., Holst-Christensen, J., Korner, B., and Liehr, H.,** Portal venous and systemic endotoxaemia in patients without liver disease and systemic endotoxaemia in patients with cirrhosis, *Scand J. Gastroentaerology,* 11, 857, 1976.
36. **Wilkinson, S. P., Moodie, H., Stamatakis, J. D., Kakkar, V. V., and Williams, R.,** Endotoxaemia and renal failure in cirrhosis and obstructive jaundice, *Brit. Med. J.,* 2, 1415, 1976.
37. **Brigham, K. L. and Meyrick B.,** Endotoxin and lung injury, *Am. Rev. Respir. Dis.,* 133, 913, 1986.
38. **Herget, J., Palecek, F., Preclik, P., Cermakova, M., Vizek, M., and Petrovicke, M.,** Pulmonary hypertension induced by repeated pulmonary inflammation in the rat, *J. Appl. Physiol.,* 51(3), 755, 1981.
39. **Kirton, O. O., and Jones, R.,** Rat pulmonary artery restructuring and pulmonary hypertension induced by continuous *Escherichia coli* infusion, *Lab. Invest.,* 56(2), 198, 1987.
40. **Meyrick B. and Brigham, K.,** Repeated inflammation of the lung by *E. coli* endotoxin leads to structural and functional changes of sustained pulmonary hypertension, *Am. Rev. Respir. Dis.,* 131, 4398, 1985.
41. **Reeves, J. T., Daoud, F. S., and Estridge, M.,** Endotoxin: a cause of spontaneous pulmonary hypertension in cattle?, *Am. J. Vet. Res.,* 34, 1573, 1973.
42. **Reeves, J. T., Daoud, F. S., and Estridge, M.,** Pulmonary hypertension caused by minute amounts of endotoxin in calves, *J. Appl. Physiol.,* 33, 739, 1971.
43. **Kuida, H., Hinshaw, L. B., Gilert, R. P., and Visscher, M. B.,** Effect of gram negative endotoxin on the pulmonary circulation, *Am. J. Physiol.,* 192, 335, 1958.
44. **Maitra, S. K., Rachmilewitz, D., Eberle, D., and Kaplowitz, N.,** The hepatocellular uptake and biliary excretion of endotoxin in the rat, *Hepatology,* 1(5), 401, 1981.
45. **Kerbel, N. C.,** Pulmonary hypertension and portal hypertension, *Can. Med. Assoc. J.,* 87, 1022, 1962.
46. **Geggel, R. L., Carvalho, A. C., Hoyer, L. W., Reid, L. M.,** Von Willebrand factor abnormalities in primary pulmonary hypertension, *Am. Rev. Respir. Dis.,* 135, 294, 1987.
47. **Kruskal, J. B., Robson, S. C., Kirsch, R. E.,** An analysis of fibrin and fibrinogen related antigens in liver disease, *S. Afr. Med. J.,* 72, 67, 1987.
48. **Franks, W. T. and Kirsch, R. E.,** unpublished data.
49. **Eisenberg, P. R., Rich, S., Kaufmann, L., and Jaffe, A. S.,** Evidence for increased thrombin activity in patients with primary pulmonary hypertension, *Circulation,* 76, 1246, 1987.
50. **Franz, R. C., Ziady, F., Coetzee, W. J. C., and Hugo, N.,** A possible relationship between defective fibrinolusis and pulmonary hypertension, *S. Aft. Med. J.,* 55, 170, 1979.
51. **Reid, L. M.,** The pulmonary circulation: remodelling in growth and disease; The 1978 J. Burns Amberson Lecture, *Am. Rev. Respir. Dis.,* 119, 531, 1979.
52. **Geer, J. C., Glass, B. A., Albert, H. M.,** The morphogenesis and reversibility of experimental hyperkinetic pulmonary vascular lesions in the dog, *Exp. Mol. Pathol.,* 4, 399, 1965.
53. **Kay, J. M. and Heath, D.,** Observations on the pulmonary arteries and heart weight of rats fed on *Crotolaria spectabilis* seeds, *J. Pathol. Bact.,* 92, 385, 1966.
54. **Heath, D. and Kay, J. M.,** Medial thickness of pulmonary trunk in rats with cor pulmonale induced by ingestion of *Crotolaria spectabilis* seeds, *Cardiovasc. Res.,* 1, 74, 1967.
55. **Kay, J. M., Harris, P., and Heath, D.,** Pulmonary hypertension produced in rats by ingestion of *Crotolaria spectabilis* seeds, *Thorax,* 22, 176, 1967.
56. **Meyrick B. and Reid, L.,** Development of pulmonary arterial changes in rats fed *Crotolaria spectabilis, Am J. Pathol.,* 94, 37, 1979.
57. **Burns, J.,** The heart and pulmonary arteries in rats fed on *Senechio jacobaea. J. Pathol.,* 106, 187, 1972.
58. **Smith, P., Moosavi, H., Winson, M., and Heath, D.,** The influence of age and sex on the response of the right ventricle, pulmonary vasculature and carotid bodies to hypoxia in rats, *J. Pathol.,* 112, 11, 1974.
59. **Rabinovitch, M., Gamble, W., Nadas, A., Miettinen, O. S., and Reid, L.,** Rat pulmonary circulation after chronic hypoxia: hemodynamic and structural features, *Am. J. Physiol.,* 236(6), H818, 1979.

60. **Hislop, A. and Reid, L.,** New findings in pulmonary arteries of rats with hypoxia induced pulmonary hypertension, *Br. J. Exp. Pathol.,* 57, 542, 1976.
61. **Jones, R., Zapol, W. M., and Reid, L.,** Pulmonary artery remodelling and pulmonary hypertension after exposure to hyperoxia for 7 days. A morphometric and hemodynamic study, *Am. J. Pathol.,* 117, 273, 1984.
62. **Meyrick B. and Brigham, K. L.,** Repeated *Escherichia coli* endotoxin-induced pulmonary inflammation causes chronic pulmonary hypertension in sheep, *Lab. Invest.,* 55(2), 164, 1986.
63. **Sobin, S. S., Tremer, H. M., Hardy, J. D., and Chiodi, H. P.,** Changes in arteriole in acute and chronic hypoxic pulmonary hypertension and recovery in rat, *J. Appl. Physiol.,* 55(5), 1445, 1983.
64. **Edwards, W. D.,** Pathology of pulmonary hypertension, *Cardiovasc, Clinics,* 18, 321, 1988.
65. **Haworth, S. G.,** Primary pulmonary hypertension (editorial), *Br. Heart J.,* 49, 517, 1983.
66. **Haworth, S. G., Hislop, A., and Reid, L.,** Progressive pulmonary hypertension in children with portal hypertension, (editorial), *J. Pedriatrics,* 84, 783, 1974.
67. **Wilson, A. G., Harris, C. N., Lavender, J. P., and Oakley, C. M.,** Perfusion lung scanning in obliterative pulmonary hypertension, *Br. Heart H.,* 35, 917, 1973.
68. **Fishman, A. J., Moser, K. M., Fedullo, P. F.,** Perfusion lung scans vs pulmonary angiography in evaluation of suspected primary pulmonary hypertension, *Chest,* 84, 679, 1983.
69. **Chapman, P. J.,** Diagnostic, prognostic and therapeutic considerations in primary pulmonary hypertension, MMed thesis submitted to the University of Cape Town, Cape Town, 1988.
70. **Fuster, V., Steele, P. M., Edwards, W. D., Gersh, B. J., McGoon, M. D., and Frye, R. L.,** Primary pulmonary hypertension: natural history and the importance of thrombosis, *Circulation,* 70, 580, 1984.
71. **Rubri, L. J., Nicod, P., Hillis, L. D., and Firth, B. G.,** Treatment of primary pulmonary hypertension with nifedipine, *Ann. Intern. Med.,* 99, 433, 1983.
72. **Wise, J. R.,** Nifedipine in the treatment of primary pulmonary hypotension, *Am. Heart. J.,* 105, 693, 1983.
73. **Rich, S., Mortinez, J., Lam, W., and Rosen, K. M.,** Captopril as treatment for patients with pulmonary hypertension: problem of variability in assessing chronic drug treatment, *Br. Heart J.,* 48, 272, 1982.
74. **Berkenboom, G., Sobolski, J., Stoupel. E.,** Failure of Nifedipine treatment in primary pulmonary hypertension, *Br. Heart H.,* 42, 511, 1982.
75. **Lupi-Herrera, E., Biolostozky, D., and Sobruvo, A.,** The role of isoproterenol in pulmonary artery hypertension of unknown etiology (primary), *Chest,* 79, 292, 1981.
76. **Pearl, R. G., Rosenthal, M. H., Schroeder, J. S., and Ashtar, J. P. A.,** Acute hemodynamic effects of nitroglycerin in pulmonary hypertension, *Ann. Intern. Med.,* 99, 9, 1983.
77. **Rubov, L. J. and Peter, R. H.,** Oral hydralazine therapy for primary pulmonary hypertension, *N. Engl. J. Med.,* 302, 69, 1980.
78. **Hall, D. R. and Petch, M.,** Remission of primary pulmonary hypertension during treatment with diazoxide, *Br. Med. J.,* 282, 1118, 1981.
79. **Lupi-Herrera, E., Sandoval, J., Seoane, M., and Biolostozky, D.,** The role of hydralazine therapy for pulmonary arterial hypertension of unknown cause, *Circulation,* 65, 645, 1982.
80. **Comerini, F., Alberti, E., Klugmann, S., and Salvi, A.,** Primary pulmonary hypertension: effects of nifedipine, *Br. Heart J.,* 44, 352, 1980.
81. **DeFeyter, P. J., Kerkkamp, H. J. J., and DeJong, J. P.,** Sustained beneficial effect of nifedipine in primary pulmonary hypertension, *Am. Heart J.,* 105, 333, 1983.
82. **Pacher, M., Greenberg, B., Massie, B., and Dash, H.,** Deleterious effects of hydralazine in patients with pulmonary hypertension, *N. Engl. J. Med.,* 306, 1362, 1982.
83. **Kronzon, I., Cohen, M., and Wiver, H. E.,** Adverse effect of hydralazine in patients with primary pulmonary hypertension, *JAMA,* 247, 3112, 1982.
84. **Daoud, F. S., Kelly, D. B., and Reeves, J. T.,** Isoproterenol as a potential pulmonary vasodilator in primary pulmonary hypertension, *Am. J. Cardiol.,* 42, 817, 1978.
85. **Kambara, H., Fujimoto, K., Wakabayashi, A., and Kawai, C.,** Primary pulmonary hypertension: beneficial therapy with diltiazem, *Am. Heart J.,* 101, 230, 1981.
86. **Leier, C. Y., Bambach, D., Nelson, S. et al.,** Captopril in primary pulmonary hypertension, *Circulation,* 67, 155, 1983.
87. **Buch, J. and Wennevold, A.,** Hazards of diazoxide in pulmonary hypertension, *Br. Heart J.,* 46, 401, 1981.
88. **Higenbottam, T., Wheeldon, D., Wells, F., and Wallwark, J.,** Long-term treatment of primary pulmonary hypertension with continuous intravenous epeprostenol (prostacyclin), *Lancet,* i, 1046, 1984.
89. **Fluckiger, M.,** Vorkommen von trommelschlageformigen Fingerendphalangen ohne chronische Veranderungen an den Lungen oder am Herzen, *Wien. Med. Wochenschr.,* 34, 1458, 1988.
90. **Snell, A. M.,** The effects of chronic disease of the liver on the composition and physicochemical properties of blood: Changes in the serum proteins, reduction in the oxygen saturation of the arterial blood, *Ann. Int. Med.,* 9, 960, 1935.

91. **Keys, A. and Snell, A. M.**, Respiratory properties of arterial blood in normal man and patients with disease of the liver: position of the oxygen dissociation curve, *J. Clin. Invest.*, 17, 59, 1938.

92. **Rodman, R., Sobel, M., and Close, H.**, Arterial oxygen unsaturation and the ventilation-perfusion defect of Laennecs cirrhosis, *N. Engl. J. Med.*, 263(2), 73, 1960.

93. **Furukuwa, T., Hara, N., Yasumoto, K., and Inokuchi, K.**, Arterial hypoxemia in patients with hepatic cirrhosis, *Am. J. Med., Sci.*, 287(3), 10, 1984.

94. **Kennedy, T. C. and Knudson, R. J.**, Exercise aggravated hypoxemia and orthodeoxia in cirrhosis, *Chest*, 72, 305, 1977.

95. **Robin, E. D., Horn, B., Goris, M. L., Theodore, J., Van Kessel, A., Mazoub, J., and Tilkian A.**, Detection, quantification and pathophysiology of lung "spiders", *Trans. Assoc. Am. Phys.*, 88, 202, 1975.

96. **Robin, E. D., Laman, D., Horn, B. R., and Theodore, J.**, Platypnea related to orthodeoxia caused by true vascular lung shunts, *N. Engl. J. Med.*, 294, 941, 1976.

97. **Krowka, M. J. and Cortese, D. A.**, Severe hypoxemia associated with liver disease: Mayo clinic experience and experimental use of almitrine bismesylate, *Mayo Clin. Proc.*, 62, 164, 1987.

98. **Bank, E. R., Thrall, J. H., and Dantzker, D. R.**, Radionuclide demonstration of intrapulmonary shunting in cirrhosis, *Am. J. Radiol.*, 140, 967, 1983.

99. **Davis, H. H., Schwartz, D. J., Lefrak, S. S., Susman, N., and Shainker, B. A.**, Alveolar-capillary oxygen dysequilibrium in hepatic cirrhosis, *Chest*, 73, 507, 1978.

100. **Shaldon, S., Caesar, J., Chiandussi, L., Williams, H. S., Sheville, E., and Sherlock, S.**, The demonstration of porta-pulmonary anastomoses in portal cirrhosis with the use of radioactive krypton, *N. Engl. J. Med.*, 265(9), 410, 1961.

101. **Stanley, N. N., Ackrill, P., and Wood, J.**, Lung perfusion scanning in hepatic cirrhosis, *Br. Med. J.*, 4, 639, 1972.

102. **Georg, J., Mellemgaard, K., Tygstrup, N., and Winkler K.**, Venoarterial shunts in cirrhosis of the liver. *Lancet*, i, 852, 1960.

103. **Mellemgaard, K., Winkler, K., Tygstrup, N., and Georg, J.**, Sources of venoarterial admixture in portal hypertension, *J. Clin. Invest.*, 42(9), 1399, 1963.

104. **Stanley, N. N. and Woodgate, D. J.**, Mottled chest radiograph and gas transfer defect in chronic liver disease, *Thorax*, 27, 315, 1972.

105. **Golding, P. L., Smith, M., and Williams, R.**, Multisystem involvement in chronic liver disease: studies on the incidence and pathogenesis, *Am. J. Med. Sci.*, 55, 772, 1973.

106. **Yao, E. H., Kong, B., Hsue, G., Zhou, A., and Wang, H.**, Pulmonary function changes in cirrhosis of the liver. *Am. J. Gastroenterology*, 1987, 81(4), 352.

107. **Funuhashi, A., Ahamed, V., Kutty, V. P., and Prater, S. L.**, Hypoxemia and cirrhosis of the liver, *Thorax*, 31, 303, 1976.

108. **Ruff, F., Hughes, J. M. B., Stanley, D., McCarthy, D., Greene, R., Aronoff, A., Clayton, L., and Milic-Emili, J.**, Regional lung functions in patients with hepatic cirrhosis, *J. Clin. Invest.*, 1971, 50, 2403.

109. **Hansoti, R. C., and Shah, N. J.**, Cirrhosis of liver simulating congenital heart disease, *Circulation*, 1966, 33, 71.

110. **El Gamal, M., Stoker, J. B., Spiers, E. M., and Whitaker, W.**, Cyanosis complicating hepatic cirrhosis. Report of a case due to multiple arteriovenous fistulas, *Am. J. Cardiol.*, 25, 490, 1970.

111. **Heinemann, H. O., Emirgil, C., and Mijnssen, J. P.**, Hyperventilation and arterial hypoxemia in cirrhosis of the liver, *Am. J. Med.*, 28, 239, 1960.

112. **Caldwell, P. R. B., Fritts, H. W., and Cournard, A.**, Oxy-hemoglobin dissociation curve in liver cirrhosis, *J. Appl. Physiol.*, 20, 316, 1965.

113. **Astrup, J. and Rorth, M.**, Oxygen affinity and red cell 2,3 diphosphoglycerate in cirrhosis, *Scan. J. Clin. Lab. Invest.*, 31, 311, 1973.

114. **Rodman, T., Hurwitz, J. K., Pastor, B. H., and Close, H. P.**, Cyanosis and clubbing associated with Laennec's cirrhosis, *Am. J. Med., Sci.*, 238, 534, 1959.

115. **Balzer, G., Auer, H., Arndt, H., Englhardt, A., and Martini, G. A.**, Die intraerythrocytare Koncentration von 2,3 Diphosphoglycerat und ihre Beziehung zur Lage der O_2 Dissoziationskurve bei Patienten mit Leberzirrhose, *Verh. Dtsch. Ges. Inn. Med.*, 78, 249, 1972.

116. **Chiesa, A., Ciappi, G., Balbi, L., and Chiandussi, L.**, Role of various causes of arterial desaturation in liver cirrhosis, *Clin. Sci.*, 37, 803, 1969.

117. **Abelmann, W. H., Kramer, G. E., Verstraeten, J. M., Gravellese, M. A., and McNeely, W. F.**, Cirrhosis of the liver and decrease arterial oxygen saturation, *Arch. Int. Med.*, 108, 34, 1961.

118. **Frothingham, J. R.**, Cirrhosis of the liver complicated by persistent right hydrothorax and ascites, *N. Engl. J. Med.*, 226, 679, 1942.

119. **Emerson, P. A. and Davies, J. H.**, Hydrothorax complicating ascites, *Lancet*, 1, 487, 1955.

120. **Williams, M. H.**, Pleural effusion produced by adomino-pleural communication in a patient with Laennec's cirrhosis of the liver, *Ann. Int. Med.*, 33, 216, 1950.

121. **Johnston, R. F. and Loo, R. V.**, Hepatic hydrothorax: studies to determine the source of the fluid and report of thirteen cases, *Ann. Int.Med.*, 61, 385, 1964.

122. **Lieberman, F. L., Hidemura, R., Peters, R. L., and Reynolds, T. B.,** Pathogenesis and treatment of hydrothorax complicating cirrhosis with ascites, *Ann. Int. Med.,* 64, 341, 1966.

123. **Vargas-Tank, L., Escobar, C., Fernandez, G., Ritter, L., Soto, J. R., Jiron, M. I., and Armas-Merino, R.,** Massive pleural effusions in cirrhotic patients with ascites, *Scand. J. Gastroenterol.,* 19, 294, 1984.

124. **McKay, D. G., Sparling, H. J., and Robbins, S. L.,** Cirrhosis of the liver with massive hydrothorax, *Arch. Int. Med.,* 79, 501, 1947.

125. **Singer, J. A., Kaplan, M. M., and Katz, R. L.,** Cirrhotic pleural effusion in the absence of ascites, *Gastroenterology,* 73, 575, 1977.

126. **Faiyaz, U. and Goyal, P. C.,** Unilateral pleual effusion without ascites in liver cirrhosis, *Postgrad. Med.,* 74, 309, 1983.

127. **Gross, P. A. and Gerding, D. N.,** Pleural effusion associated with viral hepatitis, *Gastroenterology,* 60, 898, 1971.

128. **Fujiwara, K.,** Pulmonary function in patients with cirrhosis of the liver, *Jpn. J. Chest Dis.,* 41, 422, 1982.

129. **Rydell, R. and Hoffbauer, F. W.,** Multiple pulmonary arteriovenous fistulas in juvenile cirrhosis, *A.J. Med.,* 21, 450, 1956.

130. **Calabresi, P. and Abelmann, W. H.,** Porto-caval and porto-pulmonary anastomoses in Laennec's cirrhosis and in heart failure, *J. Clin. Invest.,* 36, 1257, 1957.

131. **Berthelot, P., Walker, J. G., Sherlock S., and Reid, L.,** Arterial changes in cirrhosis of the liver:-lung spider nevi, *N. Engl. J. Med.,* 274, 291, 1966.

132. **Karlish, A. J., Marshall, R., Reid, L., and Sherlock, S.,** Cyanosis with hepatic cirrhosis. A case with arteriovenous shunting, *Thorax,* 22, 555, 1967.

133. **Hutchison, D. C. S., Sapru, R. P., Summerling, M. D., Donaldson, G. W. K., and Richmond, J.,** Cirrhosis, cyanosis and polycythemia: multiple pulmonary arteriovenous anastomoses. Case Report, *Am. J. Med.,* 45, 139, 1968.

134. **Silverman, A., Cooper, M. D., Moller, J. H., Good, R. A.,** Syndrome of cyanosis, digital clubbing, and hepatic disease in siblings, *Pediatrics,* 72, 70, 1968.

135. **Kravath, R. E., Scarpelli, E. M., and Bernstein, J.,** Hepatogenic cyanosis: arteriovenous shunts in chronic active hepatitis, *J. Pediatr.,* 78, 238, 1971.

136. **Whitaker, W.,** Cyanosis complicating hepatic cirrhosis. Report of a case due to multiple arteriovenous fistulas, *Am. J. Cardiol.,* 25, 490, 1970.

137. **Robin, E. D., Laman, P. D., Goris, M. L., and Theodore, J.,** A shunt is (not) a shunt is (not) a shunt (Editorial), *Am. Rev. Respir. Dis.,* 115, 553, 1977.

138. **Murray, J. F., Dawson, A. M., and Sherlock S.,** Circulatory changes in chronic liver disease, *Am. J. Med.,* 24, 358, 1958.

139. **Willaims, M. H.,** Hypoxemia due to venous admixture in cirrhosis of the liver, *J. Appl. Physiol.,* 15(2), 253, 1960.

140. **Schomerus, H., Buchta, I., and Arndt, H.,** Pulmonary function studies and oxygen transfer in patients with liver cirrhosis and different degrees of portasystemic encephalopathy, *Respiration,* 32, 1, 1975.

141. **Dal Palu, C., Donaggio, G., Dal Zotto, I., and Pessina, A. C.,** Arteriovenous shunts in cirrhotic patients studied with human serum albumin macroaggregates tagged with ^{131}I (MAA^{131}I), *Scand. J. Gastroent.,* 3, 425, 1968.

142. **Wolfe, J. D., Tashkin, D. P., Brachman, M. B., and Genovesi, M. G.,** Hypoxemia of cirrhosis. Detection of abnormal pulmonary vascular channels by a quantitative radionuclide method, *Am. J. Med.,* 63, 746, 1977.

143. **Andersen, B. L., Gordon, L., and Buse, M. G.,** Intrapulmonary shunting associated with cirrhosis: Incidental diagnosis by perfusion lung scan, *Clin. Nucl. Med.,* 7, 108, 1982.

144. **Cotes, J. E., Field, G. B., Brown, G. J. A., and Read, A. E.,** Impairment of lung function after portacaval anastomosis, *Lancet,* i, 952, 1968.

145. **Keren, G., Boichis, H., Zwas, T. S., and Frand, M.,** Pulmonary arterio-venous fistulae in hepatic cirrhosis, *Arch. Dis. Child.,* 58, 302, 1983.

146. **Sang, O. K., Bender, T. M., Bowmen, A., and Kledesma-Medina, J.,** Plain radiographic, nuclear medicine and angiographic observations of hepatogenic pulmonary angiodysplasia, *Pediatr. Radiol.,* 13, 111, 1983.

147. **Kowalski, H. J., and Abelmann, W. H.,** The cardiac output at rest in Laennec's cirrhosis, *J. Clin. Invest.,* 32, 1025, 1953.

148. **Williams, J. H. and Abelmann, W. H.,** Portopulmonary shunts in patients with portal hypertension, *J. Lab. Clin. Med.,* 62,(5), 715, 1963.

149. **Nakamura, T., Nakamura, S., Tazawa, T., Abe, S., Aikawa, T., and Tokita, K.,** Measurement of blood flow through portapulmonary anastomosis in portal hypertension, *J. Lab. Clin. Med.,* 65(1), 114, 1965.

150. **Khaliq, S. U., Kay, J. M., and Heath, D.,** Porta-pulmonary venous anastomoses in experimental cirrhosis of the liver in rats, *J. Pathol.*, 107, 167, 1972.
151. **Fitts, H. W., Hardewig, A., Rochester, D. F., Durand, J., and Cournard, A.,** Estimation of pulmonary arteriovenous shunt flow using intravenous injections of T1842 dye and ^{85}Kr, *J. Clin. Invest.*, 39, 1841, 1960.
152. **Seward, J. B., Hayes, D. L., Smith, H. C., Williams, D. E., Rosenow, E. C., Reeder, G. S., Piehler, J. M., and Tajik, A. I. et al.,** Platypnoea-orthodeoxia: clinical profile, diagnostic workup, management, and report of 7 cases, *Mayo Clin. Proc.*, 59, 221, 1984.
153. **Seward, J. B., Tajik, A. J., Hagler, D. J., and Rittner, D. G.,** Peripheral venous contrast echocardiography, *Am. J. Cardiol.*, 39, 202, 1977.
154. **Bussitil, R. W.,** Preoperative concerns and surgical technique, in Liver transplantation today, Bussitil, R. W., Moderator, *Ann Int Med*, 104, 377, 1986.
155. **Van Thiel, D. H., Schade, R. R., Gavaler, J. S., Shaw, B. W., Iwatsuki, S., and Starzl, T. E.,** Medical aspects of liver transplantation, *Hepatology*, 4 (Suppl.), 79, 1984.
156. **Iwatsuki, S., Shaw, B. W., and Starzl, T. E.,** Current status of hepatic transplantation, *Semin. Liver Dis.*, 3, 173, 1983.
157. **Starzl, T. E., Koep, L. J., Halgrimson, C. G., Hood, J., Schroter, G. P. J., Porter, K. A., and Weil, R.,** Fifteen years of liver transplantation, *Gastroenterology*, 77, 375, 1979.
158. **Hagenah, C. and Sybrecht, G. W.,** Disturbances of respiration of patients before and after liver transplantation, *Respiration*, 52, 290, 1987.
159. **Ikezoe, J., Morimoto, S., Arisawa, J., Takashima, S., Tomado, K., Nakanishi, K., Kodawaki, K., Kozuka, T., Shiozaki, H., and Ogawa, Y.,** Computed tomography following endoscopic sclerotherapy of esophageal varices, *Acta Radiol.*, 28, 415, 1987.
160. **Saks, B. J., Kilby, A. E., Dietrich, P. A., Coffin, L. H., and Krawitt, E. L.,** Pleural and mediastinal changes following endoscopic injection sclerotherapy of esophageal varices, *Radiology*, 149, 639, 1983.
161. **Connors, A. F., Bacon, B. R., and Miron, S. D.,** Sodium morrhuate delivery to the lung during endoscopic variceal sclerotherapy, *Ann. Int. Med.*, 105, 539, 1986.
162. **Monroe, P., Morrow, C. F., Millen, J. E., Fairman, R. P., and Glauser, F. L.,** Acute respiratory failure after sodium morrhuate esophageal sclerotherapy, *Gastroenterology*, 85, 693, 1983.
163. **Cacciola, E., Guistolisi, R., and Musso, R.,** Activation of contact phase of blood coagulation can be induced by the sclerosing agent polidocanol: possible additional mechanism of adverse reaction during sclerotherapy, *J. Lab. Clin. Med.*, 109, 225, 1987.
164. **Musso, R., Guistolisi, R., and Cacciola, E.,** Acute respiratory distress after sclerotherapy for esophageal varices, *Ann. Int. Med.*, 106, 640, 1987.
165. **Dewhurst, N. G., Colledge, N. R., and Miller, H. C.,** Severe pulmonary hypertension and multiple left coronary arterial fistulas in association with congenital hepatic fibrosis, *Br. Heart J.*, 58, 525, 1987.
166. **Lal, S. and Fletcher, E.,** Pulmonary hypertension and portal venous system thrombosis, *Br. Heart J.*, 1968, 723, 30.
167. **Pare, P. D., Chan, Yan, C., Wass, H., Hooper, R., and Hogg, J. C.,** Portal and pulmonary hypertension with microangiopathic hemolytic anemia, *Am. J. Med.*, 74, 1093, 1983.
168. **Bower, J. S., Danzker, D. R., and Naylor, B.,** Idiopathic pulmonary hypertension associated with nodular pulmonary infiltrates and portal venous thrombosis, *Chest*, 78, 111, 1980.
169. **Reinhard, E. H.,** discussant, Clinicopathological conference, Aach, R. and Kissane, J., Moderators, A fifty-six year old woman with jaundice and pulmonary hypertension, *Am. J. Med.*, 47, 287, 1969.
170. **Chun, P. K. C., San Antonio, R., Davia, J. E.,** Laennec's cirrhosis and pulmonary hypertension, *Am. Heart J.*, 99, 779, 1980.
171. **Pierce, J.,** discussant, in Clinicopathological conference, Cryer, P. E. and Kissane, J. M., Moderators, Chronic active hepatitis and pulmonary hypertension, *Am. J. Med.*, 63, 604, 1977.
172. **Adam, A. and Pattersen, D. L. H.,** Pulmonary hypertension associated with hepatic cirrhosis and primary acrocyanosis, *J. Roy. Soc. Med.*, 74, 689, 1981.
173. **Molden, D. and Abraham, J. L.,** Pulmonary hypertension: its association with hepatic cirrhosis and iron accumulation, *Arch. Pathol. Lab. Med.*, 106, 328, 1982.
174. **Bernthal, A. C., Eybel, C. E., and Payne, J. A.,** Primary pulmonary hypertension after portocaval shunt, *J. Clin. Gastroenterol.*, 5, 353, 1983.
175. **Alagille, D.,** Alpha-1 antitrypsin deficiency, *Hepatology*, 4, 115, 1984.
176. **Glasgow, J. F. T., Lynch, M. J., Hercz, A.,** Alpha-1 antitrypsin deficiency in association with both cirrhosis and chronic obstructive lung disease in two sibs, *Am. J. Med.*, 54, 181, 1973.
177. **Sharp, H. L.,** The current status of alpha-1 antitrypsin, a protease inhibitor, in gastrointestinal disease, *Gastroenterology*, 70, 611, 1976.
178. **Cohen, K. L., Rubin, P. E., and Echevarria, R. E.,** Alpha-1 antitrypsin deficiency, emphysema, and cirrhosis in an adult, *Ann. Int. Med.*, 78, 227, 1973.
179. **Rubel, L. R., Ishak, K. G., and Benjamin, S. B.,** *Arch. Pathol. Lab. Med.*, 106, 678, 1982.

180. **Bass, N. M., Burroughs, A. K., Scheur, P. J., Geraint-James, D., and Sherlock, S.,** Chronic intrahepatic cholestasis due to sarcoidosis, *Gut,* 23, 417, 1982.
181. **Golding, P. L., Smith, M., and Williams, R.,** Multisystem involvement in chronic liver disease: studies on the incidence and pathogenesis, *Am. J. Med., Sci.,* 55, 772, 1973.
182. **Weissman, E. and Becker, N. H.,** Interstitial lung disease in primary biliary cirrhosis, *Am. J. Med., Sci.,* 285(3), 21, 1983.
183. **Uddenfeldt, P., Bjerle, P., Danielsson, A., Nystromm, L., and Stjernberg, N.,** Lung function abnormal in patients with primary biliary cirrhosis, *Acta Med. Scand.,* 223, 549, 1988.
184. **Rodriguez-Roisin, R., Pares, A., Bruguera, M., Coll, J., Picardo, C., Agusti-Vidal, A., Burgos, F., Rodés, J.,** Pulmonary involvement in primary biliary cirrhosis, *Thorax,* 36, 208, 1981.
185. **Turner-Warwick, M.,** Fibrosing alveolitis and chronic liver disease, *Q. J. Med.,* 37, 133, 1968.
186. **Helman, C. A., Keeton, G. R., Benatar, S. R.,** Lymphoid interstitial pneumonia with associated chronic active hepatitis and renal tubular acidosis, *Am. Rev. Respir. Dis.,* 115, 161, 1977.
187. **Butland, R. J. A., Cole, P., Citron, K. M., Turner-Warwick M.,** Chronic bronchial suppuration and inflammatory bowel disease, *Q. J. Med.,* 50, 63, 1981.
188. **Pang, J. A. and Vicary, F. R.,** Carcinoma of the colon, sclerosing cholangitis, pericholangitis, and bronchiectasis in a patient with chronic ulcerative colitis, *J. Clin. Gastroenterology,* 6, 361, 1984.
189. **Andrade, Z. A. and Andrade, S. G.,** Pathogenesis of schistosomal pulmonary arteritis, *Am. J. Trop. Med. Hyg.,* 19, 305, 1970.
190. **Cheever, A. W.,** Pathology in Schistosome infection in humans: perspectives and recent findings, Nash, T. E., moderator, *Ann. Int. Med.,* 97, 740, 1982.
191. **Brisbane, J. U., Howell, D. A., and Bonkowsky, H. L.,** Pulmonary hypertension as a presentation of hepatocarcinoma. Report of a case and brief review of the literature, *Am. J. Med.,* 68, 466, 1980.
192. **Willet, I. R., Sutherland, R. C., O'Rourke, M. F., and Dudley, F.,** Pulmonary hypertension complicating hepatocellular carcinoma, *Gastroenterology,* 87, 1180, 1984.

Chapter 7

RENAL CIRCULATION AND PATHOGENESIS OF FUNCTIONAL RENAL FAILURE IN CIRRHOSIS*

Vicente Arroyo, Pere Ginés, and Wladimiro Jimenez

TABLE OF CONTENTS

* This work was supported by grant PA86-0405 from the Secretaria de Estado de Universidades e Investigación.

I. INTRODUCTION

Functional renal failure (FRF), a syndrome characterized by the spontaneous development of a marked reduction of renal blood flow and GFR, oliguria, and dilutional hyponatremia in the absence of significant histological abnormalities of the kidney, is a major complication of cirrhotics with ascites. FRF was first recognized by Hecker and Sherlock in 1956[1] in nine patients with hepatic cirrhosis or virus hepatitis who developed azotemia, hyponatremia, and oliguria in the setting of a severe hepatic insufficiency. All patients died during hospitalization without recovering renal function despite treatment with plasma volume expanders and vasoactive drugs. Postmortem examination of the kidneys showed normal histology. Since patients had arterial hypotension, increased cardiac output, and highly oxygenated peripheral venous blood, these authors speculated that the initial mechanism of FRF was a reduced arterial pressure secondary to peripheral arteriolar vasodilation. Following the pioneer report of Hecker and Sherlock, numerous investigators, particularly hepatologists, nephrologists, and clinical physiologists, became interested in FRF. Several reasons explain this multidisciplinary interest. First, FRF is a common complication of patients with cirrhosis and ascites. Retrospective studies indicate that this syndrome is present in approximately 17% of cirrhotics with ascites admitted to hospital and in more than 50% of the cirrhotic patients who die.[2,3] A recent study estimated that the probability of developing FRF 2 and 5 years after the onset of ascites in patients with cirrhosis is 32% and 41%, respectively[4] (Figure 1). Second, impaired renal hemodynamics probably represent the most accurate prognostic index in patients with cirrhosis and ascites. Patients with FRF usually die within weeks or months after the onset of renal failure independently of the degree of hepatic insufficiency[4-6] (Figure 2). Third, most cirrhotics with refractory ascites, i.e., the ascites that cannot be mobilized by medical treatment, have FRF, as manifested by abnormally high plasma levels of blood urea nitrogen (BUN) and serum creatinine concentration.[5] Finally, cirrhosis with ascites and FRF represents a unique condition to investigate the relationship between impaired systemic hemodynamics, endogenous vasoactive systems (renin-angiotensin system, sympathetic nervous system, antidiuretic hormone, natriuretic hormone, atrial natriuretic peptide, renal prostaglandins and leukotrienes, renal kallikrein-kinin system, etc.), and renal function in man. This broad interest in FRF, together with the great advances made during the last three decades in the physiology of the systemic and renal circulation, have led to a better understanding of the pathogenesis of the syndrome. Unfortunately, this has not been followed by any improvement in the treatment of cirrhotics with FRF, with the prognosis of these patients nowadays being as poor as it was 35 years ago.

The aim of the current chapter is to review the pathogenesis of the renal circulatory abnormalities and FRF in cirrhosis. The chapter has been arranged into three sections. The first deals with the clinical characteristics, prognosis and differential diagnosis of FRF in cirrhosis. In the second section, the neurohumoral factors that may be involved in the pathogenesis of FRF are discussed. Finally, the third section reviews the relationship between systemic and renal hemodynamic disturbances in cirrhosis and proposes a sequence of events to explain why patients with advanced cirrhosis develop FRF.

II. FUNCTIONAL RENAL FAILURE IN CIRRHOSIS: CLINICAL FEATURES

From a clinical point of view, there are two distinct types of FRF in cirrhosis.[7] The first is characterized by a rapid increase in BUN and serum creatinine concentration, which reach extremely high levels within days after the onset of renal failure (over 100 mg/dl and 5 mg/, respectively), progressive oliguria, profound dilutional hyponatremia (often below 120 mEq/l), and hyperkalemia. This progressive FRF (also called hepatorenal syndrome)

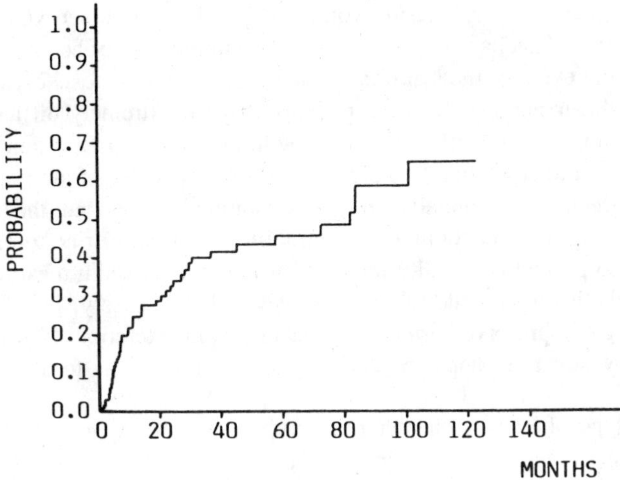

FIGURE 1.   Probability of developing FRF in a series of 136 patients with cirrhosis admitted to hospital for the treatment of an episode of ascites. (From Girés, P., Arroyo, V., and Rodés, J., in *Therapy of Liver Diseases,* Davis, M., Ed., W. B. Saunders, London, 1989, 165. With permission.)

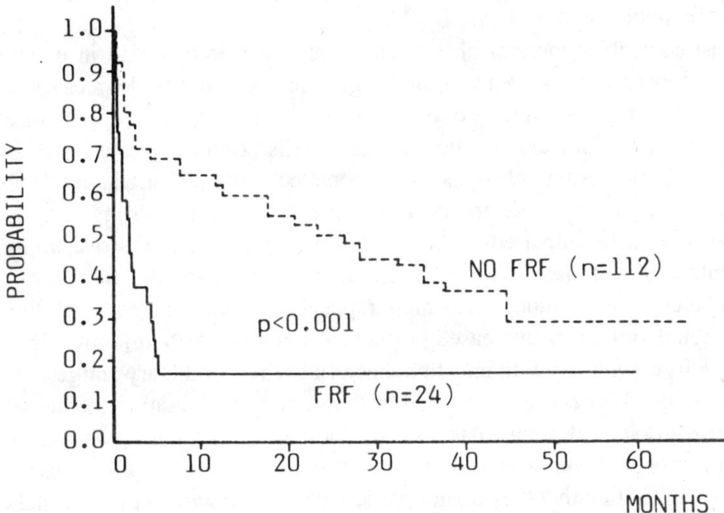

FIGURE 2.   Probability of survival in a series of 136 patients with cirrhosis and ascites classified according to the presence or absence of FRF. (From Ginés, P., Arroyo, V., and Rodés, J., in *Therapy of Liver Diseases,* Davis, M., Ed., W. B. Saunders, London, 1989, 165. With permission.)

always occurs in patients with extremely poor hepatic function who, in addition to ascites, present other complications of the underlying cirrhosis such as jaundice or hepatic encephalopathy. In our experience, progressive FRF is commonly observed in alcoholic cirrhotics with superimposed severe alcoholic hepatitis or in any etiologic type of cirrhotic with ascites in whom hepatic function deteriorates rapidly as a consequence of a serious bacterial infection, a gastrointestinal hemorrhage, or a major surgical procedure. The development of progressive FRF in a cirrhotic patient carries with it an ominous prognosis, since most of these patients die within days or weeks after the onset of the syndrome independently of the therapy used (hemodialysis, plasma volume expansion, peritoneo-venous shunt, vaso-active agents), with the mechanism of death being a combination of hepatic and renal failure and the precipitating event of the syndrome. The differential diagnosis between progressive FRF and acute tubular necrosis in these patients may be extremely difficult and in some cases even impossible. First, cirrhotic patients with progressive FRF often present complications that may lead to acute tubular necrosis, namely, episodes of arterial hypotension or serious infections requiring potentially nephrotoxic antibiotics. Second, the traditional markers of tubular integrity (urinary sodium concentration <10 mEq/l, urine-to-plasma creatinine ratio >30, urine-to-plasma osmolality ratio>1, and fractional sodium excretion<1%) may be present in cirrhotics with acute tubular necrosis and, conversely, progressive FRF may occur in the setting of a preserved urine volume and sodium excretion.[8-10] Finally, as pointed out by several investigators, hepatorenal syndrome may progress to acute tubular necrosis.[11-13]

The second type of FRF is characterized by a moderate increase in BUN and serum creatinine concentration (usually lower than 60 and 2 mg/l, respectively) which remain steady for months.[7] It is important to remark, however, that the inverse relationship between serum creatinine or BUN and GFR is hypervolic, which means that a small increase of BUN or serum creatinine represents a marked fall in GFR. In fact, GFR in patients with steady FRF is reduced by more than 50%. Steady FRF usually occurs in cirrhotics with a relatively preserved hepatic function whose main clinical problem is an ascites refractory to diuretic treatment.[5,14] The survival of these patients, however, is considerably lower than that of nonazotemic cirrhotics with ascites.

Minor histological glomerular abnormalities are frequently found in patients with cirrhosis.[15] They consist in an increase in mesangial matrix, varying degrees of thickening of the capillary walls, a modest increase in cell size and number, and deposits of electrodense material in the mesangium and in the capillary walls. Immunofluorescence studies have shown that these glomerular changes are associated with mesangial and subendothelial deposits of IgA as well as of IgG and complement, and it has been suggested that they may be a consequence of the impaired ability of the cirrhotic liver to remove inmunoglobulins or antigen-antibody complexes from the circulation.[16-20] With the failure of the hepatic reticuloendothelial system function, which represents more than 90% of the total body reticuloendothelial system, or increased portacaval shunting, or both, either IgA originating from the gut or its complexes with intestinal bacterial, viral, or dietary antigens would escape to the general circulation and be deposited in the glomeruli, initiating the above mentioned lesions.[15] These histological glomerular abnormalities, which are not accompanied by changes in urine sediment or proteinuria, have been observed independently of the presence of ascites or renal failure, indicating that they do not participate in the pathogenesis of renal dysfunction in cirrhosis.[15] Rarely, however, glomerular IgA and complement deposits in cirrhosis are associated with proliferative changes, giving rise to a rapidly progressive glomerulonephritis, with hematuria, proteinuria and progressive renal failure.[16,17,20] Interestingly enough, many of these patients have asymptomatic cirrhosis, the diagnosis of the liver disease being made during the assessment of the renal problem.[18] Differentiation between IgA-associated glomerulonephritis and progressive FRF is very easy, since proteinuria and hematuria are not prominent features in the latter condition. The explanation for the variability in the severity of IgA-associated glomerular lesion in cirrhotics is unknown. Glomerular tubular reflux, a histological lesion characterized by the reflux of proximal convoluted tubular epithelium into the Bowman's space, is another glomerular abnormality frequently observed in cirrhotic patients, particularly in those with FRF.[21] Glomerular-tubular reflux, however, is a consequence rather than a cause of renal failure in cirrhosis, since it has been observed in other clinical and experimental conditions associated with impaired renal perfussion. It affects less than 15% of the glomeruli, is not present in all cirrhotics with renal failure and may be observed in patients with normal serum creatinine concentration.[21]

In contrast, there is a great amount of evidence indicating that renal failure in cirrhosis is functional in nature and related to disturbances in systemic hemodynamics and renal perfusion.

1.   GFR in patients with cirrhosis and ascites correlates closely with renal blood flow, patients with FRF being those with lower renal perfusion.[22] Renal arteriographic studies have shown that impaired renal perfusion in patients with FRF is secondary to an active vasoconstriction of the renal arteries, which takes place not only in the small arterioles but also in the large intrarenal arteries, including the primary branches of the main renal artery and the interlobar and proximal arcuate arteries.[23]
2.   FRF in cirrhotics may disappear after the expansion of the circulating blood volume that follows the insertion of a peritoneo-venous shunt, following the surgical correction of portal hypertension by a side-to-side portacaval anastomosis, or after a successful liver transplantation.[24-28]
3.   Finally, the kidneys of patients with FRF are able to work normally when transplanted to patients with chronic renal failure.[29]

III. ENDOGENOUS VASOACTIVE SYSTEMS AND IMPAIRED RENAL HEMODYNAMICS IN CIRRHOSIS

Several neurohumoral systems and endogenous substances with vasoactive properties have been implicated in the pathogenesis of active vasoconstriction causing FRF in cirrhosis, including the renin-angiotensin and sympathetic nervous systems,[30] renal prostaglandins,[31-33] leukotrienes,[34] renal kallikrein-kinin system,[35] antidiuretic hormone,[36] glomerulopresin,[37] endotoxin,[38] and false neurotransmitters.[39] It is important to point out, however, that more than 100 different vasoactive compounds have been isolated in human urine.[40] Therefore, the above-cited vasoactive systems and substances probably represent only a small fraction of the humoral factors that may affect the renal circulation in cirrhosis with ascites. The current section will summarize the extensive data presently available implicating the renin-angiotensin system, sympathetic nervous system, antidiuretic hormone and arachidonic acid metabolites in the pathogenesis of FRF in cirrhosis. The reader is referred to other review articles that discuss the role of other endogenous vasoactive substances in this syndrome.[41-43]

A.   RENIN-ANGIOTENSIN SYSTEM*

Renin is produced in the kidney by specialized cells of the juxtaglomerular apparatus which is in intimate contact with the vascular pole of the glomerulus and convoluted distal tubule. Renin is an enzyme with no biological activity and acts on an alpha-globulin (renin substrate or angiotensinogen) synthesized by the liver, releasing the inactive decapeptide angiotensin I. At least three mechanisms control renin release from the kidney:[44-46] (1) the renal baroreceptor mechanism, sensitive to changes in renal perfusion pressure; (2) the macula densa mechanism, which responds to changes in sodium delivery or transport within the distal tubule; and (3) the renal sympathetic nervous activity, which directly stimulates renin release by operating upon beta-1-adrenergic receptors present in the juxtaglomerular apparatus. These three mechanisms are not mutually exclusive, but rather they probably operate in concert since they are influenced in the same direction when there are changes in effective circulating blood volume or arterial pressure. Angiotensin I is subsequently transformed to the octapeptide angiotensin II by the action of the specific converting enzyme dipeptidyl carboxypeptidase. Since the largest concentration of this converting enzyme is found in the lung, until recently it was believed that conversion of angiotensin I to angiotensin II occurred only there[47] and, therefore, that the function of angiotensin II was primarily systemic rather

* See also Chapter 18.

than intrarenal. However, subsequent investigations, demonstrating that the converting enzyme is also present in the juxtaglomerular apparatus, and that significant amounts of angiotensin II are generated locally within the kidney[49,50] suggest that this vasoactive compound is released immediately adjacent to the afferent and efferent glomerular arterioles. It is, therefore, very likely that renal hemodynamics could be influenced not only by the angiotensin II reaching the kidney via the renal artery, but also by that locally generated within or near the juxtaglomerular apparatus. Angiotensin II is among the most active endogenous vasoconstrictor agents so far identified. The arteriolar vasoconstrictor effect of angiotensin II is mediated by an interaction with specific receptors located directly on the vascular smooth muscle cells, the result of which is an elevation of cytosolic calcium levels and contraction of these cells, by a stimulation of specific receptors in the area postrema of the central nervous system, resulting in an increase in the sympathetic nervous activity and by an enhancement of neurotransmission at the peripheral noradrenergic neuroeffector junction.[51] The renal vasculature is especially sensitive to the vasoconstrictor effect of angiotensin II since a striking reduction of renal blood flow occurs with doses of angiotensin II well below those required to induce a pressor response.[52,53] Angiotensin II also reduces GFR. This latter effect is related to both a decrease in renal perfusion and to a direct contracting effect on glomerular mesangial cells.[54]

For many years, the physiological role of the renin-angiotensin system could only be evaluated by measuring the plasma levels of renin or angiotensin II in several physiological and pathological conditions. These studies demonstrated that the renin-angiotensin system is stimulated whenever the "effective" arterial blood volume (a term that defines the fullness of the arterial vascular circulation) and, therefore, the arterial blood pressure are compromised, either because cardiac output is decreased (low sodium diet, upright posture, hemorrhagic hypotension, low output heart failure, nephrotic syndrome) or because peripheral vascular resistance is reduced (high output heart failure, arteriovenous fistula, drug-induced arterial hypotension).[44-46] Since renal blood flow and GFR are also reduced in these circumstances, the increased activity of the renin-angiotensin system was initially interpreted as a consequence of a stimulation of the baroreceptor mechanism secondary to impaired renal hemodynamics. The introduction of pharmacological agents that interrupt the renin-angiotensin system (inhibitors of the converting enzyme and structural analogs that competitively antagonize angiotensin II at the vascular receptor) have made it possible to better define the role of endogenous angiotensin II as a determinant of the state of the systemic and renal circulation.[55] Inhibition of the endogenous renin-angiotensin system by the i.v administration of converting-enzyme inhibitors (captopril) or specific competitive antagonists (saralasin) in men and experimental animals with "effective" arterial hypovolemia is associated with a marked reduction of peripheral vascular resistance and arterial pressure.[55] Moreover, in experimental models with increased activity of the renin-angiotensin system, the intrarenal infusion of these agents at doses not producing arterial hypotension increases or totally normalizes renal blood flow and GFR.[56] These findings, therefore, indicate that the increased activity of the renin-angiotensin system in conditions of "effective" arterial hypovolemia is a homeostatic response to maintain arterial pressure within normal limits and that angiotensin II plays a contributory role in the impairment in renal perfusion and GFR in these circumstances.

Some patients with decompensated cirrhosis show high levels of plasma renin activity and plasma concentration of renin and angiotensin II[57-59] (Figure 3). The hepatic clearance of renin in these patients has been shown to be normal or only moderately decreased.[60-62] In contrast, the renal production of renin is increased and correlates closely with the plasma concentration of renin.[57] Hyperreninemia in cirrhosis, is, therefore, due to an increased secretion rather than to an impaired metabolism. Studies in nonazotemic cirrhotics with ascites have clearly demonstrated that the activity of the renin-angiotensin system (as esti-

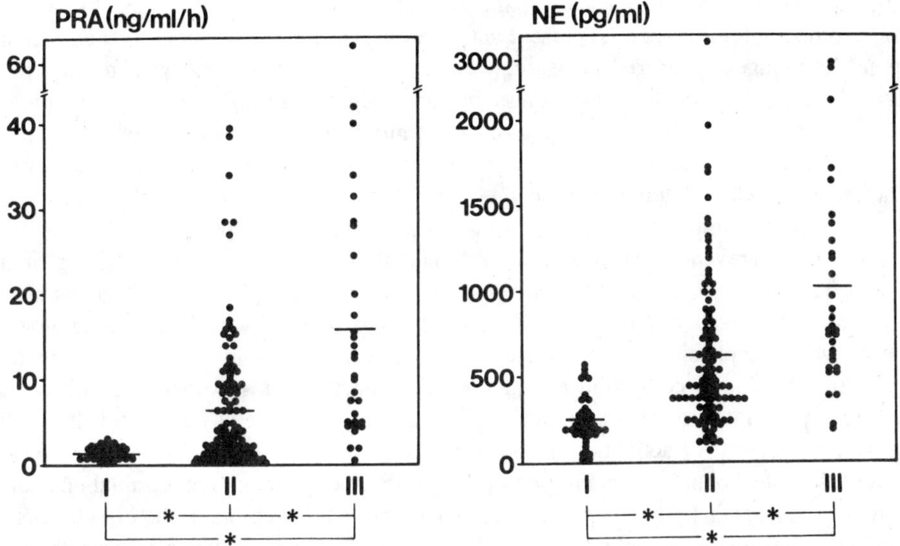

FIGURE 3.   Plasma renin activity (PRA) and plasma norepinephrine concentration in normal subjects (I), nonazotemic patients with cirrhosis and ascites (II), and cirrhotic patients with FRF (III); *p <0.001. (From Arroyo, V., Ginés, P., Rimola, A., and Gaya, J., *Am. J. Med.*, 81 (Suppl. 2B), 104, 1986. With permission.)

mated by plasma renin concentration and by the renal renin release) may be increased in patients with normal renal blood flow and GFR, indicating that alterations in total renal perfusion are not major determinants of renin secretion in cirrhotics with ascites.[57] There is evidence that overactivity of the renin-angiotensin-aldosterone system plays a role in the pathogenesis of sodium retention and ascites formation.[57,63,64] Among cirrhotics with ascites, plasma renin activity and concentration are particularly elevated in patients with FRF[35,65-67] (Figure 3). Therefore, it is reasonable to presume that endogenous angiotensin II is also involved in the pathogenesis of active vasoconstriction causing FRF in cirrhosis. Nevertheless, at present there is no direct evidence supporting this contention.

A series of studies using pharmacological agents that inhibit the renin-angiotensin system have been performed to assess the role of this system in the systemic and renal hemodynamic abnormalities in cirrhosis with ascites. The i.v administration of saralasin, a specific antagonist of angiotensin II, to patients with cirrhosis and ascites is associated with a marked decrease in arterial pressure and peripheral resistance, in patients with very high plasma renin levels.[68,69] The increased activity of this system in patients with cirrhosis and ascites is, therefore, an important mechanism in maintaining arterial pressure within normal or near normal limits. The inhibition of the renin-angiotensin system with specific antagonists of angiotensin II or converting enzyme inhibitors in patients with cirrhosis, ascites, and impaired renal perfusion has not been followed by an improvement in GFR.[68,70-74] However, this observation should not be interpreted as indicating that endogenous angiotensin II does not contribute to the active vasoconstriction causing FRF in cirrhosis, since in these studies the arterial hypotension invariably produced by these agents could have masked the renal vascular effect of angiotensin II inhibition.

B. SYMPATHETIC NERVOUS ACTIVITY*

The sympathetic nervous system is another important endogenous mechanism controlling systemic hemodynamics and renal function in man.[75,76] This system is activated through

* See also Chapter 4.

high-pressure baroreceptors located in the carotid sinus and aortic arch and low-pressure baroreceptors (volume receptors) present in the cardiac atria.[75,76] High-pressure baroreceptors respond to changes in arterial pressure, which modify the transmural wall tension of the arteries holding the receptors. Low-pressure baroreceptors are influenced by alterations in intravascular volume, which modify atrial transmural pressure. Afferent impulses arising from these structures travel via the glossopharyngeal and vagus nerves to an integrative site in the medulla, which alters the sympathetic nervous outflow according to the information received. Afferent impulses from high-and low-pressure baroreceptors are also sent to the supraoptic and paraventricular nuclei of the hypothalamus, thus modifying antidiuretic hormone secretion.[78,79] Recent studies suggest that baroreceptors may also exist within the intrahepatic sinusoidal circulation.[80] Contrary to what occurs with the renin-angiotensin system, which is physiologically active only in circumstances in which the "effective" intraarterial volume is compromised, in normal subjects the sympathetic nervous system continuously operates to maintain arterial pressure and heart rate at normal levels.[75-77] The hemodynamic effects of activation of the sympathetic nervous system result from the direct action of the catecholamines (mainly norepinephrine) released from the terminal ends of the postsynaptic sympathetic neurons upon the alpha- and beta-receptors in the effector organs. Norepinephrine release stimulates beta-1-receptors in the heart, causing increased cardiac rate and contractility. This catecholamine also causes vasoconstriction in the peripheral arterioles via stimulation of alpha-receptors. In addition to these direct effects, the sympathetic nervous system also influences systemic hemodynamics by modifying the degree of activity of the renin-angiotensin system and antidiuretic hormone secretion.[44-46,78]

The kidney is richly innervated by sympathetic noradrenergic fibers which reach the afferent and efferent arterioles, juxtaglomerular apparatus, proximal and distal convoluted tubules, thick ascending limb of the loop of Henle and collecting tubules.[81-83] In contrast, there is neither physiologic nor anatomic evidence supporting the existence of sympathetic cholinergic vasodilator fibers in the kidney.[84] Direct electric stimulation of the renal nerves produces a decrease in renal blood flow and GFR and stimulates sodium reabsorption in the proximal tubule, loop of Henle, and distal nephron.[83-85] These effects, which can also be observed when the renal sympathetic nervous system is reflexly activated through high- and low-pressure baroreceptors, are mediated by alpha-1-adrenergic adrenoreceptors.[83-85]

The most commonly used method to assess the sympathetic nervous activity in man is by measuring the plasma levels of norepinephrine, since the majority of the norepinephrine circulating in plasma is derived from that released as a transmitter at postsynaptic sympathetic nerve terminals.[83] At present numerous investigations have been published using this method in patients with cirrhosis with and without ascites or renal failure. These studies demonstrate general agreement that plasma norepinephrine concentration in peripheral venous samples is normal in compensated cirrhotics and is usually increased in patients showing sodium retention and ascites[35,65,86-94] (Figure 3). Arterial plasma norepinephrine concentration is also increased in the latter group of patients and correlates with the corresponding values obtained in venous samples.[90,95] To investigate whether the elevated plasma norepinephrine concentration in cirrhotics with ascites is due to an increased rate of release or to a decreased rate of degradation, several studies have examined the rate of secretion vs. clearance in these patients.[88,92] These investigations have conclusively shown that the elevated circulating plasma norepinephrine concentration is due to an increased release and not to an impaired degradation. In normal subjects, the plasma concentration of norepinephrine in samples obtained from the renal vein is similar to or lower than that measured in arterial samples, the renal venous-arterial difference for norepinephrine concentration being, therefore, zero or slightly negative. In contrast, in cirrhotics with ascites this difference is usually positive indicating an increased activity of the renal sympathetic nervous system.[86,89,90,92] Some investigators have even suggested that the increased plasma norepinephrine concentration in peripheral venous samples in cirrhotics with ascites may not reflect a general activation of the sympathetic nervous system but that it may be a consequence of the release of large amounts of norepinephrine into the general circulation by the kidneys due to a selective activation of the renal sympathetic nervous activity.[96] However, by using radio tracer techniques, other investigators have observed that both total body and renal norepinephrine release were elevated in parallel in these patients.[92]

Since the sympathetic nervous system stimulates tubular sodium reabsorption and has vasoconstrictor properties upon the renal circulation, it is not surprising that it has been considered as being involved in the pathogenesis of sodium retention, ascites formation, and FRF in cirrhotics. In fact, there is indirect evidence supporting this contention. As previously mentioned, plasma norepinephrine concentration is normal in compensated cirrhotics and increased in patients with sodium retention and ascites. In this latter group of patients, urinary sodium excretion correlates inversely with plasma norepinephrine.[87] Finally, among cirrhotics with ascites, patients with FRF are those with the highest plasma norepinephrine concentration[35,65] (Figure 3). Experimental studies have provided some direct evidence supporting the contention that the sympathetic nervous system is involved in sodium retention in cirrhosis. Acute bilateral surgical denervation has been followed by an increase in urine volume and sodium excretion in bile duct-ligated miniature swine with ascites and by an improvement in the renal ability to excrete both an intravenous and an oral sodium load in conscious rats with decompensated cirrhosis due to common bile duct ligation.[97,98] Such direct evidence, however, is presently lacking with respect to the possible relationship between the sympathetic nervous system and renal hemodynamics in cirrhosis.

C. ANTIDIURETIC HORMONE

In addition to reduced renal blood blow and GFR and marked sodium retention, cirrhotics with ascites and FRF are unable to generate free water after a water overload.[22,99] Traditionally, this impairment in free water excretion has been considered to be secondary to a reduced delivery of fluid to the diluting segment of the nephron (ascending limb of the loop of Henle) due to low filtered sodium and increased sodium reabsorption in the proximal tubule.[101] However, recent studies showing that plasma antidiuretic hormone is elevated in cirrhotics with ascites suggest that this hormone could also be involved in the pathogenesis of water retention and dilutional hyponatremia in these patients.[87,102-104] Antidiuretic hormone secretion is mainly influenced by changes in plasma osmotic pressure (plasma osmolality) and in blood volume and/or arterial pressure.[78] Plasma osmolality influences autidiuretic hormone secretion via osmoreceptors concentrated in the anterior hypothalamus near the supraoptic nuclei. Hemodynamic influences on antidiuretic hormone secretion are mediated largely, if not exclusively, by neurogenic stimulus that arise in high- and low-pressure baroreceptors. Cirrhotics with ascites and elevated plasma levels of antidiuretic hormone present hyponatremia and hypoosmolality.[87,102,104] On the other hand, the increased plasma antidiuretic hormone concentration in these patients does not decrease after reducing plasma osmolality by a water overload.[102,103] Antidiuretic hormone hypersecretion in cirrhotics with ascites is therefore mediated by nonosmotic stimuli. The physiological effects of antidiuretic hormone depends on its interaction upon two different types of receptors, the V-1 receptors located in the vascular smooth muscle cells and the V-2 receptors present in the collecting tubule epithelial cells.[105-107] Interaction of antidiuretic hormone with V-1 receptors results in an increase in cytosolic free calcium and vasoconstriction. This vasoactive effect of antidiuretic hormone is particularly striking in the splanchnic, muscular, and cutaneous arteriolar vasculature, with renal circulation being much less sensitive to the vasoconstrictor action of this hormone.[108] Interaction of antidiuretic hormone with V-2 receptors is followed by an increased generation of cyclic AMP within the tubular cells which mediates the antidiuretic effect. For a long time, it has been accepted that the physiological role of

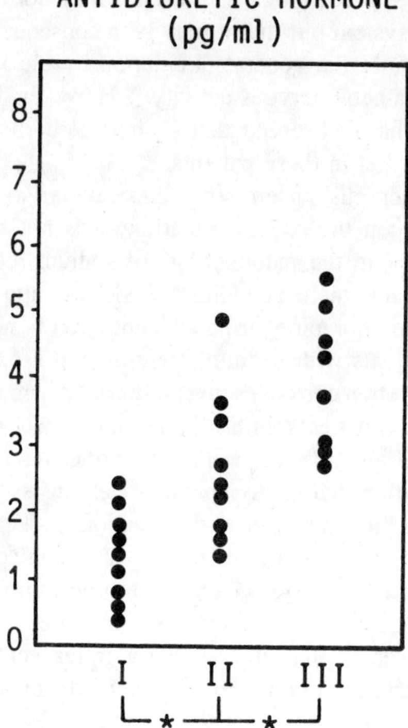

FIGURE 4.   Plasma antidiuretic hormone concentration after a
water overload of 20 ml/kg of body weight in normal subjects
(I), nonazotemic patients with cirrhosis and ascites (II), and cirrhotic patients with functional renal failure (III) CH_2O, $p < 0.05$.
(From Perez-Ayuso, R. M., Arroyo, V., Camps, J., Rimola, A.,
Gaya, J., Costa, J., Rivera, F., and Rodés, J., *Kidney Int.*, 26,
72, 1984. With permission.)

antidiuretic hormone was solely related to its antidiuretic action and cardiovascular effects
were thought to be elicited only by high pharmacological doses and to be physiologically
irrelevant. However, recent studies showing that specific V-1 receptor antagonists reduce
arterial pressure and peripheral resistance in patients with congestive heart failure and experimental animals with heart failure or hemorrhagic hypotension[109,110] and increase renal
blood flow and GFR in conscious dogs with partial obstruction of the inferior vena cana
and ascites,[36] circumstances associated with high plasma levels of antidiuretic hormone,
indicate that this hormone contributes significantly to the maintenance of arterial pressure
and to the impairment of renal hemodynamics in conditions of "effective hypovolemia".

There are indirect data as well as direct evidence indicating that antidiuretic hormone
plays an important role in the impairment of free water excretion in cirrhosis. Plasma
antidiuretic hormone concentration in cirrhotics with ascites correlates closely with the renal
ability to excrete free water.[87,102,103] On the other hand, longitudinal studies in rats with
experimental cirrhosis and ascites have shown that the impairment of water excretion appears
in close chronological relationship with the onset of antidiuretic hormone hypersecretion.[111]
Finally, the blockade of V-2 receptors normalizes the impaired renal water excretion in this
experimental model.[112] Plasma levels of antidiuretic hormone in patients with cirrhosis and
ascites also correlate with renal plasma flow and GFR, cirrhotics with FRF being those with
higher levels of this hormone[102] (Figure 4). However, at present it is not known if antidiuretic
hormone contributes to the active renal vasoconstriction present in these patients.

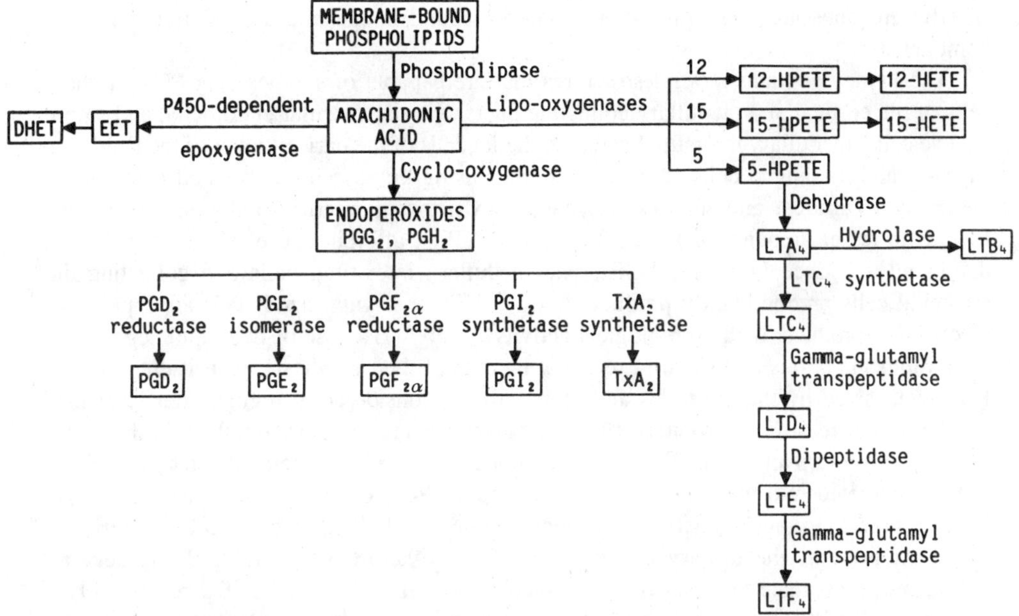

FIGURE 5. General scheme of arachidonic acid metabolism. PG, prostaglandin; HPETE, hydroperoxyeicosatetranoic acid; HETE, hydroxyeicosatetranoic acid; LT leukotriene; EET, epoxyeicosatrienoic acid; DHet, dihydroeicosatrienoic acid.

In summary, three powerful endogenous vasoconstrictor systems, the renin-angiotensin system, the sympathetic nervous system, and antidiuretic hormone, are stimulated in cirrhotics with ascites, especially in patients with FRF. There is direct evidence that the overactivity of these systems in cirrhosis is a compensatory phenomenon to maintain arterial pressure within normal limits and that they are important mediators in sodium and water retention and ascites formation. Endogenous angiotensin II, norepinephrine, and antidiuretic hormone may also be involved in the pathogenesis of FRF in these patients, although at present there is no direct evidence supporting this contention. Future research on the mechanisms of the impaired renal hemodynamics in cirrhosis is limited by the lack of experimental models of cirrhotic FRF and by the absence of specific antagonists of the renal vascular effect of these endogenous vasoconstrictors with no action on the systemic circulation.

D. ARACHIDONIC ACID METABOLITES

The kidneys are able to synthesize vasodilator substances that act locally regulating renal blood flow and GFR. Among these substances, the most extensively studied are prostaglandins (PGs) which are derived from arachidonic acid metabolism. The initial step in the formation of these compounds is the interaction of a stimulus, commonly a hormone, with a receptor in the cell surface[113] (Figure 5). This leads to an activation of phospholipase A_2, which, in combination with diglyceride lipase releases arachidonic acid from membrane phospholipids. The net effect of this process is an increase in free arachidonic acid concentration, normally quite low, within the cell. The second step in PG formation is the synthesis of the endoperoxides PGG_2 and PGH_2 from arachidonic acid. This is a complex process that is mainly catalyzed by a cyclooxygenase. Nonsteroidal anti-inflammatory drugs (NSAIDs) are powerful inhibitors of this enzyme.[114,115] The final process in PG synthesis is the conversion of PGH_2 into the active compounds $PGF_{2\alpha}$, PGE_2, PGI_2 (or prostacyclin), PGD_2, and thromboxane A_2 (TxA_2) by the action of specific enzymes[113] Cyclooxygenase and these specific enzymes are membrane bound and are found in the microsomal fraction of cell homogenates.

The kidney contains several structures that are capable of synthesizing PGs: epithelial cells of the cortical and medullary collecting ducts, arterial vascular endothelial and smooth muscle cells, medullary interstitial cells, epithelial cells of the parietal layer of the Bowman's capsule, and mesangial cells.[116] *In vitro* studies using kidney slices, isolated nephron segments, cell cultures, and microsomes have shown that glomeruli predominantly produce PGI_2 with lesser amounts of PGE_2, TxA_2, and $PGF_{2\alpha}$, afferent and efferent arterioles predominantly produce PGI_2 and PGE_2, and medullary interstitial cells and collecting duct epithelial cells predominantly produce PGE_2.[117-120] Once synthesized, PGs are rapidly metabolized to products with no biological activity.[113,117,121] Because of this rapid degradation, the biological actions of PGs are exerted at the site of their synthesis. Consistent with this, PGs synthesized by the arterioles and glomeruli are considered to regulate renal perfusion and GFR, whereas those produced by the tubular cells are probably involved in the tubular handling of sodium and water.[113,114,121-124] Although most PGE_2 is metabolized by the kidney, some is excreted into the urine. In contrast, neither PGI_2 or TxA_2 is detected in the urine because both are rapidly inactivated to more stable metabolites, such as 6-keto-$PGF_{1\alpha}$ and TxB_2. At present, the urinary excretion of PGE_2, 6-keto-$PGF_{1\alpha}$, and TxB_2 is generally considered to estimate the total renal production of PGE_2, PGI_2 and TxB_2, respectively.[125] However, from these measurements, it is impossible to assess the relative contribution of arterioles, glomeruli, renal tubules, and interstitial cells to the urinary PG concentration.

Several lines of evidence indicate that PGs play a major role in the homeostasis of renal hemodynamics. Renal artery infusion of PGE_2, PGI_2, and PGD_2 increases renal blood flow.[114,122-124,126-129] $PGF_{2\alpha}$ has no essential effect on renal hemodynamics.[129] TxA_2 is known to cause contraction of the isolated vascular smooth muscle *in vitro* and, consequently, is presumed to induce renal vasoconstriction.[129] In addition to directly dilating the renal vasculature, both PGE_2 and PGI_2 minimize the reduction of renal blood flow induced by angiotensin II, norepinephrine, and renal nerve stimulation.[90,91] Moreover, the activity of phospholipase A_2 and, therefore, the renal synthesis of PGs, is enhanced by angiotensin II, antidiuretic hormone, norepinephrine, and direct renal nerve stimulation[113,123,124,126-128,132] These data indicate that endogenous vasoconstrictors stimulate the renal synthesis of vasodilator PGs, which in turn antagonize the renal vascular effect of these compounds.

The concept that PGs modulate the renal vascular effect of endogenous vasoconstrictors is also supported by studies using NSAIDs to inhibit the renal synthesis of PGs. PG inhibition with NSAIDs potentiates the renal vasoconstrictor effect of angiotensin II, norepinephrine, and renal nerve stimulation.[113,134] On the other hand, NSAIDs induce a decrease in renal blood flow and glomerular filtration rate in circumstances of low sodium diet, hemorrhagic hypovolemia, congestive heart failure, nephrotic syndrome, surgical stress, and renal failure.[114,135,136] These conditions have two features in common. First, the activity of the renin-angiotensin system and sympathetic nervous system and antidiuretic hormone secretion are elevated; second, the renal production of PGs is increased, probably as a response to this stimulation of the endogenous neurohumoral renal vasoconstrictor systems.

The urinary excretion of PGE_2 and 6-keto-$PGF_{1\alpha}$ is generally increased in cirrhotics with ascites and preserved renal blood flow and GFR, while it is normal or reduced in patients with FRF[35,65,137-140] (Figure 6). In patients with compensated cirrhosis (patients without sodium retention), the urinary excretion of PGs is normal.[65,139] Although it is difficult to ascertain whether the reduced PG excretion in patients with FRF is a cause or a consequence of renal impairment, the increased urinary excretion of PGs in cirrhotics with ascites without FRF is generally considered as an indication that renal synthesis of PGs is increased in this group of patients. A recent study using immunofluorescence techniques showed that the content of PGH_2 synthetase in medullary collecting tubules is markedly reduced in kidney

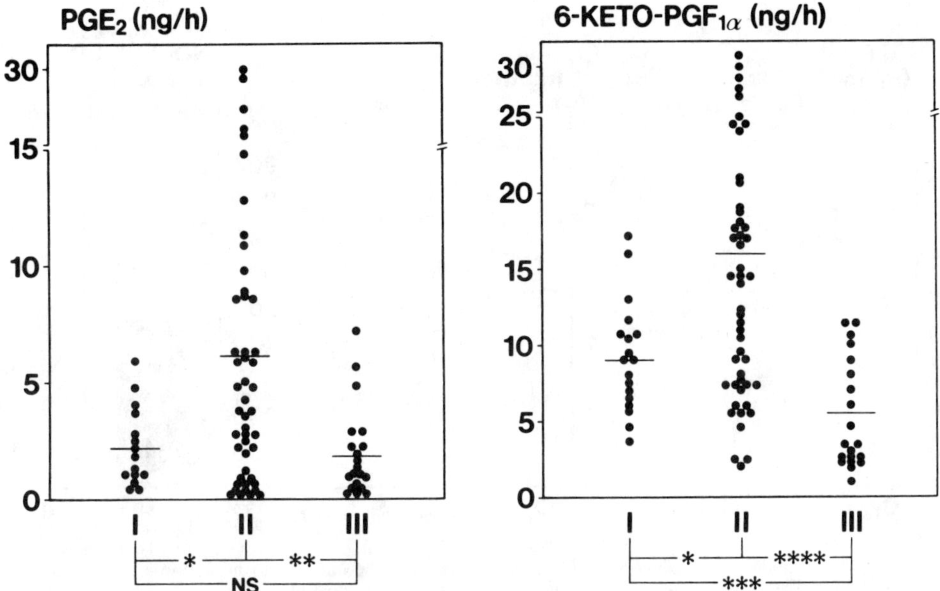

FIGURE 6. Urinary excretion of PGE$_2$ and 6-keto-PGF$_{1\alpha}$ in normal subjects (I), nonazotemic patients with cirrhosis and ascites (II), and cirrhotic patients with FRF (III). NS, not significant; *p <0.05; **p <0.02; ***p <0.01; ****p <0.001. (From Rimola et al., *J. Hepatol.*, 3, 111, 1986. With permission.)

samples from cirrhotic patients with hepatorenal syndrome as compared with that found in cirrhotics with ascites and preserved renal hemodynamics and in noncirrhotic patients with acute tubular necrosis and acute tubulo-interstitial nephritis,[141] This suggests that a loss of renal PG synthetase activity might be the cause of the diminished urinary excretion of PGs in cirrhotics with FRF.

In addition to the increased urinary excretion of PGE$_2$ and 6-keto-PGF$_{1\alpha}$, cirrhotics with ascites without FRF also show high urinary excretion of TxB$_2$ and PGF$_{2\alpha}$,[137-139] which indicates that the stimulus promoting PG synthesis in these patients acts at the initial step of the arachidonic acid cascade, thus increasing the synthesis of all PGs. Longitudinal studies in rats with carbon tetrachloride-induced cirrhosis and in chronic bile duct ligated dogs have shown a close chronological relationship between the increase in urinary PG excretion and the onset of hyperaldosteronism and sodium retention.[142,143] Therefore, it is very probable that the high renal PG synthesis in cirrhotics with ascites and preserved renal hemodynamics is a homeostatic response to the increased activity of the endogenous vasoconstrictor systems.

The most extensive hypothesis to explain the above-mentioned findings suggests that the increased renal PGE$_2$ and PGI$_2$ synthesis in nonazotemic cirrhotics with ascites, by antagonizing the renal vascular effect of endogenous angiotensin II, norepinephrine, and antidiuretic hormone, plays a critical role in the maintainance of renal blood flow and GFR. In patients with FRF, the impaired renal hemodynamics could be a consequence of an impaired renal production of PGs in the setting of a marked activation of endogenous vasoconstrictor systems.[114-146] The administration of indomethacin, ibuprofen, sulindac, or lysine acetylsalicylate induces a profound decrease in renal blood flow and GFR in nonazotemic cirrhotics with increased activity of the renin-angiotensin and sympathetic nervous systems and marked sodium retention (Figure 7), but not in compensated cirrhotics or in patients with ascites and normal or low plasma renin activity and plasma norepinephrine concentration.[65,140,147-151] These findings are the most persuasive arguments supporting renal PGs as being important factors in the maintenance of renal hemodynamics in nonazotemic cirrhotics with ascites and that an equilibrium between the degree of activity of endogenous

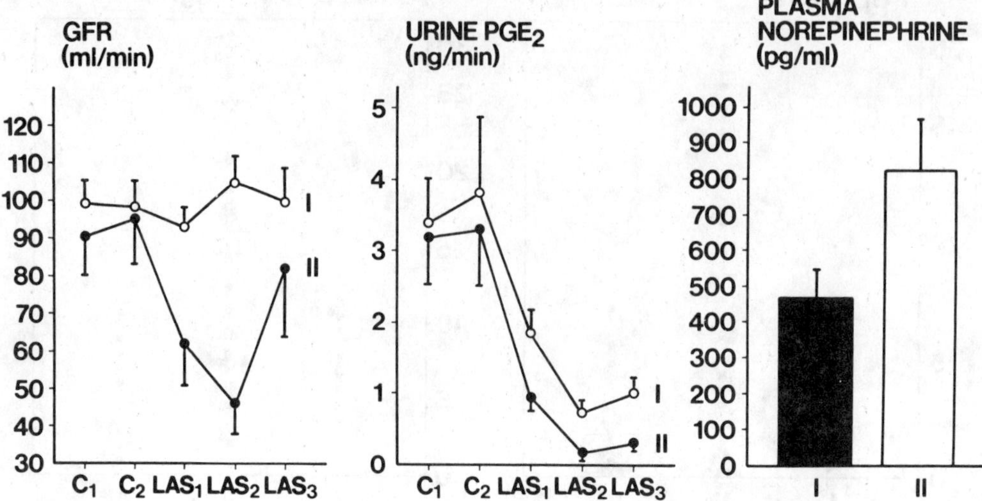

FIGURE 7.   GFR and urinary excretion of PGE$_2$ before and after the intravenous injection of 450 mg of lysine acetylsalicylate in 19 patients with cirrhosis and ascites. Patients are divided into two groups according to whether (II, eleven patients) or not (I, eight patients) renal insufficiency developed after administraion of the drug. C$_1$ and C$_2$ represent two 30-min control periods before the administration of lysine acetylsalicylate. LAS$_1$, LAS$_2$, and LAS$_3$ represent three 30-min control periods after the administration of lysine acetylsalicylate. Values of plasma norepinephrine correspond to samples obtained before lysine acetylsalicylate injection. Values are mean ± the standard error of the mean (bars). (From Arroyo et al., *Eur. J. Clin. Invest.*, 13, 271, 1983. With permission.)

vasoconstrictors and the renal synthesis of vasodilator PGs is of crucial importance in the homeostasis of renal blood flow and GFR in these patients. The observation that the decline in renal perfusion and GFR induced by indomethacin in cirrhosis with ascites could be prevented by prior administration of saralasin or converting enzyme inhibitors is consistent with this hypothesis.[152]

The initial observation of an increased urinary excretion of TxB$_2$ in cirrhotics with hepatorenal syndrome leads to the hypothesis that the impaired renal hemodynamics in these patients could be a consequence of a decrease in the ratio of the vasodilator prostaglandins PGE$_2$ and PGI$_2$ to the vasoconstrictor prostaglandin TxA$_2$.[153] However, subsequent studies have shown that, similarly to other PGs, the urinary excretion of TxB$_2$ is increased in nonazotemic cirrhotics and reduced in patients with FRF.[137-139] Moreover, the administration of thromboxane inhibitors to patients with alcoholic cirrhosis and FRF was not associated with an improvement in renal function.[154]

In addition to the synthesis of the classical PGs, two other major pathways of arachidonic acid metabolism have been described which lead to additional compounds of potential biological activity[155] (Figure 5). The first pathway involves the lypooxygenase enzymes and leads to a series of leukotrienes (LTs). The second uses cytochrome P-450-dependent enzymes and generates a series of epoxygenase products. LTs are synthesized predominantly by macrophages, including Kupffer cells, in response to several chemotactic stimuli (bacterial endotoxins, platelet-activating factor, complement component C5a). Circulating LTs are rapidly taken up and partially metabolized by the liver and the kidney, which release active and inactive compounds into the bile and urine.[34] There is *in vitro* evidence that lipooxygenase products may also be produced within the kidney, since 12-HPETE and 15-HPETE have been clearly documented in rabbit renal medulla and in rat and human glomeruli incubated with arachidonic acid, and recent studies have demonstrated that the isolated perfused rat kidney and the rat glomeruli produce LTC$_4$, LTD$_4$, and LTB$_4$.[155] LTs (LTC$_4$, LTD$_4$, and LTE$_4$) are potent vasoconstrictors. Infusions of these compounds within the renal artery increase renal vascular resistance in animals.[156,157] *In vitro*, these LTs also cause glomerular contraction.[158] Two recent investigations showing that the urinary excretion of LTE_4 and *N*-acetyl-LTE_4 are markedly increased in cirrhotics with FRF as compared to normal controls and patients with compensated cirrhosis suggest that LTs may participate in the pathogenesis of this syndrome.[159,160] Whether the increased urinary excretion of LTs in cirrhotics with FRF is a consequence of an increased renal production, representing a shift of the arachidonic acid metabolic pathway from the synthesis of vasodilator PGs to that of vasoconstrictor LTs, or is secondary to increased plasma levels, and therefore renal excretion of LTs due to impaired hepatic clearance of these compounds, is unknown. Future studies assessing the effect of specific antagonists of LTs, which are at present in various stages of development, on renal function in cirrhotics are essential to understand the role of these endogenous substances on FRF.

IV. PATHOGENESIS OF FRF IN CIRRHOSIS

Many data from experimental and human studies indicate that effective arterial blood volume is reduced in patients with hepatic cirrhosis and ascites and this intravascular underfilling occurs not because the circulating blood volume is reduced, but rather because the arterial intravascular compartment is enlarged. Cirrhotics with ascites are usually hypotensive,[88,161-165] yet the plasma volume and cardiac index may be considerably increased in this type of patients.[166-171] Thus, the low arterial blood pressure is a consequence of a reduced peripheral arteriolar vascular resistance. This hemodynamic derangement would be much more intense if the stimulated endogenous vasoconstrictor systems were not acting in the peripheral vasculature, as indicated by studies using specific angiotensin II antagonists and clonidine. The acute blockade of endogenous angiotensin II in cirrhotic patients with ascites and high plasma renin activity produces a dramatic fall of arterial pressure secondary to arteriolar vasodilation.[68,69] A similar observation has been made after normalizing plasma norepinephrine spillover with clonidine in cirrhotics with ascites and increased sympathetic nervous activity.[172] The overactivity of the renin-angiotensin and sympathetic nervous systems in cirrhotics with ascites is therefore a compensatory response to maintain systemic hemodynamics within levels compatible with life. Unfortunately, this homeostatic response also promotes renal sodium and water retention that accumulate in the abdominal cavity in the form of ascites.

Another outstanding observation in cirrhotic patients with ascites is that sinusoidal portal hypertension correlates with the degree of stimulation of the endogenous vasoconstrictor systems. In a large series of cirrhotic patients with and without ascites, Bosch et al. reported that sinusoidal portal pressure, as estimated by the free-to-wedged hepatic venous pressure gradient, correlated closely with urinary sodium excretion, plasma renin activity, and plasma renin and aldosterone concentrations, patients with more severe portal hypertension being those with higher plasma levels of renin and aldosterone and lower urinary sodium excretion[166] (Figure 8). Henriksen et al. showed that in cirrhotic patients there is also a positive correlation between portal pressure and sympathetic nervous activity.[173] Finally, since the plasma concentration of antidiuretic hormone correlates closely with plasma renin and norepinephrine concentrations in cirrhotic patients with ascites,[87,102] it is likely that antidiuretic hormone release and water retention also correlate with sinusoidal portal pressure in these patients.

Recent studies in experimental animals showing that portal hypertension induces a profound alteration in the splanchnic arteriolar circulation may be the key for understanding the complex interrelationships between sinusoidal portal hypertension, systemic hemodynamic abnormalities, overactivity of endogenous vasoconstrictor systems, and renal dysfunction in patients with cirrhosis and ascites. Traditionally portal hypertension has been considered secondary solely to an increased resistance to portal venous flow. However,

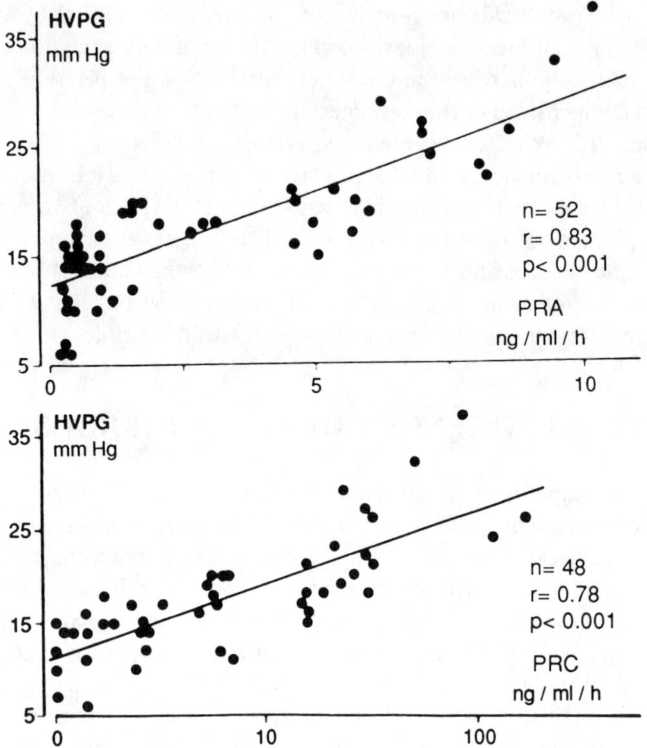

FIGURE 8.   Relationship between the hepatic venous pressure gradient (HVPG) and plasma renin activity (PRA) (top) and plasma renin concentration (PRC) (Bottom) in patients with cirrhosis. (From Bosch, J. et al., *Gastroenterology*, 78, 92, 1980. With permission.)

investigations performed in portal vein-stenosed rats and in rats with carbon tetrachloride-induced cirrhosis have shown that the pathogenesis of portal hypertension is much more complex and that an increased portal venous inflow secondary to a generalized splanchnic arteriolar vasodilation also plays an important role in the increased portal pressure.[174-178] This increased portal venous inflow may explain why portal hypertension remains elevated in cirrhosis despite the development of marked collateral circulation. How portal hypertension induces splanchnic arteriolar vasodilation is not known; however a feedback mechanism from the liver to the splanchnic arteriolar vascular bed as a compensatory measure against the loss of portal flow through the collateral circulation has been postulated.[175] Alterations in vasoactive humoral systems, such as glucagon, have also been proposed.[179] There is indirect evidence that splanchnic arteriolar vasodilation also occurs in patients with cirrhosis. Under normal conditions, almost all the blood circulating in the splanchnic bed reaches the liver, so the hepatic blood flow equals the splanchnic blood flow. In cirrhosis, because there is important shunting of blood through the portasystemic venous collateral circulation, the hepatic blood flow represents only a part of the splanchnic blood flow. Studies by Cohn et al. and Groszmann et al. have demonstrated that 60 and 80% of the mesenteric and splenic blood flow, respectively, are shunted through collateral circulation in cirrhotic patients,[180,181] Since several investigations have shown that the hepatic blood flow is normal or even increased in most cirrhotic patients,[166,167] it seems that a marked increase in splanchnic blood flow secondary to arteriolar vasodilation has to occur in these patients.

A recent study by Fernandez-Seara et al.,[161] investigating systemic and regional hemodynamics in patients with cirrhosis, ascites, and FRF, is important regarding the mechanism

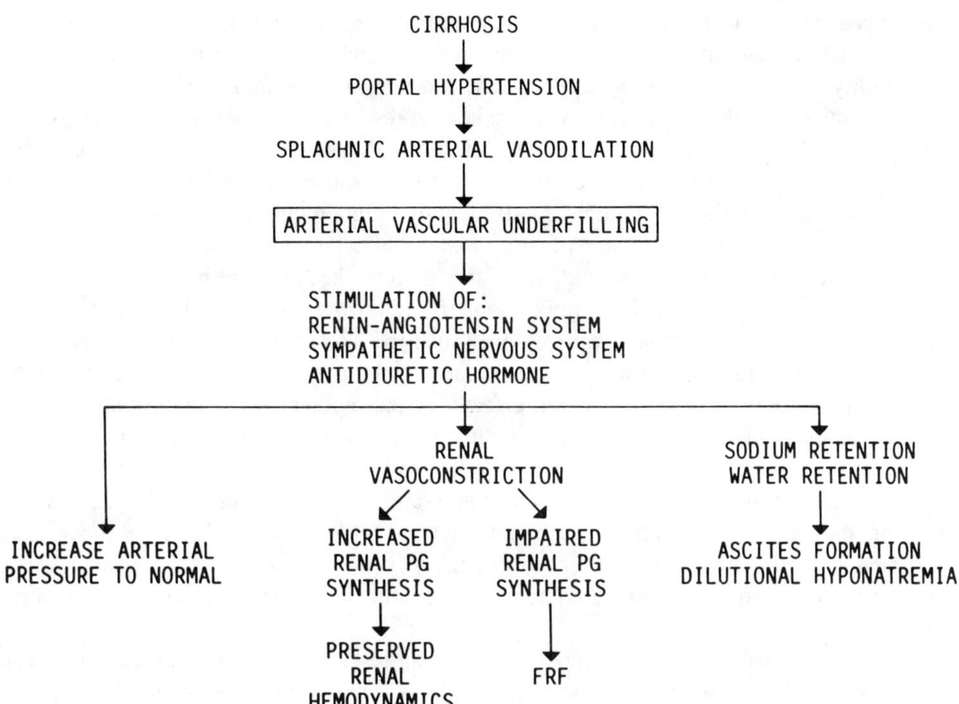

FIGURE 9.   Pathogenesis of functional renal failure in cirrhosis of the liver.

of the altered systemic circulation present in these patients. As previously reported by other studies, these investigators found that patients with FRF had lower mean arterial pressure and peripheral resistance and higher plasma renin activity than nonazotemic cirrhotics with ascites, the plasma volume and cardiac index being similarly increased in both groups of patients as compared with normal subjects. This reduction in peripheral resistance could not be accounted for by an arteriolar vasodilation in the muscular or cutaneous vascular beds since the blood flow to the legs, estimated by the doppler technique, was significantly reduced in these patients in comparison with cirrhotics without renal failure or normal subjects, probably as a consequence of the higher stimulation of endogenous vasoconstrictor systems. The renal blood flow was also markedly reduced in patients with FRF. Therefore, the only major vascular territory where arteriolar vasodilation could take place was the splanchnic vascular bed.

Considering all of these data, sodium and water retention and FRF in cirrhosis could be explained by a unifying hypothesis in which portal hypertension would be the initial event, splanchnic arteriolar vasodilation causing intravascular underfilling and stimulation of endogenous vasoconstrictor systems the intermediate step, and renal dysfunction the final consequence[182] (Figure 9). Sinusoidal portal hypertension, by an unknown mechanism, produces splanchnic arteriolar vasodilation which tends to reduce the arterial pressure. Automatically, there is a stimulation of the endogenous vasoconstrictor systems that returns the arterial pressure to normal or near normal values. When sinusoidal portal pressure is moderately increased, the systemic hemodynamic disturbance is corrected by transient sodium and water retention induced by these systems. The fluid retained by the kidneys would remain in the intravascular compartment, increase the intravascular volume and cardiac output, refill the dilated vascular bed, suppress the signals that stimulate the endogenous vasoactive systems, and normalize sodium and water excretion. This sequence of events probably explains what occurs in patients with compensated cirrhosis, who have moderate portal hypertension; increased plasma volume and cardiac index; reduced peripheral resistance; normal concentrations of renin, norepinephrine, and antidiuretic hormone; preserved renal ability to excrete sodium and free water; and normal GFR and renal blood flow.

Nonazotemic cirrhotic patients with ascites represent a more advanced stage on the continuum in the process of portal hypertension-induced vascular underfilling. At this stage of cirrhosis, the increase in cardiac output and blood volume secondary to the transient sodium and water retention is no longer sufficient to maintain circulatory homeostasis. This is probably related to the progression of sinusoidal portal hypertension which causes a greater splanchnic arteriolar vasodilation and, most importantly, because the high pressure in the hepatic sinusoids gives rise to extravasation of fluid from the sinusoidal lumen to the peritoneal cavity. The arterial baroreceptors sense the vascular underfilling, activate the endogenous vasoconstrictor systems, and promote sodium and water retention. The fluid retained by the kidneys, however, is not effective in correcting the circulatory abnormality because most of this fluid accumulates in the abdominal cavity in form of ascites. The activity of the renin-angiotensin and sympathetic nervous systems and antidiuretic hormone release remains increased to maintain arterial pressure, thus perpetuating sodium and water retention and ascites formation. Renal blood flow and GFR are normal or only moderately decreased in these patients, despite the overactivity of these vasoconstrictor systems since they are antagonized by an increased renal production of the vasodilating prostaglandins PGE_2 and PGI_2.

FRF of cirrhosis represents the most extreme manifestation of underfilling of the arterial circulation. Arterial pressure in patients with FRF is lower than in nonazotemic cirrhotics with ascites. On the other hand, the plasma concentration of the three major vasoconstrictors in patients with FRF are among the highest observed in patients with cirrhosis and ascites. An attractive theory suggests that FRF in these patients with extreme vascular underfilling occurs as a consequence of an imbalance between the activity of endogenous vasoconstrictor systems, which is very much increased, and the renal synthesis of vasodilating PGs, which may be reduced. Nevertheless, the diminution in the urinary excretion of PGs or the low renal PGH_2 synthetase activity reported in patients with FRF, which are the most important arguments supporting this hypothesis, might be a result of the decline in renal function rather than a contributory mechanism of the impaired renal hemodynamics.

REFERENCES

1. **Hecker, R. and Sherlock S.,** Electrolyte and circulatory changes in terminal liver failure, *Lancet,* 2, 1221, 1956.
2. **Bosch, J.,** Tipos de insuficiencia renal asociados a la cirrosis hepática, doctoral thesis, University of Barcelona, Barcelona, 1973, 77.
3. **Rodés, J., Bruguera, M., Terés, J., and Bordas, J. M.,** La insuficiencia renal funcional terminal de la cirrosis hepática con ascitis, *Rev. Clin.,* 117, 475, 1970.
4. **Ginés, P., Arroyo, V., and Rodés, J.,** Treatment of ascites and renal failure in cirrhosis, in *Therapy of Liver Diseases,* Davis, M., Ed., Ballière's Clinics in Gastroenterology, W. B. Saunders, London, in press.
5. **Arroyo, V. and Rodés, J.,** A rational approach to the treatment of ascites, *Postgrad, Med. J.,* 51, 558, 1975.
6. **Llach, J., Ginés, P., Arroyo, V., Rimola, A., Tito, L., Badalamenti, S., Jiménez, W., Gaya, J., Rivera, F., and Rodés, J.,** Prognostic value of arterial pressure, endogenous vasoactive systems and renal function in cirrhosis with ascites, *Gastroenterology,* 94, 482, 1988.
7. **Rodés, J., Bosch, J., and Arroyo, V.,** Clinical types and drug therapy of renal impairment in cirrhosis, *Postgrad, Med. J.,* 55, 492, 1975.
8. **Cabera, J., Arroyo, V., Ballesta, A. M., Rimola, A., Gual, J., and Rodés, J.,** Aminoglycoside nephrotoxicity in cirrhosis. Value of urinary beta-2 microglobulin to discriminate functional renal failure from acute tubular damage, *Gastroenterology,* 82, 97, 1982.

9. **Dudley, F. J., Kanel, G. C., Wood, L. J., and Reynolds, T. B.,** Hepatorenal syndrome without sodium retention, *Hepatology,* 6, 251, 1986.
10. **Diamond, J. R. and Yoburn, D. C.,** Nonoliguric acute renal failure associated with low fractional sodium excretion, *Ann. Intern. Med.,* 96, 597, 1982.
11. **Wilkinson, S. P.,** *Hepatorenal Disorders,* Marcel Dekker, New York, 1982.
12. **Wilkinson, S. P., Hirst, D., Day, D. W., and Williams, R.,** Spectrum of renal tubular damage in renal failure secondary to cirrhosis and fulminant hepatic failure, *J. Clin. Pathol.,* 31, 101, 1978.
13. **Solez, K., Racusen, L. C., and Jewell, L. D.,** Pathology of acute renal failure occurring in liver disease. in *The Kidney in Liver Disease,* 3rd ed., Epstein, M., Ed., Williams & Wilkins, Baltimore, 1988, 182.
14. **Arroyo, V., Epstein, M., Gallus, G., Gentillini, P., Ring-Larsen, H., and Salerno, F.,** Refractory ascites in cirrhosis. Mechanism and treatment, *Gastroenterology Int.,* in press.
15. **Eknoyan, G.,** Glomerular abnormalities in liver disease, in *The Kidney in Liver Disease,* 3rd ed., Epstein, M., Ed., Williams & Wilkins, Baltimore, 1988, 154.
16. **Nochy, D., Callard, P., Bellon, B., Bariety, J., and Druet, P.,** Association of overt glomerulophritis and liver disease: a study of 34 patients, *Clin. Nephrol.,* 6, 422, 1976.
17. **Callard, P., Feldmann, G., Prandi, D., Bellair, M. F., Manoet, G., Weiss, Y., Druet, P., Benhamou, J. P., and Bariety, J.,** Immunocomplex type glomerulonephritis in cirrhosis of the liver, *Am. J. Pathol.,* 80, 329, 1975.
18. **Berger, J., Yaneva, H., and Nabarra, B.,** Glomerular changes in patients with cirrhosis of the liver, *Adv. Nephrol.,* 7, 3, 1978.
19. **Montoliu, J., Darnell, A., Torras, A., and Revert, L.,** Glomerular disease in cirrhosis of the liver: low frequency of IgA deports, *Am. J. Nephrol.,* 6, 199, 1986.
20. **Praga, M., Costa, J. R., Shandas, G. J., Martínez, M. A., Miranda, B., and Rodicio, J. C.,** Acute renal failure in cirrhosis associated with macroscopic hematuria of glomerular origin, *Arch. Intern. Med.,* 147, 173, 1987.
21. **Kanel, G. C. and Peters, R. L.,** Glomerular tubular reflux—A morphologic renal lesion associated with the hepatorenal syndrome, *Hepatology,* 4, 242, 1984.
22. **Shear, L., Hall, P. W., and Gabuzda, G. J.,** Renal failure in patients with cirrhosis of the Liver. II. Factors influencing maximal urinary flow rate, *Am. J. Med.,* 39, 199, 1965.
23. **Epstein, M., Berk, D. P., Hollenberg, N. K., Adams, D. F., Chalmers, T. C., Abrams, H. L., and Merrill, J. P.,** Renal failure in the patient with cirrhosis. The role of active vasoconstriction, *Am. J. Med.,* 49, 175, 1970.
24. **Walpnick, S., Grosberg, S., Kinney, M., and LeVeen, H. H.,** Continuous peritoneal-jugular shunt. Improvement of renal function in ascitic patients, *JAMA,* 237, 131, 1977.
25. **Schroeder, E. T., Anderson, G. H., and Smulyan, H.,** Effects of portacaval or peritoneovenous shunt on renin in the hepatorenal syndrome, *Kidney Int.,* 15, 54, 1979.
26. **Wood, R. P., Ellis, D., and Starzl, T. E.,** The reversal of the hepatorenal syndrome in four pediatric patients following successful orthotopic liver transplantation, *Ann. Surg.,* 205, 415, 1987.
27. **Iwatsuki, S., Popovtzer, M. M., Corman, J. L., Ishikawa, M., Putnam, C. W., Katz, F. H., and Starzl, T. E.,** Recovery from hepatorenal syndrome after orthotopic liver transplantation, *N. Engl. J. Med.,* 289, 1155, 1973.
28. **Schroeder, E. T., Numann, P. J., and Chamberlain, B. E.,** Functional renal failure in cirrhosis. Recovery after portacaval shunt, *Ann. Intern. Med.,* 72, 923, 1970.
29. **Koppel, M. H., Coburn, J. N., Mims, M. M., Goldstein, H., Boyle, H., and Rubini, M. E.,** Transplantation of cadaveric kidneys from patients with hepatorenal syndrome. Evidence for the functional nature of renal failure in advanced liver disease, *N. Engl. J. Med.,* 280, 1367, 1969.
30. **Zipser, R. D., Little, T., Ziperouich, H., and Duke, R.,** The role of arachidonic acid metabolites in the functional renal impairment associated with liver disease, *Prostaglandins and the Kidney,* Dunn, M. J., Patrono, C., and Cinotti, Eds., Plenum Medical Books, New York, 1983, 263.
31. **Arroyo, V., Ginés, P., Rimola, A., and Gaya, J.,** Renal function abnormalities, prostaglandins and effects of non-steroidal antiinflammatory drugs in cirrhosis with ascites. An overview with emphasis on pathogenesis, *Am. J. Med.,* 81 (Suppl. 2B), 104, 1986.
32. **Zipser, R. D.,** Role of renal prostaglandins and the effects of non-steroidal anti-inflammatory drugs in patients with liver disease, *Am. J. Med.,* 81 (Suppl. 2B), 95, 1986.
33. **Epstein, M. and Lifschitz, M.,** Renal eicosanoids as determinants of renal function in liver disease, *Hepatology,* 7, 1359, 1987.
34. **Keppler, D., Hagmann, W., Rapps, S., Denzlinger, C., and Koch, H. K.,** The relation of leukotrienes to liver injury, *Hepatology,* 5, 883, 1985.
35. **Pérez Ayuso, R. M., Arroyo, V., Camps, J., Rimola, A., Costa, J., Gaya, J., Ribera, F., and Rodés, J.,** Renal kallikrein excretion in cirrhotics with ascites: relationship to renal hemodynamics, *Hepatology,* 4, 247, 1984.

36. **Vari, R. C., Freeman, R. H., Davis, J. O., and Sweet, W. D.,** Systemic and renal hemodynamic response to vascular blockade of vasopressin in conscious dogs with ascites, *Proc. Soc. Exp. Biol. Med.,* 179, 192, 1985.

37. **Alverstrand, A. and Bergstrom, J.,** Glomerular hyperfiltration after protein ingestion during glucagon ingestion, and in insulin-dependent diabetes is induced by a liver hormone: deficient production of this hormone in hepatic failure causes hepatorenal syndrome, *Lancet,* 1, 195, 1984.

38. **Wilkinson, S. P. and Williams, R.,** Renal failure in cirrhosis: current views and speculations, *Adv. Nephrol.,* 7, 15, 1978.

39. **Fisher, J. E. and Baldessarani, R. J.,** False neurotransmitters and hepatic failure, *Lancet,* 2, 75, 1971.

40. **Solez, K. and Heptinsall, R. H.,** The renal circulation: physiology and hormonal control, in *Structure and Function of the Circulation,* Schwartz, C. J., Werthessen, N. T., and Wolf, S., Eds., Plenum Press, New York, 1980, 661.

41. **Levy, M.,** Hepatorenal syndrome, in *The Kidney: Physiology and Pathology.* Seldin, D. W. and Giebish, G., Eds., Raven Press, New York, 1985, 1945.

42. **Epstein, M.,** Hepatorenal syndrome, in *The Kidney in Liver Disease,* 3rd ed., Epstein, M., Williams & Wilkins, Baltimore, 1988, 89.

43. **Bourgoigne, J. J. and Valle, G. A.,** Endotoxins and renal dysfunction in liver disease, in *The Kidney in Liver Disease,* 3rd ed., Epstein, M., Ed., Williams & Wilkins, Baltimore, 1988, 486.

44. **Davis, J. O. and Freeman, R. H.,** Mechanism regulatoring renin release, *Physiol. Rev.,* 56, 1, 1976.

45. **Peach, M. J.,** Renin-angiotensin system: biochemistry and mechanism of action, *Physiol. Rev.,* 57, 313, 1977.

46. **Reid, J. A., Morris, B. J., and Ganong, W. F.,** The renin-angiotensin system. *Annu. Rev. Physiol.,* 40, 377, 1978.

47. **Knof, N. G., Vane, J. R.,** Conversion of angiotensin I to angiotensin II, *Nature,* 216, 762, 1967.

48. **Granger, P., Dalheim, H., and Thurau, K.,** Enzyme activities of the single juxtaglomerular apparatus in the rat kidney, *Kidney Int.,* 1, 78, 1972.

49. **Disalvo, J., Peterson, A., Montefusco, C., and Menta, M.,** Intrarenal conversion of angiotensin I to angiotensin II in the dog, *Cir. Res.,* 29, 398, 1971.

50. **Bailie, M. D., Rector, F. C. J., and Seldin, D. W.,** Angiotensin II in arterial and renal venous plasma and renal lymph in the dog, *J. Clin. Invest.,* 50, 119, 1971.

51. **Jackson, E. K., Branch, R. A., Margolius, H. S., and Oates, J. A.,** Physiological function of the renal prostaglandin, renin and kallikrein systems, in *The Kidney: Physiology and Pathophysiology,* Seldin, D. W. and Giebisch, G., Eds., Raven Press, New York 1985; 613-644.

52. **Debon, E., Lee, G. J., Mottram, F. R., Pickering, G. W., Brown, J. J., Keen, J., Peart, W. S., and Sanderson, P. H.,** The action of angiotensin in man, *Clin. Sci. Mol. Med.,* 25, 123, 1963.

53. **Hollenberg, N. K., Chenitz, W. R., Adams, D. F., and Williams, G. H.,** Reciprocal influence of salt intake on adrenal glomerulosa and renal vascular responses to angiotensin II in normal man, *J. Clin. Invest.,* 54, 34, 1974.

54. **Blantz, R. C., Konnen, K. S., and Tucker, B. J.,** Angiotensin II effects upon the glomerular microcirculation and ultrafiltration coefficient of the rat, *J. Clin. Invest.,* 57, 419, 1976.

55. **Hollenberg, N. K.,** Pharmacologic interruption of the renin-angiotensin system, *Annu. Rev. Pharmacol. Toxicol.,* 19, 559, 1979.

56. **Hollenberg, N. K.,** Renin, angiotensin and the kidney: assesment by pharmacological interruption of the renin-angiotensin system. in *The Kidney in Liver Disease,* 3rd ed., Epstein, M., Ed., Williams & Wilkins, Baltimore, 1988, 374.

57. **Arroyo, V., Bosch, J., Mauri, M., Viver, J., Mas, A., Rivera, F., and Rodés, J.,** Renin, aldosterone and renal hemodynamics in cirrhosis with ascites, *Eur. J. Clin. Invest.,* 9, 69, 1979.

58. **Wernze, H., Spech, H. J., and Muller, G.,** Studies on the activity of the renin-angiotensin-aldosterone system (RAAS) in patients with cirrhosis of the liver, *Klin. Wochenschr.,* 56, 389, 1978.

59. **Rosoff, L., Jr., Zia, P., Reynolds, T. B., and Horton, R.,** Studies on renin and aldosterone in cirrhotic patients with ascites. *Gastroenterology,* 69, 698, 1975.

60. **Bosch, J., Ginés, P., Arroyo, V., Navasa, M., and Rodés, J.,** Hepatic and systemic hemodynamics and the neurohumoral systems in cirrhosis, in *The Kidney in Liver Disease,* 3rd ed., Epstein, M., Ed., Williams & Wilkins, Baltimore, 1988, 286.

61. **Mitch, W. E., Whelton, P. K., Cooke, C. R., Walker, W. G., and Maddrey, W. C.,** Plasma levels and hepatic extraction of renin and aldosterone in alcoholic liver disease, *Am. J. Med.,* 66, 84, 1979.

62. **Wernze, H., Seki, A., Schneider, K. W., and Jesse, K.,** Hepatische Extraktion und Clearance von Renin bei Lebercirrhosen, *Klin. Wochenschr.,* 50, 302, 1972.

63. **Pérez, Ayuso, R. M., Arroyo, V., Planas, R., Gaya, J., Bory, F., Rimola, A., Rivera, F., and Rodés, J.,** Randomized comparative study of efficacy of furosemide versus spironolactone in nonazotemic cirrhosis with ascites, *Gastroenterology,* 84, 961, 1984.

64. **Campra, J. L. and Reynolds, T. B.**, Effectiveness of high-dose spironolactone therapy in patients with chronic liver disease and relatively refractory ascites, *Digest Dis. Sci.*, 23, 1025, 1978.
65. **Arroyo, V., Planas, R., Gaya, J., Deulofeu, R., Rimola, A., Pérez-Ayuso, R. M., Rivera, F., and Rodés, J.**, Sympathetic nervous activity, renin-angiotensin system and renal excretion of prostaglandin E_2 in cirrhosis. Relationship to functional renal failure and sodium and water excretion, *Eur. J. Clin. Invest.*, 13, 271, 1983.
66. **Schroeder, E. T. Eich, R. H., Smulyan, H., Gould, A. B., and Gabuzda, G. J.**, Plasma renin levels in hepatic cirrhosis. Relation to functional renal failure, *Am. J. Med.*, 49, 186, 1970.
67. **Barnardo, D. E., Summerskill, W. H. J., Strong, C. G., and Baldus, W. P.**, Renal function, renin activity and endogenous vasoactive substances in cirrhosis, *Am. J. Dig. Dis.*, 15, 419, 1970.
68. **Schroeder, E. T., Anderson, G. H., Goldman, S. H., and Streeten, D. H. P.**, Effect of blockade of angiotensin II on blood pressure, renin and aldosterone in cirrhosis, *Kidney Int.*, 9, 511, 1976.
69. **Arroyo, V., Bosch, J., Mauri, M., Rivera, F., Navarro-López, S., and Rodés, J.**, Effect of angiotensin II blockade on systemic and hepatic hemodynamics and on the renin-angiotensin-aldosterone system in cirrhosis with ascites, *Eur. J. Clin. Invest.*, 11, 221, 1981.
70. **Arroyo, V., Bosch, J., Rivera, F., and Rodés, J.**, The renin-angiotensin system in cirrhosis. Its relation to functional renal failure, in *Hepato-renal Syndrome.* Bartoli, E. and Chiandusi, L. Eds., Piccin Medical Books, Padova, 1979, 202.
71. **Pariente, E. A., Bataille, C., Bercoff, E., and Lebrec, D.**, Acute effects of captopril on systemic and renal hemodynamics and on renal function in cirrhotic patients with ascites. *Gastroenterology*, 88, 1255, 1985.
72. **Lobden, I., Shore, A., Wilkinson, R., and Record, C. O.**, Captopril in the hepatorenal syndrome, *J. Clin. Gastroenterol.*, 7, 354, 1985.
73. **Wood, L. J., Stockigt, J., and Dudley, F. J.**, Adverse effects of captopril in the treatment of resistant ascites (abstract), *Gastroenterology*, 88, 1635, 1985.
74. **MaKay, I. G., McNicol, A., Finlayson, N. D. C., and Watson, M. L.**, Renal hemodynamic response to captopril in decompensated cirrhosis (abstract), *Clin. Sci.*, 68, 12, 1985.
75. **Sagawa, K., Kumada, M., and Schramm, L. P.**, Nervous control of the circulation MTP, *Int. Rev. Sci.*, 1, 197, 1974.
76. **Kopp, V. C. and Dibona, G. F.**, Neural control of volume homeostasis, in *Body Fluid Homeostasis.* Brenner, B. M. and Stein, J. H., Eds., Churchill Livingstone, New York, 1987, 185.
77. **Ludbrook, J.**, Regulation of arterial blood flow, pressure and resistance in the systemic circulation, in *Structure and Function of the Circulation,* Volume Schwartz, V. C. J, Werthessen, N. T., and Wolf, S., Eds., 1, Plenum Press, New York, 1980, 587.
78. **Robertson, G. L.**, Regulation of vasopressin secretion, in *The Kidney: Physiology and Pathophysiology,* Seldin, D. W. and Giebish, G., Eds., Raven Press, New York, 1985, 869.
79. **Swachenko, P. E. and Swanson, L. W.**, Central noradrenergic pathways for the integration of hypothalamic neuroendocrine and autonomic responses, *Science,* 214, 685, 1981.
80. **Kostreva, D., Castañer, A., and Kampine, J.**, Reflex effects of hepatic baroreceptors on renal and cardiac sympathetic nerve activity, *Am. J. Physiol.*, 238, R390, 1980.
81. **Barajas, L. and Mueller, J.**, The innervation of the juxtaglomerular apparatus and surrounding tubules. A quantitative analysis by serial section electron microscopy, *J. Ultrastruct. Res.* 43, 107, 1973.
82. **Mueller, J. and Barajas, L.**, Electron microscopic and histochemical evidence for a tubular innervation in the renal cortex of the monkey, *J. Ultrastruct. Res.*, 41, 533, 1973.
83. **Di Bona, G. F.**, The function of renal nerves, *Rev. Physiol. Biochem. Pharmacol.*, 94, 75, 1982.
84. **Gottschalk, C. W., Moss, N. G., and Colindres, R. E.**, Neural control of renal function in health and disease, in *The Kidney: Physiology and Pathophysiology,* Seldin, D. W. and Giebisch, G., Eds., Raven Press, New York, 1985, 581.
85. **Di Bona, G. F.**, Neurogenic regulation of renal tubular sodium reabsorption, *Am. J. Physiol.*, 233, F73, 1977.
86. **Ring-Larsen, H., Hesse, B., and Henriksen, J. H., Christensen, N. J.**, Sympathetic nervous activity and renal and systemic hemodynamics in cirrhosis: plasma norepinephrine concentration, hepatic extraction and renal release, *Hepatology,* 2, 304, 1982.
87. **Bichet, D. G., Van Putten, V. J., and Schrier, R. W.**, Potential role of increased sympathetic activity in impaired sodium and water excretion in cirrhosis, *N. Engl. J. Med.*, 307, 1552, 1982.
88. **Nicholls, K. M., Shapiro, M. D., Van Putten, V. J., Kluge, R., Chung, H. M., Bichet, D. G., and Schrier, R. W.**, Elevated plasma norepinephrine concentrations in decompensated cirrhosis: Association with increased secretion rate, normal clearance rate and suppressibility by central blood volume expansion, *Circ. Res.*, 56, 457, 1985.
89. **Henriksen, J., Christensen, N., and Ring-Larsen, H.**, Noradrenaline and adrenaline concentrations in various vascular beds in patients with cirrhosis. Relation to haemodynamics, *Clin. Physiol.*, 1, 293, 1981.

90. **Henriksen, J., Ring-Larsen, H., Kanstrup, I. L., and Christensen, N. J.,** Splanchnic and renal elimination and release of catecholamines in cirrhosis. Evidence of enhanced sympathetic nervous activity in patients with decompensated cirrhosis, *Gut,* 25, 1034, 1984.

91. **Bernardi, M., Santini, C., and Trevisani, F.,** Renal function impairment induced by change in posture in patients with cirrhosis and ascites, *Gut,* 26, 629, 1985.

92. **Willet, I., Esler, M., Burke, F., Leonard, P., and Dudley, F.,** Total and renal sympathetic nervous system activity in alcoholic cirrhosis, *J. Hepatol.,* 1, 639, 1985.

93. **Epstein, M., Larios, O., and Johnson, G.,** Effects of water immersion on plasma catecholamines in decompensated cirrhosis, *Miner, Electrolyte Metab.,* 11, 25, 1985.

94. **Burghardt, W., Wernze, H., and Diehl, K.,** Atrial natriuretic peptide in hepatic cirrhosis: relation to stage of disease, sympathoadrenal system and renin-aldosterone axis, *Klin. Wochenschr.,* 64 (Suppl. 6), 103, 1986.

95. **Henriksen, J., Ring-Larsen, H., and Christensen, N. J.,** Catecholamines in plasma from artery, cubital vein, and femoral vein in patients with cirrhosis. Significance of sampling site, *Scand. J. Clin. Lab. Invest.,* 46, 39, 1986.

96. **Henriksen, J., Ring-Larsen, H., and Christensen, N. J.,** Sympathetic nervous activity in cirrhosis. A survey of plasma catecholamine studies, *J. Hepatol.,* 1, 55, 1984.

97. **Zambraski, E.,** Effects of acute renal denervation on sodium excretion in miniature swine with cirrhosis and ascites, *Physiologist,* 28, 268, 1985.

98. **Koepke, J., Jones, S., and Dibona, G.,** Renal nerves mediate blunted natriuresis to atrial natriuretic peptide in cirrhotic rats, *Am. J. Physiol.,* 252, R1019, 1987.

99. **Papper, S. and Saxon, L.,** The diuretic response to administered water in patients with liver disease. II.Laennec's cirrhosis of the liver, *Arch. Int. Med.,* 103, 750, 1959.

100. **Sheld, H. P. and Bartter, F. C.,** An explanation for and experimental correction of abnormal water diuresis in cirrhosis, *J. Clin. Invest.,* 39, 2248, 1960.

101. **Lancestremere, R. G., Davidson, P. L., Earley, L. E., O'Brien, F. J., and Papper, S.,** Renal failure in Laennec's cirrhosis. III. Diuretic response to administered water, *J. Lab. Clin. Med.,* 60, 967.

102. **Perez-Ayuso, R. M., Arroyo, V., Camps, J., Rimola, A., Gaya, J., Costa, J., Rivera, F., and Rodés, J.,** Evidence that renal prostaglandins are involved in renal water metabolism in cirrhosis, *Kidney Int.,* 26, 72, 1984.

103. **Bichet, D., Szatalowicz, V., Chaimovitz, C., and Schrier, R. W.,** Role of vasopressin in abnormal water excretion in cirrhotic patients, *Ann. Intern. Med.,* 96, 413, 1982.

104. **Reznick, R. K., Langer, B., Taylor, B. R., Seif, S., and Blendis, L. M.,** Hyponatremia and arginine vasopressin secretion in patients with refractory ascites undergoing peritoneovenous shunting, *Gastroenterology,* 84, 713, 1983.

105. **Morel, F., Imbert-Teboul, M., and Chabardès. D.,** Receptors to vasopressin and other hormones in the mammalian kidney, *Kidney Int.,* 31, 512, 1983.

106. **Jard, S.,** Mechanism of action of vasopressin and vasopressin antagonists, *Kidney Int.,* 34 (Suppl. 26), S38, 1988.

107. **Thibonnier, M.,** Vasopressin and blood pressure, *Kidney Int.,* 34 (Suppl. 25), S52, 1988.

108. **Hofbauer, K. G., Studer, W., Mah, S. C., Michel, J. B., Wood, J. M., and Stalder, R.,** The significance of vasopressin as a pressor agent, *J Cardiovas. Pharmacol.,* 6, S429, 1984.

109. **Liard, J. F.,** Vasopressin antagonists and their use in animal studies, *Kidney Int.,* 34 (Suppl. 26), S43, 1988.

110. **Thibonnier, M.,** Use of vasopressin antagonists in human diseases, *Kidney Int.* 34 (Suppl. 26), S48, 1988.

111. **Camps, J., Solá, J., Arroyo, V., Pérez-Ayuso, R. M., Gaya, J., Rivera, F., and Rodés, J.,** Temporal relationship between the impairment of free water excretion and antidiuretic hormone hypersecretion in rats with experimental cirrhosis, *Gastroenterology,* 93, 498, 1987.

112. **Claria, J., Jiménez, W., Arroyo, V., López, C., Gaya, J., Rivera, F., and Rodés, J.,** The blockade of the hydro-osmotic effect of antidiuretic hormone normalizes renal water metabolism in experimental cirrhosis with ascites (abstr.), *J. Hepatol.,* 7 (Suppl. 1), S21, 1981.

113. **Smith, W. L.,** Renal prostaglandin biochemistry, *Miner. Electrolyte Metab.,* 6, 10, 1981.

114. **Dunn, W. J. and Zambraski, E. J.,** Renal effects of drugs that inhibit prostaglandin synthesis, *Kidney Int.,* 18, 609, 1980.

115. **Flower, R. J.,** Drugs which inhibit prostaglandin biosynthesis, *Pharmacol. Rev.,* 26, 33, 1974.

116. **Smith, W. L. and Bell, T. G.,** Immunohistochemical localization of the prostaglandin forming cyclooxygenase, *Am. J. Physiol.,* 235, F451, 1978.

117. **Sun, F. F., Taylor, B. M., McGuire, J. C., and Wong, P. Y. K.,** Metabolism of prostaglandins in the kidney, *Kidney Int.,* 19, 760, 1981.

118. **Hassid, A., Konieczkowski, M., and Dunn, M. J.,** Prostaglandin synthesis in isolated rat kidney glomeruli, *Proc. Natl. Acad. Sci., U.S.A.,* 76, 1155, 1979.

119. **Smith, W. L. and Bell, T. G.,** Immunohistochemical localization of the prostaglandins-forming cyclooxigenase in renal cortex, *Am. J. Physiol.,* 235, F451, 1978.
120. **Schlondorff, D.,** Renal prostaglandin synthesis, Sites of production and specific actions of prostaglandins, *Am. J. Med.,* 81 (Suppl. 2B), 1, 1986.
121. **Anggard, E. and Oliw, E.,** Formation and metabolism of prostaglandins in the kidney, *Kidney Int.,* 19, 771, 1981.
122. **Schnermann, J. and Briggs, P. J.,** Participation of renal cortical prostaglandins in the regulation of glomerular filtration rate, *Kidney Int.,* 19, 802, 1981.
123. **Dunn, M. J. and Hood, V. L.,** Prostaglandins and the kidney, *Am. J. Physiol.,* 233, F169, 1977.
124. **McGiff, J. C.,** Prostaglandins, prostacyclin and thromboxanes, *Annu. Rev. Pharmacol. Toxicol.,* 21, 479, 1981.
125. **Pugliese, F. and Ciabattoni, G.,** Investigations of renal arachidonic acid metabolites by radioimmunoassay, in *Prostaglandins and the Kidney,* Dunn, M. J., Patrono, C., and Cinotti, G. A., Eds., New York, Plenum Medical Book, 83, 1983.
126. **Weber, P. C., Scherer, B., Siess, W., Held, E., and Schnermann, J.,** Formation and actions of prostaglandins in the kidney, *Klin. Wochenschr.,* 57, 1021, 1979.
127. **Levenson, D. J., Simmons, C. E. Jr., and Brenner, B. M.,** Arachidonic acid metabolism, prostaglandins and the kidney, *Am. J. Med.,* 72, 354, 1982.
128. **Frolich, J. C. and Fejes-Toth, G.,** Renal prostaglandins, *Klin. Wochenschr.,* 60, 1155, 1982.
129. **Nasjletti, A.,** The role of arachidonic acid metabolism in the modulation of renal blood flow, in *Prostaglandins and the Kidney,* Dunn, M. J., Patrono, C., Cinotti, G. A., Eds., New York, Plenum Medical Book, 1983, 111.
130. **Lonigro, A. J., Tarragno, N. A., Malik, K. V., and McGiff, J. C.,** Differential inhibition by prosta-
131. **Malik, K. V., Susic, H., and Masjletti, A.,** Modulation of adrenergic neuro-effector event in the renal vasculature: role of prostaglandins, *Prog. Biochem. Pharmacol.,* 17, 108, 1980.
132. **Hassid, A.,** Regulation of prostaglandin biosynthesis in cultured cells, *Am. J. Physiol.,* 243, C205, 1982.
133. **Lifschitz, M. D.,** Renal effects of nonsteroidal antiinflammatory agents, *J. Lab. Clin. Med.,* 102, 313, 1983.
134. **Dunn, M. J.,** Nonsteroidal anti-inflammatory drugs and renal function, *Annu. Rev. Med.,* 35, 411, 1984.
135. **Olive, D. M. and Stoff, J. S.,** Renal syndromes associated with nonsteroidal anti-inflammatory drugs, *N. Engl. J. Med.,* 310, 563, 1984.
136. **Lifschitz, M. D.,** Prostaglandin and renal blood flow: in vivo studies, *Kidney Int.,* 19, 781, 1981.
137. **Rimola, A., Ginès, P., Arroyo, V., Camps, J., Perez-Ayuso, R. M., Quintero, E., Gaya, J., Rivera, F., and Rodés, J.,** Urinary excretion of 6-keto-prostaglandin-F_1-alpha, thromboxane A_2 and prostaglandin E_2 in cirrhosis with ascites. Relationship to functional renal failure (hepatorenal syndrome), *J. Hepatol.,* 3, 111, 1986.
138. **Guarner, C., Colina, J., Guarner, F., Corzo, J., Prieto, J., and Vilardell, F.,** Renal prostaglandins in cirrhosis of the liver, *Clin. Sci.,* 70, 477, 1986.
139. **Laffi, G., La Villa, G., Pinzani, M., Ciabattoni, G., Patrignani, R., Mannelli, M., Cominelli, F., and Gentilini, P.,** Altered renal and platelet arachidonic acid metabolism in cirrhosis, *Gastroenterology,* 90, 274, 1986.
140. **Zipser, R. D., Hoefs, J. C., Speckart, R. F., Zia, P. K., and Horton, R.,** Prostaglandins: modulators of renal function and pressor resistance in chronic liver disease, *J. Clin. Endocrinol. Metab.,* 48, 895, 1979.
141. **Govindarajan, S., Nast, C. C., Smith, W. L., Koyle, M. A., Daskalopoulos, G., and Zipser, R. P.,** Immunohistochemical distribution of renal prostaglandin endoperoxide synthase and prostacyclin synthase: diminished endoperoxide synthase in the hepatorenal syndrome, *Hepatology,* 7, 654, 1987.
142. **Zambraski, E. J. and Dunn, M. J.,** Importance of renal prostaglandins in control of renal function after chronic ligation of the common bile duct in dogs, *J. Lab. Clin. Med.,* 103, 549, 1984.
143. **Sola, J., Camps, J., Arroyo, V., Guarner, F., Gaya, J., Rivera, F., and Rodés, J.,** Longitudinal study on renal prostaglandin excretion in cirrhotic rats. Relationship with the renin-aldosterone system, *Clin. Sci.,* 75, 263, 1988.
144. **Arroyo, V., Ginès, P., Rimola, A., and Gaya, J.,** Renal function abnormalities, prostaglandins, and effects of nonsteroidal antiinflammatory drugs in cirrhosis with ascites. An overview with emphasis on pathogenesis, *Am. J. Med.,* 81, (Suppl. 2B), 104, 1986.
145. **Zipser, R. D.,** Role of renal prostaglandins and the effects of nonsteroidal anti-inflammatory drugs in patients with liver disease, *Am. J. Med.,* 81, (Suppl. 2B), 95, 1986.
146. **Epstein, M. and Lifschitz, M.,** Renal eicosanoids as determinants of renal function in liver disease, *Hepatology,* 7, 1359, 1987.
147. **Boyer, T. D., Zia, P., and Reynolds, T. B.,** Effects of indomethacin and prostaglandin A1 in renal function and plasma renin activity in alcoholic liver disease, *Gastroenterology,* 77, 215, 1979.

148. **Lianos, E. A., Alavi, N., Tobin, M., Venuto, R., and Bentzel, C. J.,** Angiotensin-induced sodium excretion patterns in cirrhosis: role of renal prostaglandins, *Kidney Int.,* 21, 70, 1982.

149. **Quintero, E., Ginès, P., Arroyo, V., Rimola, A. Camps, J., Guevara, A., Gaya, J., Rodamilans, M., and Rodés, J.,** Sulindac reduces the urinary excretion of prostaglandins and impairs renal function in cirrhosis with ascites *Nephron,* 42, 298, 1986.

150. **Planas, R., Arroyo, V., Rimola, A., Perez-Ayuso, R. M., and Rodés, J.,** Acetylasalicylic acid suppresses the renal hemodynamic effect and reduces the diuretic action of furosemide in cirrhosis with ascites, *Gastroenterology,* 84, 247, 1983.

151. **Mirouze, D., Zipser, R. D., and Reynolds, T. B.,** Effects of inhibitors of prostaglandin synthesis on induced diuresis in cirrhosis, *Hepatology,* 3, 50, 1983.

152. **Levy, M., Wexler, M. J., and Fechner, C.,** Renal perfusion in dogs with experimental hepatic cirrhosis: role of prostaglandins, *Am. J. Physiol.,* 245, F521, 1983.

153. **Zipser, R. D., Radvan, G., Kronborg, J., Duke, R., and Little, T.,** Urinary thromboxane B2 and prostaglandin E2 in the hepatorenal syndrome: evidence for increased vasoconstrictor and decreased vasodilator factors, *Gastroenterology,* 84, 697, 1982.

154. **Zipser, R. D., Kronborg, J., Rector, W., Reynolds, T., and Daskalopoulos, G.,** Therapeutic trial on thromboxane synthesis inhibition in the hepatorenal syndrome, *Gastroenterology,* 87, 1128, 1984.

155. **Ardaillou, R., Baud, L., and Sraer, J.,** Leukotrienes and other lipoxigenase products of arachidonic acid synthesized in the kidney, *Am. J. Med.,* 81 (Suppl 2B), 12, 1986.

156. **Rosenthal, A. and Pace-Asciak, C. R.,** Potent vasoconstriction of the isolated perfused rat kidney by the leukotrienes C_4 and D_4, *Can. J. Physiol. Pharmacol.,* 61, 325, 1983.

157. **Piper, P. J., Stanton, A. W. B., and McLeod, L. J.,** The actions of leukotrienes C4 and D4 in the porcine renal vascular bed, *Prostaglandins,* 29, 61, 1985.

158. **Barnett, R., Goldwasser, P., and Scharschmidt, L. A.,** Effects of leukotrienes on isolated rat glomeruli and cultured mesangial cells, *Am. J. Physiol.,* 250, F838, 1986.

159. **Huber, K., Kastner, S., Scholmerich, J., and Keppler, D.,** Enhanced urinary excretion of cysteinyl leukotrienes in patients with hepatorenal syndrome (abstract), *J. Hepatol.,* 5 (Suppl. 1), S34, 1987.

160. **Moore, K. P., Taylor, G. W., Maltby, N., Siegers, D., Dollery, C. T., and Williams, R.,** Increased urinary excretion of cysteinyl-leukotrienes in decompensated liver disease and hepatorenal syndrome (abstract), *J. Hepatol.,* 7 (Suppl. 1), S61, 1988.

161. **Fernández-Seara, J., Prieto, J., Quiroga, J., Zozaya, J. M., Cobos, M. A., Rodriguez Aire, J. L., Garcia Plaza, A., and Leal, J.,** Systemic and regional hemodynamics in patients with liver cirrhosis and ascites with and without functional renal failure, *Gastroenterology,* 97, 1304, 1989.

162. **Henriksen, J., Ring-Larsen, H., and Christensen, N.,** Circulating noradrenaline and central hemodynamics in patients with cirrhosis, *Scand. J. Gastroenterol.* 20, 1185, 1985.

163. **Shapiro, M. D., Nichols, K. M., Groves, B. M., Kluge, R., Chung, H. M., Bichet, D. G., and Schrier, R. W.,** Interrelationship between cardiac output and vascular resistance as determinants of effective arterial blood volume in cirrhotic patients, *Kidney Int.,* 28, 206, 1985.

164. **Nichols, K. M., Shapiro, M. D., Kludge, R., Chung, H. M., Bichet, P., and Schrier, R. N.,** Interrelationship between cardiac output and vascular resistance as determinants of effective arterial blood volume in cirrhotic patients, *Kidney Int.,* 28, 206, 1985.

165. **Bichet, D. G., Groves, B., and Schrier, R. W.,** Mechanism of improvement of water and sodium excretion by immersion in decompensated cirrhotic patients, *Kidney Int.,* 24, 788, 1783.

166. **Bosch, J., Arroyo, V., Betriu, A., Mas, A., Carrilho, F., Rivera, F., Navarro, F., and Rodés, J.,** Hepatic hemodynamics and the renin-angiotensin-aldosterone system in cirrhosis, *Gastroenterology,* 78, 92, 1980.

167. **Bosch, J., Mastai, R., Kravetz, D., Bruix, J., Rigau, J., and Rodés, J.,** Measurement of azygous venous blood flow in the evaluation of portal hypertension in patients with cirrhosis. Clinical and haemodynamic correlations in 100 patients, *J. Hepatol.,* 1985, 1, 125.

168. **Kotelanski, B., Groszmann, R. J., and Cohn, J. N.,** Circulation times in the splanchnic and hepatic beds in alcoholic liver disease. *Gastroenterology* 1972, 63, 102-111.

169. **Kontos, H. H., Shapiro, W., Mauck, H. P., and Patterson, J. L.,** General and regional circulatory alterations in cirrhosis of the liver. *Am. J. Med.,* 37, 526, 1964.

170. **Lieberman, F. L., Denison, E. K., and Reynolds, T. B.,** The relationship of plasma volume, portal hypertension, ascites, and renal sodium retention in cirrhosis. The "overflow" theory of ascites formation, *Ann. N.Y. Acad. Sci.,* 170, 202, 1970.

171. **Lieberman, F. L. and Reynolds, T. B.,** Plasma volume in cirrhosis of the liver: its relation to portal hypertension, ascites and renal failure, *J. Clin. Invest.,* 46, 1297, 1967.

172. **Willett, J. R., Jennings, G., Esler, M., and Dudley, F. J.,** Sympathetic tone modulates portal venous pressure in alcoholic cirrhosis, *Lancet,* 2, 939, 1986.

173. **Henriksen, J. H., Ring-Larsen, H., Kanstrup, I. L., Christensen, N. J.,** Sympathetic nervous activity and renal and systemic hemodynamics in cirrhosis: plasma norepinephrine concentration, hepatic extraction and renal release, *Hepatology,* 1982, 2, 304.

174. **Benoit, J. M. and Granger, N.**, Splanchnic hemodynamics in chronic portal hypertension, *Sem. Liver Dis.*, 6, 287, 1986.
175. **Vorobioff, J., Bredfelt, J. E., Groszmann, R. J.**, Hyperdynamic circulation in portal-hypertensive rate model: a primary factor for maintenance of chronic portal hypertension, *Am. J. Physiol.*, 244, G52, 1983.
176. **Vorobioff, J., Bredfelt, J. E., and Groszmann, R. J.**, Increased blood flow through the portal system in cirrhotic rats, *Gastroenterology*, 87, 1120, 1984.
177. **Blanchet, L. and Lebrec, D.**, Changes in splanchnic blood flow in portal hypertensive rats, *Eur. J. Clin. Invest.*, 12, 327, 1982.
178. **Bosch, J., Enriquez, R., Groszmann, R. J., and Storer, E. H.**, Chronic bile duct ligation in the dog: hemodynamic characterization of aportal hypertension model, *Hepatology*, 3, 1002, 1983.
179. **Benoit, J. N., Barrowman, J. A., Harper, S. L., Kvietys, K. R., and Granger, N. D.**, Role of humoral factors in the intestinal hyperemia associated with chronic portal hypertension, *Am. J. Physiol.*, 247, G486, 1984.
180. **Cohn, J. N., Khatri, J. M., Groszmann, R. J., and Kotelanski, B.**, Hepatic blood flow in alcoholic liver disease measured by an indicator dilution technique, *Am. J. Med.*, 53, 704, 1972.
181. **Groszmann, R. J., Kotelanski, B., Cogn, J. N., and Katri, J. M.**, Quantitation of portasystemic shunting from the splenic and mesenteric beds in alcoholic liver disease, *Am. J. Med.*, 53, 715, 1972.
182. **Schrier, R. W., Arroyo, V., Bernardi, M., Epstein, M., Henriksen, J. H., and Rodés, J.**, Peripheral vasodilation hypothesis. A proposal for the initation of renal sodium and water retention in cirrhosis, *Hepatology*, 8, 1151, 1988.

Chapter 8

HEPATIC CIRCULATION IN CIRRHOSIS

Daphna Fenyves, Pierre Michel Huet, and J. P. Villeneuve

TABLE OF CONTENTS

I. INTRODUCTION

Cirrhosis is characterized by fibrosis with loss of the normal hepatic architecture, nodule formation, and regeneration. The process is accompanied by disturbances of both the macro- and microcirculation of the liver. The evolution of the disease leads to eventual development of hepatic failure and portal hypertension, with major clinical consequences.

This chapter will deal with the vascular anomalies which have been described in the setting of cirrhosis and their potential functional implications, the current concepts of the mechanisms involved in the development of portal hypertension, and finally the pharmacological approach to the management of portal hypertension.

II. NORMAL HEPATIC CIRCULATION

A. ANATOMICAL DATA

The liver is the largest organ in the body, weighing 1200 to 1800 g, and having the largest blood flow (approximately 100 ml/min/100 g of liver or 25 to 30% of the cardiac output). It possesses a dual blood supply: the portal vein, which drains the spleen and splanchnic organs, provides 70 to 80% of the blood flow; the hepatic artery, which carries well-oxygenated blood, provides the remainder. Both the terminal portal venules and hepatic arterioles end in sinusoids through which all afferent blood must flow before reaching the effluent vessels, the terminal hepatic venules.

Since the work of Rappaport,[1] the circulation within the normal liver has been relatively well understood. Blood from a terminal branch of the portal vein flows to at least two different terminal hepatic venules, this via a functional microcirculatory unit known as a simple acinus. This unit consists of several single cell plates of hepatocytes, radiating from major afferent vessels toward a terminal hepatic vein. The acinus is thus subdivided into concentric areas referred to as zones 1 (periportal, situated at the periphery of the lobule), 2 and 3 (pericentral or centrilobular), each with its own metabolic activity. Terminal hepatic artery branches have a more complex distribution. Vascular casts have shown that their intralobular branches issue terminal subdivisions either directly into sinusoids or into dense peribiliary plexus.[2,3] These peribiliary vascular structures have been shown to consist of two layers: an inner network of fine capillaries formed by branches of the afferent hepatic artery drains into an outer venous layer which makes up the efferent arm of the plexus; these vessels in turn empty either directly into sinusoids or first into peribiliary portal radicals. The smaller peribiliary vascular networks consist only of a single layer of capillaries.[2,4] Therefore in normal livers, part of the blood derived from the hepatic artery must first flow through a capillary system before reaching the sinusoids.

Electron microscopic studies have shown that the portal vein has few sinusoidal connections, whereas the hepatic veins possess multiple sinusoidal outlets giving them a perforated appearance.[5,6] These sinusoids have a unique structure found in no other organ, which allows maximal contact between the hepatocytes and blood perfusing the liver. Their lining consists of endothelial cells which lack a basement membrane and are perforated by a multitude of fenestrae 50 to 200 nm in diameter.[7] These apertures can be found in isolation or more often as clusters called sieve plates.[5,7-9]

Within these sinusoids, one can find Kupffer cells. These are generally seen protruding into the sinusoidal lumen, attached to the fenestrated endothelial cells.[5,10] Behind the endothelial lining lies a large extravascular space known as the space of Disse. This space is continuous with the intercellular space up to the tight junctions of the hepatocytes which separate the extravascular space from the bile canaliculi. It normally contains some fat-storing cells (perisinusoidal or Ito cells) and a few collagen bundles.[5,6] The entire space is therefore freely accessible to molecules contained in plasma. For particles of equal or greater diameter, however, the fenestrae act as a filtering mechanism. For example, although small chylomicrons do pass through the pores, the larger particles (>300 nm) are normally denied access to the space of Disse,[11-13] and their effect might be important in overall fat and cholesterol metabolism and by consequence, may also play a role in the development of atherosclerosis.[13,14]

Moreover, fenestrae are dynamic structures which have been shown to vary in size in response to various stimuli. Exposure to alcohol leads to a reduction in the number of openings, accompanied by a dilatation of the remaining pores and decreased porosity (% fenestrated area with respect to the total area of sinusoidal lining).[15-18] It has been suggested that such enlarged fenestrae may admit dietary fats normally excluded from the extravascular space by virtue of their size, and thus play a role in the development of alcohol-induced fatty liver.[15] Hepatic venous outflow obstruction with venous congestion,[19] high perfusion pressure,[20] and CCl_4[16] have all been reported to increase pore size.

Serotonin has also been shown to alter the diameter of endothelial fenestrations;[21] epinephrine (see other chapters) causes a reduction in pore size in association with sinusoidal contraction and diminished sinusoidal blood flow;[22] and acetylcholine and bethanechol induce an increase in pore diameter, with sinusoidal dilatation and increased sinusoidal blood flow.[23] The mechanisms responsible for these alternations are poorly understood, but the lining endothelium has been shown to contain microtubules and filaments,[9] and more recently, actin and myosin.[23,24] In addition, sphincter-like structures devoid of smooth muscle have been described at the junction of the sinusoids with terminal portal venules (inlet) as well as terminal hepatic radicals (outlet).[22] These narrowings appear to be due to a local circular contraction of junctional endothelial cells which possess a basement membrane and no fenestrae and which also contain microfilaments. This all suggests a role for these proteins in the contraction and relaxation of sinusoids as well as endothelial fenestrations and by consequence, regulation of blood flow as well as uptake of substrates from plasma.

Studies both in animals[6,25,26] and man[8] have demonstrated lobular gradients in endothelial fenestrations. From the periphery of the lobule centrally, this consists of a slight reduction in pore diameter which, however, is offset by an increase in frequency of the fenestrations, leading to an increased porosity from 6 to 8%. Similarly, the sinusoids are tortuous and relatively narrow at the periphery of the lobule but become straighter and wider centrally. This zonal distribution favors exchange processes centrally and may serve to counterbalance the preferential uptake of substances known to occur in the periportal area.[27]

The exchange of particles between blood and hepatocytes is further influenced by the particular structure and flexibility of the endothelial lining: this lining is thought to undergo reciprocal adaptation during the passage of blood cells, causing a stirring of the space of Disse and promoting such exchanges.[9] Both red and white blood cells are larger than periportal sinusoids[24] and need to adapt their shape to be able to travel in these channels.

As they move along, the relatively rapid pliable erythrocytes displace fluid and plasma particles which then escape into the space of Disse via the fenestrations. This "forced sieving" promotes transport of substrates to the extravascular space for subsequent uptake by the parenchymal cells. Similarly, the more rigid leukocytes "massage" the endothelial lining and underlying space of Disse as they force their way through the sinusoids, further enhancing the movement of fluid and particles toward the hepatocytes.[9,24]

Wisse et al.[24] have recently published a comprehensive review of the structure and function of the specialized sinusoidal lining.

B. PHYSIOLOGICAL DATA

The multiple indicator dilution technique proposed by Goresky[28] provides the best approach to study the unique structure of the normal sinusoidal bed and, as will be seen later, to evaluate changes caused by the anatomic alterations which have been described in long-

NORMAL LIVER

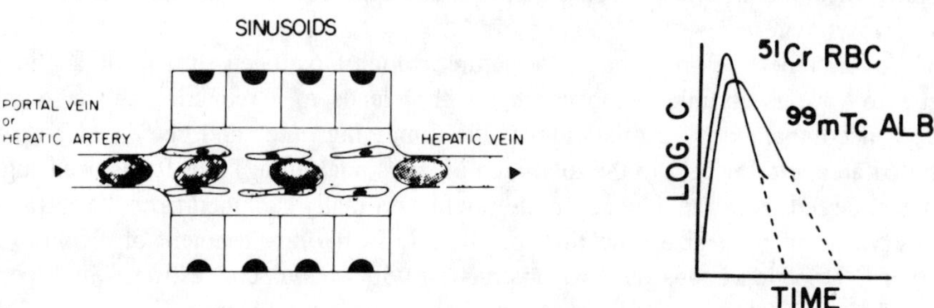

FIGURE 1. Schematic representation of the liver microcirculation in a normal liver. The entry of ^{99m}Tc albumin (^{99m}TcALB) into the space of Disse produces a major delay in and decrease in magnitude of the albumin curve with respect to that of ^{51}Cr red blood cells (^{51}CrRBC).

standing cirrhosis. This technique, as its name implies, involves the injection into the portal vein or hepatic artery of a mixture of different indicators and their subsequent recovery from the hepatic venous outflow. The indicators selected for these studies are usually labeled erythrocytes (RBC) and plasma-dissolved labeled substances not metabolized by the liver such as albumin, sucrose, and water.

In the liver, during their passage through the sinusoids, RBCs remain confined to the vascular space. The plasma-dissolved substances, however, gain access to the extravascular space of Disse through the fenestrations: albumin (69,000 mol wt) and sucrose (342 mol wt) diffuse into extravascular spaces that are inversely related to their molecular weights, and water penetrates the cellular space.[29] Following injection, the labeled particles disperse into the blood stream, their concentration in the venous effluent over time describing a dilution curve. The pattern of the curves they trace, assuming complete recovery, can thus be regarded as a reflection of the spaces they travel. The distribution (and dilution) of these plasma dissolved substances into areas larger then those of the RBCs produces a major delay in and decrease in magnitude of the peak of their outflow curves compared with that of the RBCs (Figure 1) a process that can be analyzed using the flow-limited model described by Goresky.[29] This method yields estimates of the sinusoidal blood volume (RBC volume) and of the extravascular volume of distribution of the diffusible substances, measured from the displacement of their outflow curves in relation to that of the RBCs (peak-time volume). This approach assumes that the distribution of plasma-dissolved substances in the extravascular space is flow-limited in the absence of a diffusion barrier and depends on the symmetry both in time and concentration for the distortion in shape of the diffusible label curve when compared to that of the RBCs.

Using the same dilution curve principle, one can evaluate the presence and magnitude of intrahepatic shunts, one of the major anatomical alterations described in long-standing human cirrhosis.[30] Under normal conditions, there is no direct communication between terminal portal and hepatic veins and all afferent blood has to flow through the sinusoidal bed before reaching the terminal hepatic venules. Particles larger than the diameter of normal sinusoids will therefore all be trapped within the sinusoids when delivered through the portal venous system. The passage of such particles (microspheres) through the liver and their subsequent recovery in the form of a dilution curve in the systemic circulation indicates the existence of intrahepatic porto-hepatic channels (Figure 2). Goresky's approach can also be applied, using lidocaine as a test substance, to further assess the barrier at the liver cell surface, the only one separating plasma from the interior of the hepatocytes.[31] Lidocaine,

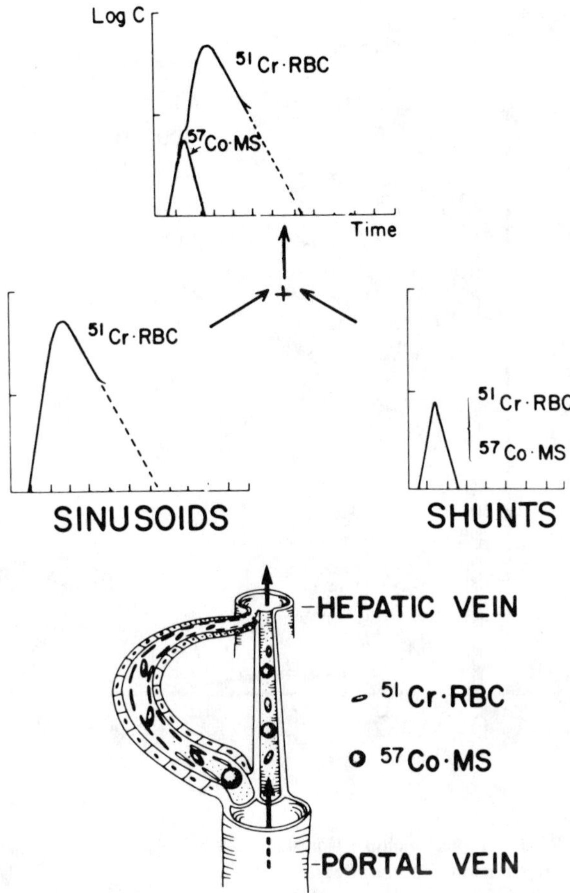

FIGURE 2.   Schematic representation of the intrahepatic microcirculation in a cirrhotic liver. The outflow pattern obtained in the hepatic vein can be resolved in two parts: An early throughput component that has come through intrahepatic shunts (right) and a later component that has come through a more normal sinusoidal bed (left). Log C: logarithm to the base 10 of the concentrations of the various markers; MS: microsphere.

a highly lipophilic substance, has been found to penetrate the liver cell membrane freely and completely during a single passage through the normal liver. Unlike labeled water, which is fully recovered in the hepatic outflow, only trace amounts of lidocaine appear in the hepatic effluent, due to its extensive intracellular binding. Since lidocaine is normally efficiently metabolized by the mixed function oxidase system, the small amount recovered unchanged in the outflow, and which emerges substantially later than labeled water, probably represents that fraction released from intrahepatic binding sites before enzymatic processing (Figure 3). By eliminating the effect of back diffusion, this phenomenon allows the evaluation of the blood to hepatocyte transfer mechanism.

In addition to the assessment of vascular and extravascular spaces, the multiple indicator dilution technique also provides an ideal approach for the study of concentrative and non-concentrative uptake processes across the liver cell membrane. This approach has been well described and reviewed by Goresky et al.[28]

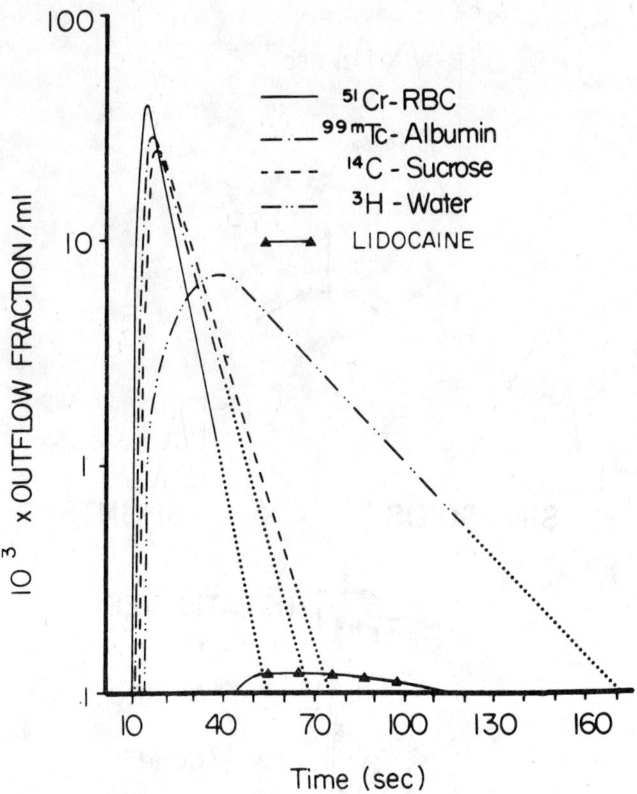

FIGURE 3.   Typical multiple indication dilution pattern obtained in an in vitro perfused normal rat liver. Relative to the intravascular marker ([51]CrRBCs) the recovery peaks of the several extravascular markers are progressively delayed and their amplitudes reduced because the space into which they distribute is progressively larger. The outflow recovery of lidocaine was 20%.

III. INTRAHEPATIC CIRCULATION IN CIRRHOSIS

A. ANATOMICAL CHANGES

Cirrhosis is characterized by destruction of the normal parenchymal architecture of the liver, development of large fibrous septae, and abnormal hepatic regeneration in the nodules.[32] The liver cell plates, which normally are one cell thick, consist of two or more rows of hepatocytes. Except for nonspecific mitochondrial alterations such as increased size, varied shapes, and paracrystalline inclusion,[33] the ultrastructural appearance of hepatocytes in the cirrhotic nodules is considered to be normal. Thus it is generally thought that cirrhosis is primarily characterized by a disturbed hepatic circulation and architecture rather than cellular alterations.

In the cirrhotic liver, both afferent (portal veins and hepatic arteries) and efferent vessels (hepatic veins) are found within the fibrous septa. Although it is thought that blood supplied to the regenerating nodules is derived mainly from the portal vein,[34] the manner in which blood leaves the nodules and drains into the hepatic veins is still not fully understood.

B. INTRAHEPATIC SHUNTS

Based on the work of Popper et al.[30] the most characteristic vascular abnormality related to cirrhosis is the development of intrahepatic porto-hepatic anastomoses.

These channels, present within fibrous septae, have been demonstrated by vascular casts which show a dense network of vessels with anastomoses (5 to 125 μm in diameter) between branches of the portal veins and hepatic veins or arteries.[30,31-37] Such connections between hepatic artery and vein radicals are rare,[34] despite the presence of a substantial arterial blood supply to this network. The enlarged arterial bed also feeds a dense pericapillary plexus which surrounds the proliferating bile ductules present in the fibrous septae.[34,37]

These anastomoses act as internal Eck fistulas shunting portal blood away from the parenchyma and regenerating nodules directly into the hepatic veins. They mostly represent remnants of previous sinusoids which have dilated and the walls of which have become thick, giving them the appearance of venous channels.[30]

The presence of large anastomoses (greater than 20 μm in diameter) between afferent and efferent vessels rests on their demonstration by vascular corrosion casts obtained at necropsy. Adequate penetration of the entire vascular system requires the injection of gelatin, latex, or plastic substances at high pressures. Extrapolation of such findings to the *in vivo* situation should therefore be viewed with caution.

C. CAPILLARIZATION AND COLLAGENIZATION

In addition to intrahepatic shunts, other structural changes have been reported in cirrhotic nodules. Schaffner and Popper[38] were the first to describe the development of a basement membrane at the margins of the microvascular channels in long-standing cirrhosis, with sealing of the sieve plates and transformation of sinusoids into capillary-like channels (capillarization). The endothelial cells form a continuous nonfenestrated lining separating the lumen from the space of Disse and parenchymal cells.

The space of Disse itself shows alterations, with various degrees of dilatation and increased deposits of collagen which accumulate mostly as bundles of fibrils.[33,38] Fat-storing cells are transformed into transitional cells, with gradual development of the rough endoplasmic reticulum and decrease in lipid storage.[39-41] This may be related to an increased fibrogenic activity.[40] Beneath the nonfenestrated endothelial cells, these transitional cells form several layers of subendothelial processes underlined by a discontinuous basement membrane-like material.[41]

Within the cirrhotic nodule, the number of Kupffer cells, or at least of functionally active fixed hepatic macrophages, appears to decrease in relation to the severity of liver damage.[42,43] At the vascular pole of the hepatocyte, microvilli are fewer in number and irregular in shape.[33,37]

These vascular changes tend to be regional within the cirrhotic nodule: capillarization is found mainly at the periphery of the nodule and more normal sinusoidal sieve plates are found at their centers. Capillarization probably proceeds from the periphery to the center of the nodule as the cirrhotic process evolves.[33,34]

Scanning electron microscopy should be an ideal tool in the assessment of capillarization of the microvascular bed and disappearance of fenestrae from the endothelial lining. However, using the freeze fracture technique is difficult because of the increase in fibrous tissue, and few reports are available. Henriksen et al.[45] have shown a decreased number of fenestrae in the cirrhotic human liver. Similarly, a reduction in the area of fenestrations per square nanometer of endothelial surface has been reported both in baboons chronically fed alcohol and in alcoholic patients.[17,18]

These morphologic changes, namely, intrahepatic shunts and capillarization of sinusoids, are not uniformly found in all cirrhotic livers and probably vary with etiology in man as well as experimental animals. However, the relative role of each of these changes in the impaired blood-liver exchanges in cirrhosis has not yet been evaluated.

CIRRHOTIC LIVER

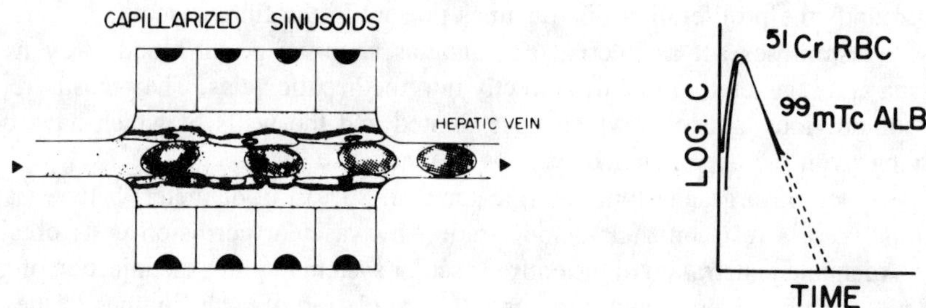

FIGURE 4.   Schematic representation of the liver microcirculation in cirrhosis. Capillarization limits the diffusion of albumin into the space of Disse and ^{99m}TcALB curve is only slightly delayed in relation to the corresponding ^{51}CrRBC curve.

IV. ASSESSMENT OF INTRAHEPATIC CIRCULATION

A. CAPILLARIZATION AND COLLAGENIZATION OF HEPATIC SINUSOIDS

The multiple indicator dilution technique (Goresky's approach) can be used to evaluate in vivo the progressive transformation of sinusoids into capillary-like channels by studying the distribution of plasma-dissolved substances into the extravascular and intracellular spaces. It can be hypothetized that in cirrhosis, the anatomic alterations will limit the spread of diffusible substances into the space of Disse by converting the microvascular bed into a two-barrier capillary system (Figure 4). Thus, in contrast to the flow-limited distribution observed in normal liver, the volume of distribution of plasma-dissolved substances should be reduced and/or their distribution in the accessible space should be limited as a function of each substance's diffusion properties with respect to the new barrier.

If diffusion into the extravascular space becomes barrier limited, the symmetry in time and concentration for the displacement of the diffusible label curves with respect to that of the RBC curve (vascular reference) will be lost, as occurs in a capillary system. Under such circumstances, estimation of the extravascular volumes of distribution of these plasma-dissolved substances as calculated from the displacement of the outflow curves in relation to that of the RBCs (peak-time method) will be incorrect and will differ systematically from those obtained in a more direct manner from the transit time (transit-time method). The latter will always be accurate, even in a system with reduced permeability, provided all the injected label is recovered at the outflow.

Such studies were carried out using the multiple indicator dilution technique in isolated perfused livers of rats with cirrhosis induced by chronic carbon tetrachloride and pheno-barbital exposure.[31] This model produces a micronodular cirrhosis akin to the human disease[46] with a finely nodular liver and connective tissue septa surrounding nodules of regenerating hepatocytes. In cirrhotic rats, the vascular space as well as the extravascular space accessible to albumin was found to be significantly reduced when compared to control rats. The profile of the albumin curves, however, remained compatible with a flow-limited diffusion, indicating that despite the reduction in size of this space, diffusion of albumin into its accessible interstitial space was not altered.

Similar studies were undertaken in cirrhotic patients undergoing hemodynamic assessment of portal hypertension.[47] A wide range of outflow dilution patterns was obtained: at one extreme, a pattern similar to that expected in the normal liver was found, with clear separation of the labeled RBC and albumin curves and a large space ratio for albumin (albumin to vascular space ratio: γ ALB); at the other end of the spectrum, the labeled albumin curve approached that of the labeled RBCs, with very small γ ALB estimates, suggesting that the vasculature had changed and become almost impermeable to albumin during a single transit. Intermediate values were probably related to the regional nature of the ultrastructural vascular changes within the cirrhotic nodules. In most patients, however, the data were still compatible with a flow-limited diffusion.

In the same group of patients, the relationship between the albumin space ratio and the disposition of indocyanine green (ICG), a molecule bound to plasma proteins, was then explored. Were the protein carrying the ICG unable to reach the liver surface due to the new barrier, a reduction in ICG elimination would be expected.[48] Indeed, a tight correlation was observed between γ ALB and the ICG extraction ratio such that as the albumin space ratio decreased, so did the ICG extraction.[47] Thus, the reduced ICG clearance may be accounted for by impaired access of the protein-bound dye to its site of uptake and disposition (the hepatocytes) due to collagenization of the space of Disse and capillarization of sinusoids in the setting of cirrhosis.

The diffusion of small molecules such as labeled sucrose and water into their respective distribution spaces is more difficult to analyze. Data obtained in cirrhotic rats following portal vein injection showed that, in some cirrhotic animals, both labeled sucrose and water dilution curves displayed a unimodal pattern. The diffusion of sucrose and water in these rats was still compatible with a flow-limited distribution, and the total space accessible to sucrose and water did not differ from that measured in noncirrhotic rats.[31] Thus, it appears that sucrose and water, which are much smaller molecules than albumin, were still able, unlike albumin, to diffuse into a near-normal extravascular space. In other cirrhotic rats, labeled sucrose and water curves showed a bimodal pattern and their diffusion was no longer compatible with a flow-limited process: the volumes of distribution calculated from peak-time concentrations (peak-time method) differed systematically from those based on the transit-times (transit-time method). In cirrhotic patients in whom sucrose studies were performed mainly following hepatic artery injection, the labeled sucrose curve did not have the form expected for flow-limited distribution into the extravascular space.[47] The time-concentration symmetry for distortion of the sucrose outflow curve was lost when compared to that of the RBC curve: the delay in peak concentration time was less than anticipated and the magnitude of the peak concentration was lower than expected. The changes in shape appeared to be systematically related to changes in the albumin space ratio (γ ALB): the peak of the labeled sucrose curve advanced in time and decreased in magnitude with the decrease in the γ ALB values.

In both patients and cirrhotic rats, these changes were compatible with those predicted when the permeability of a limiting exchange barrier is progressively decreased:[49] the form of the outflow curves indicated a major limitation in the diffusive exchange of labeled sucrose (and water in rats) across the walls of the microvasculature. At the same time, the potential contribution of intrahepatic shunts is difficult to appraise and has to be evaluated, since similar patterns could also have resulted from the transit through such channels.

B. INTRAHEPATIC SHUNTS

In 1976, Ueda et al.[50] first proposed the use of large albumin macroaggregates (20 to 50 μm in diameter) to evaluate the abnormal hepatic circulation in cirrhotic patients. Labeled macroaggregates were injected into the spleen through percutaneous puncture and the presence of collateral vessels bypassing the hepatic sinusoids was calculated from the relative amount of macroaggregates entering the systemic circulation and trapped in the pulmonary capillaries as evaluated by combined liver-lung scintigrams. This technique, as well as the one modified by Syrota et al.,[51] does not really differentiate extra- from intrahepatic shunting.

In order to measure intrahepatic shunts only, studies have been undertaken using direct injection of particulate matter into the main portal vein distal to the origin of extrahepatic portosystemic collaterals, either via umbilical vein catheterization[52] or more recently, by the percutaneous transhepatic approach.[53] Shunts between the portal vein and systemic circulation, ranging from 1 to 78%, have thus been reported in cirrhotic patients.[52,54] Significant shunts between the hepatic artery and systemic circulation using the same liver-lung scintigram approach following injection of labeled macroaggregates into the hepatic artery have also been reported.[55] These findings could not however be confirmed in a group of 16 cirrhotic patients evaluated by Ohnishi et al.[54] Several potential sources of error may account for the discrepancies. In these studies, contamination of the calculated shunts from extra-hepatic anastomoses through distal portal vein collaterals such as seen in the Cruveihlier-Baumgarten syndrome cannot be excluded, and scintillation counting over the liver and lungs can only provide indirect estimates of questionable accuracy. Another potential problem might be the nonhomogenous size of commercial macroaggregates used previously and the possible presence (or formation) of particles smaller than the normal sinusoids.

Some of these technical pitfalls were recently addressed by Hoefs et al.[56] These investigators suggested assessing the importance of large intrahepatic shunts (IHS) by the injection of labeled albumin microspheres (25 ± 5 μm in diameter) into small portal vein branches (using a thin needle) with labeled albumin being the dilution indicator.[56] IHSs were measured by comparing the relative amounts of both labels recovered in hepatic vein (or inferior vena cava) samples, after the start of a 20-sec portal vein infusion of the indicators. This method minimizes the contaminating effects of extrahepatic shunting but limits the assessment of the IHSs to the small portion of liver perfused through the distal branch of the portal vein in which the thin needle is placed (10 to 50% of the liver). Although this approach can only provide rough estimates of the transit of both labels through the portion of liver studied (particularly because of the injection and sampling procedures), it underlines an important finding in cirrhosis, that is, the relatively low frequency of large IHSs: only a few patients had an intrahepatic porto-hepatic shunt index higher than 20%. The investigators discussed the discrepancy between the relatively rare occurrence of large IHS presumably located in fibrous septa (extra-acinar IHS) and the large decrease in hepatic drug extraction found in cirrhotic patients. They related this discrepancy to abnormalities in the microcirculation within the regenerative nodules (intra-acinar IHS) due either to narrow shunts or to alterations limiting diffusion into the space of Disse (capillarization of sinusoids).[56]

However, most labeled particles, whether albumin macroaggregates (20 to 50 μm); albumin microspheres (25 μm) used in human studies; or nondegradable microspheres (15 to 20 μm) used in experimental studies, are larger than the normal sinusoids and cannot detect the possible existence of small intrahepatic shunts with a diameter in the range of that of sinusoids.[30]

We have recently reported an alternative approach, using a modification of Goresky's multiple indicator dilution technique.[29] This approach involves the injection into the portal vein of a mixture containing ^{51}Cr-labeled RBCs and ^{57}Co-labeled microspheres (MS: 15 μm in diameter) and their subsequent collection from a large hepatic vein. The hepatic venous samples were collected at rates of one sample per 1 or 2 sec, with a peristaltic pump set at a fixed flow for 40 to 60 sec following the portal vein injection. The outflow activity was divided by the total amount injected in order to provide a basis for comparison between labels, yielding a pattern expressed in terms of the outflow fraction per milliliter of blood. Linear extrapolation of the downslope to infinity was carried out on a semilogarithmic plot, and the areas under the time outflow fraction per milliliter curves (AUC) were calculated. Large IHSs (%) were calculated from the microsphere recovery as: (^{57}Co MS·AUC/^{51}Cr RBC·AUC) × 100. This approach was first applied in normal rats[31] following portal vein injections. Small amounts of ^{57}Co activity were recovered in hepatic vein samples (less than

1%) but did not attain the profile of an indicator dilution curve. This activity probably represents breakdown products smaller than the sinusoidal diameter or possibly free isotope that might be misinterpreted as shunts in the absence of the RBC reference curve.

We further assessed diffusion of lidocaine across the liver cell membrane in these normal animals in a separate set of experiments.[31] For this purpose, the injection mixture consisted of ^{51}Cr RBC, ^{3}H-labeled water, and cold lidocaine (1 mg). Following injection into the portal vein, samples were collected from the hepatic venous outflow and separated into two parts: one for the determination of gamma and beta activity, processsed as previously described,[31] and the other for unchanged lidocaine determination.[58]

The outflow activity or concentration was expressed in terms of the outflow fraction per milliliter of blood, and the AUCs were calculated as previously described. Lidocaine recovery (percent) was calculated as (lidocaine·AUC/^{51}Cr RBC·AUC) × 100. In all cases, small amounts of unchanged lidocaine emerged substantially later than the labeled water curve and its outflow fraction per milliliter increased to a much later and lower peak. Lidocaine recovery was always less than 1.5% in these normal rats.

In the presence of intrahepatic shunts in a cirrhotic liver, the hepatic outflow pattern can be expected to result from transit of blood via two different pathways: a first component related to that part of the blood flowing through intrahepatic shunts, considered to be poorly permeable, short-circuit type channels; and a second or later component, related to that part of the blood coming through the sinusoids. When considering blood passing through intrahepatic shunts, no significant exchange should occur for ^{51}Cr RBCs, ^{3}H-water, and lidocaine during the time of a single passage, and these substances can be expected to flow together without separation. Whether labeled microspheres should accompany the other test substances or not depends on their diameter relative to that of the intrahepatic shunts. When considering blood flowing through the sinusoidal bed, labeled RBCs should emerge first, followed by labeled water and, substantially later, by a small amount of lidocaine released from the liver. The additional effects of capillarization on the behavior of these test substances will be discussed later.

To evaluate this methodology and test our hypothesis, we used rats with phenobarbital and carbon tetrachloride (CCl$_4$)-induced cirrhosis.[31] On histologic examination, in some nodules, capillary-like channels were found within some thin fibrotic bands. These vascular channels were similar in diameter to more normal sinusoids, a finding confirmed by ultrastructural examination.[31,59] In addition, most of the hepatic sinusoids remained structurally unaltered, although the space of Disse was widened with collagen deposition.

Unimodal labeled RBC curves were obtained in all cirrhotic rats. In most of them, labeled water curves were unimodal and slightly delayed in relation to RBC curves; however, in a few, the labeled water upslope was almost superimposed on that of the labeled RBC and the downslope exhibited a bi-exponential character. In all rats, the lidocaine outflow pattern had the form of a dilution curve; the upslope was slightly delayed in relation to that of labeled RBCs, the peak concentration was lower and appeared earlier than that of labeled water, and the downslope exhibited a bi-exponential characteristic (Figure 5). This pattern differed systematically from that observed in noncirrhotic rats, in which unchanged lidocaine emerged substantially later than labeled water and was found only in trace amounts. Lidocaine recovery covered a wide range of values in cirrhotic rats from 2.1 to 53.9%[31] In contrast, the microsphere recovery was very low (never greater than 1.2%) and did not differ from that found in noncirrhotic rats. This finding was surprising, particularly since the existence of large intrahepatic shunts (more than 20 µm diameter) between afferent and efferent vessels has been reported in cirrhotic rats, using vascular corrosion casts.[30,34]

It appeared that lidocaine was no longer able to penetrate the liver cell membranes freely and completely and that a substantial proportion emerged in the outflow related in time to the peak of the RBC curve. The early peak of unchanged lidocaine can be interpreted as

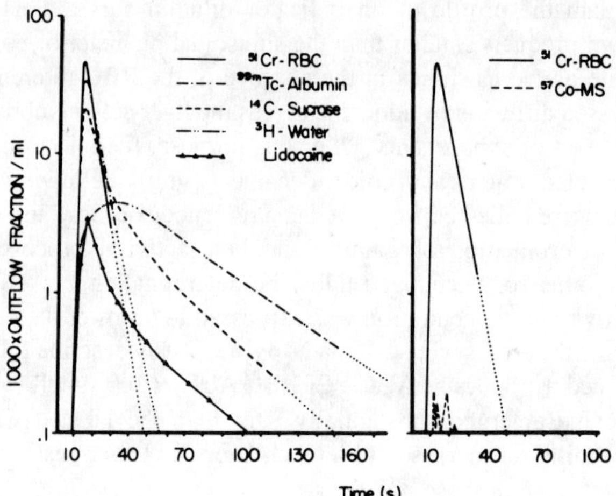

FIGURE 5.   Typical multiple indicator dilution patterns (left) and outflow recovery of microsphere (MS) (right) obtained in cirrhotic rats: the lidocaine outflow recovery was 41.4% and that of MS, 1.17%.

part of the substance flowing through a poorly permeable vascular bed, but the size of these capillarized channels was too narrow to allow the passage of large microspheres (more than 15 μm in diameter).[31] Thus, in rats with CCl_4-induced cirrhosis, lidocaine data were compatible with the development of small intrahepatic shunts (less than 15 μm). These findings are in agreement with the anatomic changes found in such rat livers, in which occasional small channels (7 to 10 μm in diameter) were found in fibrotic bands dissecting the nodules.

The throughput lidocaine may also have resulted from complete capillarization and collagenization of all sinusoids, changing the liver microcirculation into a well-capillarized system. Light and electron microscopic studies of the livers, however, did not demonstrate significant alterations of the sinusoids.

This approach was then applied to cirrhotic patients at the time of portal hypertension assessment.[60] In 35 patients, the right hepatic vein and common hepatic artery were catheterized by the Seldinger technique and, in 20 of these patients, transhepatic portal vein cannulation was successfully achieved. The injection mixture consisted of ^{51}Cr RBCs, ^{99m}Tc albumin microspheres (20 μm in diameter), and in some cases, 30 mg of lidocaine in a protein-free solution. The tracers were injected in the hepatic artery and the portal vein when available, in random order. In none of the patients did labeled microspheres appear in the hepatic effluent following injection into the hepatic artery. In all cases in which lidocaine was used, the outflow curve for unchanged lidocaine increased to a much later and lower peak than that of RBCs. In most cases, the downslope extrapolation for lidocaine could not be carried out because of recirculation, preventing lidocaine recovery determination. In contrast, following portal vein injection, an early peak of microspheres and of lidocaine appeared simultaneously with RBCs in the hepatic outflow of seven of the 20 patients (three with micronodular cirrhosis and four with macronodular cirrhosis) (Figure 6). In these seven patients, large intrahepatic shunts ranged from 2 to 65%. When shunting was important, ^{51}Cr RBC curves were bimodal, with an early component appearing in the hepatic vein simultaneously with the microspheres.

In patients without large intrahepatic shunts, the outflow curves for unchanged lidocaine were similar to those obtained following hepatic artery injection. These findings suggest that in cirrhotic patients, intrahepatic porto-hepatic shunts, when present, have a large diameter (more than 20 μm) and are probably located in the broad bands of fibrous septa.

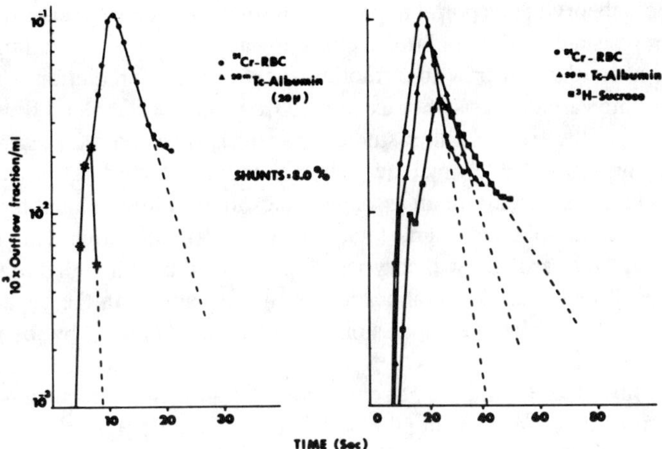

FIGURE 6. Typical multiple indicator dilution patterns (left) and outflow recoveries of microsphere (MS) (right) obtained in a cirrhotic patient. Large intrahepatic shunts were demonstrated, 8% of MS appearing in the hepatic effluent.

In human cirrhosis, small shunts as detected by lidocaine in rats, do not appear to be present following either portal vein or hepatic artery injection.

No correlation was found between the degree of shunting and the ICG extraction in the seven patients with significant shunting. However, the decreasing ICG extraction appeared larger than could be accounted for by the reduction in the albumin space ratio (γ ALB) in the same patients.[60]

C. SUMMARY

Using the multiple indicator dilution approach, events occurring in the microvascular bed can be characterized in both experimental animals and in man.

Intrahepatic shunts can be found shunting blood away from sinusoids in both cirrhotic patients and cirrhotic animals. Such channels were present in about one-third of cirrhotic patients with portal hypertension, and occurred mainly between the portal and hepatic veins. In cirrhotics, porto-hepatic anastomoses are usually large (more than 20 μm in diameter).

Although collagenization of the space of Disse and the progressive transformation of sinusoids into capillary-like channels decreased the extravascular space accessible to albumin and probably other large molecules and protein-bound substances, these sinusoidal changes do not appear to limit the diffusion of sucrose, water, and lipophilic substances, such as lidocaine into the extravascular and intracellular spaces.

V. PHYSIOPATHOLOGY OF PORTAL HYPERTENSION: "BACKWARD" AND "FORWARD" FLOW THEORIES

The pathophysiologic mechanisms involved in the development and maintenance of portal hypertension are complex. Attempts to better understand the events involved have led to the formulation of the "backward" and "forward" flow theories of portal hypertension.

In the setting of cirrhosis, the intrahepatic vascular tree is distorted by factors such as fibrosis, compression by regenerating nodules, and collagen accumulation in the space of Disse, as well as occlusive venous lesions such as are seen in alcoholic liver disease. Such distortion results in an increased resistance to the flow of blood within the liver. The ''backward'' flow theory views portal hypertension solely as a consequence of this increased hepatic vascular resistance. This traditional concept was based on early findings of a reduced portal and total hepatic blood flow in cirrhotic patients[61-63] and predictions of an associated increased splanchnic vascular resistance as derived from such portal blood flow measurement obtained proximal to the liver.[63] Other studies, however, revealed the presence of a hyperdynamic circulatory state[64-67] characterized by an increased cardiac output and reduced peripheral vascular resistance, with an associated elevation in forearm and hand blood flow, as well as an increased splenic[68-70] and total splanchnic[71] blood flow. This resulted in the formulation of the ''forward'' flow theory which proposes that although portal hypertension develops as a result of increased intrahepatic vascular resistance in the cirrhotic liver, it is thereafter maintained, despite decompression via collateral channels, by the presence of an elevated splanchnic blood flow.

Evidence in favour of an important contribution by an increased splanchnic blood flow derives mainly from experiments using the portal vein-ligated (PVL) rat model of prehepatic portal hypertension.[72] The production of a graded (75%) portal vein stenosis[73] in the rat results in the consistent development of portal hypertension in association with a high degree of porto-systemic shunting, an elevated splanchnic blood flow, and a reduced splanchnic arteriolar resistance[74] as measured using the γ-labeled microsphere technique.[75] Sikuler et al.[76] followed the chronology of these events to show that portal vein ligation is followed by portal hypertension within 2 d, initially accompanied by an increased portal vascular resistance. The subsequent development of a collateral circulation is then associated with a progressive reduction in portal vascular resistance towards normal in conjunction with an increase in portal venous inflow (total flow in all splanchnic organs) and reduction in splanchnic arteriolar resistance (forward flow theory). The relative contribution of these factors to the production and maintenance of portal hypertension in this model has been further evaluated.[77-79] Removal of the ligature in portal hypertensive PVL-rats, with elimination of the portal resistance so induced, resulted in a normalization of portal venous pressure despite persistence of an elevated portal venous inflow.[77] Thus, in the presence of a low resistance vascular bed, an increased splanchnic blood flow is not enough to raise portal pressure. Similarly, Kroeger et al.[78] demonstrated that in portal hypertensive PVL-rats β-adrenergic blockade corrected splanchnic blood flow but did not return portal pressure to normal values. Benoit et al.[79] predicted that in this model of portal hypertension, increased splanchnic flow (forward flow) contributes approximately 40% of the rise in portal venous pressure, whereas the elevated portal vascular resistance accounts for the remaining 60%.

In the PVL-rat, portal hypertension is prehepatic. Extrapolation of these findings to the situation of liver cirrhosis were the resistance to portal blood flow in mainly intrahepatic (sinusoidal)[80,81] may not be appropriate. However, the presence of hyperdynamic splanchnic circulation has been demonstrated in man[68,69,71] as well as in portal hypertensive rats and dogs with cirrhosis induced either by CCl_4 or chronic common bile duct ligation, respectively,[82-84] attesting to the universality of this phenomenon. Thus the PVL-rat model remains a valuable tool for the study of the hyperdynamic circulation in the setting of portal hypertension.

Benoit et al.[85] conducted a series of experiments to better define the factors responsible for the intestinal hyperemia in this model. They ruled out neural mediation, demonstrated that the possible opening of intestinal anastomoses could at best account for 2% of the observed reduced splanchnic resistance, and suggested that local metabolic factors were unlikely to be of significance, since O_2 consumption in the portal hypertensive rats was no different than controls. They finally proposed a major role for circulating humoral factors as suggested by cross-perfusion studies in which the small intestine of control rats perfused with blood from portal hypertensive PVL-animals showed a 30% elevation in blood flow. A dilution effect during the cross-perfusion studies may explain the fact that this represents only half the increase in splanchnic blood flow observed in the portal hypertensive animals.

Of the vasodilator candidates, glucagon has thus far received the most attention. It is a known intestinal vasodilator,[86] and has been shown to be elevated both in PVL-rats and portal hypertensive cirrhotic patients with porto-systemic shunts.[87,88] This increase is due not to reduced catabolism but rather to a hypersecretory state.[87,88] In addition, there appears to be an impaired vascular sensitivity to endogenous vasoconstrictors,[89,90] and glucagon was shown to alter the splanchnic vascular response to endogenous and exogenous sympathetic stimulation.[91] Benoit et al.[85] infused glucagon to achieve circulating concentrations equal to those encounted in the portal hypertensive PVL-rats, producing a reduction in intestinal vascular resistance. They calculated that this hormone could account for 40% of the drop in intestinal vascular resistance observed following portal vein ligation. On the other hand, Sikuler et al.[92] found that the elevated levels of circulating glucagon were not related to the presence of a hyperdynamic splanchnic circulation. Furthermore, in a group of parabiotic rats, they were unable to reproduce the hyperdynamic systemic and splanchnic circulatory state from the portal hypertensive to the control animal, and thus corroborate the above findings.[93] In a more recent study, the same group [94] demonstrated the disappearance of the hyperdynamic circulatory state in long-term portal hypertensive PVL-rats (6 months), despite the presence of increased circulating glucagon levels equal to those seen in the short-term portal hypertensive rats (3 weeks) in which a hyperdynamic circulation was evident. This "adaptation" in the long-term portal hypertensive PVL-rat, however, now puts into question the relevance of this model to the portal hypertensive cirrhotic patient in whom the hyperdynamic circulatory state persists.

Recently, Ohnishi et al.[95] evaluated portal hypertension in a group of Japanese patients with idiopathic portal hypertension. Based on estimates using Doppler flowmetry, they identified a subgroup of patients with an elevated portal flow and suggested that in a later stage of the disease, this may be a contributing factor to the maintenance of portal hypertension in these patients. Unfortunately, Doppler flowmetry is fraught with many potential sources of error[96] and one has to be careful with the interpretation of the data obtained.

In summary, it seems that portal hypertension is triggered by the increased resistance to portal vascular flow within the cirrhotic liver (backward flow), but it is the presence of a hyperdynamic splanchnic circulation which contributes to the maintenance of this portal hypertension despite the development of portosystemic collaterals which should decompress the system (forward flow). The factors responsible for the increased splanchnic blood flow and decreased resistance remain elusive and although some studies suggest an important role for a circulating vasodilator such as glucagon, results remain conflicting. The above findings should be corroborated in an experimental model of cirrhosis before the data can be extrapolated to the development of portal hypertension in human cirrhosis. In addition, refinements of noninvasive techniques such as Doppler flowmetry may allow us to further study portal hypertension directly in man.

VI. TREATMENT

The pharmacologic approach to the treatment of portal hypertension is based on the pathophysiologic mechanisms described above. Its aims are to reduce portal venous pressure by decreasing either portal venous inflow and/or vascular resistance to that flow. Thus, drugs used in the treatment of portal hypertension can be divided into two major groups: (1) the vasoconstrictors (vasopressin and its analogues, somatostatin, β-adrenergic blockers) which act by causing splanchnic vasoconstriction thus reducing portal venous inflow, and (2) vasodilators (nitrates, prazosin, sodium nitroprusside, serotonin antagonists) which may act by reducing intrahepatic resistance, although their mechanism of action might ultimately prove to be splanchnic vasoconstriction in response to the vasodilatation they induce in other regional beds.

Acute variceal hemorrhage is a major complication of portal hypertension and a leading cause of death in cirrhotics. As such, it remains the main target in the treatment of portal hypertension. Its medical management can be divided into two broad categories: maneuvers directed at controlling the acute bleeding episode and therapy aimed at preventing rebleeding in a patient with a previous variceal rupture or even preventing an initial hemorrhage in a person with no antecedent bleeding episode.

This section will be restricted to the treatment of portal hypertension by pharmacologic manipulation, with particular reference to the impact on management of esophageal varices.

A. ACUTE VARICEAL HEMORRHAGE
1. Vasopressin and Its Analogues

Vasopressin, a naturally occurring nonapeptide, has been widely used for the initial control of variceal hemorrhage in portal hypertensive patients. It lowers portal venous pressure by virtue of its potent vasoconstrictive action on the splanchnic circulation, which results in a reduced portal venous inflow. In addition, it has recently been shown to decrease azygous blood flow.[97] Since all gastroesophageal collaterals drain into the azygous vein system, this suggests that vasopressin reduces flow through these vessels.

The vasoconstrictive action of vasopressin, however, is not restricted to the splanchnic circulation. Its widespread effects are responsible for a reduced cardiac output and coronary blood flow which can lead to serious complications including myocardial ischemia and infarction, heart failure and arythmias.[98-100] Other untoward effects include peripheral vasoconstriction, hypertension, bradycardia, cerebrovascular accidents, and mesenteric infarctions. In clinical trials, major complications, mostly ischemic in nature, occurred in 25% of patients. Attempts to avoid these systemic effects of vasopressin and possibly increase the efficacy of treatment led to the use of localized intraarterial (superior mesenteric artery) rather than peripheral intravenous infusion of the drug. Unfortunately, controlled trials failed to demonstrate any significant advantage of mesenteric arterial versus intravenous infusion.[101-106] Intraarterial infusion did not prevent the unwanted systemic effects of vasopressin, and was accompanied by additional catheter-related complications.

Clinical trials of vasopressin suggest a 44 to 71% success rate in initial hemostasis, although even its efficacy over that of a placebo is questionable.[107,108] Similarly, vasopressin offered no advantage to balloon tamponade in controlling bleeding from ruptured esophageal varices.[109]

This, coupled with a high rebleeding rate (50%) upon cessation of the infusion and the lack of improvement on survival has prompted a search for alternative therapeutic agents.

Terlipressin (triglycylysine-vasopressin), a long-acting analogue of vasopressin, became an alternative candidate. Upon intravenous injection, it is enzymatically cleaved, resulting in gradual release of the vasopressin molecule. It is thought that this prevents the systemic and particularly cardiac effects seen with the administration of an equivalent dose of vasopressin. An early uncontrolled study reported that terlipressin decreased the wedge hepatic venous pressure without any untoward effect on cardiac output, and appeared to reduce both the duration and mortality of the bleeding episode compared to a placebo.[110]

Two controlled trials have since suggested that terlipressin may indeed be more effective than vasopressin and devoid of its major side effects.[111,112] However, the study by Freeman et al.[111] included only a small number of patients and had an abysmal response rate for vasopressin (9%), and the study of Walker et al.[112] is difficult to interpret since some patients were also subjected to balloon tamponade and sclerotherapy.

Furthermore, two other studies in dogs[113] and in man[114] have failed to reveal a difference between the systemic and splanchnic effects of vasopressin and its long-acting analogue except for preservation of hepatic blood flow during terlipressin infusion. Whether this can translate into a real clinical advantage remains to be determined.

In yet another attempt to benefit from the splanchnic vasoconstrictive properties of vasopressin, Grozsmann et al.[115] conducted a trial of vasopressin and nitroglycerin, in the hope that the combination may counteract the unwanted effects of vasopressin. They demonstrated that addition of the nitrate prevents the cardiotoxicity of vasopressin. Moreover, nitroglycerin enhances the portal hypotensive action of vasopressin by reducing the increase in portal venous resistance it induces. A more recent study in hypertensive cirrhotics demonstrates that sublingual nitroglycerin lowers the hepatic portal venous gradient, mostly as a result of a reduction in wedged hepatic venous pressure and independent of any effect on azygous blood flow which itself shows a variable response to the drug.[116]

Two controlled trials comparing the use of vasopressin alone and in combination with nitroglycerin demonstrated the superiority of the latter regimen in markedly reducing the untoward effects of vasopressin (69 vs. 44% and 89 vs. 35%, respectively, for vasopressin alone or in combination with nitroglycerin).[117,118] In addition, the study of Tsai et al.[118] suggested a trend towards an improved control of hemorrhage with the combined therapy (45 vs. 21% for vasopressin alone), and Gimson et al.[117] demonstrated a clear advantage of combined therapy in cessation of variceal hemorrhage (68 vs. 44% with vasopressin alone). Unfortunately, neither study showed a benefit of combined therapy with respect to survival.

Similarly, nitroprusside has been used in conjunction with vasopressin.[119] Although it prevents the adverse action of vasopressin on cardiac output, contractility and arterial pressure, it does not protect against the deleterious effects of vasopressin on coronary blood flow.[120]

2. Somatostatin

Somatostatin, a tetradecapeptide with widespread inhibitory effects on gastrointestinal hormones and secretions, has attracted the interest of hepatologists since it has been shown to reduce splanchnic blood flow.[121-124] This has been reported in healthy subjects[122,124] as well as cirrhotic patients[125,126] and is associated with a fall in portal pressure, in the absence of any untoward systemic hemodynamic effects. Unfortunately, two further studies in cirrhotic patients failed to corroborate these findings,[127,128] and yet another report demonstrated untoward consequences on both systemic hemodynamics and blood oxygenation.[129]

Several reports had described a beneficial effect of somatostatin in the control of hemorrhage due to ruptured esophageal varices[130-132] while one letter to the NEJM stated that in five patients, this hormone failed to control bleeding.[133] Two recent controlled trials suggest that somatostatin may be equal[134] or superior to[135] vasopressin in controlling acute variceal hemorrhage, and this with a much lower rate of complications.

A further study looked at the potential use of a long-acting analogue of somatostatin (SMS 201-995) in cirrhotic rats, and suggests this agent may be of similar benefit than somatostatin but without the technical difficulties surrounding administration of the parent compound.[136] All in all, most studies suggest a mild to moderate reduction in portal pressure, but the role of somatostatin and its analogues in the treatment of portal hypertension remains to be defined.

3. Summary

For management of the acute bleeding episode, pharmacologic therapy is a second choice to much more effective hemostatic procedures.

The modified four-lumen Sengstaken-Blakemore tube remains a most useful tool, providing immediate control of hemorrhage in over 90% of patients.[137,138] It is associated with a 14% rate of major complications and a 3% mortality rate, but its major shortcoming is the high rate of rebleeding (close to 50%) which follows removal of the tube. Thus, it is an effective but merely temporizing measure.

Emergency sclerotherapy has gained increasing popularity in recent years as a first-line hemostatic procedure. It controls bleeding in 90% of cases, and decreases short-term mortality with a 10% rate of major complications.[139-145] One study suggests it may favorably influence long-term survival.[146] Although helpful during the acute episode, emergency sclerotherapy must be followed by further management to prevent recurrence of bleeding.

Decompression of the portal system by surgical means offers an alternative to medical management, but emergency portocaval shunt surgery is not greeted with enthusiasm. It carries a high mortality (42%) and is associated with a significant incidence of postoperative encephalopathy (31%).[147] In patients with severe liver disease, it offered no advantage to sclerotherapy with respect to survival,[148] although it may be a more viable alternative under more selective conditions, in patients with mild to moderate disease.[149]

Thus, in our institution, emergency sclerotherapy is presently the first-line treatment for acute variceal rupture. If the procedure is unsuccessful in hemorrhage control, or if it is technically not feasible due to the severity of the bleed, the Blakemore tube is applied for primary hemostasis. Balloon tamponade is used as a temporary measure and injection of ·the varices reattempted soon thereafter. If sclerotherapy fails, patients with mild to moderate liver disease (Child A and B) are offered portocaval shunt therapy.

B. PREVENTION OF REBLEEDING
1. Propranolol and Other Beta-Blockers

Patients who rebleed from varices always have a significant degree of portal hypertension as evidenced by a portal vein or wedged hepatic vein pressure gradient of at least 12 mmHg.[150,151] Attempts to find a portal venous pressure lowering agent suitable for long-term use led Lebrec et al. in 1980[152] to try oral propranolol in patients with cirrhosis and portal hypertension. These authors demonstrated a beneficial effect of beta-blockade with a reduction of the portal pressure gradient, sustained on prolonged administration.[153] Since then, other studies have suggested that this reduction in porto-hepatic gradient is much smaller in magnitude than initially thought (10 to 15%) and not seen consistently (with up to one third of patients showing no response).[154-156]

This effect of propranolol was initially thought to result from the reduction in cardiac output and subsequent fall in hepatic blood flow and portal pressure. However, cardioselective beta-blockers such as atenolol and metoprolol are less effective than propranolol in reducing portal pressure.[157,158] Thus splanchnic vasoconstriction as a result of beta-2-receptor blockade or unopposed alpha-receptor action may play an important role by inducing a preferential reduction in portal blood flow and portal pressure. Furthermore, it has been shown that propranolol decreases azygous blood flow,[156,159] and that this effect is of greater magnitude than the aforementioned reduction in cardiac output and porto-hepatic pressure gradient. These data suggest that propranolol's action on portal and collateral blood flow may be more important than its influence on portal pressure per se.

There have been four placebo-controlled trials evaluating the efficacy of propranolol in preventing rebleeding in patients who presented with a variceal hemorrhage. The initial study of Lebrec et al.[160,161] was promising and showed a 48% reduction in the risk of rebleeding compared to controls. A subsequent trial by Burroughs et al.[162] failed to demonstrate any such benefit. This discrepancy was thought to be related to the different study populations (in Lebrec's study: no severe liver disease, more alcoholics, inclusion of patients bleeding from portal hypertensive gastritis), differences in compliance, length of time between the index bleed and randomization, and small sample size. A larger, more recent, controlled trial by Villeneuve et al.[163] again showed that propranolol is not superior to placebo in the prevention of rebleeding in a population of unselected cirrhotics with severe liver disease. Furthermore, analysis of the data related only to the patients with mild or moderate liver disease also failed to demonstrate any benefit for this subgroup of patients. Queuniet et al.[164] also reported that propranolol is ineffective in preventing rebleeding.

Other beta-blockers have been reported to lower portal pressure: nonselective blockers (nadolol, mepindolol, and sotalol),[165-167] beta-1 selective blockers (metoprolol and atenolol),[157,168-171] and a selective beta-2-blocker (ICI-11851).[172]

2. Other Drugs

Cimetidine was initially reported to reduce hepatic blood flow.[173] These results, however, were based on incorrect methodology, and subsequent studies have shown that cimetidine does not alter liver blood flow or portal pressure[174-176] and does not prevent recurrent variceal hemorrhage.[177]

Other candidates for the medical treatment of portal hypertension include the long-acting nitrates,[178] prazosin,[170] metoclopramide and domperidone,[179] calcium channel blockers,[180] and serotonin antagonists.[181] Additional information is required before considering these drugs for clinical use.

3. Summary

Pharmacologic manipulation remains a potentially useful tool in the control of portal hypertension and any candidates should be vigorously evaluated. While the search for the miracle drug continues, however, endoscopic sclerotherapy is gaining the upper hand as the treatment of choice in the prevention of rebleeding. Studies published to date suggest that serial sclerotherapy is effective in preventing recurrent hemorrhage in patients who have previously bled.[144-146,182-185] Although the risk of rebleeding persists during the initial 3 to 4 months until all varices are eradicated, once total obliteration has been achieved, rebleeding is reduced to a rate of approximately 10 to 30% per year. In addition, the severity of rebleeding may be less in these patients.

Unfortunately, the benefit of such serial sclerotherapy with respect to long-term survival is less clear. Of the trials published to date, four demonstrate an improvement in long-term survival following sclerotherapy,[144-146,182] whereas the remaining three studies fail to show such a benefit.[183-185] Close analysis of these trials, however, does suggest long-term improvement in survival in those patients treated with serial sclerotherapy.

Portocaval shunt surgery prevents recurrent bleeding in 90% of cases, but hepatic encephalopathy remains a major problem and survival is either worsened or only minimally improved.[186-189] Decompression via a distal splenorenal rather than a central shunt offers no advantage with respect to rebleeding or survival, and does not consistently result in a lower incidence of postoperative encephalopathy.[190-191] Esophageal transection with devascularization procedure has been very successful in Japanese hands, but the impressive results remain to be reproduced on this continent.

If one is to make an impact on the overall prognosis of these patients, the need to prevent the initial episode of esophageal hemorrhage with its attendant high mortality persists. Efforts should concentrate on preventing the initial rupture in patients with portal hypertension and varices who have never had a bleed. Trials appearing in the literature suggest that prophylactic sclerotherapy[192-193] and beta-blockers[194] may improve survival but further studies are needed.

Thus, sclerotherapy with serial injections aimed at eradicating all varices is the treatment of choice in our institution. If such treatment fails, Child A and B patients are offered shunt surgery. The management of patients with severe Child's C liver disease and variceal hemorrhage is limited by the fact that their survival is primarily dependent on the extent of the underlying liver disease, irrespective of the therapy applied. The prognosis is very poor, and it is unlikely that any long-term treatment will improve their outlook. Sclerotherapy seems a simple measure to prevent rebleeding but will not benefit survival. If the patient survives the bleeding episode and is a good candidate, liver transplantation should now be considered an appropriate alternative.

VII. OVERVIEW

Cirrhosis of the liver is characterized by major changes in the intrahepatic circulation. Shunts of various degrees can be found in approximately one third of patients; they occur mainly between the portal and hepatic veins, and provide an "escape" route bypassing normal sinusoids and parenchymal cells. Progressive capillarization of sinusoids and collagenization of the space of Disse form a barrier to the free movement of molecules from plasma to the hepatocytes. Although the diffusion of sucrose, water, and highly lipophilic substances such as lidocaine does not seem to be hindered, movement of large molecules such as albumin, lipoproteins, and probably substances bound to them, is impaired. The multiple indicator dilution technique has provided us with a means of studying these phenomena and the exchange processes at the plasma-hepatocyte surface.

Portal hypertension is a hallmark of advanced cirrhosis. The process results from an increased intrahepatic vascular resistance but may be perpetuated, despite the development of portosystemic collaterals which should decompress the system, by the presence of a hyperdynamic circulation. The relative contribution of these two components, and the factors responsible for the observed hyperdynamic state remain to be better defined. Refinement of noninvasive blood flow measurement techniques (Doppler flowmetry) may open new horizons for the further study of portal hypertension in man. In addition, such technology provides a useful tool in the evaluation of new drugs used in the control of portal hypertension.

The advent of endoscopic sclerotherapy in recent years has markedly improved our ability to effectively control acute variceal rupture and prevent recurrence of hemorrhage, but patients remain at risk of bleeding until all varices have been eradicated and survival remains primarily dependent on the severity of the underlying liver disease. The need to prevent the initial variceal rupture with its associated high mortality persists. Pharmacologic manipulation with sustained reduction of portal venous pressure seems a logical goal in the primary and secondary prophylaxis of gastroesophageal variceal rupture but other parameters such as azygous blood flow and intravariceal pressure may better correlate with a clinical response. Although propranolol did not turn out to be the panacea in the treatment of portal hypertension, its introduction as a portal pressure lowering agent has stimulated much research in the pharmacologic approach to the management of portal hypertension. New and exciting developments in the search for the miracle drug and a better understanding of the pathophysiology of portal hypertension are eagerly awaited.

REFERENCES

1. **Rappaport, A. M.,** The Acinus-microcircular unit of the liver, in *Hepatic Circulation in Health and Disease*, Lautt, W. W., Ed., Raven, New York, 1981, 175.
2. **Ohtani, O. and Murakami, T.,** Peribiliary portal system in the rat liver as studied by the injection replica scanning electron microscope method, *Scanning Electron Microscopy*, 11, 241, 1978.
3. **Nopanitaya, W., Grisham, J. W., Aghajanian, J. G., and Carson, J. L.,** Intrahepatic microcirculation: SEM study of the terminal distribution of the hepatic artery, *Scanning Electron Microscopy*, 11, 837, 1978.
4. **Cho, K. J. and Lunderquist, A.,** The peribiliary vascular plexus: the microvascular architecture of the bile duct in the rabbit and in clinical cases. *Radiology*, 147, 357, 1983.
5. **Motta, P., Muto, M., and Fujita, T.,** The liver, in *Atlas of Scanning Electron Microscopy*, Igaky-Shoin, Tokyo, 1978.
6. **Wisse, E., De Zanger, R. B., Jacobs, R., and McCuskey, R. S.,** Scanning electron microscope observations on the structure of portal veins, sinusoids and central veins in rat liver, *Scanning Electron Microscopy*, 111, 1441, 1983.
7. **Gendrault, J. I., Montecino-Rodriguez, F., and Cinqualbre, J.,** Structure of the normal human liver sinusoid after perfusion fixation, in *Sinusoidal Liver Cells*, Knook, D. L. and Wisse, E., Eds., Elsevier, Amsterdam, 1982, 93.

8. **Horn, T., Henriksen, J. H., and Christoffern, P.,** The sinusoidal lining cells in "normal" human liver. A scanning electron microscopic investigation, *Liver*, 61, 98, 1986.

9. **Wisse, E.,** An electron microscopic study of the fenestrated endothelial lining of rat liver sinusoids, *J. Ultrastruct. Res.*, 31, 125, 1970.

10. **Jones, A. L. and Schmucker, D. L.,** Current concepts of liver structure as related to function, *Gastroenterology*, 73, 833, 1977.

11. **Naito, M. and Wisse, E.,** Filtrating effect of endothelial fenestrations on chylomicron transport in the neonatal rat liver sinusoids, *Cell Tissue Res.*, 190, 371, 1978.

12. **De Zanger, R. B. and Wisse, E.,** The filtration of rat liver fenestrated sinusoidal endothelium on the passage of (remnant) chylomicrons to the space of Disse, in *Sinusoidal Liver Cells*, Knook, D. L. and Wisse, E., Eds., Elsevier, Amsterdam, 1982, 69.

13. **Fraser, R., Bosanquet, A. G., and Day, W. A.,** Filtration of chylomicrons by the liver may influence cholesterol metabolism and atherosclerosis, *Atherosclerosis*, 29, 113, 1978.

14. **Wright, P. L., Smith, K. F., Day, W. A., and Fraser, R.,** Small liver fenestrae may explain the susceptibility of rabbits to atherosclerosis, *Arteriosclerosis*, 3, 344, 1983.

15. **Fraser, R., Bowler, L. M., and Day, W. A.,** Damage of rat sinusoidal endothelium by ethanol, *Pathology*, 12, 371, 1980.

16. **Fraser, R., Bowler, L. M., De Zanger, R. B., and Wisse, E.,** Agents related to fibrosis such as alcohol and carbon tetrachloride, acutely affect endothelial fenestrae which may cause fatty liver, *Connective Tissue of the Normal and Fibrotic Human Liver*, Thieme Verlag, Stuttgart, 1982, 159.

17. **Mak, K. M. and Lieber, C. S.,** Alterations in endothelial fenestrations in liver sinusoids of baboons fed alcohol: a scanning electron microscopic study, *Hepatology*, 4, 386, 1984.

18. **Horn, T., Christofferson, P., and Henriksen, JH.,** Alcoholic liver injury: defenestration in non-cirrhotic livers — a scanning electron microscopic study, *Hepatology*, 7, 77, 1987.

19. **Napanitaya, W., Lamb, J. C., Grisham, J. W., and Carson, J. L.,** Effects of hepatic venous outflow obstruction on pores and fenestrations in sinusoidal endothelium, *Br. J. Exp. Pathol.*, 57, 604, 1976.

20. **Fraser, R., Bowler, L. M., Day, W. A., Dobbs, B., Johnson, H. D., and Lee, D.,** High perfusion pressure damages the sieving ability of sinusoidal endothelium in rat livers, *Br. J. Exp. Pathol.*, 61, 222, 1980.

21. **Arias, I. M., Gatmaitan, Z., Mikkelson, R., Penman, S., and Fay, E.,** On the dynamic nature of hepatic endothelial cell fenestrae, *Hepatology*, 6, 1222, 1986.

22. **Oda, M., Nakamura, M., Watanabe, N., Ohya, Y., Sekizuka, E., Tsukada, N., Yonei, Y., Komatsu, H., Nagata, H., and Tsuchiya, M.,** Some dynamic aspects of the hepatic microcirculation demonstration of sinusoidal endothelial fenestrae as a possible regulatory factor, in *Intravital Observation of Organ Microcirculation*, Tsuchiya, M. et al., Eds., Exerpta Medica Foundation, The Hague, 1983, 105.

23. **Oda, M., Tsukada, N., Komatsu, H., Yonei, Y., Ronda, K., and Tsuchiya, M.,** Mechanism of contraction and dilatation of sinusoidal endothelial fenestrae in the liver, *Hepatology*, 6, 771, 1986.

24. **Wisse, E., De Zanger, R. B., Charels, K., Van Der Smissen, P., and McCushey, R. S.,** The Liver Sieve: considerations concerning the structure and function of endothelial fenestrae, the sinusoidal wall and the space of Disse, *Hepatology*, 5, 683, 1985.

25. **Wisse, E., De Zanger, R., and Jacobs, R.,** Lobular gradients in endothelial fenestrae and sinusoidal diameter favour centrolobular exchange process: a scanning EM study, in *Sinusoidal Liver Cells*, Knooks, D. L. and Wisse, E., Eds., Elsevier, Amsterdam, 1982, 61.

26. **Vidal-Vanaclocha, F. and Barbera-Guillem, E.,** Fenestration patterns in endothelial cells of rat liver sinusoids, *J. Ultrastruct. Res.*, 90, 995, 1985.

27. **Gumucio, J. J. and Miller, D. L.,** Liver cell heterogeneity, in *The Liver: Biology and Pathobiology*, Arias, I. M., Popper, H., Schacter, D. and Shafritz, D. A., Eds., Raven Press, New York, 1982, 647.

28. **Goresky, C. A., Huet, P. M., and Villeneuve, J. P.,** Blood-tissue exchange and blood flow in the liver, in *Hepatology. A Textbook of Liver Disease*, Zakim, D. and Boyer, T. D., Eds., W. B. Saunders, Philadelphia, 1982, 32.

29. **Goresky, C. A.,** A linear method for determining liver sinusoidal and extravascular volumes, *Am. J. Physiol.*, 204, 626, 1963.

30. **Popper, H., Elias, H., and Petty, D. E.,** Vascular pattern of the cirrhotic liver, *Am. J. Clin. Pathol.*, 22, 717, 1952.

31. **Varin, F. and Huet, P. M.,** Hepatic microcirculation in the perfused cirrhotic rat liver, *J. Clin. Invest.*, 76, 1904, 1985.

32. **Conn, H. O.,** Cirrhosis, in *Diseases of the Liver*, Shiff, L. and Schiff, E. R., Eds., J. B. Lippencott, Philadelphia, 1982, 847.

33. **Lapis, K.,** Cirrhosis, in *Electron Microscopy in Human Medicine*, Johannessen, J. E., Ed., McGraw-Hill, New York, 1979, 158.

34. **Mitra, S. K.,** Hepatic vascular changes in human and experimental cirrhosis, *J. Path. Bact.*, 92, 405, 1966.

35. **Hales, M. R., Alan, J. S., and Hall, E. M.,** Injection-corrosion studies of normal and cirrhotic livers, *Am. J. Pathol.,* 35, 909, 1959.

36. **Nakamura, T., Nakamura, S., and Suzuki, T.,** Studies on cirrhosis of the liver, IX. structure of shunted blood vessels in the autopsied cirrhotic liver, *Tohoku J. Exp. Med.,* 75, 1, 1961.

37. **Baldus, W. P. and Hoffbauer, F. W.,** Vascular changes in the cirrhotic liver as studied by the injection technique, *Am. J. Dig. Dis.,* 8, 689, 1963.

38. **Schaffner, F. and Popper, H.,** Capillarization of hepatic sinusoids in man, *Gastroenterology,* 44, 239, 1963.

39. **Kent, G., Gay, S., Inouye, T., Bahu, R., Minick, O. T., and Popper, H.,** Vitamin A-containing lipocytes and formation of type III colagen in liver injury, *Proc. Natl. Acad. Sci. U.S.A.,* 73, 3719, 1976.

40. **Minato, Y., Hasumara, Y., and Takeuchi, J.,** The role of fat-storing cells in Disse space fibrogenesis in alcohol liver disease, *Hepatology,* 3, 559, 1983.

41. **Lamouliatte, H., Dubroca, J., Quinton, A., Balabaud, C., and Bioulac-Sage, P.,** Sinusoids in human cirrhotic nodules: better identification with the perfusion fixation technique, *J. Submicrosc. Cytol.,* 17, 279, 1985.

42. **Mannifold, I. H., Triger, D. R., and Underwood, J. C. E.,** Kupffer cell depletion in chronic liver disease: implication for hepatic carcinogenesis, *Lancet,* 2, 431, 1983.

43. **Mills, L. R. and Scheuer, P. J.,** Hepatic sinusoidal macrophages in alcoholic liver disease, *J. Pathol.,* 147, 127, 1985.

44. **Phillips, M. J. and Steiner, J. W.,** Electron microscopy of liver cells in cirrhotic nodules, *Am. J. Pathol.,* 46, 985, 1965.

45. **Henriksen, J. H., Horn, T., and Christoffersen, P.,** The blood-lymph barrier in the liver. A review based on morphological and functional concepts of normal and cirrhotic liver, *Liver,* 4, 221, 1984.

46. **Proctor, E. and Chatamra, K.,** High yield micronodular cirrhosis in the rat, *Gastroenterology,* 83, 1183, 1982.

47. **Huet, P. M., Goresky, C. A., Villeneuve, J. P., Marleau, D., and Lough, J. O.,** Assessment of liver microcirculation in human cirrhosis, *J. Clin. Invest.,* 80, 1234, 1982.

48. **Forker, E. L. and Luxon, B. A.,** Albumin-mediated transport of rose bengal by perfused rat liver. Kinetics of the reaction of the cell surface, *J. Clin. Invest.,* 72, 1764, 1983.

49. **Goresky, C. A., Ziegler, W. M., and Bach, G. G.,** Capillary exchange modeling barrier-limited and flow-limited distribution, *Circ. Res.,* 27, 739, 1970.

50. **Ueda, H., Kitani, K., Kameda,, H., Yamada, H., and Ho, M.,** Detection of hepatic shunts by the use of ^{131}I-macroaggregated albumin, *Gastroenterology,* 52, 480, 1967.

51. **Syrota, A., Vinot, J. M., Parat, A., and Roucayrol, J. C.,** Scintillation splenoportography: hemodynamic and morphological study of the portal circulation, *Gastroenterology,* 71, 652, 1976.

52. **Gross, G., Babel, J. F., Ritschard, J., Megevand, R., Rohner, A., Donath, A., Perrier, C. V.,** Quantification of intrahepatic porta-systemic shunting in cirrhotic patients: possible relevance to the problem of indication for surgical procedure, in *The liver. Quantitative Aspects of Structure and Function,* Preisig, R., Bircher, J. and Paumgartner, G., Eds., Cantor, Aulendorf, 1976, 159.

53. **Okuda, D., Suzuki, K., Musha, H., and Arimizu, N.,** Percutaneous transhepatic catheterization of the portal vein for the study of portal hemodynamics and shunts, *Gastroenterology,* 73, 279, 1977.

54. **Ohnishi, K., Chin, N., Sugita, S., Saito, M., Tanaka, H., Terabayashi, H., Iida, S., Nonura, F., and Okuda, K.,** Quantitative aspects of portal systemic and arterio-venous shunts within the liver in cirrhosis, *Gastroenterology,* 93, 135, 1987.

55. **Groszmann, R. J., Kravetz, D., and Parysow, O.,** Intrahepatic arteriovenous shunting in cirrhosis of the liver, *Gastroenterology,* 73, 201, 1977.

56. **Hoefs, J. C., Reynolds, T. B., Pare, P., and Sakimura, I.,** A new method for the measurement of intrahepatic shunts, *J. Lab. Clin. Med.,* 103, 446, 1984.

57. **Chojkier, M. and Groszmann, R. J.,** Measurement of portal-systemic shunting in the rat by using co-labeled microspheres, *Am. J. Physiol.,* 240-G371, 1981.

58. **Huet, P. M. and Villeneuve, J. P.,** Determinants of drug disposition in patients with cirrhosis, *Hepatology,* 3, 913, 1983.

59. **Stenger, R. J.,** Hepatic sinusoids in carbon tetrachloride induced cirrhosis, *Arch. Pathol.,* 81, 439, 1966.

60. **Huet, P. M., Villeneuve, J. P., Pomier-Layrargues, G., and Marleau, D.,** Hepatic circulation in cirrhosis, *Clinics in Gastroenterology,* 14, 155, 1985.

61. **Bradley, S. E., Ingelfinger, F. J., and Bradley, G. P.,** Hepatic circulation in cirrhosis of the liver, *Circulation,* 5, 419, 1952.

62. **Moreno, A. H., Rousselot, L. M., Panke, W. F., Panke, W. F., and Burke, M. L.,** The rate of hepatic blood flow in normal subjects and in patients with portal hypertension, *Surg. Gynecol. Obstet.,* 111, 443, 1960.

63. **Moreno, A. H., Burchell, A. R., Rousselot, L. M., Panke, W. F., Slafsky, S. F., and Burke, M. L.,** Portal blood flow in cirrhosis of the liver, *J. Clin. Invest.,* 46, 436, 1967.

64. **Kawalski, H. J. and Abelmann, W. H.**, The cardiac output at rest in Laennec's cirrhosis, *J. Clin. Invest.*, 32, 1025, 1953.
65. **Claypool, J. G., Delp, M., and Lin, T. K.**, Hemodynamic studies in patients with Laennec's cirrhosis, *Am. J. Med. Sci.*, 234, 48, 1957.
66. **Murray, J. F., Dawson, A. M., and Sherlock, S.**, Circulatory changes in chronic liver disease, *Am. J. Med.*, 24, 358, 1958.
67. **Kontos, H. A., Shapiro, W., Mauck, H. P., and Patterson, J. L.**, General and regional circulatory alterations in cirrhosis of the liver, *Am. J. Med.*, 37, 526, 1964.
68. **Williams, R., Condon, R. E., Williams, H. S., Blendis, L. M., and Kreel, L.**, Splenic blood flow in cirrhosis and portal hypertension, *Clin. Sci.*, 34, 441, 1968.
69. **Gitlin, N., Grahame, G. R., Kreel, L., Williams, H. S., and Sherlock, S.**, Splenic blood flow and resistance in patients with cirrhosis before and after portocaval anastomoses, *Gastroenterologoy*, 59, 208, 1970.
70. **Witte, C. L., Witte, M. H., Renert, W., and Corrigan, J. J.**, Systemic circulatory dynamics in congestive splenomegaly, *Gastroenterology*, 67, 498, 1974.
71. **Kotelanski, B., Groszmann, R., and Cohn, J. N.**, Circulation times in the splanchnic and hepatic beds in alcoholic liver disease, *Gastroenterology*, 63, 102, 1972.
72. **Benoit, J. N. and Granger, D. N.**, Splanchnic hemodynamics in chronic portal hypertension, *Sem. Liv. Dis.*, 6, 287, 1986.
73. **Halvorsen, J. F. and Myking, A. O.**, Prehepatic portal hypertension in the rat. Immediate and long-term effects on portal vein and aortic pressure of a graded portal vein sclerosis, followed by occlusion of the portal vein and splenorenal collaterals, *Eur. Surg. Res.*, 11, 89, 1979.
74. **Vorobioff, J., Bredfeldt, J. E., and Groszmann, R. J.**, Hyperdynamic circulation in portal hypertensive rat model: a primary factor for maintenance of chronic portal hypertension, *Am. J. Physiol.*, 244, G52, 1983.
75. **Groszmann, R. J., Vorobloff, J., and Riley, E.**, Splanchnic hemodynamics in portal hypertensive rats: measurement with x-labeled microspheres, *Am. J. Physiol.*, 242, G156, 1982.
76. **Sikuler, E., Kravetz, D., and Groszmann, R. J.**, Evolution of portal hypertension and mechanisms involved in its maintenance in a rat model, *Am. J. Physiol.*, 248, G618, 1985.
77. **Sikuler, E. and Groszmann, R. J.**, Interaction of flow and resistance in maintenance of portal hypertension in a rat model, *Am. J. Physiol.*, 250, G205, 1986.
78. **Kroeger, R. D. and Groszmann, R. J.**, Increased portal venous resistance hinders portal pressure reduction during administration of B-adrenergic blocking agents in a portal hypertensive model, *Hepatology*, 5, 97, 1985.
79. **Benoit, J. N., Womack, W. A., Hernandez, L., and Granger, D. N.**, "Forward" and "backward" flow mechanisms of portal hypertension. Relative contributions in the rat model of portal vein stenosis, *Gastroenterology*, 89, 1092, 1985.
80. **Shibayama, Y. and Nakata, K.**, Localization of increased hepatic vascular resistance in liver cirrhosis, *Hepatology*, 5, 643, 1985.
81. **Moriyasu, F., Nishida, O., Ban, N., Nakamura, T., Miura, K., Sakai, M., Miyake, T., and Uchino, H.**, Measurement of portal vascular resistance in patients with portal hypertension, *Gastroenterology*, 90, 710, 1986.
82. **Vorobioff, J., Bredfeldt, J. E., and Groszmann, R. J.**, Increased blood flow through the portal system in cirrhotic animals, *Gastroenterology*, 87, 1120, 1984.
83. **Arderiu, M. T., Bosch, J., and Rodés, J.**, Increased vascular resistance to portal blood flow is the primary factor promoting portal hypertension in CCl_4-cirrhotic rats, *J. Hepatol.*, 2, S200, 1986.
84. **Bosch, J., Enriquez, R., Groszmann, R. J., and Sturer, E. H.**, Chronic bile duct ligation in the dogs hemodynamic characterization of a portal hypertensive model, *Hepatology*, 3, 1002, 1983.
85. **Benoit, J. N., Barrowman, J. A., Harper, S. L., Kvietys, P. R., and Granger, D. N.**, Role of humoral factors in the intestinal hyperemia associated with chronic portal hypertension, *Am. J. Physiol.*, 247, G486, 1984.
86. **Richards, P. D. I. and Withrington, R.**, Liver blood flow. II. Effects of drugs and hormones on liver blood flow, *Gastroenterology*, 81, 356, 1981.
87. **Sherwin, R., Joshi, P., Handler, R., Selig, P., and Shepherd, A. P.**, Hyperglucagonemia in Laennec's cirrhosis, *N. Engl. J. Med.*, 290, 239, 1974.
88. **Sherwin, R. S., Fischer, M., Bessoff, J., Snyder, N., Hendler, R., Conn, H. O., and Felig, P.**, Hyperglucagonemia in cirrhosis: altered secretion and sensitivity to glucagon, *Gastroenterology*, 74, 1224, 1978.
89. **Johansson, B.**, Structural and functional changes in rat portal veins after experimental portal hypertension, *Acta Physiol. Scand.*, 98, 381, 1976.
90. **Kiel, J. W., Pitts, V., Benoit, J., Granger, N., and Shepherd, A. P.**, Reduced vascular sensitivity to norepinephrine in portal hypertensive rats, *Am. J. Physiol.*, 248, G192, 1985.

91. **Kock, N. G., Tibblin, S., and Schenk, W. G.,** Modification by glucagon of the splanchnic vascular responses to activation of the sympathoadrenal system, *J. Surg. Res.,* 1, 12, 1971.

92. **Sikuler, E., Vorobioff, J., Hendler, R., and Groszmann, R. J.,** Systemic and portal glucagon levels in two rat models of portal hypertension. The relation to portal systemic shunting and portal venous inflow, *Hepatology,* 4, 1040, 1984.

93. **Sikuler, E. and Groszmann, R. J.,** Hemodynamic studies in a parabiotic model of portal hypertension, *Experientia,* 41, 1323, 1985.

94. **Sikuler, E. and Groszmann, R. J.,** Hemodynamic studies in long and short term portal hypertensive rats: the relation of systemic glucagon levels, *Hepatology,* 6, 414, 1986.

95. **Ohnishi, K., Saito, M., Sato, S., Terabayashi, H., Iida, S., Nomura, F., Nakano, M., and Okuda, K.,** Portal hemodynamics in idiopathic portal hypertension (Banti's syndrome). Comparison with chronic persistent hepatitis and normal subjects, *Gastroenterology,* 92, 751, 1987.

96. **Burns, P., Taylor, K., and Blei, A. T.,** Doppler flowmetry and portal hypertension, *Gastroenterology,* 92, 824, 1987.

97. **Bosch, J., Mastai, R., Kravetz, D., Bruix, J., Rigau, J., and Rodes, J.,** Measurement of azygous venous blood flow in the evaluation of portal hypertension in patients with cirrhosis. Clinical and Haemodynamic correlations in 100 patients, *J. Hepatol.,* 1, 125, 1985.

98. **Silva, Y. J., Moffat, R. C., and Watt, A. J.,** Vasopressin effect on portal and systemic hemodynamic studies in intact unanesthetized humans, *JAMA,* 210, 1065, 1969.

99. **Corliss, R. J., McKenna, D. H., Sialer, S., O'Brien, G. S., and Bowe, J. J.,** Systemic and coronary hemodynamic effects of vasopressin, *Am. J. Med. Sci.,* 256, 293, 1968.

100. **Conn, H. O., Ramsby, G. R., Storer, E. H., Mutchnick, M. G., Joshi, P., Phillips, M. M., Cohen, G. A., Fields, G. N., and Petroski, D.,** Intra-arterial vasopressin in the treatment of upper gastrointestinal hemorrhage: a prospective controlled trial, *Gastroenterology,* 68, 211, 1975.

101. **Johnson, W. C., Widrich, W. C., Ansell, J. E., Robbins, A. H., and Nasbeth, D. C.,** Control of bleeding varices by vasopressin: a prospective randomized study, *Ann. Surg.,* 186, 369, 1977.

102. **Chojkier, M., Groszmann, R. J., Atterbury, C. E., Bar-Meir, S., Blei, A. T., Frankel, J., Glickman, M. G., Kniaz, J. C., Schade, R., Taggart, G. J., and Conn, H. O.,** A controlled comparison of continuous intra-arterial and intravenous infusion of vasopressin in hemorrhage from esophageal varices, *Gastroenterology,* 77, 540, 1979.

103. **Clanet, I., Tournut, R., Fourtanier, C., Joncquiert, F., and Pascal, J. P.,** Traitement par la pitressine des hémorrhagie par rupture de varices oesophagiennes chez les cirrhotiques, *Acta Gastro-Enterol. Belg.,* 41, 539, 1978.

104. **Mallory, A., Schaefer, J. W., Cohen, J. R., Holt, S. A., and Norton, L. W.,** Selective intra-arterial vasopressin infusion for upper gastrointestinal tract hemorrhage. A controlled trial, *Arch. Surg.,* 115, 30, 1980.

105. **Millette, B., Huet, P. M., Lavoie, P., and Viallet, A.,** Portal and systemic effects of selective infusion of vasopressin into the superior mesenteric artery in cirrhotic patients, *Gastroenterology,* 69, 6, 1975.

106. **Barr, J. W., Hakin, R. C., and Bosch, J.,** Similarity of arterial and intravenous vasopressin on portal and systemic hemodynamics, *Gastroenterology,* 69, 13, 1975.

107. **Merigan, T. C., Plotkin, G. R., and Davidson, C. S.,** The effect of intravenous pituitrin on hemorrhage from bleeding esophageal varices. A controlled evaluation, *N. Engl. J. Med.,* 266, 134, 1962.

108. **Fogel, M. R., Knauer, C. M., Andres, L. L., Mahal, A. S., Stein, D. E. T., Kemeny, J. J., Rinki, M. M., Walker, J. E., Siegmund, D., and Gregory, P. B.,** Continuous intravenous vasopressin in active upper gastrointestinal bleeding. A placebo-controlled trial, *Ann. Int. Med.,* 96, 565, 1982.

109. **Correia, J. P., Alves, M. M., Alexandrino, P., and Silveira, J.,** Controlled trial of vasopressin and balloon tamponade in bleeding esophageal varices, *Hepatology,* 4, 885, 1984.

110. **Vosmik, J., Jedlicka, K., Mudler, J., and Cort, J. H.,** Action of the triglycyl hormogen of vasopressin (glypressin) in patients with liver cirrhosis and bleeding esophageal varices, *Gastroenterology,* 72, 605, 1977.

111. **Freeman, J. G., Cobden, I., Lishman, A. H., and Record, C. O.,** Controlled trial of terlipressin ("Glypressin") versus vasopressin in the early treatment of esophageal varices, *Lancet,* 2, 66, 1982.

112. **Walker, S., Stiehl, A., Raedsch, R., and Kommerell, B.,** Terlipressin in bleeding esophageal varices: a placebo-controlled, double-blind trial, *Hepatology,* 6, 112, 1986.

113. **Blei, A. T., Groszmann, R. J., Gusberg, R., and Conn, H. O.,** Comparison of vasopressin and triglycyl-lysine vasopressin on splanchnic and systemic hemodynamics in dogs, *Dig. Dis. Sci.,* 25, 688, 1980.

114. **Valla, D., Lee, S. S., Moreau, R., Hadenge, A., Sayegh, R., and Lebrec, D.,** Effets de la glypressine sur la circulation splanchnique et systémique des malades atteints de la cirrhose, *Gastroenterol. Clin. Biol.,* 9, 877, 1985.

115. **Groszmann, R. J., Kravetz, D., Bosch, J., Glickman, M., Bruix, J., Bredfeldt, J., Conn, H. O., Rodes, J., and Storer, E. H.,** Nitroglycerin improves the hemodynamic response to vasopressin in portal hypertension, *Hepatology,* 2, 757, 1982.

116. **Garcia-Tsao, G. and Groszmann, R. J.,** Portal hypodynamics during nitroglycerin administration in cirrhotic patients, *Hepatology,* 7, 805, 1987.
117. **Gimson, A. E. S., Westaby, D., Hegarty, J., Watson, A., and Williams, R.,** A randomized trial of vasopressin plus nitroglycerin in the control of acute variceal hemorrhage, *Hepatology,* 6, 410, 1986.
118. **Tsai, Y. T., Lay, C. S., Lai, K. H., Ng, W. W., Yeh, Y. S., Wang, J. Y., Chiang, T. T., Lee, S. D., Chiang, B. N., and Lo, K. J.,** Controlled trial of vasopressin plus nitroglycerin vs. vasopressin alone in the treatment of bleeding esophageal varices, *Hepatology,* 6, 406, 1986.
119. **Gelman, S. and Ernst, E. A.,** Nitroprusside prevents adverse hemodynamic effects of vasopressin, *Arch. Surg.,* 113, 1465, 1980.
120. **Zito, R. A., Diez, A., and Groszmann, R. J.,** Comparative effects of nitroglycerin and nitroprusside on vasopressin-induced cardiac dysfunction in the dog, *J. Cardiovasc. Pharmacol.,* 5, 586, 1983.
121. **Jaspan, J., Polonsky, J., Lewis, M., and Moossa, R.,** Reduction of portal vein blood flow by somatostatin, *Diabetes,* 28, 888, 1979.
122. **Wahren, J. and Felig, P.,** Influence of somatostatin on carbohydrate disposal and absorption in diabetes mellitus, *Lancet,* 2, 1213, 1976.
123. **Samnegard, H., Thulin, L., Tyden, A. G., Samnegard, H., Thulin, L., Andreen, M., Tyden, G., Hallberg, D., and Efendie, S.,** Circulatory effects of somatostatin in anesthetized dogs, *Acta Chir. Scand.,* 145, 209, 1979.
124. **Tyden, S., Samnegard, H., Thulin, L., Tyden, G., Samnegard, H., Thulin, L., Muhrbeck, O., and Efendie, S.,** Circulatory effects of somatostatin in anesthetized man, *Acta Chir. Scand.,* 145, 443, 1979.
125. **Bories, P., Pomier-Layrargues, G., Chotard, J. P., Jacob, C., and Michel, H.,** La somatostatine diminue l'hypertension portale chez le cirrhotique, *Gastroenterol. Clin. Biol.,* 4, 616, 1980.
126. **Bosch, J., Kravetz, D., and Rodes, J.,** Effects of somatostatin on hepatic and systemic hemodynamics in patients with cirrhosis of the liver: comparison with vasopressin, *Gastroenterology,* 80, 518, 1981.
127. **Sonnenberg, G. E., Keller, J., Perruchoud, A., Burckhardt, D., and Gyr, K.,** Effects of somatostatin on splanchnic hemodynamics in patients with cirrhosis of the liver and in normal subjects, *Gastroenterology,* 80, 526, 1981.
128. **Merkel, C., Gatta, A., Zuin, R., Finucci, G. F., Nosadini, R., and Ruol, A.,** Effect of somatostatin on splanchnic hemodynamics in patients with liver cirrhosis and portal hypertension, *Digestion,* 32, 92, 1985.
129. **Naeije, R., Hallemans, R., Mols, P., Melot, C., and Reding, P.,** Effects of vasopressin and somatostatin on hemodynamics and blood gases in patients with liver cirrhosis, *Crit. Care Med.,* 10, 578, 1982.
130. **Tyden, G., Samnegard, H., Thulin, L., Frimon, L., and Efendie, S.,** Treatment of bleeding esophageal varices with somatostatin, *N. Engl. J. Med.,* 299, 1466, 1978.
131. **Thulin, L., Tyden, G., Samnegard, H., Muhrbeck, O., and Efendie, S.,** Treatment of bleeding esophageal varices with somatostatin, *Acta Chir. Scand.,* 145, 395, 1979.
132. **Limberg, B. and Kommerell, B.,** Treatment of acute bleeding esophageal varices with somatostatin, *IRCS Medical Science,* 10, 542, 1982.
133. **Raptis, S. and Zoupas, C.,** Somatostatin not helpful in bleeding esophageal varices, *N. Engl. J. Med.,* 300, 736, 1979.
134. **Kravetz, D., Bosch, J., Teres, J., Bruix, J., Rimola, A., and Rodes, J.,** Comparison of intravenous somatostatin and vasopressin infusion in treatment of acute variceal hemorrhage, *Hepatology,* 4, 442, 1984.
135. **Jenkins, S. A., Baxter, J. N., Corbett, W. A., Devitt, P., Ware, J., and Schields, R.,** A prospective randomized controlled clinical trial comparing somatostatin and vasopressin in controlling acute variceal hemorrhage, *Br. Med. J.,* 290, 275, 1985.
136. **Jenkins, S. A., Baxter, J. N., Corbett, W. A., and Shields, R.,** The effects of a somatostatin analogue SMS 201-995 on hepatic hemodynamics in the rat, *Br. J. Surg.,* 72, 864, 1985.
137. **Teres, J., Cecilia, A., Bordas, J., Rimola, A., Bru, C., and Rodes, J.,** Esophageal tamponade for bleeding varices. Controlled trial between the Sengstaken-Blakemore tube and the Linton-Nachlas tube, *Gastroenterology,* 75, 566, 1978.
138. **Hunt, P. S., Korman, M. G., Hansky, J., and Parkin, W. G.,** An 8-year prospective experience with balloon tamponade in emergency control of bleeding esophageal varices, *Dig. Dis. Sci.,* 27, 413, 1982.
139. **Lewis, J. W., Chung, R. S., and Allison, J. G.,** Injection sclerotherapy for control of acute variceal hemorrhage, *Am. J. Surg.,* 142, 592, 1981.
140. **Kjaergaard, J., Fischer, A., Miskowiak, J., Lindahl, F., and Baden, H.,** Sclerotherapy of bleeding esophageal varices, *Scand. J. Gastroenterol.,* 17, 363, 1982.
141. **Stray, N., Jacobsen, C. D., and Rosseland, A.,** Injection sclerotherapy of bleeding oesophageal and gastric varices using a flexible endoscope, *Acta Med. Scand.,* 311, 125, 1982.
142. **Takase, Y., Ozadi, A., Orii, K., Nagoshi, K., Okamura, T., and Iwasaki, Y.,** Injection sclerotherapy of esophageal varices for patients undergoing emergency and elective surgery, *Surgery,* 92, 474, 1982.
143. **Soehendra, N., de Heer, K., Kempeneers, I., and Runge, M.,** Sclerotherapy for esophageal varices: acute arrest of gastrointestinal hemorrhage or long-term therapy, *Endoscopy,* 15, 125, 1983.

144. **Barsoum, M. S., Bolous, F. I., El-Rooby, A. A., Rizk-Allah, M. A., and Ibrahim, A. S.,** Tamponade and injection sclerotherapy in the management of bleeding oesophageal varices, *Br. J. Surg.,* 69, 76, 1982.

145. **Paquet, K. J. and Feussner, H.,** Endoscopic sclerosis and esophageal balloon tamponade in acute hemorrhage from esophageal gastric varices: a prospective controlled randomized trial, *Hepatology,* 5, 580, 1985.

146. **The Copenhagen Esophageal Varices Sclerotherapy Project,** Sclerotherapy after first variceal hemorrhage in cirrhosis. A randomized multicenter trial, *N. Engl. J. Med.,* 311, 1594, 1984.

147. **Orloff, W. J., Bell, R. H., Hyde, P. V., and Skivolocki, W. P.,** Long-term results of emergency portacaval shunts for bleeding esophageal varices in unselected patients with alcoholic cirrhosis, *Ann. Surg.,* 192, 325, 1980.

148. **Cello, J. P., Grendell, J. H., Crass, R. A., Trunkey, D. D., Cobb, E. E., and Heilbron, D. C.,** Endoscopic sclerotherapy versus portacaval shunt in patients with severe cirrhosis and variceal hemorrhage, *N. Engl. J. Med.,* 311, 1589, 1984.

149. **Villeneuve, J. P., Pomier-Layrargues, G., Duguay, L., Lapointe, R., Tanguay, S., Marleau, D., Willems, B., Huet, P. M., Infante-Rivard, C., and Lavoie, P.,** Emergency portocaval shunt for variceal hemorrhage: a prospective study, *Ann. Surg.,* 206, 48, 1987.

150. **Viallet, A., Marleau, D., Huet, P. M., Martin, F., Farley, A., Villeneuve, J. P., and Lavoie, P.,** Hemodynamic evaluation of patients with intrahepatic portal hypertension: relationship between bleeding varices and the portohepatic gradient, *Gastroenterology,* 69, 1297, 1975.

151. **Garcia-Tsao, G., Groszmann, R. J., Fischer, R. L., Conn, H. O., Atterbury, C. E., and Glickman, M.,** Portal pressure, presence of gastroesophageal varices and variceal bleeding, *Hepatology,* 5, 419, 1985.

152. **Lebrec, D., Nouel, O., Corbic, M., and Benhamou, J. P.,** Propranolol — a medical treatment for portal hypertension?, *Lancet,* 1, 180, 1980.

153. **Lebrec, D., Hillon, P., Munoz, C., Goldfarb, G., Nouel, O., and Benhamou, J. P.,** The effect of propranolol on portal hypertension in patients with cirrhosis. A Hemodynamic study, *Hepatology,* 2, 523, 1982.

154. **Rector, W. G.,** Propranolol for portal hypertension, *Hepatology,* 2, 678, 1982.

155. **Nakayama, T., Ohnishi, K., Saito, M., Hatano, H., Nomura, F., Kono, K., and Okuda, K.,** Effects of propranolol on portal vein pressure, portal blood flow, hepatic blood flow and cardiac output in patients with chronic liver disease, *Hepatology,* 3, 812, 1983.

156. **Bosch, J., Mastai, R., Kravetz, D., Bruix, J., Gaya, J., Rigau, J., and Rodes, J.,** Effects of propranolol on azygos venous blood flow and hepatic and systemic hemodynamics in cirrhosis, *Hepatology,* 4, 1200, 1984.

157. **Hillon, P., Lebrec, D., Munoz, C., Jungers, M., Goldfarb, G., and Benhamou, J. P.,** Comparison of the effects of a cardioselective and a nonselective β-blocker on portal hypertension in patients with cirrhosis, *Hepatology,* 2, 528, 1982.

158. **Westaby, D., Bihari, D. J., Gimson, A. E. S., Crossley, I. R., Williams, R., Crossley, I. R., and Williams, R.,** Selective and nonselective beta-receptor blockade in the reduction of portal pressure in patients with cirrhosis and portal hypertension, *Gut,* 25, 121, 1984.

159. **Cales, P., Braillon, A., Jiron, I., and Lebrec, D.,** Superior porto-systemic collateral circulation estimated by azygos blood flow in patients with cirrhosis. Lack of correlation with eosophageal varices and gastrointestinal bleeding. Effect of propranolol, *J. Hepatology,* 1, 37, 1984.

160. **Lebrec, D., Poynard, T., Hillon, P., and Benhamou, J. P.,** Propranolol for the prevention of recurrent gastrointestinal bleeding in patients with cirrhosis. A controlled study, *N. Engl. J. Med.,* 305, 1371, 1981.

161. **Lebrec, D., Poynard, T., Bernuau, J., Bercoff, E., Nouel, O., Capron, J. P., Poupon, R., Bouvry, M., Rueff, B., and Benhamou, J. P.,** A randomized controlled study of propranolol for prevention of recurrent gastrointestinal bleeding in patients with cirrhosis: a final report, *Hepatology,* 4, 355, 1984.

162. **Burroughs, A. K., Jenkins, W. J., Sherlock, S., Dunk, A., Walt, R. P., Osuafor, T. O. K., Mackie, S., and Dick, R.,** Controlled trial of propranolol for the prevention of recurrent variceal hemorrhage in patients with cirrhosis, *N. Engl. J. Med.,* 309, 1539, 1983.

163. **Villeneuve, J. P., Pomier-Layrargues, G., Infante-Rivard, C., Willems, B., Huet, P. M., Marleau, D., and Viallet, A.,** Propranolol for the prevention of recurrent variceal hemorrhage: a controlled trial, *Hepatology,* 6, 1239, 1986.

164. **Queuniet, A. M., Czernichow, P., Lerebours, E., Ducrotte, P., Transvouez, J. L., and Colin, R.,** Etude contrôlée du propranolol dans la prévention des récidives hémorragiques chez les patients cirrhotiques, *Gastroenterol. Clin. Biol.,* 4, 41, 1987.

165. **Gatta, A., Sacerdoti, D., Merkel, C., Milani, L., Battaglia, G., and Zuin, R.,** Effects of nadolol treatment on renal and hepatic hemodynamics and function in cirrhotic patients with portal hypertension, *Am. Heart. J.,* 108, 1167, 1984.

166. **Gatta, A., Sacerdoti, D., Merkel, C., Rossoni, R., Finusci, G., Bolognesi, M., and Zuin, R.,** Use of a non-selective beta-blocker, nadolol in the treatment of portal hypertension in cirrhotics, *Int. J. Clin. Pharmacol. Res.,* 5, 413, 1985.

167. **Wink, K.,** Acute and chronic effects of the beta-receptor blocker mepindolol on hemodynamics and the portal circulation, *Int. J. Clin. Pharmacol. Ther. Toxicol.,* 22, 447, 1984.

168. **Deflandre, J., Pirotte, J., Allaf, B., and Carlier, J.,** Effet du sotalol sur l'hypertension portale du cirrhotique. Résultats préliminaires d'une étude hémodynamique cardiaque et hépatique, *Biomed. Pharmacother.,* 40, 154, 1986.

169. **Zoli, M., Marzocchi, A., Marchesini, G., Marrozzini, C., Dondi, C., and Pisi, E.,** Atenolol in portal hypertension: a hemodynamic study, *Ital. J. Gastroenterol.,* 17, 252, 1985.

170. **Mills, I. R., Rae, A. P., Farah, D. A., Russel, R. I., Lorimier, A. R., and Carter, D. C.,** Comparison of three adrenoreceptor-blocking agents in patients with cirrhosis and portal hypertension, *Gut,* 25, 73, 1984.

171. **Butzow, G. H., Remmecke, J., and Brauer, A.,** Metoprolol in portal hypertension: a controlled study, *Klin. Wochenschr.,* 60, 1311, 1982.

172. **Bihari, D., Westaby, D., Simson, A., Crossley, I., Harry, J., and Williams, R.,** Reductions in portal pressure by selective beta-2-adrenoceptor blockade in patients with cirrhosis and portal hypertension, *Br. J. Clin. Pharmacol.,* 17, 753, 1984.

173. **Feely, J., Wilkinson, G. R., and Wood, A. J. J.,** Reduction of liver blood flow and propranolol metabolism by cimetidine, *N. Engl. J. Med.,* 304, 692, 1981.

174. **Burroughs, A. K., Walt, R., Dunk, A., Jenkins, W., Sherlock, S., Mackie, S., and Dick, R.,** Effect of cimetidine on portal hypertension in cirrhotic patients, *Br. Med. J.,* 284, 1159, 1982.

175. **Henderson, J. M., Ibrahim, S. Z., Millikan, W. J., Santi, M., and Warren, W. D.,** Cimetidine does not reduce liver blood flow in cirrhosis, *Hepatology,* 3, 919, 1983.

176. **Herz, R., Rossle, M., Bonzel, T., Keller, E., and Gerok, W.,** Effect of cimetidine on the hepatic extraction of Indocyanine green, the portal pressure and the systemic circulation in patients with cirrhosis of the liver, *Klin. Wochenschr.,* 62, 759, 1984.

177. **MacDougall, B. R. D. and Williams, R.,** A controlled clinical trial of cimetidine in the recurrence of variceal hemorrhage: implications about the pathogenesis of hemorrhage, *Hepatology,* 3, 69, 1983.

178. **Hallemans, R., Naeije, R., Mols, P., Melot, C., and Reding, P.,** Treatment of portal hypertension with isosorbide dinitrate alone and in combination with vasopressin, *Crit. Care Med.,* 11, 536, 1983.

179. **Mastai, R., Grande, L., Bosch, J., Bruix, J., Rigau, J., Kravetz, D., Navasa, M., Pera, C., and Rodes, J.,** Effects of metoclopramide and domperidone on azygous venous blood flow in patients with cirrhosis and portal hypertension, *Hepatology,* 6, 1244, 1986.

180. **Kong, C. W., Lay, C. S., Tsai, Y. T., Yeh C-L, Lai, K. M., Lee, S. D., Lo, K. J., and Chiang, B. N.,** The hemodynamic effect of verapamil on portal hypertension in patients with post-necrotic cirrhosis, *Hepatology,* 6, 423, 1986.

181. **Mastai, R., Rocheleau, B., and Huet, P. M.,** Ritanserin, a serotonin antagonist: a new approach in the pharmacological treatment of portal hypertension, *Hepatology,* 7, 1030, 1987.

182. **Westaby, D., MacDougall, B. R. D., and Williams, R.,** Improved survival following injection sclerotherapy for esophageal varices: final analysis of a controlled trial, *Hepatology,* 5, 827, 1985.

183. **Terblanche, J., Bornman, P. C., Kahn, D., Janker, M. A. T., Campbell, J. A. H., Wright, J., and Kirsh, R.,** Failure of repeated injection sclerotherapy to improve long-term survival after esophageal bleeding, *Lancet,* 2, 1328, 1983.

184. **Korula, J., Balart, L. A., Radvan, G., Zweiban, B. E., Larson, A. Q., Kao, H. W., and Yamada, S.,** A prospective, randomized controlled trial of chronic esophageal variceal sclerotherapy, *Hepatology,* 5, 584, 1985.

185. **Söderlund, C. and Ihre, T. H.,** Endoscopic sclerotherapy vs. conservative management of bleeding esophageal varices, *Acta Chir. Scand.,* 151, 449, 1985.

186. **Jackson, F. C., Perrin, E. B., Felix, W. R., and Smith, A. G.,** A clinical investigation of the portacaval shunt V: survival analysis of the therapeutic operation, *Ann. Surg.,* 174, 672, 1971.

187. **Resnick, R. H., Iber, F. L., Ishihara, A. M., Chalmers, T. C., Zimmerman, H., and the Boston InterHospital Liver group,** A controlled study of the therapeutic portacaval shunt, *Gastroenterology,* 67, 843, 1974.

188. **Rueff, B., Prandi, D., Degos, F., Sicot, J., Degos, J. D., Sicot, C., Maillard, J. N., Fauvert, R., and Benhamou, J. P.,** A controlled study of therapeutic portocaval shunt in alcoholic cirrhosis, *Lancet,* 1, 655, 1976.

189. **Reynolds, T. B., Donovan, A. J., Mikkelsen, W. P., Redeker, A. G., Rurrill, F. W., and Weiner, J. M.,** Results of a 12-year randomized trial of portocaval shunt in patients with alcoholic liver disease and bleeding varices, *Gastroenterology,* 80, 1005, 1981.

190. **Langer, B., Taylor, B. R., Mackenzie, D. R., Gilas, T., Stone, R. M., and Blendis, L.,** Further report of a prospective randomized trial comparing distal splenorenal shunt with end-to-side portacaval shunt. An analysis of encephalopathy, survival and quality of life, *Gastroenterology,* 88, 424, 1985.

191. **Conn, H. O., Resnick, R. H., Grace, N. D., Atterbury, C. E., Horst, J., Groszmann, K. J., Gazmuri, P., Gusberg, R. J., Thayer, B., Berk, D., Wright, S. C., Vollman, R., Tilson, D. M., McDermott, W. V., Cohen, J. A., Kerstein, M., Toole, A. L., Maselli, J. P., Razvi, S., Ishihara, A., Stern, H., Trey, C., O'Hara, E. T., Widrich, W., Aiserberg, H., Stansel, C., and Zinny, M.,** Distal splenorenal shunt vs. portal systemic shunt: Current status of a controlled trial, *Hepatology,* 1, 151, 1981.
192. **Paquet, K. J.,** Prophylactic endoscopic sclerosing treatment of the esophageal wall in varices. A prospective controlled randomized trial, *Endoscopy,* 80, 1005, 1981.
193. **Witzel, L., Wolbergs, E., and Merki, H.,** Prophylactic endoscopic sclerotherapy of esophageal varices, *Lancet,* 1, 773, 1985.
194. **Pascal, J. P., Cales, P., and a Multicenter study group,** Propranolol in the prevention of first upper gastrointestinal tract hemorrhage in patients with cirrhosis of the liver and esophageal varices, *N. Engl. J. Med.,* 317, 856, 1987.

Chapter 9

SPLANCHNIC HEMODYNAMICS IN ACUTE AND CHRONIC PORTAL HYPERTENSION

Joseph N. Benoit, Ronald J. Korthuis, D. Neil Granger, and Harold D. Battarbee*

TABLE OF CONTENTS

*   J. N. Benoit is supported by a Grant-in-Aid from the American Heart Association, LA, Inc. R. J. Korthuis is the recipient of an Established Investigator Award from the American Heart Association.

I. INTRODUCTION

There is a growing body of evidence which indicates that microcirculatory disturbances play an important role in the pathogenesis of a variety of gastrointestinal disorders. The intimate relationship between gastrointestinal pathology and the circulation has primarily been emphasized in ischemic disorders, presumably due to the well-defined influence of tissue hypoxia on cell function and survival. Less emphasis has been devoted to the possible role of microcirculatory disturbances in the pathogenesis of gastrointestinal diseases characterized by an increased blood flow. While excess delivery of blood to tissues is not generally viewed as being detrimental to parenchymal cell function, it does impose a mechanical stress on the vasculature, which can lead to pathologic elevations in intravascular pressure. Indeed, such a link between excess delivery of blood and gastrointestinal pathology appears to exist in conditions associated with chronic portal hypertension. In this chapter, we summarize evidence that supports the view that the hyperdynamic circulation of chronic portal hypertension plays a major role in increased intravascular pressure. Emphasis is also placed on intestinal transvascular exchange and mechanisms responsible for the alterations in gastrointestinal blood flow that accompany acute and chronic portal hypertension.

II. REGULATION OF GASTROINTESTINAL BLOOD FLOW

Moment to moment control of splanchnic blood flow is accomplished through integration of intrinsic and extrinsic control systems. These systems serve to maintain blood flow at a constant level and to modulate blood flow in various physiological and pathological conditions. Although it is not within the realm of this review to present a detailed discussion of splanchnic blood flow regulation, a brief treatment of this topic is necessary to understand the factors that may contribute to the hemodynamic alterations associated with portal hypertension. For more in-depth information regarding the regulation of gastrointestinal blood flow, the reader is referred to several excellent reviews.[1-5]

The ability of gastrointestinal organs to instantaneously modulate blood flow is most often explained by the presence of local (intrinsic) regulatory mechanisms. Intrinsic regulation of splanchnic blood flow is exemplified by the presence of blood flow autoregulation, reactive hyperemia, hypoxic vasodilation and functional hyperemia in denervated preparations. To explain the aforementioned phenomena, two theories of local blood flow regulation (i.e., metabolic and myogenic) have been proposed. According to the metabolic theory, blood flow is dependent on the metabolic activity of the tissue. Increases in tissue oxygen demand or decreases in oxygen delivery lead to the release of vasodilator metabolites into the interstitial fluid. These vasodilator metabolites cause relaxation of vascular smooth muscle which serve to return blood flow and oxygen delivery towards normal. Therefore, according to the metabolic theory, tissue pO_2 is regulated, and changes in blood flow maintain an adequate supply of oxygen to the tissue. Although several substances have been proposed as metabolic vasoregulators, hydrogen ions, potassium ions, interstitial osmolality, adenosine and the adenine nucleotides remain the most likely candidates.

Myogenic control represents the other major theory of local blood flow regulation. According to this theory, vascular resistance is related to arteriolar transmural pressure and the effect of stretch on vascular smooth muscle tone. In essence, the myogenic theory proposes the existence of receptors in the walls of arterioles and precapillary sphincters that are responsive to changes in wall tension. Wall tension increases as intravascular pressure increases, since tension is the product of pressure and radius. The increased wall tension elicits constriction of arterioles and precapillary sphincters, thereby reducing vascular radius and returning wall tension towards normal. Thus, according to the myogenic theory, vascular wall tension is the regulated variable and changes in arteriolar diameter maintain wall tension constant as vascular transmural pressure changes.

An important criterion for determining whether metabolic or myogenic mechanisms predominate in the local blood flow control is the effects of acute venous pressure elevation. According to the metabolic theory, venous pressure elevation initially reduces blood flow (by reducing the pressure gradient driving flow) and tissue pO_2. As a consequence of the reduction in flow, vasodilator metabolites accumulate in the interstitial space and vasodilation ensues. Blood flow and tissue pO_2 are therefore returned towards control values. On the other hand, the myogenic theory predicts that vascular resistance increases in response to increases in transmural pressure produced by venous pressure elevation. Many splanchnic organs respond to acute venous hypertension in a fashion consistent with a myogenic mechanism (i.e., vasoconstriction). This response to acute venous pressure elevation differs drastically from chronic venous hypertension, which is characterized by an intense splanchnic vasodilation.

In addition to local regulatory systems, splanchnic blood flow is influenced by several extrinsic factors such as nerve activity and hormones. The splanchnic vasculature is richly innervated by both sympathetic and parasympathetic fibers.[6] Stimulation of sympathetic nerves at varying frequencies results in a frequency-dependent increase in vascular resistance. With continued stimulation, intestinal resistance begins to decrease and intestinal blood flow returns toward normal. This phenomenon of autoregulatory escape only occurs in the small intestine and is not well understood. Greenway[7] has postulated that the escape is mediated by the release of an antagonist to norepinephrine, while Crissinger et al.[8] report that the escape can be attenuated by adenosine deaminase which prevents adenosine accumulation during ischemia. Parasympathetic innervation of the gastrointestinal tract originates from the vagus and pelvic splanchnic nerves. While these fibers are thought to mediate several systemic cardiovascular reflexes of splanchnic origin,[9] they appear to have little or no direct influence on intestinal blood flow.

The splanchnic circulation may also be modulated by numerous endogenous blood-borne substances. These vasoactive agents can alter blood flow by directly affecting vascular smooth muscle or indirectly by changing nerve activity. Table 1 lists several endogenous substances that modulate splanchnic blood flow and their effects on splanchnic vascular resistance.

III. HEMODYNAMIC RESPONSE TO PORTAL HYPERTENSION

The responses of the splanchnic circulation to elevations in portal pressure have been extensively characterized during the past decade. In the sections that follow, we will describe the hemodynamic responses of the gastrointestinal tract to both acute and chronic venous hypertension. Special emphasis will be placed on the small intestine, since the majority of information in the literature is derived from this organ.

A. ACUTE PORTAL HYPERTENSION

The gastrointestinal circulation responds to acute venous pressure elevation in a manner consistent with the myogenic theory of blood flow control. In the small intestine of cats and dogs,[10] acute venous hypertension increases total vascular resistance, reduces capillary density and redistributes blood flow from the mucosa-submucosa to the muscularis. Similar results have been reported for the dog colon.[5] This increase in vascular resistance results from intense precapillary constriction[11] and involves active vascular smooth muscle contraction since the increased vascular resistance caused by venous pressure elevation is abolished by cyanide.[12]

Recently, Davis and Gore[13] conducted a systematic study of intestinal microvascular responses during acute venous pressure elevation. Their results (Figures 1 and 2) indicate that graded increments in venous pressure result in constriction of submucosal arterioles (i.e., first, second and third order) and dilation of muscularis arterioles (i.e., fourth and

TABLE 1
Blood-Borne Modulators of Gastrointestinal Blood Flow

Agent	Splanchnic vascular action
Catecholamines	
Epinephrine	Vasodilation, β-adrenergic
	Vasoconstriction, α-adrenergic
Norepinephrine	Vasoconstriction, α-adrenergic
Autacoids	
Histamine	Vasodilation, H_1 receptor
Serotonin	Vasodilation
	Vasoconstriction
	No effect
Bradykinin	Vasodilation
Prostaglandins	
PGI_2	Vasodilation
PGE_2	Vasodilation
PGA_1	Vasodilation
PGA_2	Vasodilation
PGF_2	Vasoconstriction
PGD_2	Vasoconstriction
Thromboxane B_2	Vasoconstriction
Bile Acids	Vasodilation
Gastrointestinal peptides	
Cholecystokinin[a]	Vasodilation
Secretin[a]	Vasodilation
Gastrin	Vasodilation
Neurotensin	Vasodilation
Glucagon	Vasodilation
Substance P[a]	Vasodilation
Somatostatin	Vasoconstriction
Vasoactive intestinal peptide	Vasoconstriction (low dose)
	Vasodilation (high dose)

[a] Vasoactive only at supraphysiological concentrations.

Compiled from References 1, 2, 3, 4, 65.

fifth order). In addition, the diameters of capillaries of the muscularis externa as well as postcapillary venules (i.e., first, second, third and fourth order) are increased. These findings are consistent with both a myogenic flow mechanism and flow redistribution to the muscularis. It is unclear why the terminal arterioles of the muscularis respond differently from the larger arterioles. Davis and Gore[13] suggested that either local metabolic factors override the myogenic response, or a neural reflex may account for these differences.

Granger et al.[14] has recently used a theoretical analysis to investigate the possibility that larger arterioles are under different control systems than the smaller arterioles. His early models of skeletal muscle hemodynamics were based on the assumption that large arterioles are under myogenic control while small arterioles are under metabolic control. More recently, Granger proposed a three-compartment model of intestinal blood flow regulation[80] with the assumption that the submucosal arterioles (i.e., first, second and third order) are under myogenic control and mucosal arterioles are under metabolic control. Although Granger's model does not allow for a complete analysis of the muscularis arteriolar response (muscularis arterioles were assumed to react passively) it is conceivable that the differential response of submucosal and muscularis arterioles observed by Davis and Gore[13] may be explained by Granger's model if muscularis arterioles are also under metabolic control. In any instance, it is evident that future studies designed to evaluate differences in the intestinal microvascular responses to acute venous pressure elevation are warranted.

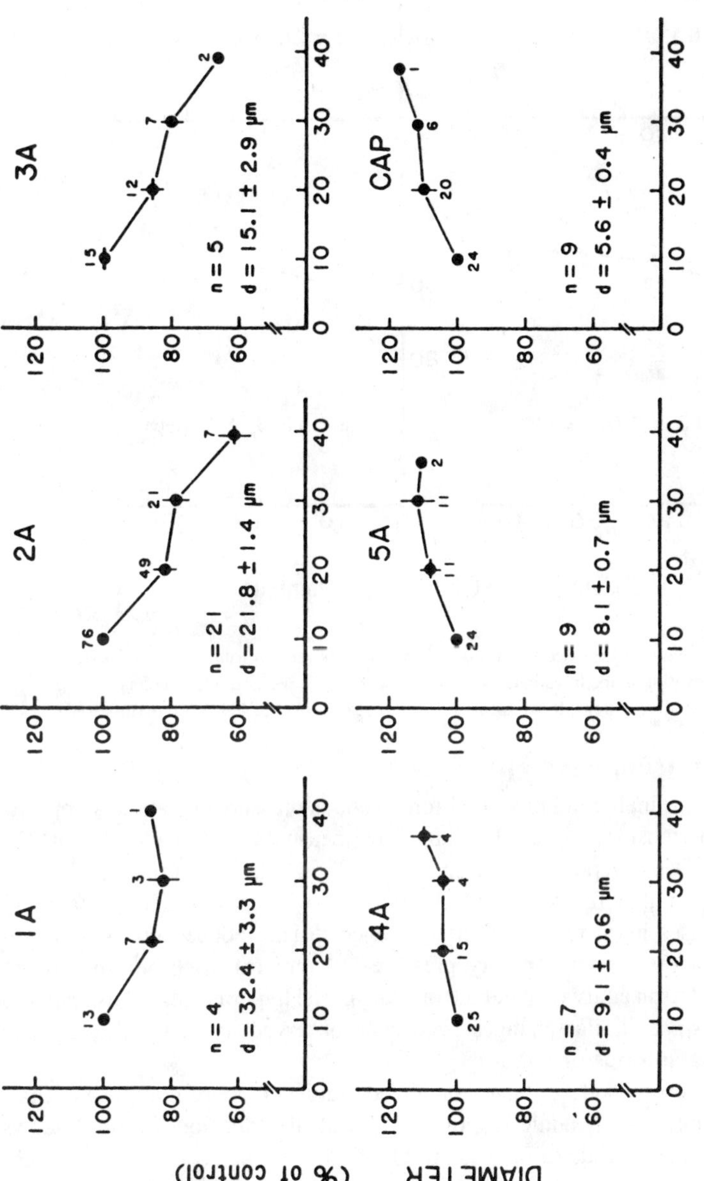

FIGURE 1. Change in diameter of first, second, third, fourth and fifth order arterioles as well as capillaries of the muscularis externa following brief periods of acute venous pressure elevation in the intestine. All submucosal vessels (i.e., 1A, 2A, and 3A) constricted while muscularis vessels (4A, 5A, and CAP) dilated as venous pressure was elevated. (From Davis, M. J. and Gore, R. W., *Am. J. Physiol.*, 249, H174, 1985. With permission.)

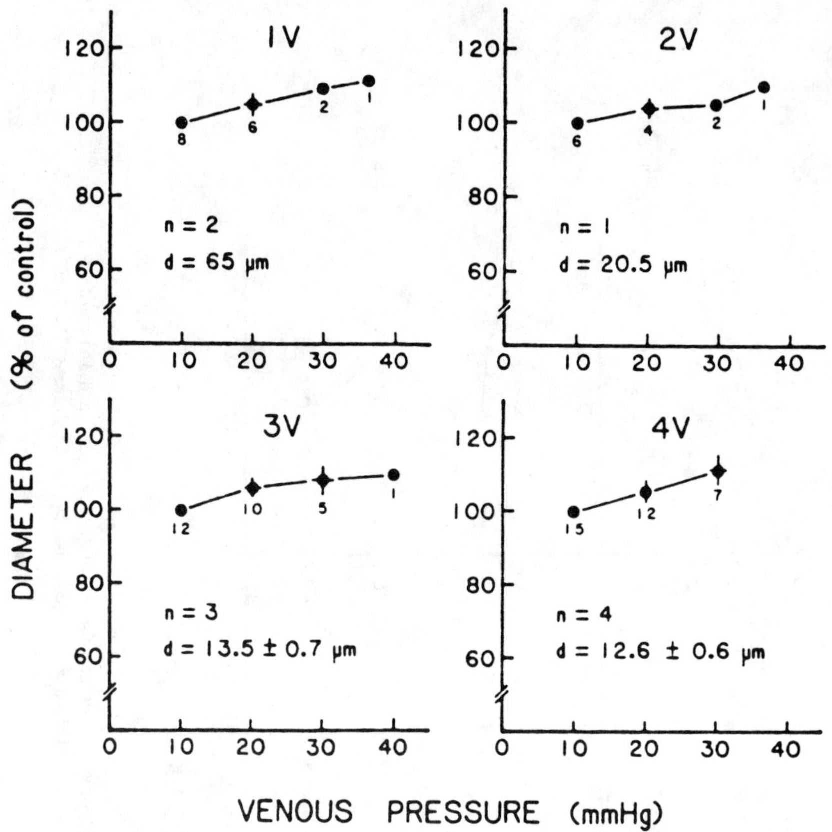

FIGURE 2.   Change in diameter of first, second, third and fourth order venules following brief periods of acute venous pressure elevation in the intestine. Diameters of all venules increased as venous pressure was elevated. (From Davis M. J. and Gore, R. W., *Am. J. Physiol.*, 249, H174, 1985. With permission.)

B. CHRONIC PORTAL HYPERTENSION

The response of the intestinal circulation to chronic venous pressure elevation is opposite that of acute venous hypertension. Figure 3 summarizes measurements of blood flow and whole organ capillary pressure reported by Benoit et al.[15] in rats with prehepatic portal hypertension. As shown in this figure, intestinal blood flow increases and precapillary vascular resistance decreases in portal hypertensive subjects. The reduced precapillary resistance is responsible for the higher capillary pressure (10 mmHg) in chronic portal hypertension when compared to an equivalent degree of acute portal hypertension. This response is not restricted to rats, since similar changes have been observed in man and dogs with intrahepatic and extrahepatic forms of portal hypertension.[16]

Recently, Benoit and co-workers,[17] have conducted studies to more completely characterize the gastrointestinal hemodynamic response to portal hypertension. Table 2 shows that chronic portal hypertension leads to increase in blood flow in the esophagus, stomach, duodenum, jejunum, ileum and colon. Furthermore, Benoit et al.[17] have used nonradioactive microspheres to determine whether chronic portal hypertension is associated with a redistribution of blood flow in the wall of the gastrointestinal organs. These results, summarized in Table 3, indicate that portal hypertension does not significantly alter the transmural distribution of blood flow in the esophagus, duodenum, jejunum and colon. However, there is a redistributuion of blood flow from the muscularis to the submucosal and mucosal layers of the stomach. This observation in the stomach is consistent with the data of Kitano et al.[18,19] that gastric mucosal vasodilation occurs in cirrhotic rats with portal hypertension.

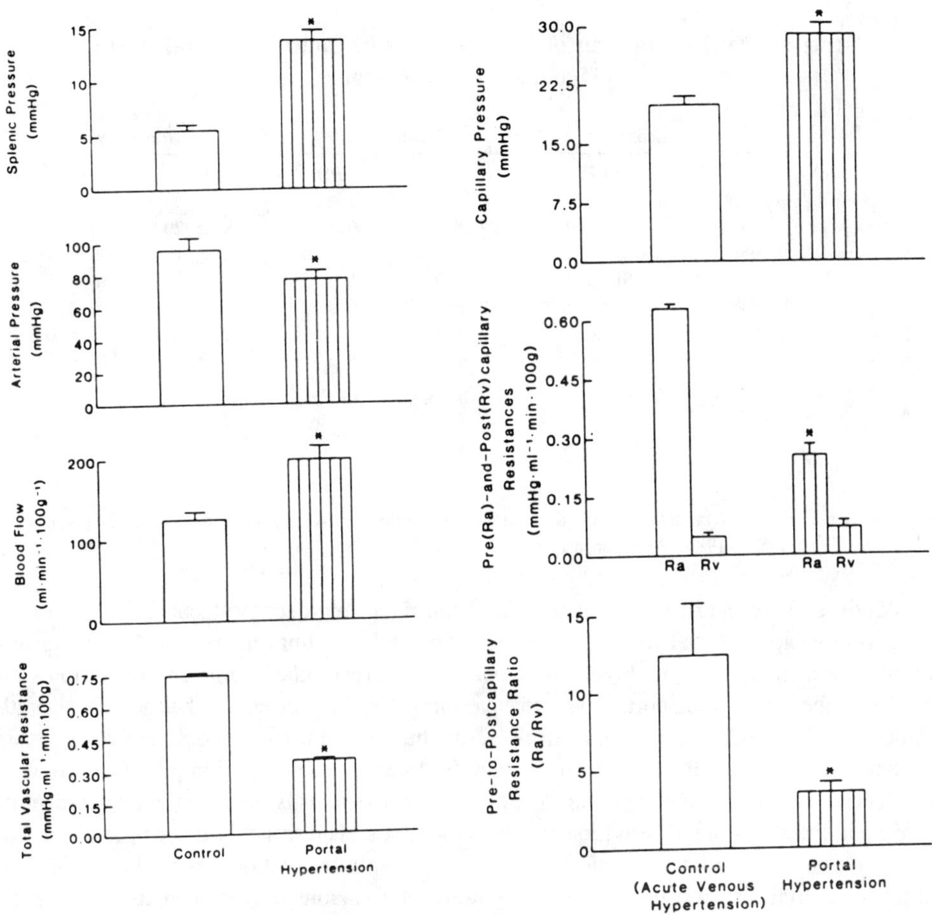

FIGURE 3. Effects of chronic portal hypertension on portal pressure, arterial pressure, intestinal blood flow, vascular resistance, and capillary pressure. (From Benoit, J. N. et al., *Am. J. Physiol.*, 247, G486, 1984. With permission.)

TABLE 2
Effects of Chronic Portal Hypertension on Gastrointestinal Blood Flow

	Blood Flow (ml/min/100 g)	
Organ	**Control**	**Portal hypertensive**
Esophagus	14.4 ± 1.6	23.9 ± 3.6[a]
Stomach	31.5 ± 3.7	63.8 ± 6.3[a]
Duodenum	141.8 ± 11.0	202.0 ± 14.1[a]
Jejunum	118.2 ± 11.6	179.5 ± 12.4[a]
Ileum	68.3 ± 10.8	105.0 ± 15.5[a]
Colon	40.2 ± 3.3	71.9 ± 10.0[a]

Note: Values are means ± S.E.

[a] $p < 0.05$.

From Benoit, J. N., Womack, W. A., Korthuis, R. J., Wilborn, W. H., and Granger, D. N., *Am. J. Physiol.*, 230, G535, 1986. With permission.

TABLE 3
**Intramural Distribution of Microspheres in Control (C) and Portal
Hypertensive (PH) Rats**

Organ	Mucosa		Submucosa		Muscularis	
	C	PH	C	PH	C	PH
Esophagus	3 ± 2	1 ± 0.5	27 ± 18	20 ± 4	70 ± 20	79 ± 4
Stomach	95 ± 1	89 ± 2[a]	2 ± 0.4	4 ± 0.4[a]	3 ± 1	6 ± 2[a]
Duodenum	84 ± 2	88 ± 2	12 ± 2	6 ± 2	4 ± 2	6 ± 3
Jejunum	84 ± 3	88 ± 2	12 ± 1	10 ± 3	5 ± 3	2 ± 0.3
Ileum	82 ± 3	77 ± 15	14 ± 2	22 ± 15	4 ± 2	1 ± 0.5
Colon	63 ± 10	56 ± 8	30 ± 6	25 ± 11	7 ± 7	24 ± 14

Note: Values are mean ± S.E.

[a] $p < 0.05$.

From Benoit, J. N., Womack, W. A., Korthuis, R. J., Wilborn, W. R., and Granger, D. N., *Am. J. Physiol.*, 230, G535, 1986. With permission.

Benoit and Granger[20] have recently used intravital microscopic techniques and the rat portal vein stenosis model to determine the segmental intestinal microvascular response to chronic portal hypertension. Figure 4 shows the microvascular diameter of arterioles and venules in the intestine of portal hypertensive rats. Portal hypertension had no effect on the diameter of first and second order arterioles of the intestinal submucosa. However, a significant increase in the diameter of the third order arterioles was noted in portal hypertensive rats. It is interesting to note that dilation of third order arterioles is consistent with a transmural increase in intestinal blood flow, inasmuch as these vessels ultimately determine blood flow to both the mucosa and muscularis.[21] A more important observation lies in the fact that the submucosal arterioles did not follow the pattern of vasoconstriction seen in acute venous pressure elevation.[13] Therefore, it appears that the myogenic response observed in the normal rat intestine is abolished or overridden by extrinsic factors in the portal hypertensive rat. It is unlikely that the observed arteriolar dilation can be explained on the basis of a metabolic override of the myogenic response because intestinal oxygen consumption is unaffected by chronic portal hypertension.[15] More likely, neural or humoral factors are involved.

IV. VENOUS HYPERTENSION AND MICROVASCULAR EXCHANGE

Under normal physiological conditions, a balance exists between steady-state transvascular (J_v) and lymphatic (J_L) fluid fluxes exists such that:

$$J_v = K_f[(P_c - P_t) - \sigma(\pi_c - \pi_t)] = J_L$$

where K_f represents the microvascular filtration coefficient (which, in turn, represents a product of microvascular surface area and permeability to filtered fluid), P_c represents microvascular hydrostatic pressure, P_t represents interstitial fluid pressure, σ represents the osmotic reflection coefficient for total plasma proteins (a measure of vascular permeability), π_c and π_t represent the colloid osmotic pressure of the plasma and interstitial fluid, respectively. From a consideration of the Starling equation, it is apparent that venous pressure elevation should increase the rate of transcapillary fluid filtration (via increased capillary pressure) and lymph flow. Indeed, a major consequence of elevated portal venous pressure

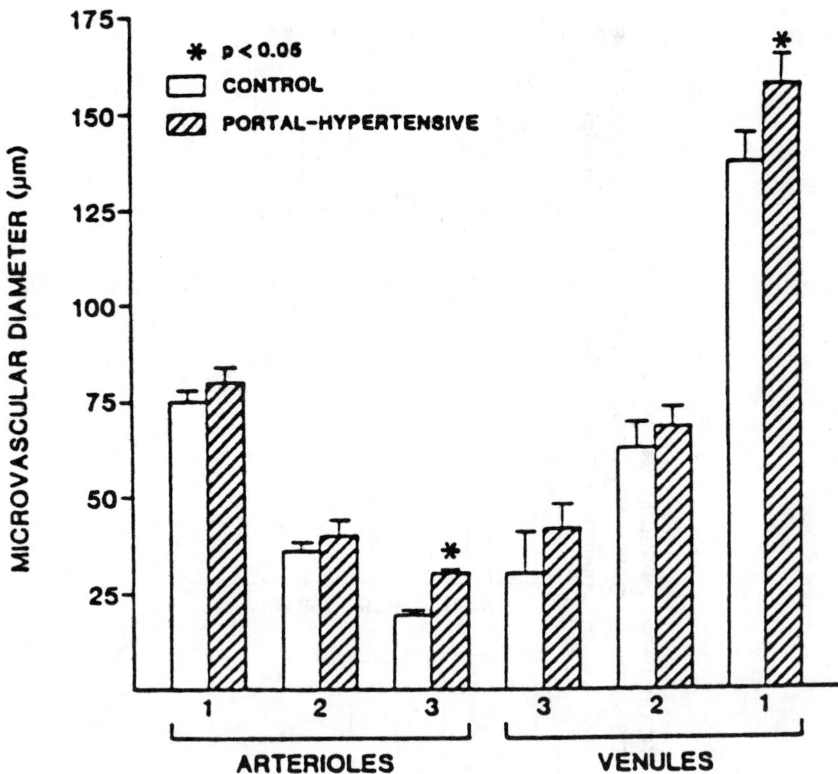

FIGURE 4.   Diameter of arterioles and venules in the submucosa of control and portal hypertensive rats. Chronic portal hypertension was associated with a dilation of third order arterioles and first order venules. (From Benoit, J. N. and Granger, D. N., *Gastroenterology*, 94, 471, 1988. With permission.)

is enhanced transcapillary fluid filtration, with subsequent accumulation of interstitial fluid (edema).

The severity of edema produced by portal hypertension is, to a large extent, determined by the site of portal vein obstruction.[16] For example, the formation of edema in prehepatic portal hypertension is primarily localized in the mucosal layer.[22,23] However, in patients with chronic portal hypertension associated with cirrhosis (sinusoidal or postsinusoidal venous obstruction), this excessive accumulation of interstitial fluid has been noted in the mucosal, muscular, and serosal layers of the bowel wall.[24-26] The serosal edema is manifested as a five-fold increase in the thickness of jejunal peritoneum in cirrhotic patients relative to controls.

The formation of edema in acute and chronic portal hypertension appears to be related, at least in part, to a dramatic increase in intestinal capillary pressure that accompanies the rise in portal pressure (Figure 5). However, since precapillary resistance is reduced in chronic portal hypertension, the increment in capillary pressure produced by chronic elevations in portal pressure is greater than that produced by acute elevations in portal pressure of equivalent magnitude in control animals (Figure 5).[16,27] Analysis of the microvascular pressure distribution for control and portal hypertensive rats (Figure 6) indicates that, despite systemic hypotension, intravascular pressure is elevated from third order arterioles to the portal vein in rats with chronic portal hypertension.[20] Thus, a greater portion of arterial pressure is transmitted to the capillaries in chronic portal hypertension.

The observation that intestinal capillary pressure is elevated in chronic portal hyperten-

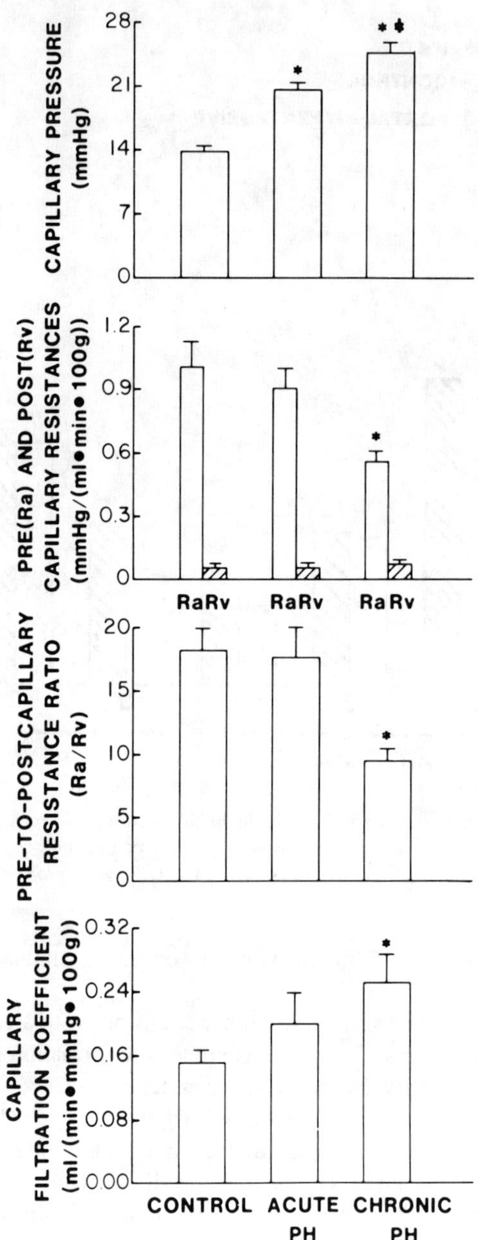

FIGURE 5.   Effects of acute and chronic portal hypertension of the same magnitude on intestinal capillary pressure, pre- and postcapillary resistances, pre-to-post resistance ratio and the capillary filtration coefficient. (From Korthuis, R. J. et al., *Am. J. Physiol.*, 254, G339, 1988. With permission.)

sion is especially interesting in view of the hypothesis put forward by Williamson and Kilo[28] and Parving et al.[29] These investigators proposed that increased capillary pressure in diabetes mellitus and congestive heart failure may act as an important initiating event for the thickening of capillary basement membranes which occurs in these disorders. Since intestinal capillary pressure is also increased in chronic portal hypertension, it is conceivable that capillary

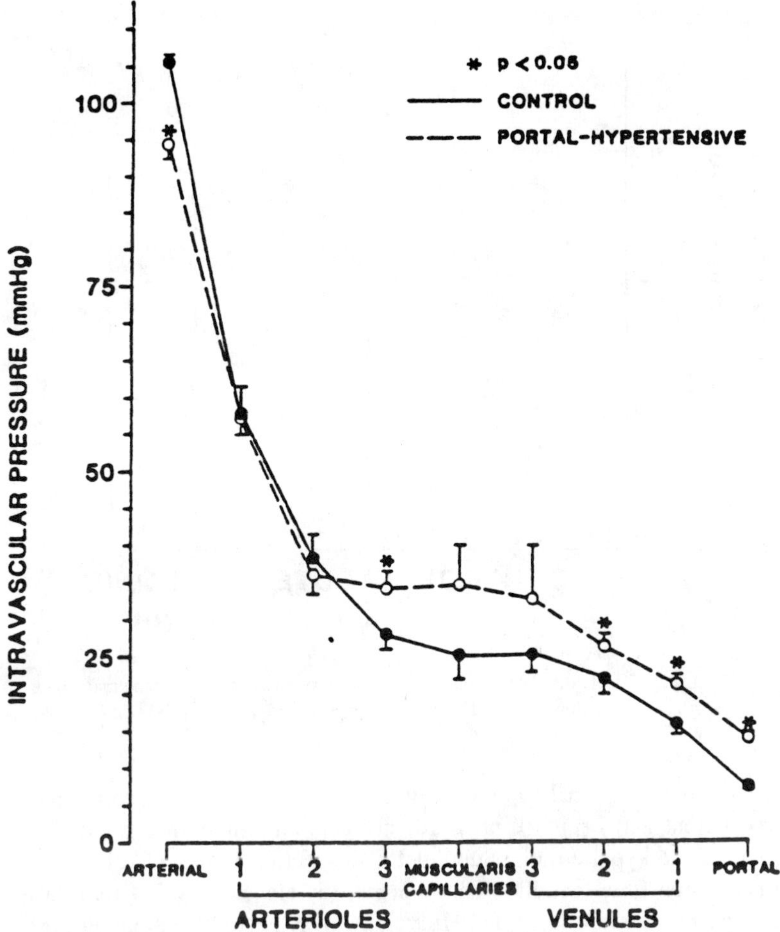

FIGURE 6. Microvascular pressure distribution in arterioles, capillaries and venules of control and portal hypertensive rats. Chronic portal hypertension was associated with a consistent elevation in pressure from the third order arterioles to the portal vein when compared to control. (From Benoit, J. N. and Granger, D. N., *Gastroenterology*, 94, 471, 1988. With permission.)

basement membrane thickness of intestinal microvessels may also be increased. However, measurements of intestinal capillary basement membrane thickness indicate that no change in basement membrane thickness occurred in response to chronic portal hypertension.[27] This may be due to the relatively short duration of the model of portal hypertension (10 d) used in these studies. Indeed, capillarization of the hepatic sinusoids occurs in long standing cirrhosis.[30] Furthermore, Granger et al.[31] have shown that the liver becomes less permeable to plasma proteins in dogs with posthepatic portal hypertension.

An important factor governing the rate of fluid movement from the vascular to extravascular compartment is the capillary filtration coefficient. Whereas acute elevations in portal pressure are generally associated with decreases in the capillary filtration coefficient,[32-34] chronic portal hypertension is associated with an increase in the capillary filtration coefficient.[27] With acute venous hypertension, the reduction in the filtration coefficient limits the excessive accumulation of interstitial fluid that might otherwise occur following an acute elevation of venous pressure. However, the increase in the capillary filtration coefficient that accompanies chronic portal hypertension serves to amplify the effect of increased cap-

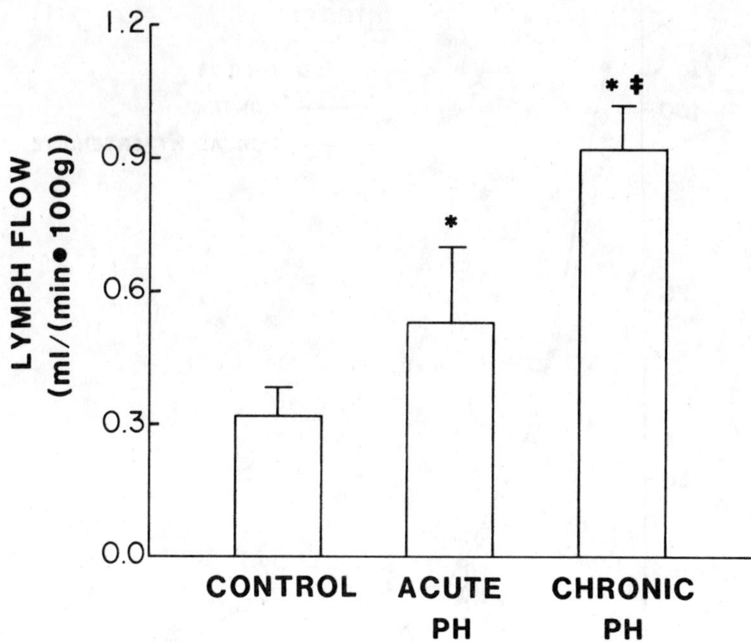

FIGURE 7. Effects of acute and chronic portal hypertension of the same magnitude on intestinal lymph flow. (From Korthuis, R. J. et al., *Am. J. Physiol.*, 254, G339, 1988. With permission.)

illary pressure. Since intestinal capillary filtration rate is proportional to the product of the filtration coefficient and capillary pressure, net capillary fluid flux should be greater in chronic versus acute hypertension. Support for this notion is provided by the observation that intestinal lymph flow (capillary filtration rate) is elevated by 2.9 fold during chronic elevations in portal pressure to 15 mmHg.[27] However, acute elevations in portal pressure of equivalent magnitude increase intestinal lymph flow by only 1.7 fold (Figure 7).

The increase in the capillary filtration coefficient with chronic portal hypertension is consistent with the actions of the proposed mediators (increased plasma glucagon and reduced vascular sensitivity to norepinephrine) of the intestinal hemodynamic response to chronic elevations in portal pressure.[15,35] For example, it is well established that elevated plasma glucagon levels increase the capillary filtration coefficient.[36] Although the effect of reduced vascular sensitivity to norepinephrine is more difficult to predict, it is known that denervation of the intestine produces an increase in the filtration coefficient.[36] This finding indicates that the sympathetic fibers innervating precapillary sphincters are tonically active. Thus, one might expect an increase in the capillary filtration coefficient when vascular sensitivity to norepinephrine is reduced.

It has been suggested that the increased capillary filtration rate in cirrhosis with portal hypertension arises as a consequence of reduced plasma oncotic pressure and increased portal pressure.[37] However, it has recently been shown that interstitial oncotic pressure is decreased to an even greater extent than is plasma oncotic pressure. Thus, the oncotic pressure gradient is decreased in most cirrhotic patients despite the reduction in plasma oncotic pressure.[38-40] The decreased oncotic pressure gradient would tend to oppose further capillary fluid filtration. Thus, the marked increase in intestinal capillary filtration rate in cirrhosis with portal hypertension is caused primarily by increased capillary pressure and capillary filtration coefficient which arises as a consequence of reduced precapillary resistance and increased portal venous pressure.[15,20,27,41]

Intestinal lymph flow is increased approximately two- to four-fold by acute and chronic

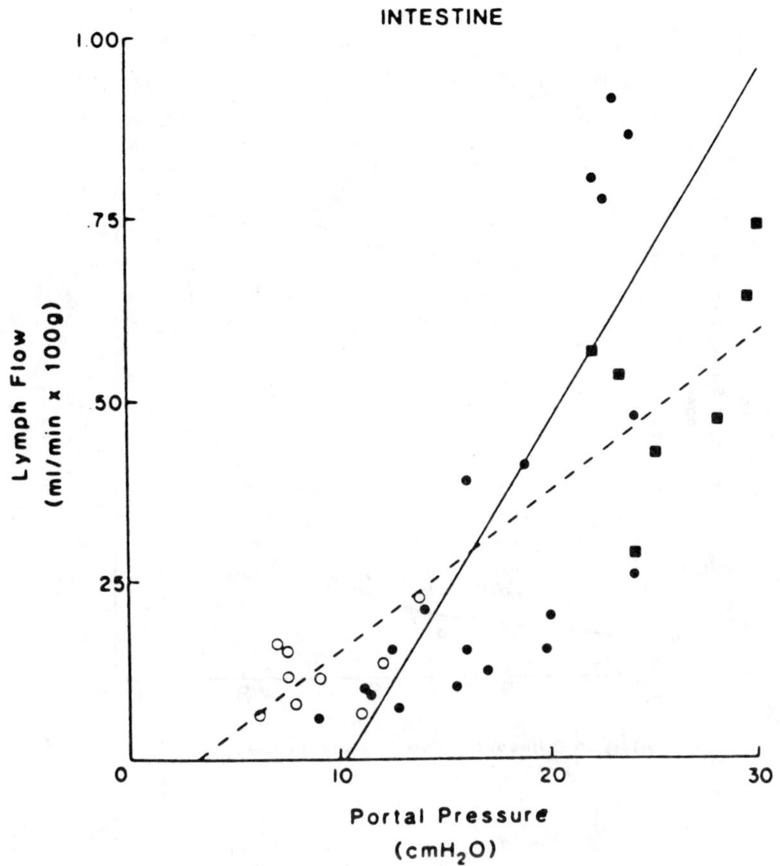

FIGURE 8. Relationship between intestinal lymph flow and portal pressure for control (open circles, dashed line) and cirrhotic rats (closed circles, solid line). (From Barrowman, J. A. and Granger, D. N., *Gastroenterology*, 87, 165, 1984. With permission.)

elevations of portal pressure to 15 mmHg (Figure 7). Similar increments in intestinal lymph flow have been noted in cirrhotic animals and man[41,42] when compared with normal subjects. These large increases in lymph flow may account for the observations that: (1) partial occlusion of the portal vein is associated with pronounced dilation of mucosal lymphatics,[22,23] and that (2) the portal hypertension of cirrhosis is associated with marked dilation of the lymphatics in the mucosal and serosal layers as well as the major collecting lymphatics of the small bowel.[43]

The magnitude of the rise in intestinal lymph flow is well correlated with portal pressure in cirrhotic animals (Figure 8). However, the relationship between lymph flow and portal pressure in cirrhotic rats is not significantly different from the relationship obtained in control animals (Figure 8).[42] Analysis of the lymph: plasma protein concentration ratio at various lymph flows is consistent with a capillary osmotic reflection coefficient of approximately 0.80 (Figure 9).[42] Inasmuch as a comparable value for the reflection coefficient is predicted from the L/P ratio and lymph flow in control animals,[27,44,45] intestinal capillary permeability does not appear to be altered by the chronic portal hypertension associated with carbon tetrachloride-induced cirrhosis. In contrast, the liver vasculature becomes less permeable to macromolecules in cirrhosis and other forms of posthepatic portal hypertension.[30,31]

The large increments in intestinal lymph flow associated with acute and chronic portal hypertension indicate that capillary fluid filtration is markedly increased during these perturbations. However, several compensatory edema safety factor mechanisms are available

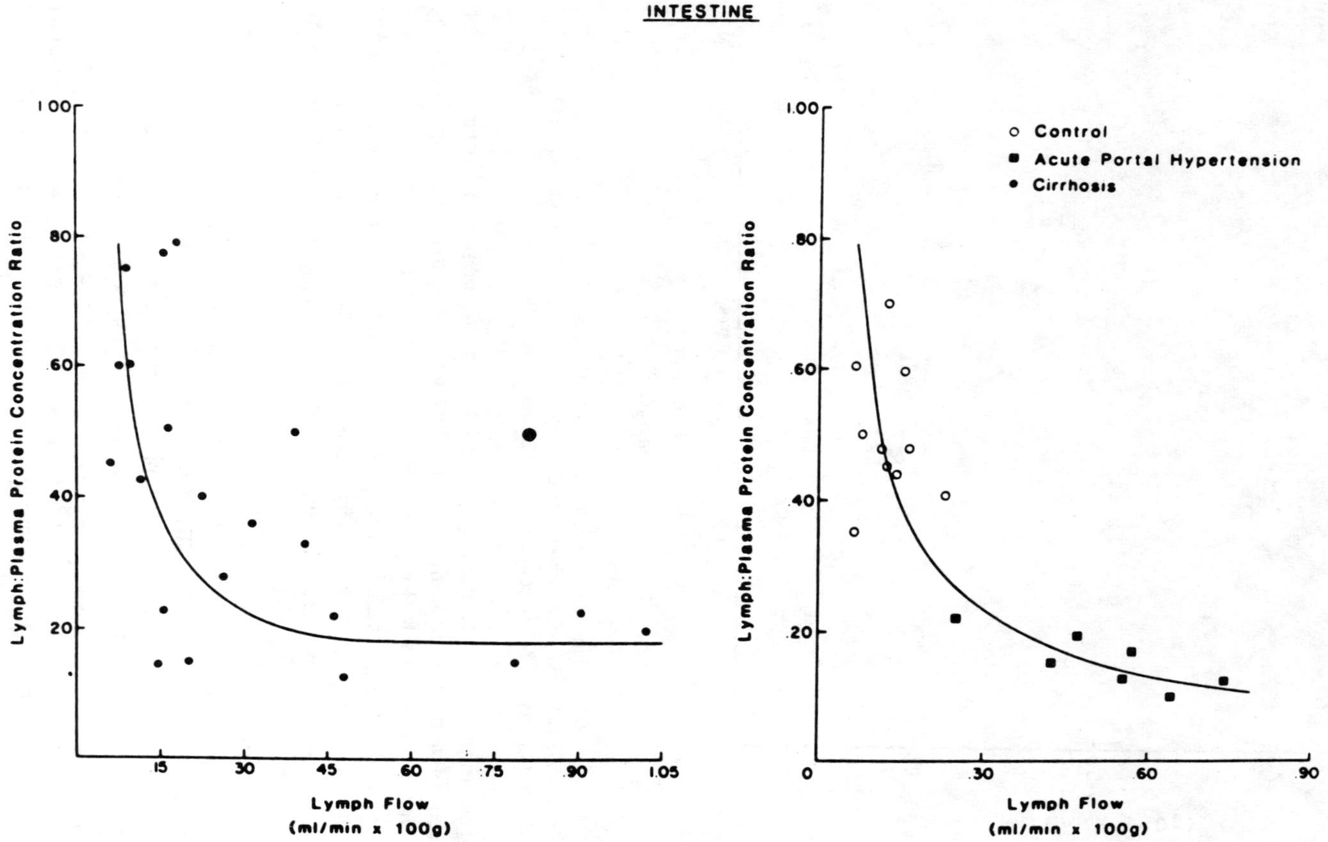

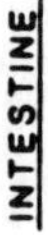

FIGURE 9.   Relationships between lymph:plasma protein concentration and lymph flow during acute (right panel) and chronic (left panel) elevation in portal pressure. (From Barrowman, J. A. and Granger, D. N., *Gastroenterology*, 87, 165, 1984. With permission.)

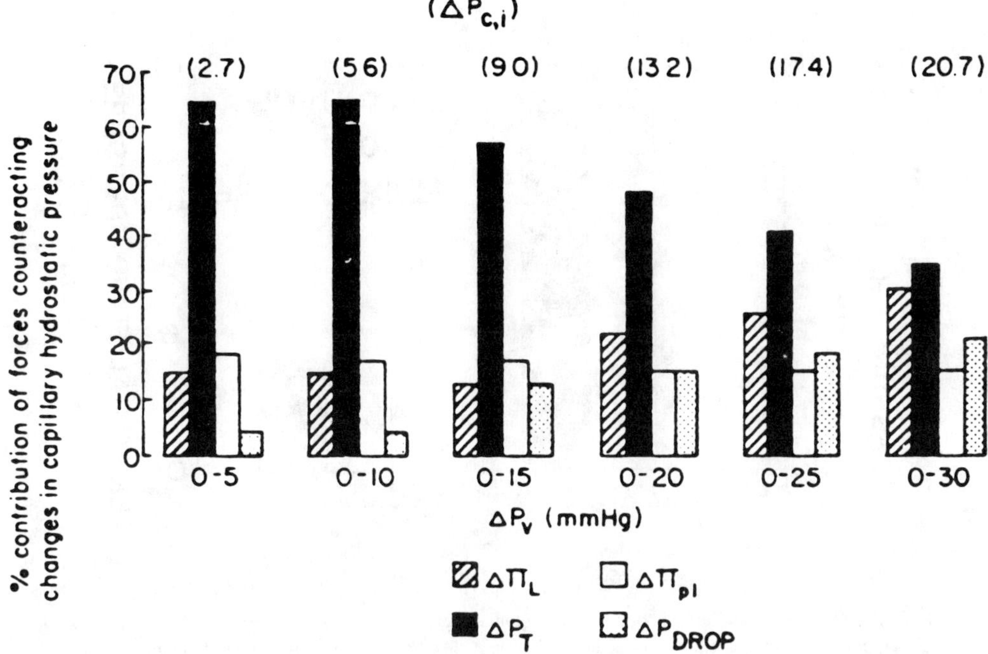

FIGURE 10.   Changes in lymph oncotic pressure (π_L), plasma oncotic pressure (π_{pl}), interstitial hydrostatic pressure (P_T) and capillary hydrostatic pressure (P_{Drop}) that occur following acute venous pressure elevation in the small intestine. (From Mortillaro, N. A. and Taylor A. E., *Circ. Res.*, 39, 348, 1976. With permission.)

in the intestine to prevent the excessive accumulation of interstitial fluid following elevation of venous pressure. These compensatory adjustments include increased tissue fluid pressure, decreased tissue oncotic pressure, elevated lymph flow, and myogenic constriction of arterioles and precapillary sphincters.

Wallentin[46] and Johnson[47] were the first to propose that accumulation of interstitial fluid in response to acute venous hypertension produces compensatory adjustments in the interstitial forces that allow the intestine to regain an isogravimetric state (no net fluid movement). Wallentin[46] suggested that changes in interstitial fluid pressure represented the major factor opposing excessive capillary filtration following venous pressure elevation. However, others[10,48] have proposed that reductions in tissues oncotic pressure constitute the major force adjustment caused by elevated capillary pressure.

Mortillaro and Taylor[34] were first to systematically analyze the interactions of the capillary and interstitial forces and lymph flow in response to acute venous pressure elevation. In their study, estimates of capillary pressure, interstitial fluid pressure, capillary filtration coefficient, transcapillary oncotic pressure gradient and net transcapillary fluid filtration (lymph flow) were obtained over a range of venous pressures (0—30 mmHg) in the cat small intestine. Their results indicate that venous pressure elevations induce increases in both transvascular filtration rate and lymph flow. Accompanying these changes were progressive increases in interstitial fluid pressure and the transcapillary oncotic pressure gradient. In addition, venous pressure elevation was associated with a progressive reduction in the capillary filtration coefficient and increase in precapillary resistance. These results were interpreted to suggest that myogenic arteriolar and precapillary sphincter constriction occurred in response to venous pressure elevation. Arteriolar constriction serves to prevent dramatic alterations in capillary pressure following elevation of venous pressure while myogenic reduction of the number of open capillaries decreases the available surface area for fluid exchange. Thus, a rise in capillary pressure secondary to acute elevations in venous pressure can be offset by myogenic, interstitial, and lymphatic compensations (Figure 10).

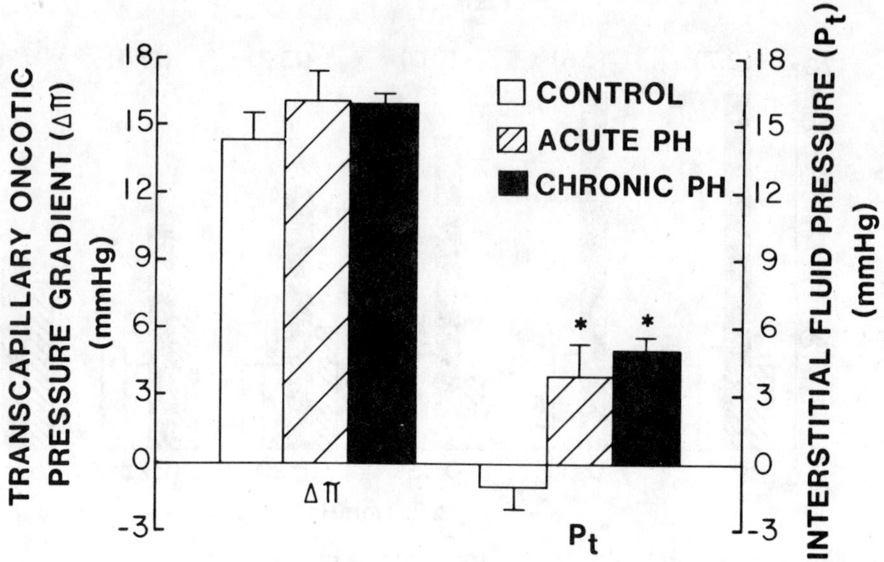

FIGURE 11.   Transcapillary oncotic pressure gradient and interstitial fluid pressure in the intestine during normal as well as equivalent acute and chronic elevations in portal pressures. Interstitial fluid pressure was increased during acute and chronic portal hypertension while the transcapillary oncotic pressure gradient was unaltered. (From Korthuis, R. J. et al., *Am. J. Physiol.*, 1987, 254, G339, 1988. With permission.)

Interstitial fluid pressure and lymph flow also increase in response to chronic portal hypertension.[27] However, the magnitude of these increases is greater in chronic vs. acute portal hypertension (Figures 7 and 11). Since the capillary filtration coefficient increases in response to chronic portal hypertension, myogenic reduction in the surface area available for fluid exchange seems unlikely.[27] However, there is an increase in the number of lymphatic vessels in the mesentery with chronic portal hypertension[43] which may represent a specific adaptation to longstanding edemagenic stress.

Based on interstitial compliance values for the small intestine,[34,36] one would predict that an increase in interstitial fluid volume of approximately 25% and 40%, respectively, would be required to produce the changes in interstitial fluid pressure associated with acute and chronic portal hypertension (Figure 11). This corresponds to a 80 to 160 ml increase in intestinal interstitial fluid volume in a 70-kg man when portal pressure is acutely elevated to the levels measured in chronic portal hypertension. Chronic elevations in portal pressure would be associated with an even more dramatic elevation in intestinal interstitial fluid volume (160 to 320 ml).

Edema of the gut is a common feature of chronic portal hypertension.[23-26] While interstitial edema of the intestine is not generally life threatening, it is likely to compromise the function of the delicate intestinal mucosa, especially absorptive function. One would expect that the high capillary filtration rate, coupled with the fact that a portion of the safety factor against edema is exhausted (increased interstitial fluid pressure and lymph flow),[27] predisposes the intestine of patients and experimental animals with portal hypertension to interstitial edema, filtration-secretion and diarrhea. Although acute elevations of portal pressure (25 mmHg increment) are associated with filtration-secretion, edema, and diarrhea,[36] diarrhea is not a prominent feature in patients with cirrhosis despite portal pressures as high as 55 mmHg. Estimates of absorptive and secretory water fluxes in cirrhotic patients suggest that filtration-secretion may occur.[26] However, an increased absorptive flux may compensate for the secretory flux, thereby preventing net fluid secretion in the small bowel.[26] Furthermore,

Lifson[49] proposed that the resistance of the mucosa to the detrimental effects of elevated interstitial fluid pressure may be increased as an adaptive response to the elevated portal pressure in cirrhosis.

It is tempting to propose that the alterations in the dynamics of intestinal capillary fluid exchange in chronic prehepatic (i.e., portal vein stenosis) and intrahepatic portal hypertension (i.e., cirrhosis) may contribute to the formation of ascites. However, in contrast to the portal hypertension associated with cirrhosis (i.e., intrahepatic), prehepatic portal hypertension produces only a transient and moderate ascites.[22,23,50] Although partial occlusion of the portal vein produces pronounced mucosal interstitial edema and a striking dilation of mucosal lymphatics,[22,23] no major changes are observed in the serosal and muscular layers of the intestine. This latter observation probably accounts for the relatively infrequent occurrence of ascites in patients and experimental animals with partial occlusion of the portal vein.

V. MECHANISM OF THE SPLANCHNIC VASCULAR RESPONSE TO CHRONIC PORTAL HYPERTENSION

The observation that chronic portal hypertension results in vasodilation in the gastrointestinal tract, muscle and kidneys has spurred much research aimed at identifying the mechanism responsible for this phenomenon.[16,51] Many studies have addressed the potential roles of physical, metabolic, humoral, and neural factors in initiating and maintaining the splanchnic vasodilation of portal hypertension.

A possible role of physical factors in mediating the reduced gastric vascular resistance was first proposed by Hashizume et al.[52] These investigators demonstrated 15- to 50 μm arteriovenous connections in the gastric submucosa of man with cirrhosis and portal hypertension. Hashizume et al.[52] concluded that a portion of the reduced gastric vascular resistance (and increased blood flow) observed in portal hypertension could be related to these shunts. While this mechanism may be important in the stomach, we do not believe that it is the major factor involved in the small intestinal hyperemia associated with chronic portal hypertension. This contention is based on the observation that the arteriovenous shunting of 15-μm microspheres increases only slightly in the portal hypertensive rat. Benoit et al.[15] have estimated that this slight, yet significant increase in A—V shunting accounts for less than 2% of the reported 50% decrease in intestinal vascular resistance commonly observed in the rat portal vein stenosis model.

Another possible explanation for the intestinal vasodilation of chronic portal hypertension is the release of vasodilator metabolites from the tissue since acute portal hypertension is known to increase oxygen consumption in the small intestine of both dogs[53] and cats.[54] To test the possibility that an increased metabolic activity may account for the intestinal vasodilation, Benoit et al.[15] measured intestinal oxygen consumption in normal and portal hypertensive rats. These results indicate that intestinal metabolic demand is unaltered in chronic portal hypertension. Therefore, it seems unlikely that the response of the intestinal vasculature to chronic portal hypertension could be explained in terms of a metabolic mechanism.

In recent years, there has been growing evidence that portal hypertension may lead to an elevation in circulating plasma levels of vasoactive substances. Indeed, increased plasma levels of substances normally metabolized or utilized by the liver (e.g., bile acids and glucagon), are commonly reported in portal hypertensive man and animals.[15,55-58] Although the reason for the elevation of these substances remains unclear, it is likely that altered hepatic clearance by a diseased liver and shunting of vasoactive compounds away from the liver (via portosystemic collaterals) are involved. The latter mechanism is of particular interest, inasmuch as More et al.[59] have been able to mimic the splanchnic vascular response to chronic portal hypertension in portacaval shunted rats without portal hypertension.

Direct evidence in support of a humoral mediator of the intestinal vasodilation in portal hypertension was first obtained by cross-perfusion studies performed by Benoit et al.[15] Figure 12 shows that intestinal blood flow to the intestine of a normal rat can be increased when it is perfused with blood from a portal hypertensive animal. Therefore, it appears that blood-borne agent(s), is responsible for a large portion of the intestinal vascular response to portal hypertension. Since this initial experiment was performed, Korthuis et al.[60] have extended this observation to the rat hindquarters (Figure 12).

A large number of humoral factors are known to be elevated in portal hypertension characterized by portosystemic shunting. Table 4 lists several likely candidates that have been evaluated and further emphasizes that the factor (or factors) responsible for the splanchnic vasodilation is not completely resolved.

Studies in many vascular beds indicate that increases in plasma osmolality can cause intense vasodilation. For example, Levine et al.,[61] have previously shown that as little as a 5% increase in plasma osmolality is capable of reducing intestinal vascular resistance by approximately 13% in the cat. Furthermore, Korthuis et al,[62] have recently proposed that the increased plasma osmolality observed in untreated diabetes mellitus may be partially responsible for the intestinal vasodilation that occurs in this condition. To test the hypothesis that portal hypertension leads to increases in plasma osmolality (secondary to portosystemic shunting and altered hepatic metabolism of absorbed nutrients), Benoit et al.[15] measured the plasma osmolality of control and portal hypertensive rats. These measurements produced negative findings, since no difference in plasma osmolality was observed between groups.

The possibility that the autacoids, histamine and serotonin, could mediate the splanchnic hyperemia of chronic portal hypertension has been investigated by Benoit[51] and others.[63,64] Studies in our laboratory failed to demonstrate any reduction of intestinal blood flow in portal hypertensive rats following simultaneous administration of the H_1 and H_2 receptor antagonists, diphenhydramine and cimetidine. These findings are further supported by Henderson et al.[63] who reported the inability of cimetidine to reduce hepatic blood flow in cirrhotic man. Recently, Cummings et al.[64] have demonstrated that intraportal administration of the serotonin antagonist, ketanserin, leads to reductions in portal pressure, cardiac output, and portal venous inflow. These investigators concluded that ketanserin caused dilation of the portal vein and venous pooling in portal hypertensive rats. The observed decrease in portal venous inflow was attributed to the decrease in cardiac output caused by venous pooling. Although untested, it is likely that blockade of serotonin receptors may directly reduce blood flow in portal hypertensive animals since serotonin is a known dilator of the splanchnic circulation.[65]

The role of prostaglandins as mediators of the splanchnic hyperemia has been investigated by several laboratories, only to yield varying results. Hamilton et al.[66] demonstrated an increased prostacyclin activity in portal vein homogenates obtained from rats with portal hypertension due to portal vein stenosis. Bruix and co-workers,[67] have shown that the cyclooxygenase inhibitor, indomethacin, decreases splanchnic blood flow, cardiac output, and portal pressure in cirrhotic man. Although these studies suggest that prostaglandins may mediate the circulatory derangements of chronic portal hypertension, considerable evidence argues against vasodilator prostaglandins. PGE_2 and 6-keto $PGF_{1\alpha}$ (a stable spontaneous metabolite of PGI_2) levels are not elevated in the portal blood of rats with prehepatic portal hypertension.[51] Furthermore, Blanchart et al.,[68] have demonstrated that chronic suppression of prostaglandin synthesis does not attenuate the splanchnic hyperemia observed in rats with portal vein stenosis.

Another class of blood-borne substances that may be involved in the portal hypertension-induced splanchnic hyperemia is the gastrointestinal peptides. In order to determine if chronic portal hypertension leads to increased plasma levels of these substances, Premen et al.[69] measured the concentration of several vasoactive peptides in control and portal vein stenosed

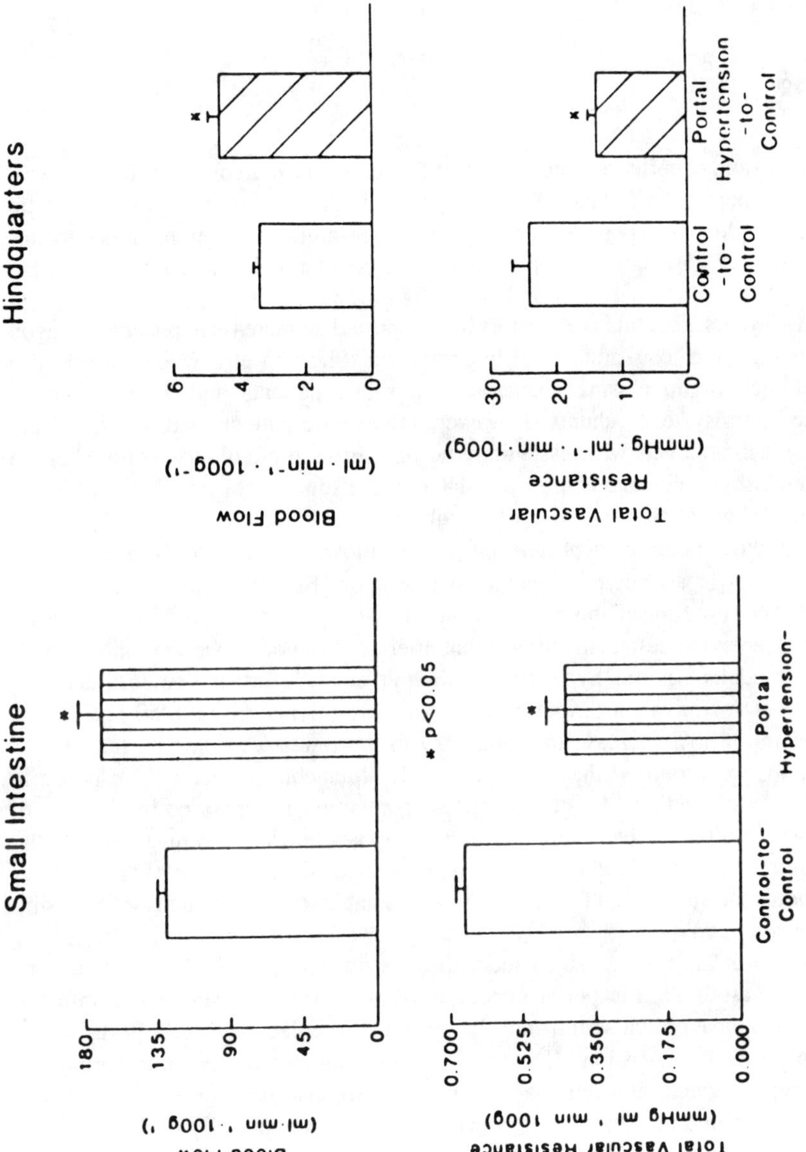

FIGURE 12. Effects of cross-perfusion of the rat intestine or hindquarters with blood from either control or portal hypertensive animals. Portal hypertensive blood increased blood flow and decreased vascular resistance in both vascular beds. (From Benoit, J. N. et al., *Int. J. Microcir. Clin. Exp.*, 3, 322, 1984; and Korthuis, R. J. et al., *Am. J. Physiol.*, 249, H 82, 1985. With permission.)

TABLE 4
Potential Humoral Mediators of the Hyperdynamic Circulation

Agent	Reported contribution	Ref.
Plasma osmolality	(−)	15
Vasodilator prostaglandins	(+/−)	51, 66, 67, 68
Histamine	(−)	51
Serotonin	(+)	64
Gastrointestinal peptides	(−)	69
Glucagon	(+)	15, 72
Bile acids	(+/?)	56, 74

rats. These investigators reported no increase in the arterial plasma concentration of vaso-active intestinal polypeptide, substance P, cholecystokinin/gastrin, neurotensin, pancreatic polypeptide, B-endorphin, and peptide histidine-isoleucine amide. Therefore, it seems un-likely that this group of gastrointestinal peptides can account for the increased splanchnic blood flow.

Over the last 15 years, several investigators have reported an increase in plasma glucagon levels in patients with cirrhosis and portal hypertension. Sherwin et al.[58] demonstrated a two- to fivefold increase in plasma glucagon in cirrhotic patients with spontaneous or surgically induced portosystemic shunts. However, in cirrhotic patients without significant portal shunting, glucagon levels were essentially normal. From these observations, Sherwin et al.[58] proposed that hyperglucagonemia was related to the shunting of portal venous blood away from the liver. This possibility was further substantiated by studies in normal pigs that demonstrated a gradual increase in plasma glucagon following portacaval anastomosis.[70] Inasmuch as glucagon is a known splanchnic vasodilator, Benoit at al.[15] measured the systemic arterial concentration of this hormone in rats with prehepatic portal hypertension (i.e., portal vein stenosis). These data indicate that arterial glucagon concentration increased threefold in this model of portal hypertension. Benoit et al.[15] further demonstrated that glucagon concentration equivalent to that measured in portal hypertension (450 pg/ml) was capable of producing a 30% increase in blood flow to the intestine of normal rats. Based on this observation, we proposed that a portion of the splanchnic hyperemic response to portal hypertension was mediated by glucagon. Our contention is supported by the data of Kravetz et al.[71] which indicate that a direct correlation exists between the magnitude of the splanchnic hyperemia and plasma glucagon levels in portacaval shunted rats (Figure 13). It is interesting to note that Sikuler and Groszmann[57] were unable to observe such a relationship in portal hypertensive rats.

Recently, Benoit et al.[72] have gained more direct evidence in support of a glucagon-induced splanchnic vasodilation in portal hypertensive rats. Figure 14 shows that infusion of a highly specific glucagon antiserum into the systemic circulation reduces portal blood flow in rats with portal hypertension. However, glucagon antiserum does not completely abolish the hyperemia, which indicates that other factors are also involved.

Another group of humoral substances that has yet to be systematically evaluated is the bile acids. Recently, Okhubo et al.[56] have measured serum bile acids in patients with cirrhosis and varying degrees of portal shunting. These investigators reported a strong positive cor-relation between the degree of portal shunting and serum bile acid concentrations. The bile acid concentrations reported by these investigators are within the vasoactive range reported by Kvietys et al.,[73] suggesting that bile acids may be involved in the splanchnic dilation associated with portal hypertension. This contention is also held by Bomzon et al.,[74] who first proposed that elevated plasma bile salts may mediate the hypotension associated with obstructive jaundice.

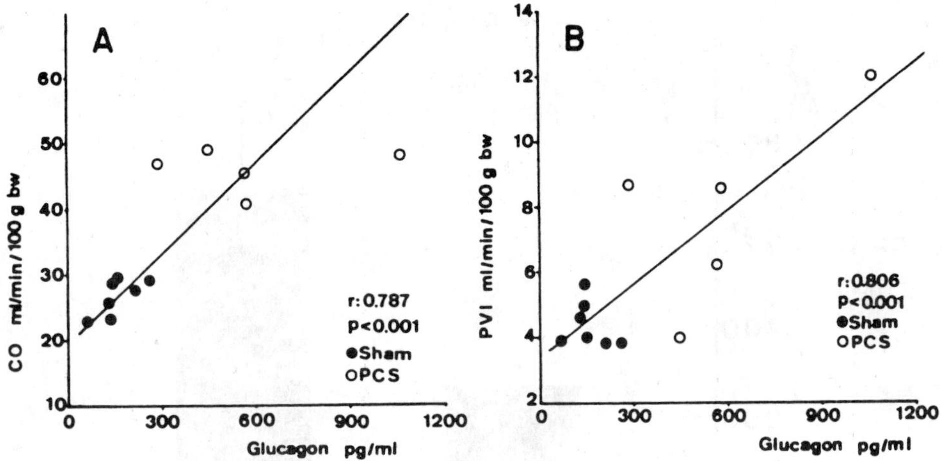

FIGURE 13. Correlation between plasma glucagon levels, cardiac output (CO) and portal venous inflow (PVI) in portacaval shunted rats. (From Kravetz, D. et al., *Am. J. Physiol.*, 252, G257, 1987. With permission.)

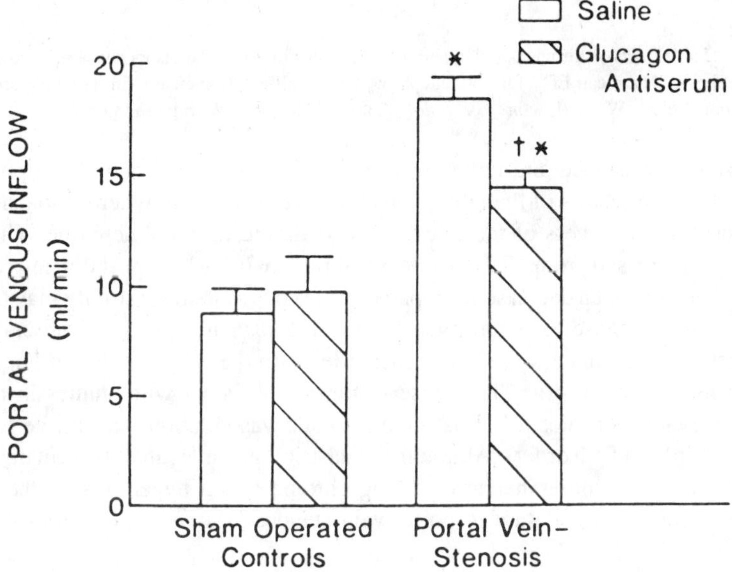

FIGURE 14. Effects of glucagon neutralization on portal venous inflow in control and portal hypertensive rats. Glucagon antiserum reduced, but did not abolish the hyperemic response to chronic portal hypertension. (From Benoit, J. M. et al., *Am. J. Physiol.*, 251, G674, 1986. With permission.)

Thus far, we have only addressed the role of circulating vasodilator substances in the splanchnic hyperemia of chronic portal hypertension. However, it is likely that the vascular sensitivity to endogenous vasoconstrictors is impaired in portal hypertensive conditions. Kitano et al.[19] have recently demonstrated a reduced sensitivity of the portal hypertensive (secondary to cirrhosis) gastric mucosa to exogenous norepinephrine. These investigators suggested that the reduced vascular sensitivity observed in the portal hypertensive rats could be responsible for the decreased vascular resistance in the stomach. In order to determine if the vascular responsiveness of the intestine to exogenous norepinephrine was altered by chronic portal vein stenosis, Kiel et al.[35] obtained cumulative dose response relationships

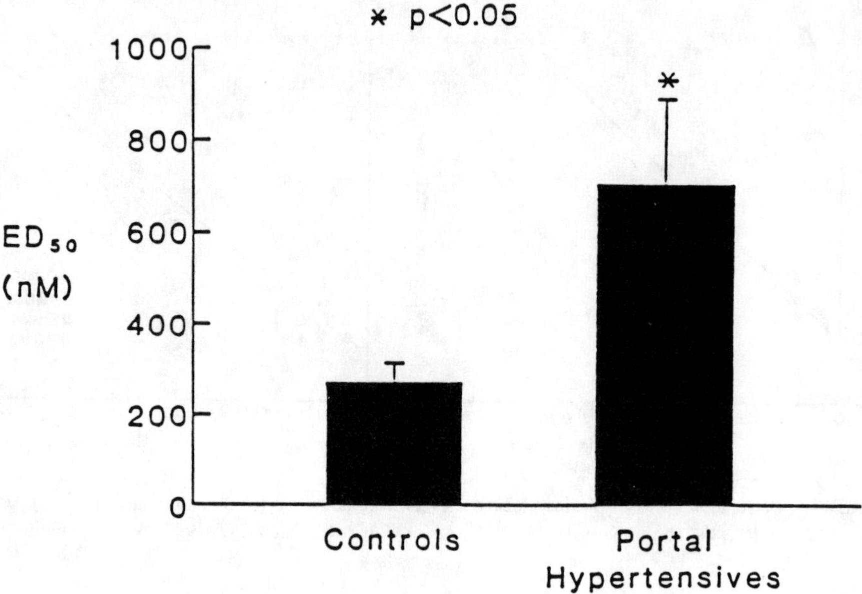

FIGURE 15.   Effects of chronic portal hypertension on intestinal vascular responsiveness to exogenous norepinephrine. The mean ED_{50} for norepinephrine was significantly increased in portal hypertensive rats. (From Kiel, J. W. et al., *Am. J. Physiol.*, 248, G192, 1985. With permission.)

between vascular resistance and norepinephrine concentration in control and portal hypertensive animals. The results of the latter study indicate that portal hypertension significantly attenuates the responsiveness of the intestinal vasculature to norepinephrine. The ED_{50} for norepinephrine increased from 271 nM in control rats to 740 nM in portal vein-stenosed rats (Figure 15). The fact that a decreased sympathetic nervous system sensitivity may be involved in the hyperemic response to portal hypertension is substantiated by the observation from our laboratory[20] that chronic portal hypertension leads to the selective dilation of third order arterioles in the small intestine. This observation is consistent with studies in the sympathetically denervated rat intestine[75] that demonstrated vasodilation only in the terminal arterioles (i.e., third and fifth order). Although the gastric[19] and intestinal[35] vasculatures become relatively insensitive to norepinephrine during chronic portal hypertension, the sensitivity of the skeletal muscle vasculature in portal vein-stenosed rats is not different from that in controls.[60]

There are several possible explanations for the reduced sensitivity of the intestinal vasculature to norepinephrine. These include receptor down-regulation and the interaction between humoral agents and the catecholamine receptor. The latter is particularly attractive for two reasons. First of all, it has been established that humoral agents, including glucagon, are primary mediators of the hyperemia. Second, pancreatic glucagon has been demonstrated to reduce the responsiveness of the hepatic arteriolar[76] and intestinal[77] vasculatures to exogenously administered norepinephrine and hepatic nerve stimulation.[78] The vascular responsiveness to other vasoconstrictors, namely, angiotensin,[76] vasopressin[76] and 5-hydroxytryptamine,[79] was also attenuated in the liver. In all instances the removal of glucagon restored vascular sensitivity to control levels.[76-79]

Elevations in serum bile salts have also been reported in patients with cirrhosis and obstructive jaundice.[56,74] Bile acids have been shown to alter transmembrane ionic movements and modify Na^+,K^+-ATPase activity. These alterations have been linked to the reduced sensitivity of vascular and extravascular smooth muscle from bile duct-ligated rats to norepinephrine.[74]

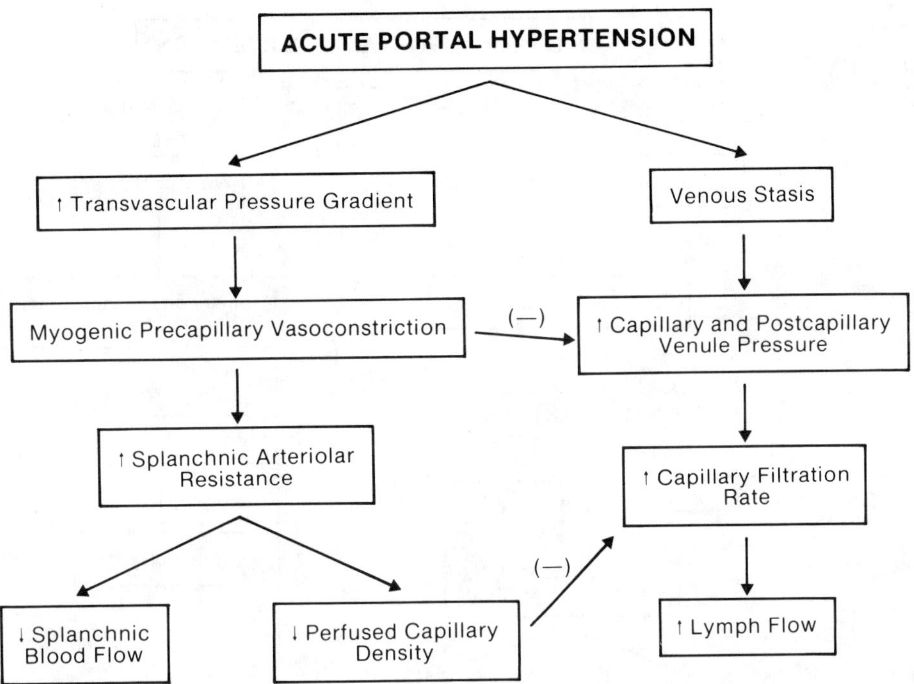

FIGURE 16.   Summary of consequences of acute venous pressure elevation on the splanchnic circulation.

The role of vagal reflexes in the intestinal hyperemia associated with chronic portal hypertension has also been evaluated. Benoit and co-workers[15] demonstrated that bilateral vagotomy fails to alter the intestinal hyperemia in portal vein-stenosed rats. This finding indicates that a vagally mediated vasodilator reflex is not responsible for the increased splanchnic blood flow associated with chronic portal hypertension.

VI. SUMMARY

The hemodynamic alterations accompanying acute and chronic portal hypertension are summarized in Figures 16 and 17. In both cases, venous pressure elevation leads to increased vascular transmural pressure and venous stasis. However, with acute elevations in portal pressure, a myogenic precapillary vasoconstriction occurs which leads to increased precapillary resistance, decreased intestinal blood flow, and a reduced number of perfused capillaries (Figure 16). The venous stasis that occurs in acute portal hypertension leads to increased capillary and postcapillary venular pressure which, in turn, increases capillary filtration rate and lymph flow. Thus, the rise in microvascular pressure produced by acute portal hypertension promotes the formation of interstitial edema. However, the excessive accumulation of interstitial fluid is opposed, in part, by a rise in precapillary resistance and a reduction in perfused capillary density associated with acute elevations in portal venous pressure.

In contrast to acute portal hypertension, chronic elevations in portal pressure result in reduced precapillary resistance and increased intestinal blood flow (Figure 17). These changes are presumably due to the onset of portosystemic shunting which results in increased plasma levels of glucagon and other dilators of the intestinal vasculature. This vasodilation may be augmented by a reduced sensitivity of the intestinal vasculature to norepinephrine and other endogenous vasoconstrictors. Like acute portal hypertension, chronic elevations in portal pressure result in increased capillary and postcapillary venular pressure, transcapillary filtration rate and lymph flow. However, the magnitude of these increases is much greater in

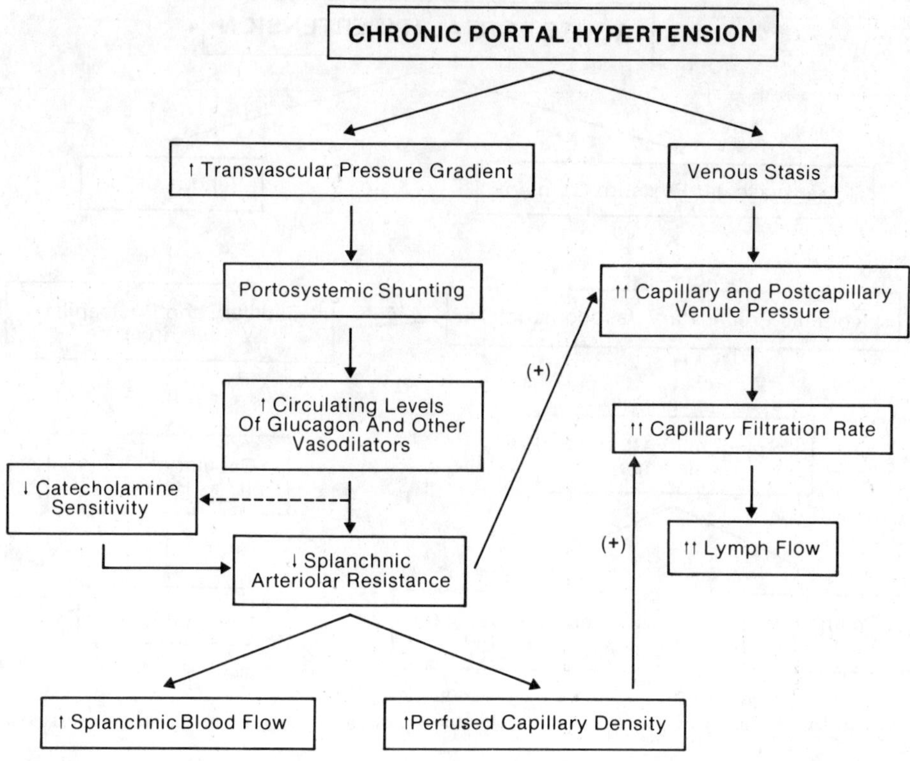

FIGURE 17.   Summary of consequences of chronic portal hypertension on the splanchnic circulation.

chronic portal hypertension, a result attributable to a reduced precapillary resistance and an increased number of perfused capillaries.

REFERENCES

1. **Granger, D. N., Richardson, P. D. I., Kvietys, P. R., and Mortillaro, N. A.,** Intestinal blood flow, *Gastroenterology,* 78, 837, 1980.
2. **Granger, D. N. and Kvietys, P. R.** The splanchnic circulation: intrinsic regulation, *Annu. Rev. Physiol.,* 43, 409, 1981.
3. **Svanvik, J. and Lundgren, O.,** Gastrointestinal Circulation, in *International Review of Physiology, Gastrointestinal Physiology, Part II,* Vol. 12, Crane, R. K., Ed., University Park Press, Baltimore, 1977, 1.
4. **Granger, D. N., Kvietys, P. R., Parks, D. A., and Benoit, J. N.,** Intestinal blood flow: relations to function, *Surv. Dig. Dis.,* 1, 217, 1983.
5. **Kvietys, P. R.** Microcirculation of the large intestine, in *The Physiology and Pharmacology of the Microcirculation, Vol. 2,* Mortillaro, N. A., Ed., Academic Press, New York, 1984, 77.
6. **Jacobwitz, D.,** Histochemical studies of the autonomic innervation of the gut, *J. Pharmacol. Exp. Ther.,* 149, 1965.
7. **Greenway, C. V.,** Neural control and autoregulatory escape, in *Physiology of the Intestinal Circulation,* Shepherd, A. P. and Granger, D. N., Eds., Raven Press, New York, 1984, 61.
8. **Crissinger, K. D., Kvietys, P. R., and Granger, D. N.,** Autoregulatory escape from norepinephrine infusion: roles of adenosine and histamine, *Am. J. Physiol.,* 1988, in press.
9. **Longhurst, J. C.,** Cardiovascular reflexes of gastrointestinal origin, in *Physiology of the Intestinal Circulation,* Shepherd, A. P. and Granger, D. N., Eds., Raven Press, New York, 1984, 165.
10. **Johnson, P. C.,** Myogenic and venous-arteriolar responses in intestinal circulation, in *Physiology of the Intestinal Circulation,* Shepherd, A. P. and Granger, D. N., Eds., Raven Press, New York, 1984, 49.

11. **Johnson, P. C.,** The myogenic response, in *Handbook of Physiology, Section II, The Cardiovascular System,* Vol. 2, *Vascular Smooth Muscle,* Bohr, D. F., Somylo, A. T., and Sparks, H. V., Eds., Williams & Wilkins, Baltimore, 1980, 409.

12. **Johnson, P. C.,** Myogenic nature of increase in intestinal vascular resistance with venous pressure elevation, *Circ. Res.,* 6, 992, 1959.

13. **Davis, M. J. and Gore, R. W.,** Capillary pressures in rat intestinal muscle and mucosal villi during venous pressure elevation, *Am. J. Physiol.,* 249, H174, 1985.

14. **Granger, H. J., Barnes, G. E., Meininger, G. A., and Goodman, A. H.,** Mathematical models of myogenic/metabolic interactions in local control of the microcirculation, *Int. J. Microcirc. Clin. Exp.,* 3, 322, 1984.

15. **Benoit, J. N., Barrowman, J. A., Harper, S. L., Kvietys, P. R., and Granger, D. N.,** Role of humoral factors in the intestinal hyperemia associated with chronic portal hypertension, *Am. J. Physiol.,* 247, G486, 1984.

16. **Benoit, J. N. and Granger, D. N.,** Chronic portal hypertension and the splanchnic circulation, in *Pathophysiology of the intestinal circulation,* Vol. 1, Kvietys, P. R., Barrowman, J. A., and Granger, D. N., Eds., CRC Press, Boca Raton, FL, 1987, 57.

17. **Benoit, J. N., Womack, W. A., Korthuis, R. J., Wilborn, W. H., and Granger, D. N.,** Chronic portal hypertension: effects on gastrointestinal blood flow distribution, *Am. J. Physiol.,* 230, G535, 1986.

18. **Kitano, S., Inokuchi, K., Sugimachi, K., and Koyanagi, N.,** Hemodynamic and morphological changes in the stomach of portal hypertensive rats, *Eur. Surg. Res.,* 13, 227, 1981.

19. **Kitano, S., Koyanagi, N., Sugimachi, K., Kobayashi, M., and Inokuchi, K.,** Mucosal blood flow and modified vascular responses to norepinephrine in the stomach of rats with liver cirrhosis, *Eur. Surg. Res.,* 14, 221, 1982.

20. **Benoit, J. N. and Granger, D. N.,** Intestinal microvascular adaptation to chronic portal hypertension in the rat, *Gastroenterology,* 1988, 94, 471, 1988.

21. **Gore, R. W. and Bohlen, H. G.,** Pressure regulation in the microcirculation, *Fed. Proc.,* 34, 1031, 1975.

22. **Verzar, F. and McDougall, E. J.,** *Absorption from the intestines,* Longmans, London, 1936.

23. **Yoffey, J. M. and Courtice, F. C.,** *Lymphatics, lymph and the lymphomyeloid complex,* Academic Press, New York, 1970.

24. **Astaldi, G. and Strosselli, E.,** Peroral biopsy of the intestinal mucosa in hepatic cirrhosis, *Am. J. Dig. Dis.,* 5, 603, 1960.

25. **Buhac, J. and Jarmolych, J.,** Histology of the intestinal peritoneum in patients with cirrhosis of the liver and ascites, *Dig. Dis.,* 23, 417, 1968.

26. **Norman, D. A., Atkins, J. A., Sielig, L. I., Gomez-Sanchez, C., and Krejs, G. J.,** Water and electrolyte movement and mucosal morphology in the jejunum of patients with portal hypertension, *Gastroenterology,* 79, 707, 1980.

27. **Korthuis, R. J., Kinder, D. A., Brimer, G. E., Slattery, K. A., Stogsdill, P., and Granger, D. N.,** Intestinal capillary filtration in acute and chronic portal hypertension, *Am. J. Physiol.,* 254, G339, 1988.

28. **Williamson, J. R. and Kilo, C.,** Current status of capillary basement-membrane disease in diabetes mellitus, *Daibetes,* 26, 65, 1977.

29. **Parving, H. H., Viberti, G. C., Keen, H., Christiansen, J. S., and Lassen, N. A.,** Hemodynamic factors in the genesis of diabetic microangiopathy, *Metabolism,* 9, 943, 1983.

30. **Schaffner, F. and Popper, H.,** Capillarization of hepatic sinusoids in man, *Gastroenterology,* 44, 239, 1963.

31. **Granger, H. J., Laine, G. A., Mackan, E. R., Richardson, M. W., and Johnson, R. L.,** Exchange of fluid and protein across hepatic sinusoids and Glisson's capsule in chronic caval hypertension, *Fed. Proc.,* 43, 417, 1984.

32. **Granger, D. N., Richardson, P. D. I., and Taylor, A. E.,** Volumetric assessment of the capillary filtration coefficient in the cat small intestine, *Pfluegers Arch.,* 381, 25, 1979.

33. **Johnson, P. C. and Hanson, K. M.,** Effect of arterial pressure on arteriolar and venous resistance of intestine, *J. Appl. Physiol.,* 17, 503, 1966.

34. **Mortillaro, N. A. and Taylor, A. E.,** Interactions of capillary and tissue forces in the cat small intestine, *Circ. Res.,* 39, 348, 1976.

35. **Kiel, J. W., Pitts, V., Benoit, J. N., Granger, D. N., and Shepherd, A. P.,** Reduced vascular sensitivity to norepinephrine in portal hypertensive rats, *Am. J. Physiol.,* 248, G 192, 1985.

36. **Granger, D. N., Kvietys, P. R., Premen, A. J., and Korthuis, R. J.,** Microcirculation of the intestinal mucosa, in *Handbook of Physiology,* Vol. 1, Part 2, Wood, J., Ed., Williams & Wilkins, Baltimore, 1989, 1405.

37. **Better, O. S. and Schrier, R. W.,** Disturbed volume homeostasis in patients with cirrhosis of the liver, *Kidney Int.,* 23, F203, 1983.

38. **Witte, C. L. and Witte, M. H.,** Physiologic factors involved in the causation of cirrhotic ascites, *Gastroeneterology,* 61, 742, 1971.

39. **Fauchild, P. and Ritland, S.,** Interstitial fluid volume, plasma volume and transcapillary colloid osmotic gradient in patients with hepatic cirrhosis and fluid retention, *Scand. J. Clin. Lab. Invest.,* 45, 553, 1985.

40. **Henriksen, J. H.,** Colloid osmotic pressure in decompensated cirrhosis, A mirror image of portal venous hypertension, *Scand. J. Gastroenterol.,* 20, 170, 1985.

41. **Witte, C. L., Witte, M. H., and Dumont, A. E.,** Estimates of net transcapillary water and protein flux in the liver and intestine of patients with portal hypertension from hepatic cirrhosis, *Gastroenterology,* 80, 265, 1981.

42. **Barrowman, J. A. and Granger, D. N.,** Effects of experimental cirrhosis of splanchnic microvascular fluid and solute exchange in the rat, *Gastroenterology,* 87, 165, 1984.

43. **Witte, C. L. and Witte, M. H.,** The circulation in portal hypertension, *Yale J. Biol. Med.,* 48, 141, 1975.

44. **Anzueto, L., Benoit, J. N., and Granger, D. N.,** A rat model for studying the intestinal circulation, *Am. J. Physiol.,* 246, G56, 1984.

45. **Granger, D. N. and Taylor, A. E.,** Permeability of intestinal capillaries to endogenous macromolecules, *Am. J. Physiol.,* 238, H457, 1980.

46. **Wallentin, I.,** Importance of tissue pressure for the fluid equilibrium between the vascular and interstitial compartments in the small intestine, *Acta Physiol. Scand.,* 68, 304, 1966.

47. **Johnson, P. C.,** Effect of venous pressure on mean capillary pressure and vascular resistance in the intestine, *Circ. Res.,* 16, 294, 1965.

48. **Yablonski, M. E. and Lifson, N.,** Mechanism of production of intestinal secretion by elevated venous pressure, *J. Clin. Invest.,* 57, 904, 1976.

49. **Lifson, N.,** Fluid secretion and hydrostatic pressure relationships in the small intestine, in *Mechanisms of Intestinal Secretion,* Binder, H. J., Ed., Alan R. Liss, New York 1979, 249.

50. **Iber, F. L.,** Normal and pathologic physiology of the liver, in *Pathologic Physiology,* Sodeman, W. A. and Sodeman, W. A., Eds., W. B. Saunders, Philadelphia, 1974, 790.

51. **Benoit, J. N. and Granger, D. N.,** Splanchnic hemodynamics in chronic portal venous hypertension, *Sem. Liv. Dis.,* 6, 287, 1986.

52. **Hashizume, M., Tanaka, K., and Inokuchi, K.,** Morphology of gastric microcirculation in cirrhosis, *Hepatology,* 3, 1008, 1983.

53. **Shepherd, A. P.,** Effect of elevated venous pressure on intestinal oxygen extraction, in *Microcirculation,* Grayson, J. and Zingg, W., Eds., Plenum Press, New York, 1976.

54. **Mortillaro, N. A. and Granger, H. J.,** Reactive hyperemia and oxygen extraction in the feline small intestine, *Circ. Res.,* 41, 859, 1977.

55. **Angelico, M., Attili, A. F., Cantaforo, A., Lombardi, M., Thau, A., and Capocaccia, L.,** Differences in serum bile acid composition between unoperated cirrhotic patients and patients with portacaval or mesocaval shunt, *Digestion,* 19, 126, 1979.

56. **Ohkubo, H., Okuda, K., Iida, S., Ohnishi, K., Ikawa, S., and Makino, I.,** Role of portal and splenic vein shunts and impaired hepatic extraction in the elevated serum bile acids in liver cirrhosis, *Gatroenterology,* 86, 514, 1984.

57. **Sikuler, E. and Groszmann, R. J.,** Hemodynamic studies in long- and short-term portal hypertensive rats: the relation to systemic glucagon levels, *Hepatology,* 6, 414, 1986.

58. **Sherwin, R., Joshi, P., Hendler, R., Felig, P., and Conn, H. O.,** Hyperglucagonemia in Laennec's cirrhosis — the role of portal systemic shunting, *N. Engl. J. Med.,* 290, 239, 1974.

59. **More, N., Lobosotomayor, G., Basse-Cathalinat, B., Christiane, B., and Balabaud, C.,** Splanchnic arterial blood flow in rats with portacaval shunts, *Am. J. Physiol.,* 246, G331, 1984.

60. **Korthuis, R. J., Benoit, J. N., Kvietys, P. R., Townsley, M. I., Taylor, A. E., and Granger, D. N.,** Humoral factors may mediate increased rat hindquarter blood flow in portal hypertension, *Am. J. Phsyiol.,* 249, H827, 1985.

61. **Levine, S. E., Granger, D. N., Brace, R. A., and Taylor, A. E.,** Effect of hyperosmolality on vascular resistance and lymph flow in the cat ileum, *Am. J. Physiol.,* 234, H14, 1978.

62. **Korthuis, R. J., Benoit, J. N., Kvietys, P. R., Laughlin, M. H., Taylor, A. E., and Granger, D. N.,** Intestinal hyperemia in experimental diabetes mellitus, *Am. J. Physiol.,* 253, G26, 1987.

63. **Henderson, J. M., Ibrahim, S. Z., Millikan, W. J., Santi, M., and Warren, W. D.,** Cimetidine does not reduce liver blood flow in cirrhosis, *Hepatology,* 3, 919, 1983.

64. **Cummings, S., Groszmann, R. J., and Kaumann, A. J.,** Hypersensitivity of mesenteric veins to 5-hydroxytryptamine- and ketanserin-induced reduction of portal pressure in portal hypertensive rats, *Br. J. Pharmacol.,* 89, 501, 1986.

65. **Chou, C. C. and Kvietys, P. R.,** Physiological and pharmacological alterations in gastrointestinal blood flow, in *Measurement of Blood Flow, Applications to the Splanchnic Circulation,* Granger, D. N. and Bulkley, G. B., Eds., Williams & Wilkins, Baltimore, 1981, 477.

66. **Hamilton, G., Phing, R. C. F., Hulton, R. A., Dandona, P., and Hobbs, K. E. F.,** The relationship between prostacyclin activity and pressures in the portal vein, *Hepatology,* 2, 236, 1982.

67. **Bruix, J., Bosch, J., Kravetz, D., Mastai, R., and Rodes, J.,** Effects of prostaglandin inhibition on systemic and hepatic hemodynamics in patients with cirrhosis of the liver, *Gastroenterology,* 88, 430, 1985.
68. **Blanchart, A., Hernando, N., Fernando-Munoz, D., Hernando, L., and Lopez-Novoa, J. M.,** Lack of effect of indomethacin on systemic and splanchnic hemodynamics in portal hypertensive rats, *Clin. Sci.,* 68, 605, 1985.
69. **Premen, A. J., Go, V. L. W., Banchs, V., Benoit, J. N., and Granger, D. N.,** Renal hyperemia in portal hypertension is not mediated by gastrointestinal peptides, *Reg. Peptides,* 16, 39, 1986.
70. **van Hoorn-Hickman, R., Vinik, A. I., and van Hoorn, W. A.,** Transhepatic hormone levels in the portacaval shunted pig — the effects upon gastrin and glucagon release *Am. J. Clin. Nutr.,* 32, 2009, 1979.
71. **Kravetz, D., Arderiu, M., Bosch, J., Fuster, J., Visa, J., Casamitjana, R., and Rodes, J.,** Hyperglucagonemia and hyperkinetic circulation after portocaval shunt in the rat, *Am. J. Physiol.,* 252, G257, 1987.
72. **Benoit, J. N., Zimmerman, B., Premen, A. J., Go, V. L. W., and Granger, D. N.,** Role of glucagon in the splanchnic hyperemia of chronic portal hypertension, *Am. J. Physiol.,* 251, G674, 1986.
73. **Kvietys, P. R., McLendon, J. M., and Granger, D. N.,** Postprandial intestinal hyperemia: role of bile salts in the ileum, *Am. J. Physiol.,* 241, G469, 1981.
74. **Bomzon, A., Finberg, J. P. M., Tovbin, D., Naidu, S. G., and Better, O. S.,** Bile salts, hypotension and obstructive jaundice, *Clin. Sci.,* 67, 177, 1984.
75. **Bohlen, H. G. and Gore, R. W.,** Comparison of microvascular pressures and diameters in the innervated and denervated rat intestine, *Microvas. Res.,* 14, 251, 1977.
76. **Richardson, P. D. I. and Withrington, P. G.,** The inhibition by glucagon of the vasoconstrictor actions of noradrenaline, angiotensin and vasopressin on the hepatic vascular bed, *Br. J. Pharmacol.,* 57, 93, 1976.
77. **Kock, N. G., Tibblin, S., and Schenk, W. G.,** Modification by glucagon of the splanchnic vascular responses to activation of the sympathicoadrenal system, *J. Surg. Res.,* 11, 12, 1971.
78. **Richardson, P. D. I. and Withrington, P. G.,** Glucagon inhibition of hepatic arterial responses to hepatic nerve stimulation, *Am. J. Physiol.,* 2, H647, 1977.
79. **Richardson, P. D. I. and Withrington, P. G.,** Responses of the simultaneously perfused hepatic arterial and portal venous vascular beds of the dog to histamine and 5-hydroxytryptamine, *Br. J. Pharmacol.,* 64, 581, 1978.
80. **Granger, H. J.,** personal communication.

Chapter 10

VASCULAR REACTIVITY IN LIVER DISEASE

Arieh Bomzon

TABLE OF CONTENTS

I. INTRODUCTION

Patients with cirrhosis, as well as jaundiced patients, tend to be hypotensive in the face of an elevated cardiac output. As indicated in Chapter 1, the basis for this hypotension is thought to be due to a fall in the total peripheral resistance with an inadequate compensatory increase in the cardiac output.[1] The pathogenesis for the fall in total peripheral resistance is unclear, but the early studies of Laragh and his colleagues[2-4] indicated that, in part, it may be due to refractoriness to endogenous vasoactive compounds such as angiotensin II. These initial observations prompted additional investigations in cirrhotic subjects into the ability of the cardiovascular system to respond to numerous stimuli, such as changes in posture or infusions of vasoactive compounds such as norepinephrine. From such studies, the concept of diminished end organ responsiveness or blunted vascular reactivity developed and currently, has become an integral component of the hyperkinetic circulation and other cardiovascular complications of liver disease. Some of these studies were directed towards the identification of the ''endogenous vasodilator'' in order to provide an explanation for the generalized vascular dilatation of liver disease. Before reviewing the data on vasular reactivity in liver disease, a brief explanation of the current understanding of smooth muscle contraction, vascular reactivity, and resistance will be presented.

II. SMOOTH MUSCLE CONTRACTION, VASCULAR REACTIVITY, AND RESISTANCE

The tone of a vascular smooth muscle cell has been shown to be dependent upon the intracellular concentration of free calcium. The concentration range of intracellular calcium over which contraction can be recorded varies between 10^{-7} to 10^{-5} M. The sources of calcium are from the intracellular stores and the extracellular environment. The sequence of events following the initiation of contraction by an agonist such as norepinephrine is an initial coupling of the agonist with its receptor. This in turn stimulates a cascade of events involving the second messenger, inositol phosphate, resulting in the release of calcium from the intracellular stores. This rise in calcium concentration is a critical factor in contraction-coupling of the vascular smooth muscle cell. Associated with receptor activation, there is a simultaneous opening of the membrane receptor-regulated calcium channels which permit the entry of extracellular calcium into the cell. At the same time, potential-regulated calcium channels may also be opened to allow an additional influx of extracellular calcium. The role of the endothelial-derived dilator or constrictor factors in the contractile response is unknown although *in vitro* studies have shown that the dilator factor(/s) are released when the muscle is stimulated. The uptake of the norepinephrine into nerve terminals (uptake$_1$) or into non-neuronal tissue (uptake$_2$) signals the cessation of contraction with subsequent sequestration of calcium into the intracellular stores or its extracellular extrusion by a membrane calcium pump, possibly linked to the enzyme, Na^+,K^+-ATPase. The intracellular events associated with direct vasodilatation such as are seen with nitrates and atrial natriuretic factor are poorly understood but appear to involve the activation of guanylate cyclase and increase the synthesis of guanosine monophosphate (cGMP) and a probable reduction in the free intracellular calcium concentration.

What then does the expression ''diminished end organ responsiveness'' in liver disease mean? The work of Laragh and his colleagues[2-4] suggested that the pressor response induced by angiotensin was reduced or not as great as one might have anticipated. Since angiotensin is a potent constrictor of resistance vessels, their observations suggest that the loss of response occurred because the transfer of information from the receptor to the contractile process did not cause an appropriate rise in the free intracellular calcium; or that there was a defect in the coupling processes of contraction; or both. With the subsequent observations that the response to other pressor stimuli were also impaired,[6-9] it became widely accepted that the basis for a reduction in total peripheral resistance was linked with an inability of vessels to respond to constrictor influences or that the vasodilatation was indirect. Alternatively, the loss of end organ response may also be associated with an excess of vasodilator compounds whose plasma concentrations might be elevated in chronic liver disease.

Turning the attention to vascular resistance, this can be defined as a measure of friction between the wall of the blood vessel and the blood and between the components of blood themselves which oppose flow. Vascular resistance depends upon the viscosity of blood and the geometry of the vessel.

Both length and radius of the blood vessel affect its resistance. The resistance to flow is directly proportional to the length of the vessel. Although tortuosity of blood vessels in portal hypertension has been described and the increase in length is difficult to quantify, this relationship will not be discussed. The relationship between the radius of a blood vessel and resistance is given by the formula which states that the resistance is inversely proportional to the fourth power of the radius of the blood vessel.

$$\text{Resistance} = \frac{1}{r^4}$$

In other words, a doubling of the radius increases the flow 16-fold. It then follows, since the length of blood vessels is constant, that the radius of arterioles constitutes the most important factor in the control of resistance to blood flow. While this relationship is important when applied to arterioles and resistance vessels, some allowances need to made when applying these principles to veins since they are capacitance vessels. In these vessels, resistance to flow is less important, although the factors that enable veins to constrict and dilate in order to accommodate for changes in plasma volume may be identical to that described for arterioles which regulate resistance.

The traditional definition of the factors that can influence the radius of blood vessels did not make any distinction between arterioles and veins. Moreover, it stated that these factors can originate from within the blood vessel itself, i.e., local controls which serve the metabolic needs of the tissue in which they occur, and from the rest of the cardiovascular system, i.e., reflex controls which integrate and coordinate the needs of the whole body. The local controls were defined as blood pH, gas tensions, and the local concentrations of "injury" agents, metabolites, and ions such as potassium. The reflex controls were a combination of the inputs of either humoral or neural origin. The humoral factors included circulating vasoactive substances such as epinephrine and angiotensin, whereas the neural factor was the sympathetic neurotransmitter, norepinephrine.

While this definition represented an apt framework in which to appreciate vascular reactivity or the regulatory processes of vessel radius, this definition has undergone considerable change since its presentation in the older texts of physiology. Today, vascular reactivity is probably best defined as those factors that can alter the intracellular concentration of free calcium within the vascular smooth muscle cell of blood vessels. Using this approach, it is no longer possible to define vascular reactivity in terms of local or reflex control, but rather as the ability of the vascular smooth muscle cell to integrate and respond to information that originates from the sympathetic nerve terminal, the endothelial cell, and the blood itself.

The disadvantage of such a unifying approach is that it does not distinguish between resistance and capacitance vessels. This may be particularly important because in cirrhosis, the cardiovascular complications are focused around systemic arteriolar hypotension, portal venous hypertension, and an altered intravascular volume. On the other hand, such an approach may be advantageous since the entire vasculature, be it arterial or venous, may be considered to be dilated, and this general phenomenon manifests itself as systemic hypotension, portal hypertension, and altered intravascular volume.

TABLE 1
List of Endogenous Compounds That Alter Vessel Radius

Neuronally Derived Compounds
    Norepinephrine
    Acetylcholine
    γ-aminobutyric acid (GABA)
    Substance P
Endothelial Cell-Derived Compounds
    Arachidonic acid derivatives (prostaglandins, leukotreines, thromboxanes)
    Endothelial-derived relaxing factor(s), e.g., EDRF
    Endothelial-derived constrictor factor(s), e.g., endothelin
Humorally Derived Compounds
    Angiotensin II
    Serotonin (5-hydroxytryptamine)
    Adenosine
    Atrial natriuretic factor (ANF)
    Vasopressin
    Vasoactive intestinal peptide (VIP)
    Bradykinin
    Glucagon
    Bile acids

It is not the purpose of this chapter to determine which of these viewpoints are correct; or to establish whether the loss of vascular reactivity or reduced resistance is due to an excess of endogenous vasodilators in the face of an adequate or inadequate concentration of vasoconstrictors and so forth; but its purpose is rather to discuss the role of each of these substances on vascular smooth muscle in liver disease. Table 1 lists the numerous endogenous compounds that can alter vascular tone and whose plasma concentrations are elevated in liver disease. It can be seen that this list contains both vasoconstrictors and vasodilator substances that at some point have been implicated as "the endogenous vasodilator". Against this background, the role of these compounds, using data obtained from both clinical and experimental observations, will be reviewed on the basis of their origin.

III. NEURONALLY DERIVED COMPOUNDS

A. NOREPINEPHRINE

It is well documented that the sympathetic nervous system activity in patients suffering from cirrhosis is increased as reflected by both an increase in the plasma concentration of norepinephrine and the urinary excretion of catecholamine metabolites.[5] Despite this increase in activity, it has been reported that the pressor response of the cardiovascular system of these patients is attenuated to intravenous infusions of norepinephrine or the local application of the amine, and to procedures that may stimulate further release of the neurotransmitter from the nerve terminals. One of the first descriptions of loss of responsiveness to norepinephrine in both jaundiced and cirrhotic patients was made by Morandini and his colleagues.[6,7] Their observations contrast with the earlier findings of Laragh's group who found that pressor responsiveness to the amine was normal.[4] Subsequent studies by Lunzer and his colleagues in 1973 and 1975 confirmed the findings that the vasculature of cirrhotic patients was refractory to endogenous as well as exogenous norepinephrine.[8,9] However, Lenz et al.[10] reported that the pressor response to norepinephrine in eleven patients with hepatic encephalopathy (nine of which had chronic liver disease) was enhanced.

Tables 2 and 3 summarize the results of *in vivo* and *in vitro* observations in the various experimental animal models of cirrhosis, portal hypertension, and jaundice. Four points are apparent from this table. First, the responsiveness of the individual animal models varies.

TABLE 2
The Summary of Experiments That Assessed the *In Vivo* Pressor Responsiveness to Norepinephrine in the Various Animal Models of Liver Disease.

Experiment	Time	Methodology	Response	Ref.
Bile Duct-Ligated Rats				
Finberg et al.	6 d	Anesthetized	Potentiated	11
Bomzon et al.	3 d	Conscious	Diminished	12
Bile Duct-Ligated Dogs				
Saito	3 weeks	Anesthetized	Normal	13
Finberg et al.	3 weeks	Conscious	Diminished	14
Bomzon et al.	3 weeks	Conscious	Diminished	15
Bomzon et al.	12 weeks	Conscious	Normal	16
Bomzon et al.	3 weeks	Anesthetized	Normal to diminished[a]	17
Carbon Tetrachloride-Induced Cirrhotic Rats				
Leehey et al.		Anesthetized	Normal[b]	18
Murray and Paller.		Conscious	Normal	19
Bomzon et al.		Conscious	Normal	20
Villamediana et al.		Conscious	Normal	21

[a] Varied according to anesthetic used.
[b] Phenylephrine, the selective α_1-adrenoreceptor agonist, was used instead of norepinephrine.

Second, loss of responsiveness occurs predominantly when the animal is in the acute phase of surgically induced jaundice. Third, there is an intact pressor and contractile response in the nonsurgical-induced models of cirrhosis. And fourth, a direct relationship between systemic hypotension and loss of pressor and contractile reactivity is not always seen in the animal models.

Do all these experimental observations mean that diminished end organ responsiveness to norepinephrine does not contribute to the reduction in total peripheral resistance in liver disease? First, it would appear that loss of responsiveness to norepinephrine occurs in the presence of hyperbilirubinemia and no doubt does contribute to the reduction in total peripheral resistance in jaundice. Furthermore, the loss is transient since intact or normal responsiveness returns once the jaundice dissipates. Second, as noted in the chapter on animal models,[37] there are inherent differences between each of the animal models and the clinical situation and such differences may explain the variability that exists between the animal experiments. Third, since a loss of pressor response to the amine is not always associated with an attenuated *in vitro* contractile response, it would suggest that the basis for the loss of response to norepinephrine may be due to factors other than its effect on resistance vessels. These other factors include the heart (where variable inotropic and chronotropic responsiveness has been observed)[38] and the lung as a potential source of inactivating norepinephrine. The pulmonary endothelium is capable of this function which would reduce the effective concentration before reaching the heart and blood vessels. In fact, Bomzon and his colleagues[39] have shown that there was a time-dependent increased inactivation of norepinephrine in isolated perfused lungs of bile duct-ligated rats.

From Table 3, it can be seen that the response of the portal or mesenteric circulation also exhibits blunted responsiveness to norepinephrine. Clinical observations such as that made by Willett et al.[40] and Lebrec and his group[41] have shown that a component of portal

TABLE 3
The Summary of Experiments That Assessed the Responsiveness of Blood Vessels or Circulations to Norepinephrine in the Various Animal Models of Liver Disease

Experiment	Time	Methodology	Response	Ref.
Bile Duct-Ligated Rats				
Naidu	6 d	Isolated perfused hind limb	Normal	22
Bomzon et al.	3 d	Portal vein	Diminished	23
Bomzon et al.	1—6 d	Aortic strip and portal vein	Transient loss of response	24
Gali et al.	1—28 d		3 days	25
Jacob and Bomzon	35 d	Aortic ring	Potentiated	26
Bile Duct-Ligated Dogs				
Bomzon et al.	3 weeks	Arterial strips	Normal	15
Bomzon et al.	12 weeks	Arterial strips	Normal	16
Carbon Tetrachloride-Induced Cirrhotic Rats				
Kitano et al.		Arterial strip and portal vein	Normal	27
Leehey et al.		Arterial ring	Normal[a]	28
Gali		Portal vein	Potentiated	29
Lopez-Novoa		Arterial strip	Normal	29
Jacob and Bomzon		Arterial ring	Normal	26
Bomzon et al.		Arterial ring	Normal	20
Villamediana et al.		Perfused hindlimb and arterial ring	Normal	21
Portal Vein-Ligated Rats				
Kiel et al.	10 d	Mesenteric perfusion	Diminished	30
Cummings et al.	14 d	Mesenteric vein	Diminished	31
		Aortic strip	Normal	
Bomzon and Blendis	10 d	Arterial strip	Normal	32
Bomzon and Blendis	21 d	Arterial strip	Diminished	32
Jacob and Bomzon	10 d	Arterial ring and portal vein	Diminished	26
Bile Duct-Ligated Baboons				
Bloom et al.	2 weeks	Cerebral circulation	Potentiated	33
Bomzon et al.	2 weeks	Renal circulation	Potentiated	34
Bomzon et al.	2 weeks	Skeletal muscle circulation	Diminished	35
Portal Vein-Ligated Rabbits				
Jensen et al.	4 weeks	Esophageal varices	Potentiated	36
		Mesenteric veins	Normal	

[a] Phenylephrine, the selective α_1-adrenoreceptor agonist, was used instead of norepinephrine.

pressure in patients with alcoholic cirrhosis is under the control of the sympathetic nervous system and is amenable to pharmacological treatment by nonselective β-adrenoreceptor antagonists and α_2-adrenoreceptor agonists. Since the mechanism of action of these two drug classes is quite different, it emphasizes an important point that certainly in the venous system, assessment of reactivity to an agonist cannot be based solely upon the ability of an agonist to induce contraction.

Measurement of venous reactivity should probably include indices of the ability of the vessel to "stretch" in order to accommodate for increases in intravenous vascular volume which does occur in portal hypertension. Such a study has been done by Jensen et al.,[36] who measured the mechanical, morphological, and pharmacological characteristics of small esophageal varices and mesenteric veins taken from portal hypertensive rabbits. In addition to finding that portal hypertension changed the mechanical and morphological properties of these two vessels (in particular, and increased thickness of the media), differences in responsiveness to norepinephrine also occurred (Table 3). Their data may explain the discrepancy between the use of sympatholytic drugs to treat portal hypertension and the experimental observations of reduced reactivity to norepinephrine of the mesenteric venous vasculature.

Returning to loss of end organ responsiveness in hyperbilirubinemia, the mechanism of this phenomenon has been investigated by Bomzon and his colleagues. From their studies, it would appear that the loss of responsiveness to norepinephrine is located at the level of the receptor and not related to transmembrane calcium flux, intracellular calcium release, the biochemistry of contraction, or re-uptake of the amine.[28,42] The mechanism of blunted response to norepinephrine in the mesenteric or systemic vasculature of the portal vein-ligated rat has not been evaluated in detail. Bomzon and Blendis[32] have shown that it may be linked to the release of calcium from the intracellular stores associated with α-adrenoreceptor activation. Their findings suggest that the mechanism of loss of end organ response in this model may be different from that seen in the jaundiced bile duct-ligated rat.

B. ACETYLCHOLINE

The role of the parasympathetic neurotransmitter, acetylcholine, as an endogenous vasodilator in liver disease has not been investigated. The reasons are threefold — resistance vessels are not innervated by the parasympathetic nervous system, and the activities or amounts of plasma and tissue cholinesterases are so high that the local vascular concentration of this compound are almost negligible. In addition, it has been claimed in chronic liver disease that the activity of the parasympathetic nervous system is decreased.[10] For these reasons, it is highly unlikely that acetylcholine has an important role to play in the pathogenesis of portal hypertension and systemic hypotension of chronic liver disease and hyperbilirubinemia.

C. GAMMA-AMINOBUTYRIC ACID (GABA)

GABA is a potent inhibitory neurotransmitter whose plasma concentrations are elevated in cirrhosis. Recently, Minuk and MacCannell[43] suggested that GABA or a GABA-mediated process might contribute to the hypotension of cirrhosis. The mechanism whereby GABA exerts its hypotensive action is not known, but it has been shown in other studies that it may induce relaxation in isolated cerebral blood vessels.[44,45] It still remains to be established whether GABA can induce the same response in other noncerebral vessels as well as to identify the intracellular mechanism of GABA-induced vasodilatation.

D. SUBSTANCE P

Substance P is one of the many peptides that have been identified in the central and peripheral nervous systems. In the peripheral nervous system, it has been found mainly in primary afferent nerves, where it may be released by antidromic activation of the afferent fibers. Since one of the principal pharmacological actions of substance P includes vasodilatation, it is not altogether surprising that it has been implicated in the pathogenesis of the cardiovascular complications of liver disease.[46] Hortnagl and colleagues measured a tenfold increase in the plasma of patients with liver failure caused by acute or chronic hepatocellular disease.[46] Although the mechanism of its action is not clarified, it should be noted that the rise in substance P occurred at end stage liver disease. Further studies are necessary to establish a more definitive role for substance P, especially in well-compensated cirrhosis before it can be classified as an "endogenous vasodilator".

IV. ENDOTHELIAL-DERIVED COMPOUNDS

A. ARACHIDONIC ACID DERIVATIVES

The emphasis of research into the role of these compounds in the complications of liver disease have largely been directed towards the kidney in liver disease, and a review of the topic was recently written by Zipser and Lifschitz.[47]

Endogenous derivatives of arachidonic acid, i.e., the prostaglandins (PG), leukotrienes (LT) and thromboxanes, have been proposed as contributing elements in the control of vascular resistance. Their cardiovascular effects are numerous and diverse and the different metabolites show different activities, both qualitatively and quantitatively. For example, PGE_2, PGD_2 and PGI_2 have been shown to induce vasodilatation, whereas thromboxane A_2, PGF_{2a} and LTC_4, LTD_4, LTE_4 are all vasoconstrictor agents. In addition to their own actions, they are capable of modulating the pressor or contractile response of other vasoactive compounds.[48]

Several studies investigated the *in vitro* synthesis of arachidonic acid derivatives in liver disease, but the studies have concentrated upon their synthesis as contributing to altered end organ responsiveness in jaundice. Heidenreich et al.[49] were unable to demonstrate either an increase or decrease in the synthesis of PGE_2, and the stable hydrolysis products of prostacyclin (PGI_2) and thromboxane A_2, namely, 6-keto-PGF_{1a} or thromobxane B_2, respectively, from aortic rings of 6-d bile duct-ligated rats. More recently, Schroeder et al.[50] demonstrated that vascular prostacyclin production was significantly decreased after incubation of rat aortic tissue with jaundiced human serum as compared with normal human serum.

In the light of these data, it would appear that arachidonic acid derivatives have little or no role in the mechanism of reduced vascular responsiveness to norepinephrine in jaundice. However, it is premature to conclude that this represents the "state of the art", because of the numerous vasoactive metabolites that may be generated. Until such time that all of the metabolites are assessed, the role of this interesting group of compounds must remain an open question.

B. ENDOTHELIAL-DERIVED RELAXING FACTOR(S)

The discovery by Furchgott and Zawadski in 1980[51] that the endothelial cell of blood vessels contained an endogenous vasodilator, subsequently named endothelial-derived relaxant factor (EDRF), has resulted in a considerable amount of research into its structure, its mechanism of release, and its action on vascular smooth muscle.[52] Moncado and Ignarro and their respective groups have identified EDRF as nitric oxide whose half-life is less than 60 seconds.[53-55] Furthermore, it would appear that the mechanism of its vasodilator action is similar to that of nitrites and nitrates in that their action on vascular smooth muscle is followed by a rise in the intracellular concentration of cGMP within the vascular smooth muscle cell.[56] Independent studies by Vanhoutte and Rubanyi[57] have suggested that there may even be more than two relaxant factors released by the endothelial cell. It has also been shown that EDRF may be released following norepinephrine-induced contraction of vascular smooth muscle.[58] Last, it has been shown that the release of EDRF is calcium-dependent and can be stimulated by acetylcholine.[51,52] In spite of all these investigations, a physiological role for this compound has yet to be established. In the absence of a definitive role for this substance, it is not surprising that investigations on EDRF in liver disease have not been undertaken.

C. ENDOTHELIAL-DERIVED CONSTRICTOR FACTORS

In 1988, a Japanese group of investigators reported that the vascular endothelial cell

TABLE 4
Summary of Experiments That Assessed the *In Vivo* Pressor Responsiveness to Angiotensin II in the Various Animal Models of Liver Disease

Experiment	Time	Methodology	Response	Ref.
Bile Duct-Ligated Rats				
Finberg et al.	6 d	Urethane anesthetized	Normal	11
Bomzon et al.	3 d	Conscious	Diminished	12
Bile Duct-Ligated Dogs				
Finberg et al.	3 weeks	Conscious	Diminished	14
Bomzon et al.	3 weeks	Conscious	Diminished	15
Bomzon et al.	12 weeks	Conscious	Diminished	16
Bomzon et al.	3 weeks	Anesthetized	Normal to diminished[a]	17
Carbon Tetrachloride-Induced Cirrhotic Rats				
Bala et al.		Urethane anesthetized; nonascitic	Normal	61
Leehey et al.		Ketamine and pentobarbital anesthetized; nonascitic	Normal	18
Murray and Paller		Conscious; nonascitic	Diminished	19
Weinbroum et al.		Conscious; nonascitic	Diminished	63

[a] Varied according to anesthetic used.

synthesized and released a potent vasoconstrictor peptide, termed endothelin.[59,60] Obviously, the physiological role of this peptide in the regulation of vascular resistance in the normal situation is unknown.

However, its discovery has no doubt focused the attention of investigators in the area of vascular reactivity on reevaluation of the role of the endothelium and the mechanisms associated with vasodilatation and vasoconstriction. The sensory inputs to the endothelial cell that result in their release and subsequent communication with the smooth muscle cell have yet to be determined. This clarification needs to be undertaken before a definitive role for these compounds as part of the generalized vascular dilatation of liver disease can be established.

V. HUMORALLY DERIVED COMPOUNDS

A. ANGIOTENSIN

The renin-angiotensin-aldosterone system in liver disease is discussed elsewhere in this book.[61] In this section, the comments will be confined to the vasoactive actions of this peptide in clinical and experimental cirrhosis.

Laragh and his colleagues[2-4] and subsequently the Italian group of Morandini and others[6,7] demonstrated that cirrhotic patients with ascites were resistant to the pressor effect of intravenously infused angiotensin. Their observations which were made in the mid-sixties have gone unchallenged to this day, although recently Lenz and his colleagues[10] found pressor supersensitivity to angiotensin in their group of hepatic encephalopathic patients.

The studies in experimental animals are more or less consistent with the clinical observations in that there is a diminished pressor responsiveness to infused angiotensin (Table 4). Anesthesia, per se, may account for some of the discrepancies in the data. However, the *in vitro* studies, although limited, are not consistent with the *in vivo* data (Table 5). In view of the very few studies, it is not possible to offer a full explanation on the inconsistency.

TABLE 5
**Summary of Experiments That Assessed the Responsiveness of
Blood Vessels to Angiotensin II in the Various Models of Liver
Disease**

Experiment	Time	Methodology	Response	Ref.
Bile Duct-Ligated Dogs				
Bomzon et al.	3 weeks	Arterial strips	Diminished	15
Bomzon et al.	12 weeks	Arterial strips	Diminished	16
Carbon Tetrachloride-Induced Cirrhotic Rats				
Leehey et al.		Arterial rings	Normal	18
Portal Vein-Ligated Rabbits				
Jensen et al.	4 weeks	Esophageal varices	Potentiated	36
		Mesenteric veins	Potentiated	

It has been suggested that diminished end organ responsiveness to angiotensin is dependent upon undefined factors other than those associated with the receptor. Murray and Paller[19] postulated that the reason for loss of pressor response to the peptide was not due to down-regulation of the receptor but rather due to an as yet undefined postreceptor factor. These other undefined factors may be the sodium or potassium status of the animal which is known to influence angiotensin responsiveness.[61]

In 1976, Schroeder et al,[64] infused saralasin, the angiotensin II antagonist, into patients with cirrhosis and ascites after 3 days of sodium restriction. Since the blood pressure fell even more after its administration, they concluded that the blood pressure of cirrhotic patients was dependent upon circulating angiotensin II levels. The observations of two Japanese groups[65,66] in the late seventies in similar groups of patients confirmed the findings of Schroeder's group, although the three groups suggested that the renin-angiotensin system might be involved in the maintenance of normal blood pressure in cirrhotic patients, or at least those patients with cirrhosis at an early stage of ascites development or sodium retention. When the angiotensin-converting enzyme inhibitor, captopril, was administered to cirrhotic patients with ascites,[67] the fall in blood pressure (possibly due to an increase in circulating bradykinin) was accompanied by antinatriuresis. This fall in blood pressure was not seen when captopril was given to carbon tetrachoride-induced cirrhotic rats, suggesting that in this animal model of cirrhosis, maintenance of blood pressure is not dependent upon angiotensin II.[19]

If the maintenance of blood pressure in cirrhotic patients is dependent upon angiotensin II, is diminished end organ responsiveness to angiotensin a fact or a myth? As already stated, the clinical and experimental observations have, by and large, shown that the pressor response to angiotensin II is depressed; and those experiments in which captopril was administered to patients and animals indicate that prior occupancy of the receptor site is not the basis for this refractoriness. If the maintenance of blood pressure is some cirrhotic patients is dependent upon angiotensin II and the *in vitro* data indicate that blood vessels can contract to the peptide, one can conclude that refractoriness to angiotensin II at the level of the resistance vessel has little or no part in the pathogenesis of a reduced total peripheral resistance in cirrhosis.

In the light of the above information, the mechanisms associated with pressor subsensitivity to angiotensin II need further investigation. Moreover, it would appear somewhat premature to implicate angiotensin refractoriness as the basis for systemic hypotension and as the ''endogenous vasodilator''.

TABLE 6
Summary of Experiments That Assessed Cardiovascular
Responsiveness to Serotonin in the Various Animal Models of
Liver Disease

Experiment	Time	Methodology	Response	Ref.
Bile Duct-Ligated Rats				
Lee et al.	3 d	Pithed rat	Diminished	69
	3 d	Aortic ring	Normal	
	3 d	Portal vein	Normal	
	35 d	Pithed rat	Diminished	
	35 d	Aortic ring	Diminished	
	35 d	Portal vein	Normal	
Carbon Tetrachloride-Induced Cirrhotic Rats				
Lee et al.		Pithed rat	Diminished	69
		Aortic ring	Potentiated	
		Portal vein	Normal	
Portal Vein-Ligated Rat				
Cummings et al.	14 d	Mesenteric vein	Potentiated	31
Jacob et al.	10 d	Pithed rat	Diminished	70
	10 d	Aortic ring	Potentiated	
	10 d	Portal vein	Normal	
Portal Vein-Ligated Rabbit				
Jensen et al.	4 weeks	Esophageal varices and mesenteric vein	Diminished relaxation	36

B. SEROTONIN

The diverse actions of serotonin on the cardiovascular system are well known.[68] This amine causes vasoconstriction, but under certain conditions, it can induce vasodilatation. In recent years, considerable attention has been focused upon this substance since it was observed that the mesenteric veins of rats with partial vein ligation exhibit *in vitro* supersensitivity to serotonin.[31] This observation thus raised the possibility that portal hypertension may be treated with serotonin antagonists such as ketanserin. The use of such antagonists are reviewed elsewhere in this book by Lebrec and Lee.[41]

While ketanserin and other serotonin (S_2) antagonists hae been used to treat portal hypertension, little is known about the cardiovasular actions of serotonin in liver disease. Table 6 summarizes the experimental *in vivo* and *in vitro* data. It can be that jaundice has no effect upon the *in vivo* pressor and *in vitro* contractile responsiveness to serotonin. Furthermore, while the pressor response is reduced in the models of portal hypertension, this loss is not always associated with *in vitro* contractile responsiveness of isolated aortic vessels. The *in vitro* data on isolated veins is conflicting and again emphasizes the use of *in vitro* contractility to an agonist as the determinant for venous reactivity.

If one compares the serotonin data with those of norepinephrine (Tables 2 and 3), it would appear that the induction of experimental liver disease differs in its effects on responsiveness at the level of the receptor to these two amines. This is indeed intriguing since both receptors utilize the same second messenger, viz., inositol phosphate, to increase the free intracellular calcium concentration. This differential effect on noradrenergic and serotonergic receptors has also been noted by Hadengue et al.[71] In patients with portal hypertension treated with propranolol and ketanserin, they observed that the effects were additive but independent.

C. ADENOSINE

In recent years, evidence has accumulated that adenosine may be important in the regulation of organ blood flow. Much of the evidence has been obtained from studies on the coronary and hepatic circulations where it acts as a vasodilator and participates in the autoregulation of blood flow in these organs.[72,73] It exerts its action through two receptors, but vasodilatation is mediated by the adenosine (A_2) receptor.[74] The cellular origin of adenosine is uncertain, but there is evidence to show that it is derived from intracellular acetate.[75] The role of adenosine in cirrhosis and portal hypertension has not yet been investigated.

D. ATRIAL NATRIURETIC FACTOR

The role of atrial natriuretic factor or peptide and its role in sodium retention in cirrhosis is discussed elsewhere in this book and much of the information pertaining to its vasodilator action on the cardiovascular system is discussed therein.[76]

E. VASOPRESSIN

In addition to its antidiuretic action, vasopressin is a general vasoconstrictor agent. Its role in cardiovascular regulation has recently been reviewed by Liard.[77] Its action on blood vessels is mediated by the vasopressin (V_1) receptor subtype.[78] The peptide and its analogues may be beneficial in the treatment of acute variceal hemorrhage in cirrhotic patients.[79] The only study on the effect of vasopressin on *in vitro* vascular reactivity in liver disease was undertaken by Groszmann and his colleagues who found that the contractile responses of mesenteric veins of portal hypertensive rats were normal when compared to sham-operated controls.[31] Their data suggests that the beneficial effects of vasopressin are not associated with its contractile effect.

F. VASOACTIVE INTESTINAL PEPTIDE

Vasoactive intestinal peptide (VIP) has been shown to be widely distributed within central and peripheral nervous systems and has been postulated to be released as a neurotransmitter or cotransmitter from nonadrenergic neurones. It is a potent vasodilator but its *in vitro* action on isolated blood vessels taken from experimental models of liver disease has not been investigated. However, it is worth noting that Levy and Finestone[80] infused VIP, as well as secretin and glucagon, into the renal artery of dogs whose bile duct had been ligated for 4 hours. Although secretin increased renal blood flow, they concluded that these vasodilator vasoactive peptides could not account for the renal vasodilatation of acute biliary obstruction.

G. BRADYKININ AND OTHER KININS

The kinins, of which bradykinin is the best-known example, are formed from plasma and tissue kallikreins. Kinins are inactivated by kinases or angiotensin-converting enzyme. Bradykinin is a potent vasodilator, but like many of the aforementioned endogenous vasodilators, little is known of their vascular effects in liver disease.

H. GLUCAGON

The role of glucagon as a blood-borne mediator of the hyperdynamic circulation associated with portal hypertension is reviewed elsewhere in this book[38,81] and it would serve little purpose to represent this information in this section.

I. BILE ACIDS

In contrast to the above-mentioned endogenous humoral vasoactive compounds, bile acids have been implicated as a potential vasodilator by acting as an α-adrenoreceptor antagonist.[82] In other words, they exert their vasodilator action indirectly. Their action on the heart has been reviewed by both Lee and Bomzon[38] and Benoit et al.[81] in their respective chapters in this book, and it is possible that the hypotensive action of bile acids is mediated through their cardiodepressive action.

VI. CONCLUSIONS

The efferent inputs to the vascular smooth muscle cell arise from three primary sources which potentially can alter muscle tone by changing the free intracellular calcium concentration. The exact details of the intracellular pathways which contribute to the regulation of the calcium concentration following stimulation by an agonist still need elucidation.

Assessment of vascular reactivity in liver disease, be it arterial or venous, to most of the compounds, has never been undertaken. Of all the compounds listed in Table 1, the reactivity of norepinephrine and angiotensin II have been evaluated to any great extent, whereas that of the remainder (with the exceptions of, in a limited sense, serotonin and glucagon) still need to be assessed. Our information is also incomplete inasmuch that no functional distinctions between arterial and venous reactivity were made by most, if not all, of the investigators. Furthermore, where altered reactivity has been described, the intracellular processes have not been elucidated.

The plasma of patients and experimental liver disease contains a plethora of substances which under circumstances have no intrinsic vasoactive activity such as bile acids, estrogen, and ammonia. This chapter has reviewed only some of many known endogenous vasoactive compounds. Their choice was determined by previous clinical and experimental observations where it has been suggested that they may be implicated in the pathogenesis of systemic hypotension. Of the compounds reviewed, bile acids may be considered to fall into the category of an endogenous substance with no known intrinsic vasoactive properties. In other words, it exerts its vasoactive action indirectly by modifying the response of an endogenous vasoactive compound. The mechanism of action of these other substances such as estrogen may act in the same manner as bile acids. Hence, they cannot be eliminated as "endogenous vasodilators", despite the different mechanism of action.

While in some instances, diminished pressor responsiveness to norepinephrine and angiotensin have been reported, these observations often do not correlate with the *in vivo* pressor and *in vitro* contractile responses observed in the animal models. The differences between the models have been discussed[37] and this probably accounts for the discrepancy and variability of the data.

As has been said previously, venous reactivity has been determined by measuring the contractile response of the splanchnic vasculature to numerous agonists without any considerations given to assess capacitance. Assuming that capacitance or "stretch" is dependent upon contraction, it is also worth noting that a direct relationship between portal hypotension and venous reactivity has still to be established.

Methodological considerations also need to be taken into account in the evaluation of diminished end organ responsiveness in liver disease. For example, the discrepancy between the *in vivo* pressor responses and the *in vitro* contractile reactivity may be in part explained by the differences in methodology associated with *in vivo* and *in vitro* techniques. In the latter situation, the vessel is isolated from its "normal" environment and its reactivity assessed. While this approach is acceptable, its major limitation is that it assumes that the isolated vessel has a "memory" which is recalled when exposed to the various agonists. This drawback can be overcome if the vessel is bathed in "abnormal" plasma instead of normal bathing media. Such an approach may satisfy the experimental prerequisites for an endogenous vasoactive compound, such as norepinephrine, but not for indirect acting substances such as bile acids. In this instances, experiments such as assessing the reactivity of normal vessel exposed to "abnormal" plasma should be undertaken. Such an experiment was reported by Schroeder and his colleagues,[50] where normal rat aortic tissue was exposed to serum obtained from jaundiced patients.

Other factors have also been implicated as reasons for diminished pressor responsiveness in patients with liver disease. These other factors include the sodium balance of the patient, the pulmonary endothelium, and the heart. The influence of each of these factors on pressor responsiveness in liver disease needs to be evaluated.

In view of the limited, and sometimes, confusing and conflicting data, as well as the species and methodological considerations, one must question the existence of the concept of diminished end organ responsiveness in liver disease. Based upon our currently available knowledge, the present concept of systemic hypotension, portal hypertension, diminished end organ responsiveness, and "endogenous vasodilators" as the pathophysiological basis for the generalized vasodilatation of liver disease is difficult to reconcile.

ACKNOWLEDGMENTS

The useful comments of Drs. L. M. Blendis, S. Lee, K. Sharkey, and K. MacCannell while the manuscript was being prepared were greatly appreciated. The typing skills and patience of Julie Walker and Diane Buzan were of enormous assistance.

REFERENCES

1. **Blendis, L. M. and Bomzon, A.,** The cardiovascular complications of cirrhosis, in *The Cardiovascular Complications of Liver Disease,* Bomzon, A. and Blendis, L. M., Eds., CRC Press, Boca Raton, FL, 1990, chap. 1.
2. **Laragh, J. H.,** Hormones and the pathogenesis of congestive heart failure: vasopressin, aldosterone and angiotensin. II. Further evidence for renal-adrenal interaction for studies in hypertension and in cirrhosis, *Circulation,* 25, 1015, 1962.
3. **Laragh, J. G., Cannon, P. J., Bentzel, C. J., Sicinski, A. M., and Melzer, J. I.,** Angiotensin II, norepinephrine and renal transport of electrolytes and water in normal man and in cirrhosis with ascites, *J. Clin. Invest.,* 42, 1179, 1963.
4. **Ames, R. P., Borkowski, A. J., Sicinski, A. M., and Laragh, J. M.,** Prolonged infusions of angiotensin II and norepinephrine and blood pressure, electrolyte balance, and aldosterone and control secretion in normal man and in cirrhosis with ascites, *J. Clin. Invest.,* 44, 1171, 1965.
5. **Henriksen, J. H., Ring-Larsen, H., and Christensen, N. J.,** Autonomic nervous function in liver disease, in *The Cardiovascular Complications of Liver Disease,* Bomzon, A. and Blendis, L. M., Eds., CRC Press, Boca Raton, FL, 1990, chap. 4.
6. **Morandini, G. and Spanedda, M.,** Contributo allo studio della reattivita vascolare periferica all'angiotensina ed all noradrenalina in corso di affezioni epatiche, *Minerva Med.,* 57, 2175, 1966.
7. **Morandini, G., Spanedda, M., and Spanedda, L.,** La riposta pressoria all'angiotensina e all noradrenalina in soggetti con affezioni epatiche, *Minerva Med.,* 58, 1794, 1967.
8. **Lunzer, M. R., Newmann, S. P., and Sherlock, S.,** Skeletal muscle blood flow and neurovascular reactivity in liver disease, *Gut,* 14, 354, 1973.
9. **Lunzer, M. R., Newman, S. P., Bernardi, A. G., Manghani, K. K., Sherlock, S., and Ginsberg, J.,** Impaired cardiovascular responsiveness in liver disease, *Lancet,* 2, 382, 1975.
10. **Lenz, K., Hortnagl, H., Magometschnigg, D., Kleinberger, G., Druml, W., and Langgner, A.,** Function of the autonomic nervous system in patients with hepatic encephalopathy, *Hepatology,* 5, 831, 1985.
11. **Finberg, J. P. M., Sideman, R., and Better, O. S.,** Cardiovascular responsiveness to vasoactive agents in rats with obstructive jaundice, *Clin. Exp. Pharmacol. Physiol.,* 9, 693, 1982.

12. **Bomzon, A., Weinbroum, A., and Kamenetz, L.,** Systemic hypotension and pressor responsiveness in cholestasis, *J. Hepatol.,* in press.
13. **Saito, H.,** Clinical and experimental studies on the hyperdynamic states in obstructive jaundice, *J. Jpn. Surg. Soc.,* 82, 483, 1981.
14. **Finberg, J. P. M., Syrop, H. A., and Better, O. S.,** Blunted pressor response to angiotensin and sympathomimetic amines in bile duct ligated dogs, *Clin. Sci.,* 61, 535, 1981.
15. **Bomzon, A., Rosenberg, M., Gali, D., Binah, O., Mordechowitz, D., Better, O. S., Greig, P. D., and Blendis, L. M.,** Systemic hypotension and decreased pressor response in dogs with chronic bile duct, (CBDL), *Hepatology,* 6, 595, 1986.
16. **Bomzon, A., Binah, O., and Blendis, L. M,,** Temporal changes in pressor and contractile responsiveness in the conscious chronic bile duct-ligated (CBDL) dog, *Hepatology,* 8(Abstr.), 1393, 1988.
17. **Bomzon, A., Monies-Chass, I., Kamenetz, L., and Blendis, L. M.,** Anesthesia and pressor responsiveness in chronic bile duct-ligated (CBDL) dogs, *Hepatology,* in press.
18. **Leehey, D. J., Daugirdas, J. T., Ing, T. S., Stanley, M. M., and Betzelos, S. J.,** Pressor sensitivity to angiotensin II and phenylephrine in cirrhotic rats, *Gastroenterology,* 88(Abstr.), 1674, 1985.
19. **Murray, B. M. and Paller, M. S.,** Decreased pressor reactivity to angiotensin II in cirrhotic rats: evidence for a post-receptor defect in angiotensin action, *Circ. Res.,* 57, 424, 1985.
20. **Bomzon, A., Weinbroum, A., and Blendis, L. M.,** Loss of cardiovascular responsiveness to norepinephrine, systemic hypotension and pressor response to PTD postural change in cirrhosis: an experimental study, *Eur. J. Clin. Invest.,* submitted.
21. **Villamediana, L. M., Dieguez, G., Santos, J. C., Garcia-Villalon, A. L., Caramelo, C., and Lopez-Novoa, J. M.,** Vascular reactivity to norepinephrine in rats with cirrhosis of the liver, *Can. J. Physiol. Pharmacol.,* 66, 667, 1988.
22. **Naidu, S.,** The effect of chronic bile duct ligation, hepatic and extrahepatic metabolites on vascular response to noradrenaline, M. Sc. thesis, University of the Witwatersrand, Johannesburg, South Africa, 1982.
23. **Bomzon, A., Finberg, J. P. M., Tovbin, D., Naidu, S. G., and Better, O. S.,** Bile salts, hypotension and obstructive jaundice, *Clin. Sci.,* 67, 177, 1984.
24. **Bomzon, A., Gali, D., Better, O. S., and Blendis, L. M.,** Reversible suppression of the vascular contractile response in rats with obstructive jaundice, *J. Lab. Clin. Med.,* 105, 568, 1985.
25. **Gali, D., Blendis, L. M., and Bomzon, A.,** Vascular reactivity in reversible experimental obstructive jaundice, *J. Surg. Res.,* 42, 242, 1987.
26. **Jacob, G. and Bomzon, A.,** unpublished data, 1988.
27. **Kitano, S., Koyonagi, N., Sugimachi, K., Kobayashi, M., and Inokuchi, K.,** Mucosal blood flow and modified vascular responses to norepinephrine in the stomach of rats with liver cirrhosis, *Eur. J. Surg. Res.,* 14, 221, 1981.
28. **Gali, D.,** Pathogenetic mechanisms of cardiovascular disturbances in liver disease, M.Sc. thesis, Faculty of Medicine, Technion-Israel Institute of Technology, Haifa, 1985.
29. **Lopez-Novoa, J. M.,** Pathophysiological features of the carbon tetrachloride/phenobarbitol model of experimental liver cirrhosis in rats, in *The Kidney in Liver Disease,* 3rd ed., Epstein, M., Ed., Williams & Wilkins, Baltimore, 1988, 309.
30. **Kiel, J. W., Pitts, V., Benoit, J. N., Granger, D. N., and Shepherd, A. P.,** Reduced vascular sensitivity to norepinephrine in portal hypertensive rats, *Am. J. Physiol.,* 248, G192, 1985.
31. **Cummings, S. A., Groszmann, R. J., and Kaumann, A. J.,** Hypersensitivity of mesenteric veins to 5-hydroxytryptamine and ketanserin induced reduction of portal pressure in portal hypertensive rats, *Brit. J. Pharmacol.,* 89, 501, 1986.
32. **Bomzon, A. and Blendis, L. M.,** Vascular ractivity in experimental portal hypertension, *Am. J. Physiol.,* 252, G158, 1987.
33. **Bloom, D. S., Eidelman, B. M., and McCalden, T. A.,** Modification of the cerebrovascular response to norepinephrine by bile duct ligation, *Gut,* 16, 732, 1975.
34. **Bomzon, A. and Kew, M. C.,** Renal blood flow in obstructive jaundice: the baboon as an experimental model, in *The Kidney in Liver Disease,* Epstein, M., Ed., Elsevier, New York, 1978, 167.
35. **Bomzon, A, Wilton, P. B., and McCalden, T. A.,** Impaired skeletal muscle vasomotor response to infused noradrenaline in baboons with obstructive jaundice, *Clin. Sci. Mol. Med.,* 55, 109, 1978.
36. **Jensen, L. S., Juhl, C. O., and Mulvany, M.,** Mechanical, morphological and pharmacological properties of esophageal varices and small mesenteric veins in portal hypertensive rabbits, *Acta Physiol. Scand.,* 130, 649, 1987.
37. **Bomzon, A. and Blendis, L. M.,** Animal models of liver disease, in *The Cardiovascular Complications of Liver Disease,* Bomzon, A. and Blendis, L. M., Eds., CRC Press, Boca Raton, Florida, 1990, chap. 2.
38. **Lee, S. S. and Bomzon, A.,** The heart in liver disease, in *The Cardiovascular Complications of Liver Disease,* Bomzon, A. and Blendis, L. M., Eds., CRC Press, Boca Raton, Florida, 1990, chap. 5.

39. **Bomzon, A., Blendis, L. M., Better, O. S., Yarhi, D., Copel, Y., and Youdin, M. B. H.,** Modification of pulmonary metabolism of noradrenaline in experimental obstructive jaundice, *Biochem. Pharmacol.*, 34, 3049, 1985.

40. **Willett, I. R., Esler, M., Jennings, G., and Dudley, F. J.,** Sympathetic tone modulates portal venous pressure in alcoholic cirrhosis, *Lancet*, 2, 939, 1986.

41. **Lebrec, D. and Lee, S. S.,** Effects of vacoactive drugs on the systemic and splanchnic circulation, in *The Cardiovascular Complications of Liver Disease*, Bomzon, A. and Blendis, L. M., Eds., CRC Press, Boca Raton, Florida, 1990, chap. 17.

42. **Sayid, O. and Bomzon, A.,** unpublished data, 1989.

43. **Minuk, G. Y. and MacCannell, K. L.,** Is the hypotension of cirrhosis a GABA-mediated process? *Hepatology*, 8, 73, 1988.

44. **Anwar, N. and Mason, D. F. J.,** Two actions of γ-aminobutyric acid on the responses of the isolated basilar artery from the rabbit, *Brit. J. Pharmacol.*, 75, 177, 1982.

45. **Edvinsson, L. and Krause, D. N.,** Pharmacological characterization of GABA receptors mediating vasodilatation of cerebral arteries, *in vivo*, *Brain Res.*, 173, 89, 1979.

46. **Hortnagl, H., Singer, E. A., Lenz, K., Kleinberger, G., and Lochs, H.,** Substance P is markedly increased in plasma of patients with hepatic coma, *Lancet*, 1, 480, 1984.

47. **Zipser, R. D. and Lifschitz, M. D.,** Protaglandins and related compounds, in *The Kidney in Liver Disease*, 3rd ed., Epstein, M., Ed., Williams & Wilkins, Baltimore, 1988, 393.

48. **Moncada, S., Flower, R. J., and Vane, J. R.,** Prostaglandins, prostacyclin, thromboxane A_2 and leukotrienes, in *The Pharmacological Basis of Therapeutics*, 7th ed., Gilman, A. G., Goodman, L. S., Rall, T. W., and Murad, F., Eds., Macmillan, New York, 1985, 660.

49. **Heidenreich, S., Brinkema, E., Martin, A., Dusing, R., Kipnowski, J., and Kramer, H. J.,** The kidney and the cardiovascular system in obstructive jaundice: functional and metabolic studies in conscious rats, *Clin. Sci.*, 73, 593, 1987.

50. **Schroeder, E. T., Finn, A. F., and Hueber, P.,** Suppression of vascular prostaglandin generation by jaundiced serum: relation to lipid peroxides, *J. Lab. Clin. Med.*, 112, 784, 1988.

51. **Furchgott, R. F. and Zawadski, J. V.,** The obligatory role of endothelial cells in the relaxation of arterial smooth muscle by acetylcholine, *Nature*, 288, 373, 1980.

52. **Vanhoutte, P. M., Rubanyi, G. M., Miller, V. M., and Houston, D. S.,** Modulation of vascular smooth muscle contraction by the endothelium, *Annu. Rev. Physiol.*, 48, 307, 1986.

53. **Palmer, R. M., Ferrige, A. G., and Moncada, S.,** Nitric oxide release accounts for the biological activity of endothelial derived relaxing factor, *Nature*, 327, 524, 1987.

54. **Ignarro, L. J., Buga, G. M., Wood, K. S., Byrns, R. E., and Chandhuri, G.,** Endothelium derived relaxing factor produced and released from artery and vein is nitric oxide, *Proc. Nat. Acad. Sci. U.S.A.*, 84, 9265, 1987.

55. **Moncada, S., Radowski, M. W., and Palmer, R. M.,** Endothelium-derived relaxant factor. Identification as nitric oxide and role in the control of vascular tone and platelet function, *Biochem. Pharmacol.*, 37, 2495, 1988.

56. **Ignarro, L. J., Byrns, R. E., and Wood, K. S.,** Endothelium dependent modulation of cGMP levels and intrinsic smooth muscle tone in isolated bovine intrapulmonary artery and vein, *Circul. Res.*, 60, 82, 1987.

57. **Rubanyi, G. M. and Vanhoutte, P. M.,** Nature of endothelium-derived relaxing factor: are there two relaxing mediators, *Circul. Res.*, 61(Suppl. II), II-61, 1987.

58. **Martin, W., Furchgott, R. F., Villani, G. M., and Jothiananden, D.,** Depression of contractile responses in rat aorta by spontaneously released endothelium-derived relaxing factor, *J. Pharmacol. Exp. Ther.*, 237, 529, 1986.

59. **Yanagisawa, M., Kurihara, H., Kimura, S., Tomobe, Y., Kobayashi, M., Mitsui, Y., Yazaki, Y., Goto, K., and Masaki, T.,** A novel potent vasoconstrictor peptide produced by vascular endothelial cells, *Nature*, 332, 411, 1988.

60. **Yanagisawa, M., Inoue, A., Ishikawa, T., Kasuya, Y., Kimura, S., Kumagaye, S., Nakajima, K., Watanabe, T. X., Sakakibara, S., Goto, K., and Masaki, T.,** Primary structure, synthesis and biological activity of rat endothelin, an endothelium-derived vasoconstrictors peptide, *Proc. Nat. Acad. Sci. U.S.A.*, 85, 6964, 1988.

61. **Bernardi, M., Trevisani, F., Gasbarrini, G.,** Renin-angiotensin-aldosterone system in liver disease, in *The Cardiovascular Complications of Liver Disease*, Bomzon, A. and Blendis, L. M., Eds., CRC Press, Boca Raton, Florida, 1990, chap. 3.

62. **Bala, S., Sharma, P. L., and Garg, K. N.,** Effect of angiotensin on blood pressure in normal and cirrhotic rats, *Jpn. J. Pharmacol.*, 23, 409, 1973.

63. **Weinbroun, A., Blendis, L. M., Pourcell, S., and Bomzon, A.,** Temporal relationships between cirrhosis, portal hypertension and systemic hemodynamics in carbon tetrachloride (CT) induced cirrhosis in rats, *Hepatology*, 6(Abstr.), 1120, 1986.

64. **Schroeder, E. T., Anderson, G. H., Goldman, S. H., and Streeten, D. H. P.,** Effect of blockade of angiotensin II on blood pressure, renin and aldosterone in cirrhosis, *Kidney Int.,* 9, 511, 1976.
65. **Hata, T., Ogihara, T., Mikami, H., Nakamura, M., Mandai, T., and Kumahara, Y.,** Blood pressure response to (1-sarcosine, 8-isoleucine) angiotensin II in patients with liver cirrhosis and ascites, *Jpn. Circul. J.,* 43, 37, 1979.
66. **Saito, I., Saruta, T., Eguchi, T., Nakamura, R., Kondo, K., Igori, S., and Kato, E.,** Role of renin-angiotensin system in the controls of blood pressure and aldosterone in patients with cirrhosis and ascites, *Jpn. Heart J.,* 19, 741, 1978.
67. **Daskalopoulos, G., Pinzani, M., Murray, N., Hirschberg, R., and Zipser, R. D.,** Effects of captopril on renal function in patients with cirrhosis and ascites, *J. Hepatol.,* 4, 330, 1987.
68. **Douglas, W. W.,** Histamine, and 5-hydroxytryptamine (serotonin) and their antagonists, in *The Pharmacological Basis of Therapeutics,* 7th ed., Gilman, A. G., Goodman, L. S., Rall, T. W., and Murad, F., Eds., MacMillan, New York, 1986, 605.
69. **Jacob, G., Bishara, B., Lee, S. S., Hilzenart, N., and Bomzon, A.,** Cardiovascular responses to serolonin in experimental liver disease, *Hepatology,* submitted.
70. **Jacob, G., Bishara, B., Lee, S. S., Helzenart, N., and Bomzon, A.,** Cardiovascular responses to serotonin in experimental liver disease, *Hepatology,* 1989, submitted.
71. **Hadengue, A., Moreau, R., Cerini, R., Koshy, A., Lee, S. S., and Lebrec, D.,** Combination of ketanserin and verapamil or propranolol in patients with alcoholic cirrhosis; search for an additive effect, *Hepatology,* 9, 83, 1989.
72. **Schutz, W. J., Schrader, J., and Gerlach, E.,** Different sites of adenosine formation in the heart, *Am. J. Physiol.,* 240, H963, 1981.
73. **Lautt, W. W. and Greenway, C. V.,** Hepatic circulation in homeostasis, in *The Kidney in Liver Disease,* 3rd ed., Epstein, M., Ed., Williams & Wilkins, Baltimore, 1988, 244.
74. **Hamilton, H. W., Taylor, M. D., Steffen, R. P., Haleen, S. J., and Bruns, R. F.,** Correlation of adenosine receptor affinities and cardiovascular activity, *Life Sci.,* 41, 2295, 1987.
75. **Carmichael, F. J., Saldivia, V., Varghese, G. A., Israel, Y., and Orrego, H.,** Ethanol-induced increase in portal blood flow: role of acetate and A_1- and A_2-adenosine receptors, *Am. J. Physiol.,* 255, G417, 1988.
76. **Campbell, P., Skorecki, K., and Blendis, L. M.,** Atrial natriuretic peptide and its role in sodium retention in cirrhosis, in *The Cardiovascular Complications of Liver Disease,* Bomzon, A. and Blendis, L. M., Eds., CRC Press, Boca Raton, FL, 1990, chap. 15.
77. **Liard, J.-F.,** Vasopressin in cardiovascular regulation, in *Vasopressin Analogs and Portal Hypertension,* Lebrec, D. and Blei, A. T., Eds., John Libbey Eurotext, Paris, France, 1987, 1.
78. **Robinson, I, C, A, F., Melin, P., and Trojnar, J.,** Some aspects of the development of potent, specific and long-lasting pressor analogues of vasopressin, in *Vasopressin Analogs and Portal Hypertension,* Lebrec, D. and Blei, A. T., Eds., John Libbey Eurotext, Paris, France, 1987, 11.
79. **Lebrec, D. and Blei, A. T., Eds.,** *Vasopressin Analogs and Portal Hypertension,* John Libbey Eurotext, Paris, France, 1987.
80. **Levy, M. and Finestone, H.,** Renal response to four hours of biliary obstruction in the dog, *Am. J. Physiol.,* 244, F516, 1983.
81. **Benoit, J. N., Korthuis, R. J., Granger, D. N., and Battarbee, H. D.,** Splanchnic hemodynamics in acute and chronic portal hypertension in *The Cardiovascular Complications of Liver Disease* Bomzon, A. and Blendis, L. M., Eds., CRC Press, Boca Raton, FL, 1990, chap.9.
82. **Better, O. S. and Bomzon, A.,** Effects of jaundice on the renal and cardiovascular systems. in *The Kidney in Liver Disease,* 3rd ed., Epstein, M., Ed., Williams & Wilkins, Baltimore, 1988, 508.

Chapter 11

OXYGEN TRANSPORT AND CONSUMPTION IN CIRRHOSIS

Richard Moreau

TABLE OF CONTENTS

I. INTRODUCTION

A hyperdynamic systemic circulation (i.e., high cardiac output and low systemic vascular resistance) is often observed in cirrhosis, especially in patients with impaired liver function.[1-3] Recently, liver failure associated-hyperkineticism was found to be accompanied, in patients with cirrhosis, by an increase in systemic oxygen (O_2) transport to the tissues (which is the product of arterial O_2 content and cardiac output; see below and Table 1), and by a paradoxical reduction in O_2 uptake (i.e., in O_2 consumption, which is the product of arteriovenous O_2 content difference and cardiac output [see below and Table 1].[4] These alterations were associated with an increase in arterial lactate concentration in patients with liver failure, thus suggesting that a subclinical tissue hypoxia might explain the low O_2 consumption observed in these patients.[3] Similar results have also been reported in patients with fulminant hepatitis.[5]

Vasoactive drugs have been used to lower portal pressure in patients with cirrhosis. Drugs such as nitroglycerin,[6,7] vasopressin[8,9] and propranolol[7,10] decrease cardiac output and thereby decrease O_2 transport. Nitroglycerin, per se, may induce a reduction in arterial oxyhemoglobin saturation which contributes to the reduction in O_2 transport.[11] Drugs may also act at the microcirculatory level, either directly or via reflex changes of sympathetic outflow so that they may alter arteriolar tone and tissue O_2 extraction.[7]

In this chapter, we summarize the available evidence for abnormal tissue oxygenation in patients with cirrhosis. Moreover, effects of widely used vasoactive drugs in these patients, on O_2 transport and utilization, are also reviewed.

II. NORMAL AND ABNORMAL RELATIONSHIP BETWEEN OXYGEN TRANSPORT AND CONSUMPTION

The formulas used for the calculation of O_2 transport (Table 1) show that it depends on cardiovascular function (principally cardiac output) as well as on respiratory and hematopoietic systems (arterial oxyhemoglobin saturation and hemoglobin concentration, respectively).[4]

In the normal resting subjects, O_2 consumption reflects O_2 demand and is constant over a wide range of O_2 transport.[12] The critical delivery below which O_2 consumption becomes linearly dependent on O_2 transport was found to be equal to about 330 ml min^{-1} m^{-2} in humans.[12] Above this critical threshold tissue, O_2 demand is satisfied by the variations of the O_2 extraction ratio which increases when O_2 transport decreases and vice versa.[13] The oxygen extraction ratio reflects tissue O_2 extraction, which in turn appears to be regulated by functional capillary density.[14] Functional capillary density modulates the surface of exchange and the distance for diffusion of O_2 from capillary to cell, which is critical for mitochondrial function.[14]

It has been suggested that perfusion of the capillary network was under control of terminal arterioles and precapillary sphincters.[15] Vascular tone of these structures might be altered by local metabolites (e.g., adenosine)[14,15] and by neurohumoral factors.[15] For instance, when tissue pO_2 falls below a critical value, some local metabolite(s) may induce a relaxation of precapillary sphincters, resulting in capillary recruitment.[15] Adequate O_2 supply to cells also supposes that the appropriate blood flow is delivered to tissues according to regional needs.[13] This is particularly important in situations characterized by values of O_2 transport approaching the critical threshold. Cain has shown that conservation of a vasoconstrictor arteriolar tone was necessary to optimize tissue O_2 extraction when O_2 transport was critically decreased.[16] Vascular smooth muscle tone of resistance vessels may be altered by neurohumoral factors and by local metabolite(s).[15]

Recently, it has been suggested that O_2 consumption was abnormally dependent on O_2

TABLE 1

Calculation and Normal Range of Oxygen (O_2)-Derived Variables

	Calculation	Normal range
Arterial O_2 content (CaO_2) (ml/dl)	$CaO_2 = ([Hb]^a \times 1.34 \times SaO_2^b) + 0.003\ PaO_2^c$	15—20
Mixed venous O_2 content ($C\bar{v}O_2$) (ml/dl)	$C\bar{v}O_2 = ([Hb] \times 1.34 \times S\bar{v}O_2) + 0.003\ P\bar{v}O_2$	10—15
Arteriovenous O_2 content difference (AVD) (ml/dl)	$AVD = CaO_2 - C\bar{v}O_2$	3.5—5.0
O_2 extraction ration (O_2 Ext) (%)	$O_2\ Ext = AVD/CaO_2$	22—30
O_2 transport (O_2 T) (ml min^{-1} m^{-2})	$O_2\ T = CaO_2 \times$ cardiac index $\times$ 10	520—720
O_2 consumption (VO_2) (ml min^{-1} m^{-2})	$VO_2 = AVD \times$ cardiac index $\times$ 10	120—160

[a]   [Hb] means hemoglobin concentration.

[b] SO_2 means measured oxyhemoglobin saturation.

[c] PO_2 means measured O_2 tension.

transport in patients with adult respiratory distress syndrome,[17] septic shock,[18] and fulminant hepatitis.[5] Indeed, O_2 consumption was found to change in the same direction as O_2 transport, whereas O_2 transport was above the value usually considered as critical.[17,18,5] This pathologic O_2 supply dependency would result from an abnormal limitation of tissue O_2 extraction, due to microcirculatory derangements whose mechanisms remain to be determined.[19,20] As a result, satisfaction of tissue O_2 needs would depend abnormally on the magnitude of the blood flow.[19] This abnormal O_2-supply dependency, by exposure to tissue hypoxia, could contribute to the multiple-organ failure observed in patients with either adult respiratory distress syndrome or severe sepsis.[21]

In patients with congestive heart failure, O_2 consumption also appears to be dependent on O_2 transport.[22] However, this O_2-supply dependency is consistent with the physiologic O_2-supply dependency rather than with the pathologic supply dependency, both described by Cain.[19] Indeed, in heart failure, it is the decreased cardiac output and O_2 transport which are the main abnormalities. Oxygen consumption becomes dependent on O_2 transport when the latter is below the critical threshold since tissue O_2 extraction is already maximal.

III. OXYGEN TRANSPORT AND CONSUMPTION IN CIRRHOSIS: EVIDENCE FOR ABNORMAL TISSUE OXYGENATION

Features compatible with tissue hypoxia have recently been observed in patients with cirrhosis and hepatic insufficiency.[3] We have studied patients with alcoholic cirrhosis and control alcoholic patients without cirrhosis.[3] There were 20 grade A (Pugh Grade),[23,24] 16 grade B, and 17 grade C and 20 controls, matched for age and sex. The main results are shown in Table 2. These results confirm previous findings which showed that O_2 transport significantly increased during deterioration of liver function.[3] This was due to the significant increase in cardiac output which offset the significant reduction of arterial O_2 content observed in grade C patients. This reduction was accounted for by the significant diminution of hemoglobin concentration (Table 4). These data also showed that O_2 consumption was significantly decreased in grade C patients as previously found.[3]

The decrease in O_2 consumption in patients with marked hepatic insufficiency might result from an overestimation of body weight and body surface area of grade C patients with ascites. This would in turn underestimate the cardiac index, and thus O_2 consumption. Such a possibility can be excluded, inasmuch as we used a corrected body weight for the determination of body surface area, i.e., the measured weight at the time of the study minus the estimated weight of ascites. One can also argue that decreased O_2 uptake was artifactual, as we used calculated (Fick principle), and not measured O_2 consumption (which is obtained by measuring the inspired and expired gas concentrations). However, our results do fit with previous findings showing that measured O_2 consumption decreased while cardiac output increased in patients with cirrhosis.[25] Chappell et al. have shown that calculated and measured O_2 consumption were significantly correlated (r = 0.9).[26] In this study, the decrease in mixed venous carbon dioxide tension (reflecting a reduced production of carbon dioxide) is consistent with the existence of a decreased metabolic activity in patients with deteriorating liver function.

Several lines of evidence support the view that low O_2 consumption resulted from O_2 deprivation, i.e., from tissue hypoxia, in grade C patients. In other words, whole-body O_2 demand in these patients appears to be unsatisfied. First, O_2 consumption increased when cardiac output and systemic O_2 transport were augmented by means of dobutamine (Table 3 and Figure 1).[7] These increases in O_2 consumption were unexpected since, usually, changes in O_2 transport, such as those observed in the latter study are not accompanied by alterations in O_2 uptake. We have shown that increases in cardiac output and systemic O_2 transport induced by dobutamine in three patients without cirrhosis were not accompanied by alterations

TABLE 2

Systemic Hemodynamics, Oxygen (O_2) Transport, and Utilization in Alcoholic Patients without Cirrhosis and in Patients with Alcoholic Cirrhosis Classified According to the Degree of Liver Failure by Means of Pugh's Classification

	Patients without cirrhosis	Patients with cirrhosis		
		Grade A	Grade B	Grade C
No. of patients	20	20	16	17
Heart rate (beats/min)	79 ± 13[a]	72 ± 19	87 ± 12[b,c]	89 ± 12 [b,c]
Mean arterial pressure (mmHg)	97 ± 12	94 ± 12	91 ± 10	89 ± 15
Cardiac index ($1\ min^{-1}\ m^{-2}$)	3.72 ± 0.88	3.78 ± 0.58	4.33 ± 1.05	5.15 ± 100[b,c]
Systemic vascular resistance index (dyne s $cm^{-5}\ m^2$)	2055 ± 489	2014 ± 440	1786 ± 577	1393 ± 429[b,c]
O_2 transport (ml $min^{-1}\ m^{-2}$)	637 ± 185	597 ± 115	644 ± 208	705 ± 186[c]
O_2 consumption (ml $min^{-1}\ m^{-2}$)	146 ± 23	141 ± 19	130 ± 23	117 ± 24[b,c]
Arteriovenous O_2 content difference (ml/dl)	4.1 ± 0.9	3.8 ± 0.7	3.1 ± 0.6[b]	2.3 ± 0.4[b,c]
O_2 extraction ratio (%)	23 ± 6	24 ± 3	21 ± 5	17 ± 3[b,c]
Arterial lactate concentration (mmol/l)	0.8 ± 0.4	0.7 ± 0.3	0.9 ± 0.4	1.5 ± 1.2[b,c]
Arterial O_2 content (ml/dl)	17.0 ± 2.0	15.8 ± 2.4	14.7 ± 2.1[b]	13.6 ± 2.0[b,c]
Arterial O_2 tension (mmHg)	86 ± 15	85 ± 10	86 ± 14	81 ± 17
Arterial oxyhemoglobin saturation (%)	92 ± 2	97 ± 1	96 ± 1	95 ± 3
Arterial carbon dioxide tension (mmHg)	37 ± 5	36 ± 3	34 ± 3	33 ± 4[c]
Mixed venous O_2 content (ml/dl)	12.9 ± 2.1	12.4 ± 1.9	11.6 ± 2.2	11.3 ± 1.9
Mixed venous O_2 tension (mmHg)	39 ± 4	40 ± 3	42 ± 4	43 ± 3
Mixed venous oxyhemoglobin saturation (%)	74 ± 6	74 ± 8	76 ± 5	80 ± 4[b,c]
Mixed venous carbon dioxide tension (mmHg)	42 ± 5	40 ± 2	37 ± 3[b]	36 ± 4[b,c]
Hemoglobin concentration (g/dl)	13.0 ± 0.5	12.1 ± 1.8	11.4 ± 1.5[b]	10.4 ± 1.6[b,c]

Note: Statistical analysis was performed by means of one-way analysis of variance with a Bonferroni correction for multiple comparisons.

[a] Mean ± SD.
[b] Significantly different from patients without cirrhosis.
[c] Significantly different from grade A patients ($p < 0.05$).

TABLE 3
Oxygen (O_2) Transport and Utilization in Patients with Alcoholic Cirrhosis Who Received Dobutamine and Propranolol

	Basal values	During dobutamine infusion[a]	After propranolol administration
Cardiac index (l min^{-1} m^{-2})	3.84 ± 0.74[b]	4.84 ± 0.90[c]	2.90 ± 0.66[c]
Systemic vascular resistance index (dyne s cm^{-5} m^2)	1752 ± 399	1324 ± 348[c]	2206 ± 452[c]
Hemoglobin concentration (g/dl)	10.1 ± 1.8	10.1 ± 1.6	10.1 ± 1.8
Arterial O_2 content (ml/dl)	14.3 ± 1.2	14.5 ± 1.5	14.0 ± 1.5
Mixed venous O_2 content (ml/dl)	11.1 ± 1.8	11.6 ± 1.8	10.1 ± 1.8[c]
O_2 extraction ratio (%)	23 ± 6	20 ± 6	28 ± 6[c]
Arterial lactate concentration (mmol/l)	1.0 ± 0.1	0.8 ± 0.1	0.9 ± 0.3

[a] The results reported are those of the 9 patients in whom dobutamine increased cardiac output. (See text and Reference 7.)

[b] Mean ± SD.

[c] Significantly different from basal values ($p < 0.05$). A Dunnett's test for multiple comparisons was used.

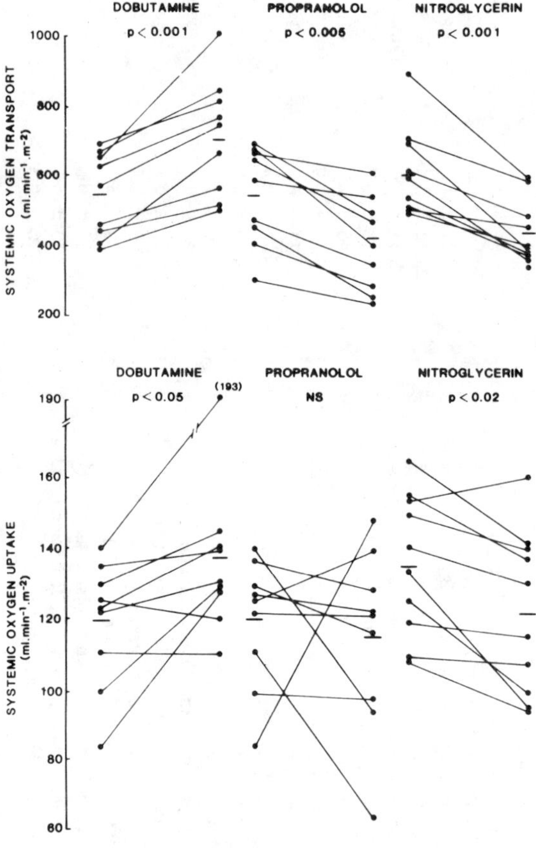

FIGURE 1.   Systemic oxygen transport and uptake before and after drug administration in patients with cirrhosis. (From Moreau, R., *Hepatology*, 9, 427, 1989. Copyright © by the American Association for the Study of Liver Diseases. With permission.)

TABLE 4
Oxygen (O_2) Transport and Utilization in Patients with Alcoholic Cirrhosis
Who Received Nitroglycerin

	Basal values	During nitroglycerin infusion
Cardiac index (l min^{-1} m^{-2})	4.60 ± 0.99[a]	3.47 ± 0.60[b]
Systemic vascular resistance index (dyne s cm^{-5} m^2)	1645 ± 417	1705 ± 426
Hemoglobin concentration (g/dl)	10.1 ± 1.5	9.9 ± 1.5
Arterial O_2 content (ml/dl)	13.4 ± 2.1	12.7 ± 1.8[b]
Mixed venous O_2 content (ml/dl)	10.3 ± 1.8	9.1 ± 1.5[b]
O_2 extraction ratio (%)	23 ± 3	28 ± 6[b]
Arterial lactate concentration (mmol/l)	0.9 ± 0.1	1.3 ± 0.3[b]

[a] Mean ± SD.
[b] Significantly different from basal values ($p < 0.05$).

in whole-body O_2 consumption.[7] In addition, O_2 consumption decreased in patients with cirrhosis when cardiac output and O_2 transport were reduced by means of nitroglycerin (Table 4 and Figure 1). In this study, O_2 transport, although decreased, was always in the normal range.[7] Taken together, these results suggested that O_2 consumption might be abnormally dependent on O_2 transport in cirrhosis.[7] This might indicate that a basal O_2 debt was repaid (at least partially) by dobutamine infusion and was worsened by that of nitroglycerin.

Second, we found that arterial lactate concentration was higher in grade C patients than in grade A patients (Table 3), thus suggesting that anaerobic metabolism occurred with hepatic insufficiency.[3,5] However, blood lactate accumulation can be ascribed to hepatic underutilization of lactate due to a reduction in gluconeogenesis by the diseased liver. Hypoglycemia and hyperlactatemia have been found in association with impaired liver function.[27] This view does not rule out the liver failure-associated tissue hypoxia hypothesis. Indeed, deranged lactate uptake by the diseased liver might be related to hepatic hypoxia.[28,29] Evidence for this was found in noncirrhotic animals, in which graded tissue hypoxia was followed by a progressive reduction in hepatic uptake of lactate, and eventually by a conversion of the liver from a lactate-consuming to a lactate-producing organ.[30] Similar findings were observed in normal humans subjected to hypoxemia.[31] Moreover, the dependence of hepatic gluconeogenesis on O_2 is well established.[32]

A decrease in hepatic O_2 consumption, assessed by organ reflectance spectrophotometry, has been described in patients with cirrhosis.[33] In the latter study, there was also a significant correlation between hepatic O_2 consumption and some liver function tests such as serum albumin concentration and prothrombin time.[33] Therefore, it may be speculated that liver failure is associated with defective lactate processing and hypoglycemia, both related to hypoxia-induced decrease in gluconeogenesis.

IV. MECHANISMS OF TISSUE HYPOXIA IN CIRRHOSIS

Three different mechanisms of tissue hypoxia are possible in cirrhosis: (1) limitation of tissue O_2 extraction; (2) Limitation of the augmentation of O_2 transport; and (3) changes in affinity of hemoglobin for O_2. Limitation of tissue O_2 extraction, due to arteriovenous shunting, is supported in our patients with impaired liver function by the low O_2 extraction ratio and the high mixed venous blood oxyhemoglobin saturation, both associated with decreased systemic vascular resistance (Table 2). In addition, systemic vascular resistance was significantly correlated in all patients with O_2 extraction ratio and with arterial lactate concentration. These results suggest that derangement of tissue oxygenation could be related to an abnormal regulation of the microcirculation. Furthermore, limitation of tissue O_2

extraction is also demonstrated by the abnormal O_2-supply dependency, evidenced by pharmacological manipulation of O_2 transport in our patients (see below). An abnormal limitation of hepatic O_2 extraction might also contribute to the decrease in the hepatic O_2 consumption previously described.[33] Intrahepatic shunts[34] and capillarization of sinusoids[34] as well as impaired control of blood flow distribution in hepatic microcirculation,[35] are well-known complications of cirrhosis that may act by augmenting the distance for diffusion of O_2 from blood to cells which is critical for mitochondrial respiration.[36]

Tissue hypoxia might be due to a limitation of O_2 transport to tissues. This, in turn, might be related to either an insufficient increase in cardiac output or to a decrease in arterial O_2 content. Recently, Mikulic et al. have shown that plasma from patients with alcoholic cirrhosis depresses contractility of cultured rat heart cells.[37] Plasma from control patients was devoid of effects on these cells.[37] This was the first study showing that plasma of patients with alcoholic cirrhosis may contain a myocardial depressant factor. Therefore, myocardial depression might hinder the augmentation of cardiac output and of O_2 transport in patients with hepatic failure. In addition, the decrease in arterial O_2 content, due to the reduction in hemoglobin concentration, also contributes to limit the increase in O_2 transport in patients with hepatic insufficiency (Table 2). Thus, it is possible that, in these patients, O_2 transport, although apparently increased, was in fact limited. This limitation together with that of tissue O_2 extraction could account for the low O_2 consumption.

Finally, a leftward shift of the oxyhemoglobin dissociation curve, by increasing the affinity of hemoglobin for O_2, might reduce O_2 unloading to tissues and thereby might contribute to decrease O_2 consumption. However, this mechanism remains questionable[38] and it is a rightward shift of the dissociation curve, which is usually observed in patients with cirrhosis.[39]

V. EFFECTS OF VASOACTIVE DRUGS ON OXYGEN TRANSPORT AND CONSUMPTION IN CIRRHOSIS

We used four different drugs to change O_2 transport in order to define the pathophysiologic derangements in O_2 utilization in cirrhosis. First, O_2 transport and consumption were increased by dobutamine. Second, O_2 transport was decreased, and tissue oxygenation was impaired by nitroglycerin and vasopressin. Third, O_2 transport was decreased and tissue oxygenation status maintained by propranolol. Although different, these situations might be explained by a common abnormality, i.e., by the fact that the O_2 consumption may be abnormally dependent on O_2 transport in patients with cirrhosis, due to a limitation of tissue O_2 extraction mainly related to the underlying disease. Drugs could unmask this abnormal relationship by altering O_2 supply to tissues through change in cardiac output, arterial oxygenation, or vascular smooth muscle tone.[7] In addition, these drugs may modify O_2 needs by changing endogenous catecholamine-induced O_2 demand.[40]

A. DOBUTAMINE

Dobutamine is a synthetic catecholamine that stimulates β_1 adrenergic receptors.[41] This drug is widely used in the treatment of circulatory failure complicating cirrhosis. It has been shown that dobutamine did not alter portal pressure in these patients.[42] We studied the effects of dobutamine on O_2 transport and consumption in cirrhosis.[7] Fourteen grade B patients[23] were studied as previously described.[7] The drug was also infused in three patients without cirrhosis (control patients).[7] The dose of dobutamine was increased until cardiac output elevation reached 15%. Doses administered ranged from 5 to 15 μg kg^{-1} min^{-1}. In nine patients with cirrhosis, dobutamine infusion was accompanied by a significant increase in cardiac output ($+21\%$), oxygen transport ($+21\%$), and in O_2 consumption ($+21\%$). The oxygen extraction ratio did not change. The results are summarized in Table 3 and Figure

1. In five cirrhotic patients, dobutamine did not significantly increase cardiac output (4.90 ± 0.89 and 4.76 ± 1.00 $l \cdot min^{-1} \cdot m^{-2}$ before and during dobutamine infusion, respectively). The corresponding values of O_2 transport were 661 ± 123 and 633 ± 104 ml min^{-1} m^{-2}, respectively. Values of O_2 consumption were 109 ± 18 and 107 ± 14 ml min^{-1} m^{-2}, respectively. No significant changes were observed in these patients. In control patients, increases in O_2 transport were not accompanied by an augmentation in O_2 consumption.

Catecholamines increase whole-body O_2 demand by a direct effect on oxidative metabolism.[21] Thus dobutamine might have increased O_2 consumption by increasing O_2 demand. However, this effect was unlikely to be the sole factor responsible for the increased O_2 consumption, since the expected elevation in O_2 extraction[43] was not observed. In addition, we have previously shown that the dobutamine-induced increase in myocardial O_2 consumption could not account for changes in whole-body O_2 consumption.[7] Therefore, it appears that the elevation in O_2 consumption probably resulted from the increase in O_2 transport. Increases in O_2 consumption were obtained only in those patients in whom O_2 transport was augmented. By contrast, when dobutamine was administered to patients without cirrhosis, O_2 consumption remained unchanged, whereas O_2 transport was increased. These results support the contention that O_2 consumption may be abnormally dependent on O_2 transport in patients with cirrhosis, and that this abnormal O_2-supply dependency was related to the underlying disease rather than to the drug itself.[7] These results also suggest that O_2 demand, in the basal conditions, was not satisfied in our patients.

B. NITROGLYCERIN

Nitroglycerin is a venodilator which has been proposed for treatment of portal hypertension in patients with cirrhosis[44] and to counteract the adverse effects of vasopressin on systemic hemodynamics.[6,45] Effects of intravenous nitroglycerin on O_2 transport and consumption in patients with cirrhosis had never been studied until recently.[7] Ten grade B patients have been investigated as previously described.[7] They received incremental doses of nitroglycerin until mean arterial pressure was decreased by about 20% during 20 min. Doses infused ranged from 25 to 75 μg/min. The results are shown in Table 4 and in Figure 1.

Nitroglycerin decreased significantly cardiac output (-21%), arterial O_2 content (-5%), O_2 transport (-26%), and O_2 consumption (-10%), while O_2 extraction ratio ($+18\%$) and arterial lactate concentration ($+31\%$) were significantly increased. The reducing effects of nitroglycerin on cardiac output[46] as well as on arterial O_2 content[11] are well-known complications in patients without cirrhosis.

It has been shown, in patients with cirrhosis, that nitroglycerin induced a significant increase in plasma norepinephrine concentration.[47] Catecholamines are known to increase whole-body O_2 demand.[21] Therefore, the nitroglycerin-associated decrease in O_2 consumption was not due to a diminution of whole-body O_2 demand.

The frank increase in arterial lactate concentration suggests that O_2 deprivation was related to an imbalance between an augmented O_2 demand and a decreased O_2 supply. Since the reduction in O_2 consumption occurred while O_2 transport, although decreased, was above the critical threshold, this shows that an abnormal limitation of tissue O_2 extraction impeded the compensation for the decrease in O_2 transport. In other words, O_2 consumption became abnormally dependent on O_2 transport. This can be ascribed to drug effects per se. Indeed, nitroglycerin is not only a venous dilator but also exerts a dilating effect on resistance vessels.[46] This would cause relative overperfusion of tissues with low O_2 requirements, during a period of limited O_2 delivery.[16] As a result, tissue O_2 extraction by actively respiring tissues could be insufficient. However, the decrease in O_2 consumption, while O_2 transport is reduced by nitroglycerin, might be explained by an abnormal limitation of tissue O_2 extraction associated with circulatory derangement of cirrhosis as discussed above. This

TABLE 5
Systemic Hemodynamics, Oxygen (O_2) Transport, and Utilization in 11 Patients with Alcoholic Cirrhosis and in Control Patients' during Vasopressin Infusion

	Patients with cirrhosis		Control patients	
	Basal values	During vasopressin infusion	Basal values	During vasopressin infusion
Heart rate (beats/min)	79 ± 18[a]	66 ± 14[b]	90 ± 12	80 ± 11
Mean arterial pressure (mmHg)	87 ± 11	98 ± 7[b]	97 ± 5	96 ± 8
Cardiac index (l min^{-1} m^{-2})	4.16 ± 0.91	3.67 ± 0.93[b]	3.58 ± 0.52	2.81 ± 0.43[b]
Systemic vascular resistance index (dyne s cm^{-5} m^2)	1699 ± 374	2111 ± 521[b]	2132 ± 357	2622 ± 479
Hemoglobin concentration (g/dl)	12.1 ± 2.0	12.0 ± 2.0	13.3 ± 1.9	13.2 ± 1.8
Arterial O_2 content (ml/dl)	15.9 ± 2.6	15.7 ± 2.8	17.6 ± 2.5	17.5 ± 2.2
Mixed venous O_2 content (ml/dl)	12.5 ± 2.0	11.9 ± 2.4[b]	13.6 ± 2.4	13.0 ± 2.7
O_2 transport (ml min^{-1} m^{-2})	655 ± 136	577 ± 178[b]	628 ± 128	497 ± 130
O_2 consumption (ml min^{-1} m^{-2})	133 ± 23	133 ± 22[b]	141 ± 12	124 ± 15
O_2 extraction ratio (%)	21 ± 3	25 ± 5[b]	22 ± 3	26 ± 6
Arterial lactate concentration (mmol/l)	0.7 ± 0.3	1.1 ± 0.2[b]	0.9 ± 0.3	1.4 ± 0.7[b]

[a] Mean ± SD.
[b] Significantly different from basal values ($p < 0.05$).

view is supported by the fact that decreases in O_2 transport and consumption have been noted in patients with chronic respiratory failure[48] in whom an abnormal O_2 supply dependency has recently been shown by nonpharmacological means.[49] By contrast, nitroglycerin decreased O_2 transport without change in O_2 consumption in patients with toxemia of pregnancy, complicated by pulmonary edema.[50] Furthermore, when nitroglycerin was given to patients with chronic heart failure, an augmentation of O_2 transport and consumption was observed.[22] Therefore, our results support the view that cirrhosis is associated with an abnormal O_2 supply dependency exposing to tissue hypoxia. Nitroglycerin could further aggravate this tissue hypoxia.

C. VASOPRESSIN

Vasopressin is a potent vasoconstrictor which stimulates V_1-receptors.[51] It is widely used for treatment of variceal hemorrhages complicating portal hypertension.[51] However, its utilization is limited by untoward effects on systemic hemodynamics related to systemic vasoconstriction and the subsequent vasopressor effect.[9]

We performed hemodynamic studies in 11 patients with alcoholic cirrhosis. There were seven grade A patients, two grade B, and two grade C patients. In addition, we had the opportunity to investigate five patients without cirrhosis (control patients).[58] All patients received intravenously 0.4 U/min of vasopressin for 30 min. In patients with cirrhosis, drug infusion was accompanied by significant decreases in cardiac output (-15%) and O_2 transport (-15%), and by significant increases in O_2 extraction ratio ($+20\%$) and arterial lactate concentration ($+50\%$). Oxygen consumption was unchanged (Table 5). Vasopressin elicited similar effects in nonalcoholic patients as well as in cirrhotic patients, with respect to cardiac output, O_2-transport, and arterial lactate concentration. However, O_2 consumption decreased in the former patients. A peak increase in arterial pressure associated with a reflex-decrease in heart rate occurred 5 to 9 min after drug infusion was started in cirrhotic and in noncirrhotic patients (data not shown). Previous hemodynamic studies in patients with cirrhosis found comparable results to ours with regard to effects of vasopressin on systemic hemodynamics, O_2 transport, and consumption.[8,52]

What are the reasons for the decline in O_2 consumption in the control patients that did not occur in patients with cirrhosis? Two factors may have contributed to this result in noncirrhotic patients. First, vasopressin, per se, could have induced an abnormal O_2-supply dependency, since in these patients, O_2 consumption decreased, while values of O_2 transport were above those usually considered as critical.[12] The abnormality of these results was evidenced by the elevation of arterial concentration lactate. Thus, vasopressin could have induced a limitation of both tissue O_2 extraction and O_2 transport. These observations are in keeping with the known effects of vasopressin on the intestinal circulation. It has been shown that vasopressin reduced intestinal O_2 uptake, by decreasing both functional capillary density (and thus O_2 extraction) and local blood flow.[53]

Second, there could have been a decrease in whole-body O_2 demand in control patients. It has been demonstrated that vasopressin augments, in normal subjects, arterial and central venous pressures, and thereby activates baroreceptors.[54,55] This activation could, in turn, induce a decrease in sympathetic outflow which is one of the regulatory responses aimed at reducing arterial pressure.[54] This decrease in sympathetic activity could account for the diminution in whole-body O_2 demand and thereby contributes to the decrease in O_2 consumption in these patients, in whom normally baroreceptor function is demonstrated by the adequate decrease in arterial pressure at 30 min. (Table 5). In our patients with cirrhosis, the frank elevation of arterial lactate concentration during vasopressin infusion resulted from O_2 deprivation. This is reinforced by the significant decrease in mixed venous pH (from 7.41 ± 0.03 to 7.39 ± 0.03, before and during drug infusion, respectively). Thus, the change in O_2 consumption during drug infusion was abnormal, that is, more O_2 should have been consumed to meet O_2 needs which were necessarily augmented by comparison with the basal conditions. Therefore, O_2 consumption should have been greater than in basal conditions, if consumable O_2 had been supplied in sufficient quantity. As these events occurred, while reduced O_2 transport was still above the critical threshold, one can conclude that our patients were in a situation of abnormal O_2-supply dependency owing to an insufficient rise in tissue O_2 extraction. This limitation of O_2 tissue extraction can be ascribed to the drug itself inasmuch as there were several grade A patients in this study who were thus comparable to control patients. The underlying disease together with vasopressin contributed to limit tissue O_2 extraction in the remaining patients. The increase in whole-body O_2 demand during drug infusion might be related to an absence of baroreflex-mediated decrease in sympathetic outflow—suggested by the persistent increase in arterial pressure in cirrhotic patients (Table 5) — along with some factors related to cirrhosis which remain to be elucidated. Therefore, vasopressin itself and the underlying disease act in concert to induce an abnormal O_2-supply dependency which is responsible for tissue hypoxia when O_2 transport is reduced by the drug.

D. PROPRANOLOL

Propranolol is a nonselective β_1 and β_2 adrenoreceptor antagonist.[10] Propranolol has been proposed by Lebrec et al. to decrease portal pressure in patients with cirrhosis.[10]

Nine grade B patients[23] were studied as previously described (see above and Reference 7). Hemodynamic studies and laboratory measures were performed 15 min. after the administration of 15 mg of propranolol intravenous. The results are shown in Table 3 and in Figure 1. Propranolol significantly decreased cardiac output (-24%), O_2 transport (-25%), and significantly increased O_2 extraction ratio $(+19\%)$, whereas O_2 consumption and arterial lactate concentration did not change.

Therefore, our patients with cirrhosis and impaired liver function appear to react to the reduction of O_2 transport in the same manner as normal subjects would be expected to. This could seem contradictory with the previously postulated abnormal O_2-supply dependency in cirrhosis.[7] However, propranolol may act on factors that contribute to abnormal O_2-supply dependency so that O_2 consumption does not decrease with O_2 transport. In this regard, propranolol may decrease whole-body O_2 demand by reducing endogenous catecholamine-related O_2 demand.[56] In addition, propranolol may improve tissue O_2 extraction. Indeed, propranolol is a vasoconstrictor agent as evidenced by the increase in systemic vascular resistance which followed its administration in our patients (Table 3). It has been shown that the increase in arteriolar tone is an important factor contributing to optimize tissue O_2 extraction when O_2 delivery is limited.[16] It must be noted that the lack of change in O_2 consumption after propranolol does not mean that O_2 debt was absent in basal conditions. Normal arterial lactate concentration does not disprove tissue hypoxia.[57] Part of basal O_2 demand might be ascribed to extramitochondrial oxidases that are sensitive to small decreases in cell PO_2.[57]

VI. CONCLUSIONS

Our results suggest that tissue hypoxia could occur in patients with cirrhosis, in association with the circulatory hyperkineticism accompanying liver failure. Oxygen deprivation appears to be due to arteriovenous shunting-induced limitation of tissue O_2 extraction. Additionally, insufficient increase in O_2 transport may contribute to impaired O_2 supply to tissues. Limitation of tissue O_2 extraction is responsible for an abnormal O_2-supply dependency which may be unmasked by using drugs such as nitroglycerin and vasopressin. These drugs, by decreasing O_2 transport and by inducing further derangement in the regulation of tissue O_2 extraction may aggravate the underlying tissue hypoxia. Propranolol, by contrast, does not appear to have similar deleterious effects.

REFERENCES

1. **Valla, D., Poynard, T., Bercoff, E., Bataille, C., Goldfarb, G., and Lebrec, D.,** Le syndorme d'hypercinésie circulatoire systémique chez les malades atteints de cirrhose. Relations avec l'insuffisance hépatocellulaire et l'hypertension portale, *Gastroentérol. Clin. Biol.,* 8, 321, 1984.
2. **Braillon, A., Cales, P., Valla, D., Gaudy, D., Geoffroy, P., and Lebrec, D.,** Influence of the degree of liver failure on systemic and splanchnic haemodynamics and on response to propranolol in patients with cirrhosis, *Gut,* 27, 1204, 1986.
3. **Moreau, R., Lee, S. S., Soupison, T., Roche-Sicot, J., and Sicot, C.,** Abnormal tissue oxygenation in patients with cirrhosis and liver failure, *J. Hepatol.,* 7, 98, 1988.
4. **Fromm, R. E., Guimond, J. G., Darby, J., and Snyder, J. V.,** The craft of cardiopulmonary profile analysis, in *Oxygen Transport in the Cricitally Ill,* Snyder, J. V. and Pinsky, M. R., Eds., Year Book Medical Publishers, Chicago, 1987, 249.
5. **Bihari, D. J., Gimson, A. E. S., and Williams, R.,** Disturbances in cardiovascular and pulmonary function in fulminant hepatic failure, in *Liver Failure,* Williams, R., Ed., Churchill Livingstone, London, 1986, 47.
6. **Westaby, D., Gimson, A., Hayes, P. C., and Williams, R.,** Haemodynamic response to intravenous vasopressin and nitroglycerin in portal hypertension, *Gut,* 29, 372, 1988.
7. **Moreau, R., Lee, S. S., Hadengue, A., Ozier, Y., Sicot, C., and Lebrec, D.,** Relationship between oxygen transport and oxygen uptake in patients with cirrhosis: effects of vasoactive drugs. *Hepatology,* 9, 427, 1989.
8. **Naeije, R., Hallemans, R., Mols, P., Mélot, C., and Reding, P.,** Effects of vasopressin and somatostatin on hemodynamics and blood gases in patients with liver cirrhosis, *Crit. Care Med.,* 10, 578, 1982.
9. **Moreau, R., Hadengue, A., Soupison, T., Méchin, G., Assous, M., Roche-Sicot, J., and Sicot, C.,** Y a-t-il intérêt à associer la trinitrine à la vasopressine chez les malades atteints de cirrhose alcoolique?, *Gastroentérol. Clin. Biol.,* (Abstr.), 13, 170, 1989.

10. **Lebrec, D., Hillon, P., Munoz, C., Goldfarb, G., Noel, O., and Benhamou, J. P.,** The effect of propranolol on portal hypertension in patients with cirrhosis: a hemodynamic study, *Hepatology,* 2, 523, 1982.

11. **Mookherjee, S., Fuleihan, D., Warner, R. A., Vardan, S., and Obeid, A. N.,** Effects of sublingual nitroglycerin on resting pulmonary gas exchange and hemodynamics in man, *Circulation,* 57, 106, 1978.

12. **Sibutani, K., Komatsu, T., Kubal, K., Sanchala, V., Kumar, V., and Bizzarri, V.,** Critical level of oxygen delivery in anesthetized man, *Crit. Care Med.,* 11, 640, 1983.

13. **Schumacker, P. T. and Cain, S. M.,** The concept of a critical oxygen delivery, *Intensive Care Med.,* 13, 223, 1987.

14. **Granger, H. J., Goodman, A. H., and Cook, B. H.,** Metabolic models of microcirculatory regulation, *Fed. Proc.,* 34, 2025, 1975.

15. **Renkin, E. M.,** Control of microcirculation and blood-tissue exchange, in *Handbook of Physiology, Section 2: The Cardiovascular System,* Vol. 4, (Part 2), American Physiological Society, Washington, D.C., 1984, 627.

16. **Cain, S. M.,** Effects of time and vasoconstrictor tone on O_2 extraction during hypoxic hypoxia, *J. Appl. Physiol.,* 45, 219, 1978.

17. **Danek, S. J., Lynch, J. P., Weg, J. G., and Dantzker, D. R.,** The dependence of oxygen uptake on oxygen delivery in the adult respiratory distress syndrome, *Am. Rev. Respir. Dis.,* 122, 387, 1980.

18. **Kaufman, B. S., Rackow, E. C., and Falk, J. L.,** The relationship between oxygen delivery and consumption during fluid resuscitation of hypovolemic and septic shock, *Chest,* 85, 336, 1984.

19. **Cain, S. M.,** Supply dependency of oxygen uptake in ARDS: myth or reality?, *Am. J. Med. Sci.,* 288, 119, 1984.

20. **Nelson, D. P., Beyer, C., Samsel, R. W., Wood, L. D. H., and Schumacker, P. T.,** Pathological supply dependence of O_2 uptake during bacteremia in dogs, *J. Appl. Physiol.,* 63, 1487, 1987.

21. **Cain, S. M.,** Peripheral oxygen uptake and delivery in health and disease, *Clin. Chest Med.,* 4, 139, 1983.

22. **Mohsenifar, Z., Amin, D., Jasper, A. C., Shah, P. K., and Koerner, S. K.,** Dependence of oxygen consumption on oxygen delivery in patients with chronic congestive heart failure, *Chest,* 92, 447, 1987.

23. **Pugh, R. N. H., Murray-Lyon, I. M., Dawson, J. L., Pietroni, M. C., and Williams, R.,** Transection of the oesophagus for bleeding oesophageal varices, *Br. J. Surg.,* 60, 646, 1973.

24. **Moreau, R. and Sicot, C.,** Évaluation du pronostic à court terme des cirrhotiques admis en réanimation, à l'aide de 4 indices de gravité, *Gastroentérol. Clin. Biol.,* 9, 871, 1985.

25. **Kowalski, H. J. and Abelmann, W. H.,** The cardiac output at rest in Laennec's cirrhosis, *J. Clin. Invest.,* 32, 1025, 1953.

26. **Chappell, T. R., Rubin, L. J., Marham, R. V., and Firth, B. C.,** Independence of oxygen consumption and systemic oxygen transport in patients with either stable pulmonary hypertension or refractory left ventricular failute, *Am. Rev. Respir. Dis.,* 128, 30, 1983.

27. **Medalle, R., Webb, R., and Waterhouse, C.,** Lactic acidosis and associated hypoglycemia, *Arch. Intern. Med.,* 128, 273, 1971.

28. **Cain, S. M.,** Appearance of excess lactate in anesthetized dogs during anemic and hypoxic hypoxia, *Am. J. Physiol.,* 209, 604, 1965.

29. **Madias, N. E.,** Lactic acidosis, *Kidney Int.,* 29, 752, 1986.

30. **Tashkin, D. P., Goldstein, P. J., and Simmons, D. H.,** Hepatic lactate uptake during decreased liver perfusion and hypoxemia, *Am. J. Physiol.,* 223, 968, 1972.

31. **Rowell, B., Brengelmann, L., Backmon, R., Twiss, D., and Kusumi, F.,** Splanchnic blood flow and metabolism in heat-stressed man. *J. Appl. Physiol.,* 24, 475, 1968.

32. **Romero, F. J., Pallardo, F. V., Bolinches, R., Roma, J., Saez, G. T., Noll, T., and DeGroot, H.,** Dependence of hepatic gluconeogenesis on PO_2: inhibitory effects of halothane, *J. Appl. Physiol,,* 63, 1776, 1987.

33. **Kamada, T., Hayashi, N., Sato, N., Kasahara, A., and Abe, H.,** Estimated hepatic oxygen consumption in patients with chronic liver diseases as assessed by organ reflectance spectrophotometry, *Dig. Dis. Sci.,* 31, 119, 1986.

34. **Huet, M., Goresky, C. A., Villeneuve, J. P., Marleau, D., and Lough, J. O.,** Assessment of liver microcirculation in human cirrhosis, *J. Clin. Invest.,* 70, 1234, 1982.

35. **Reichen, J. and Le, M.,** Verapamil favorably influences hepatic microvascular exchange and function in rats with cirrhosis of the liver, *J. Clin. Invest.,* 78, 448, 1986.

36. **Tenney, S. M.,** A theoretical analysis of the relationship between venous blood and mean tissue oxygen pressures, *Respir. Physiol.,* 20, 283, 1974.

37. **De Mikulic, L. E. P., Auclair, M. C., Vernimmen, C., Lebrec, D., and Mikulic, E.,** Plasma from cirrhotic patients induces inotropic changes on cultured rat heart cells, *Life Sci.,* 41, 2177, 1987.

38. **Ross, B. K. and Hlastala, M. P.,** Increased hemoglobin-oxygen affinity does not decrease skeletal muscle oxygen consumption, *J. Appl. Physiol.,* 51, 864, 1981.

39. **Astrup, J. and Rirth, M.,** Oxygen affinity of haemoglobin and red cell 2.3-diphosphoglycerate in hepatic cirrhosis. *Scand. J. Clin. Lab. Invest.,* 31, 311, 1973.
40. **Brent, B. N., Matthay, R. A., Mahler, D. A., Berger, H. J., Zaret, B. L., and Lister, G.,** Relationship between oxygen uptake and oxygen transport in stable patients with chronic obstructive pulmonary disease. Physiologic effects of nitroprusside and hydralazine, *Am. Rev. Respir. Dis.,* 129, 682, 1984.
41. **Leier, C. V. and Unverferth, D. V.,** Diagnosis and treatment. Drugs five years later. Dobutamine, *Ann. Intern. Med.,* 99, 490, 1983.
42. **Mikulic, E., Munoz, C., Puntoni, L. E., and Lebrec, D.,** Hemodynamic effects of dobutamine in patients with alcoholic cirrhosis. *Clin. Pharmacol. Ther.,* 34, 56, 1983.
43. **Shepherd, A. P., Granger, H. J., Smith, E. E., and Guyton, A. C.,** Local control of tissue oxygen delivery and its contribution to the regulation of cardiac output, *Am. J. Physiol.,* 225, 747, 1973.
44. **Garcia-Tsao, G. and Groszmann, R. J.,** Portal hemodynamics during nitroglycerin administration in cirrhotic patients, *Hepatology,* 7, 805, 1987.
45. **Zito, R. A., Diez, A. R., and Groszmann, R. J.,** Comparative effect of nitroglycerin and nitroprusside on vasopressin-induced cardiac dysfunction in the dog, *J. Cardiovas. Pharmacol.,* 5, 586, 1983.
46. **Needleman, P. and Johnson, E. M.,** Vasodilators and the treatment of angina, in *The Pharmacological Basis of Therapeutics,* 6th ed., Gilman, A. G., Goodman, L. S., Gilman, A., Eds., Macmillan, New York, 1980, 819.
47. **Moreau, R., Roulot, D., Braillon, A., Hadengue, A., Gaudin, C., Bacq, Y., and Lebrec, D.,** Lack of effect of low dose of nitroglycerin on splanchnic hemodynamics in patients with cirrhosis. Evidence for a decrease in cardiopulmonary baroreflex control, *Hepatology,* 9, 93, 1989.
48. **Chick, T. W., Kochukoshy, K. N., Matsumoto, S., and Leach, J. K.,** The effect of nitroglycerin on gas exchange hemodynamics transport in patients with chronic obstructive pulmonary disease, *Am. J. Med. Sci.,* 276, 105, 1978.
49. **Albert, R. K., Schrijen, F., and Poincelot, F.,** Oxygen consumption and transport in stable patients with chronic obstructive pulmonary disease, *Am. Rev. Respir. Dis.,* 134, 678, 1986.
50. **Cotton, D. B., Jones, M. M., Longmire, S., Dorman, K. F., Tessem, J., and Joyce, T. H.,** Role of intravenous nitroglycerin in the treatment of severe pregnancy-induced hypertension complicated by pulmonary edema, *Am. J. Obstet. Gynecol.,* 1954, 91, 1986.
51. **Lebrec, D.,** Vasopressin versus somatostatin or vasopressin and vasodilator, in *Methodology and Review of Clinical Trials in Portal Hypertension,* Burroughs, A. K., Ed., Elsevier Amsterdam, 1987, 81.
52. **Mols, P., Hallemans, R., Van Kuyk, M., Melot, C., Lejeune, P., Ham, H., Vertongen, F., and Naeije, R.,** Hemodynamic effects of vasopressin, alone and in combination with nitroprusside, in patients with liver cirrhosis and portal hypertension, *Ann. Surg.,* 199, 176, 1984.
53. **Kvietys, P. R. and Granger, N.,** Vasoactive agents and splanchnic oxygen uptake, *Am. J. Physiol.,* 243 (Gastrointest. Liver Physiol., 6), G1, 1982.
54. **Ebert, T. J., Cowley, A. W., and Skelton, M.,** Vasopressin reduces cardiac function and augments cardiopulmonary baroreflex resistance increases in man, *J. Clin. Invest.,* 77, 1136, 1986.
55. **Aylward, P. E., Floras, J. S., Phil, D., Leimbach, W. N., and Abboud, F. M.,** Effects of vasopressin on the circulation and its baroreflex control in healthy men, *Circulation,* 73, 1145, 1986.
56. **Cain, S. M.,** Survival time of hypoxic dogs given epinephrine or propranolol, *Am. J. Physiol.,* 225, 1405, 1973.
57. **Jones, D. P., Kennedy, F. G., Andersson, B. S., Aw, T. Y., and Wilson, E.,** When is a mammalian cell hypoxic? Insights from studies of cells versus mitochondria, *Mol. Physiol.,* 8, 473, 1985.
58. **Moreau, R.,** unpublished data.

Chapter 12

THE CEREBRAL CIRCULATION IN LIVER FAILURE

Frank L. Silver

TABLE OF CONTENTS

I. INTRODUCTION

Coma signifies severely compromised brain function. The mechanism by which coma occurs in hepatic failure remains poorly understood. The absence of macroscopic structural cerebral changes after acute hepatic failure, and the rapid neurological recovery which ensues with improved hepatic function supports a metabolic causation.

Many potentially toxic substances have been found to be increased in hepatic failure.[1] The common assumption is that the brain is exposed to toxic substances which are present in portal blood when liver function is inadequate, or when portal blood bypasses the liver to enter directly into the systemic circulation. A complete understanding of the pathogenesis of hepatic encephalopathy requires knowledge of the mechanism by which a substance interferes with cerebral function. Reversible loss of cerebral function implies interruption of neuronal transmission without the loss of structural integrity. Neurophysiologically, successful transmission requires release of neurotransmitters into the synaptic cleft, binding to postsynaptic receptors, and subsequent depolarization of the adjacent neuron. This is an energy-dependent process. Under normal conditions, neurons metabolize glucose in the presence of oxygen for energy production. Most of the resultant energy provides for synaptic transmission, with the remainder being used in other neuronal processes such as the maintenance of ionic gradients required for the membrane potential.[2]

Since the brain has no energy stores, metabolism is just sufficient to meet its immediate needs. Any interference with synaptic transmission will be instantaneously reflected by a lower cerebral uptake of glucose and oxygen, since energy requirements are reduced. Conversely, a defect in energy production will immediately result in failure of synaptic transmission and cerebral function.

The cerebral circulation is exquisitely regulated by the brain's energy requirements. Cerebral blood flow (CBF) is normally tightly coupled to cerebral metabolism (CMR) so that, as glucose or oxygen consumption falls, CBF is reduced.[3]

Decreased cerebral blood flow and metabolism in patients with hepatic failure have been described since 1956.[4,5] Animal models demonstrate that the energy state of cerebral tissue is unchanged during brain failure resulting from ammonia intoxication or portacaval shunting,[1,6,7] i.e., the level of high energy phosphates remains normal. Therefore, hepatic encephalopathy is not a consequence of a primary failure of energy metabolism. Rather, this reduction in CBF and substrate consumption reflects decreased energy demands when neuronal transmission is abolished by a primary metabolic process.

Although probably secondary in nature, the pathophysiological changes occurring in the cerebral circulation during liver failure remain important because:

1.   Any theory attempting to explain the pathogenesis of hepatic encephalopathy must account for the changes observed in cerebral blood flow and metabolism.
2.   Changes in cerebral blood flow and metabolism occur early, allowing the recognition of hepatic encephalopathy before it is clinically apparent.
3.   The determination of cerebral blood flow and metabolism allows quantitation of cerebral function, providing an accurate index to the severity of the hepatic encephalopathy.
4.   The brain appears especially sensitive to hypoxia, hypercarbia, and hypotension in liver failure, and the reasons for this may be explained by examining the factors that regulate cerebral blood flow and metabolism.

The situation of fulminant hepatic failure (FHF) requires separate attention. Although the pathogenesis of encephalopathy in fulminant and in chronic hepatic failure might be expected to be the same, there are several striking differences. A working knowledge of cerebral blood flow and metabolism is especially important since:

1. Disturbances in the cerebral circulation associated with cerebral edema and increased intracranial pressure are implicated in the death of patients with FHF.
2. Known changes in the blood brain barrier (BBB) of patients with FHF may account for the increased toxicity of some circulating substances on the central nervous system. Also, changes in the BBB may be important to the pathogenesis of chronic hepatic encephalopathy.

This chapter will briefly review the physiological parameters determining CBF and CMR. The relationships between CBF, the BBB, and intracranial pressure (ICP) will be discussed. The current methods of measuring cerebral blood flow and metabolism will be outlined. Theories on the pathogenesis of hepatic encephalopathy in chronic and fulminant hepatic failure will be reviewed separately in the context of the human and animal studies which have investigated the cerebral circulation in each. Finally, the future of research using new noninvasive means of measuring CBF and CMR in humans will be considered.

II. PHYSIOLOGICAL MECHANISMS DETERMINING CBF AND CMR

The concept that CBF is variable and regulated was not appreciated until the 1930s when Forbes and colleagues, using a skull window, observed pial arteries actively changing their caliber in response to various neuronal and hemodynamic stimuli.[8,9] The prevailing view of the time, proposed by Monro and Kellie, was that the skull was filled with three incompressible constituents: blood, cerebrospinal fluid, and cerebral tissue, and that the inflow of blood to the cranium matched outflow, leaving constant the volume of blood in the skull.[10]

Our current understanding of the physiology of the cerebral circulation required the development of methods whereby CBF and CMR could be measured in experimental situations.

A. METHODS OF MEASURING CBF AND CMR

In 1945 Kety and Schmidt developed a method of measuring human CBF using the inhalation of nitrous oxide, an inert tracer.[11] Application of this technique provided the foundation of our present knowledge of the regulation of cerebral blood flow and metabolism. The technique was not totally noninvasive since blood samples were obtained from a catheter in the internal jugular vein. Only mean CBF for the hemisphere sampled could be obtained. Hemispheric CMRgl or $CMRO_2$ could be calculated from the arterial-venous difference for glucose or O_2, respectively.

Completely noninvasive measurements of regional CBF became possible using the ^{133}Xe inhalation method.[12] Regional CBF was determined by placing many radiation detectors over the scalp and measuring the "wash out" of radioactivity after the inhalation of ^{133}Xe. Arterial blood concentrations of ^{133}Xe for the "input curve" were determined from end-tidal sampling of the subject's expired breath. CMR cannot be determined using this method.

The development of autoradiographic techniques allowed the measurement of both CBF and CMR in specific brain structures of animals,[13,14] "local" rather than "regional" best describing the small volume of tissue being examined. Autoradiography involves injecting an animal with a radioactive tracer at a known time. The animal is then sacrificed and the brain is immediately removed and frozen. The radioactive tracer is thus trapped according to the distribution of the substance being measured, allowing for adjustments as determined by a known kinetic model for that tracer. Sections of the brain are placed on a photographic plate and the resulting images are read with a densitometer to determine tissue concentrations of the tracer. An operational equation converts the tissue concentrations to actual metabolic rates. Validated methods are available for determining the local cerebral metabolic rate for glucose (lCMRgl) and for oxygen (lCMRO$_2$), and the local cerebral blood flow (lCBF).[13,14]

The last two decades have seen the development of sophisticated cameras employing computerized tomographic techniques of image reconstruction and radiopharmaceuticals which allow the principles of autoradiography to be applied to man. Noninvasive, *in vivo* measurements of lCBF and lCMR are now possible. Positron emission tomography, the method employing this advanced technology, has been used extensively for the investigation of cerebral ischemia, tumors, dementia, degenerative neurological diseases, and psychiatric disorders.[15,16]

B. FACTORS REGULATING CBF

CBF can be defined mathematically as the cerebral perfusion pressure (CPP) divided by the cerebral vascular resistance (CVR) (Equation 1). The CPP is simply the difference between mean arterial blood pressure (mABP) and the cerebral venous pressure (CVP) (Equation 2). CVP is practically the equivalent of the intracranial pressure (ICP), and therefore CBF is determined by the mABP, ICP, and the CVR (Equation 3).

$$CBF = \frac{CPP}{CVR} \tag{1}$$

$$CPP = mABP - CVP \tag{2}$$

$$CBF = \frac{mABP - ICP}{CVR} \tag{3}$$

CVR depends on the caliber of the vessels in the vascular bed and on the viscosity of the circulating blood. Since the blood viscosity is relatively constant over time, the most important mechanism controlling CBF is the ability of feeding arteries to constrict and dilate. Adjustments in the caliber of these vessels are governed by: (1) "autoregulation" in response to changes in CPP; (2) metabolic regulation in response to local tissue metabolic demands; (3) chemical regulation with changes in pCO$_2$ and pO$_2$; and (4) the requirement of keeping cerebral blood volume relatively constant.[17]

C. AUTOREGULATION

Assuming that ICP is nearly zero (as it is normally) and that CVR remains constant, CBF should vary directly with the mABP. In humans, however, changes in mABP from 50 to 170 mmHg have little effect on CBF,[18] because of autoregulation, the rapid adjustment of the caliber of resistance arteries which maintains a constant CBF. Increased perfusion pressure results in arteriolar constriction (increased CVR), and decreased perfusion pressure causes vasodilation (decreased CVR). Increasing ICP had the same effect as decreasing mABP, since both decrease CPP. A direct myogenic mechanism for autoregulation has been considered but probably is not the complete answer.[17]

When the cerebral perfusion pressure falls below the lower limit of autoregulation, CBF begins to fall. The changes which ensue have been recently reviewed,[19] and are shown diagrammatically in Figure 1. Cerebral metabolism is initially maintained, despite the lowered CBF, by increasing oxygen extraction from the blood. A high local oxygen extraction ratio (lOER) signifies this phase of "critical perfusion". Once the OER is maximal, any further decline in cerebral perfusion will result in cerebral ischemia. Neurological dysfunction occurs when CBF is insufficient to maintain synaptic function (tissue ischemia), and irreversible cell death (tissue infarction) occurs soon after CBF falls below the level required to maintain the ionic gradients which support cell membrane function.[20]

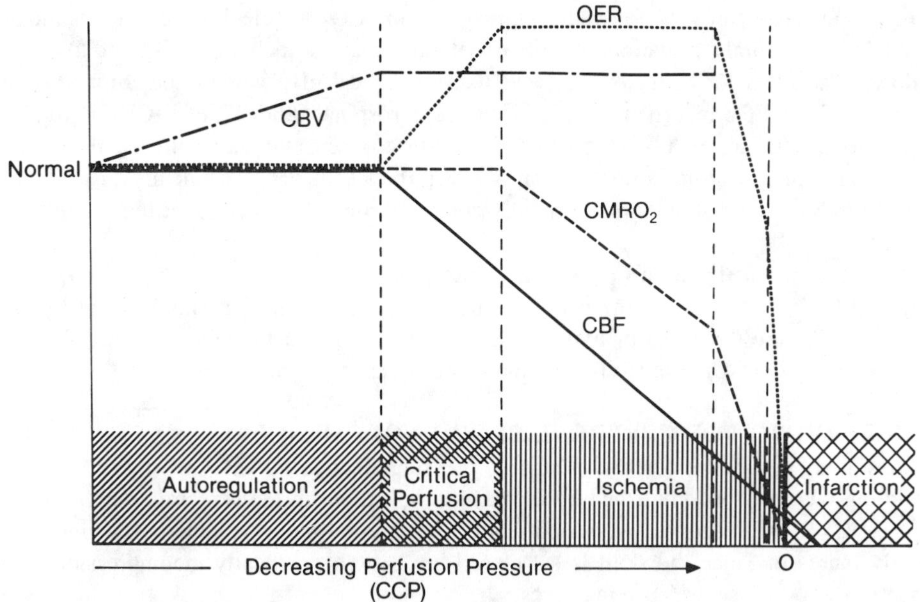

FIGURE 1. Diagram relating cerebral blood flow (CBF), cerebral blood volume (CBV), cerebral metabolic rate for oxygen (CMRO$_2$), and oxygen extraction ratio (OER) to the cerebral perfusion pressure (CPP). CBF remains constant despite the falling CPP during the phase of "autoregulation". During the phase of critical perfusion, the increased OER compensates for the falling CBF to maintain CMRO$_2$. When OER is maximal, further decline in CPP results in tissue ischemia and subsequent tissue infarction.

Therefore, autoregulation prevents the development of ischemia when the mABP falls slightly. When autoregulation becomes defective, as after head trauma or cerebral ischemia,[18] any decrease in mMABP results in decreased CBF. As a consequence, tissue ischemia occurs at a relatively higher level of mABP, or, when autoregulation fails, the brain is more susceptible to hypotension.

D. METABOLIC REGULATION

The tight coupling of cerebral blood flow and metabolism is known as the metabolic regulation of CBF. This assures that the local supply of substrates to the tissue is sufficient for its energy demands. The mechanism by which lCBF is regulated to meet metabolic demands is not understood, although local humoral factors, such as changes in extracellular K^+ and H^+, and cyclic AMP are thought to play a role.[17]

The brain is unique in terms of its functional organization. Unlike other organs (such as the liver) which are homogeneic, the brain is organized into complex functional regions. It follows that only certain brain structures are activated in response to a given task. For example, PET can demonstrate the selective increase in lCBF and lCMRgl in the visual cortex when subjects look at a picture.[21] While global measurements are of value in situations of diffuse cerebral dysfunction, as results from sedative drugs, global ischemia, or metabolic encephalopathy, local changes in CBF and CMR in response to cognitive activation will go undetected in hemispheric or whole-brain measurements.

Unfortunately, many investigators of hepatic encephalopathy have used such non-regional methods which overlook the local changes in CBF and CMR that might account for the specific clinical manifestations of hepatic encephalopathy which precede coma.

E. CHANGES IN pCO$_2$

Carbon dioxide is a potent cerebral vasodilator: within the physiological range, CBF increases approximately 4% for each 1 mmHg rise in pCO_2.[18] Teleologically this is thought to enable the cerebral circulation to remove metabolic wastes, including CO_2, and to prevent acidosis. The mediator of this response is likely the local pH, which is determined by the arterial pCO_2 and the bicarbonate level of the cerebrospinal fluid (CSF).[17] CBF normalizes with chronic changes in pCO_2, probably because compensatory adjustments in the CSF bicarbonate concentration correct the initial disturbance in pH.[18] Clinically this adaption takes 24 to 36 h, so that attempts to rapidly correct chronic hypercapnia or hypocapnia may be harmful.

Changes in pO_2 have an opposite and less potent effect on CBF. Hypoxia results in increased CBF, but not until the pO_2 has fallen below 50 mmHg.[18] This level of hypoxia corresponds to the threshold of hypoxia necessary to cause lactic acidosis. Therefore, the effect of hypoxia of CBF is likely also mediated by changes in pH.

F. RESTRICTION OF CEREBRAL BLOOD VOLUME (CBV)

Assuming a constant cerebral perfusion pressure, increasing CBF by any of the above regulating factors is accomplished by increasing the caliber of the cerebral arteries so as to decrease CVR. With progressive vasodilation, the cerebral blood volume (CBV) must necessarily increase. Since the skull is a "closed box" with practically incompressible components, ICP will rise as CBV increases.

Control of CBV is effected by the constriction of the major cerebral feeding arteries in order to regulate blood flowing into the skull and prevent unwanted increases in ICP.[17] Therefore, any conditions which increase CBF can result in higher CBV and ICP. This may be relevant to the early stages of a toxic encephalopathy when brain tissue is relatively hypermetabolic in its attempt to metabolize circulating toxins.

III. THE BLOOD BRAIN BARRIER (BBB)

Endothelial cells of cerebral capillaries have unique properties that make them impermeable to many substances and thus provide brain tissue with privileged isolation from the body's liquid milieu. They are joined to each other by tight junctions, supported by a basement membrane and enveloped by astrocytic foot processes. The continuous double membrane created by endothelial cells fused by tight junctions has been shown to be the anatomic structure responsible for the BBB.[22] Unlike endothelial cells situated elsewhere, cerebral endothelial cells have no fenestrations and pinocytic vesicles are limited (Figure 2).

Certain substances like glucose and essential amino acids can enter the brain freely via non-energy-dependent, stereospecific, and saturable transport carriers driven by concentration gradients.[23] Large neutral amino acids share a common transport carrier in the endothelial membrane. This results in competition for carrier sites when different amino acids are present in the plasma. Nonessential amino acids including γ-aminobutyric acid (GABA) and glycine are prevented from entering the brain by an intact BBB.[24] These amino acids are potent inhibitory neurotransmitters which, if allowed entry to the brain, can severely suppress cerebral function.

Loss of integrity of the blood brain barrier is important to the pathogenesis of hepatic failure. Toxic substances, normally excluded, may gain access to cerebral tissues to initiate or increase encephalopathy. In addition, the leakage of osmotically active substances from the blood into the extracellular space leads to cerebral edema. As a result, ICP progressively increases until the cerebral perfusion pressure is reduced beyond the regulating capacity of autoregulation. CBF subsequently falls and tissue ischemia ensues. In this case, the depressed cerebral metabolism is a primary disturbance, reflecting an inadequate supply of blood (CBF), rather than being secondary to a direct toxic/metabolic loss of neuronal function.

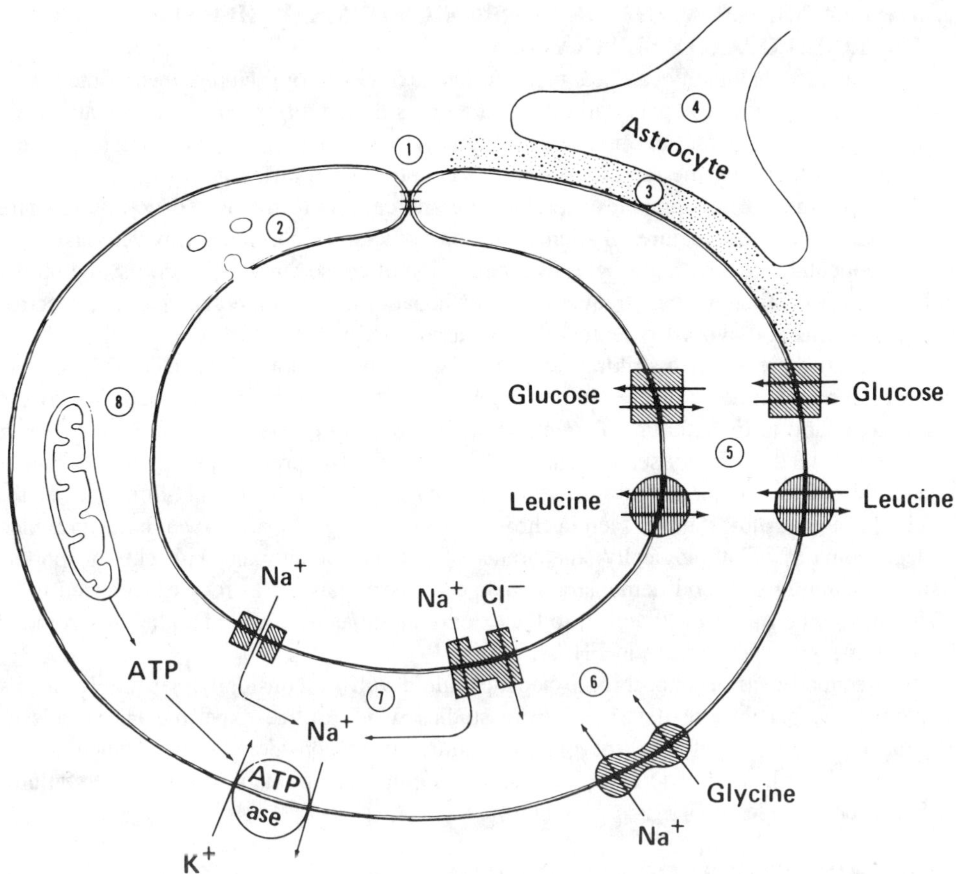

FIGURE 2.   Model of brain capillary: The tight junctions (1) that join endothelial cells in brain capillaries are continuous and complex, and limit the diffusion of large and small solutes. Very few pinocytotic vesicles (2) are found in the cytoplasm; this potential route for transendothelial transport is inoperative in normal brain capillaries. The basement membrane (3) provides structural support for the capillary and may influence endothelial cell function. Foot processes of astrocytes (4) encircle the capillary but do not create an impermeable barrier. Transport carriers (5) for glucose and essential amino acids facilitate the movement of these solutes into the brain. Active transport systems (6) appear to cause efflux of certain small amino acids from brain to blood. Na$^+$ pores and NaCl carriers on the luminal surface of the endothelial cell and Na$^+$,K$^+$-ATPase on the anteluminal surface (7) account for movement of ions across the brain capillary. Mitochondria (8) produce the adenosine triphosphatase needed for energy-dependent transport processes. Not shown are receptor sites for agents that may regulate the permeability of the barrier. (From Goldstein, G. W. and Betz, A. L., *Ann. Neurol.*, 14, 389, 1983. With permission.)

IV. CHANGES IN THE CEREBRAL CIRCULATION WITH HEPATIC ENCEPHALOPATHY

Studies of the human cerebral circulation in hepatic encephalopathy are almost exclusively confined to patients with cirrhosis and chronic portal-systemic encephalopathy. These were performed 10 to 30 years ago, using nonregional measurements of CBF and CMRO$_2$. Animal studies usually employed models of FHF such as toxin-induced liver failure or total liver devascularization. The number of animals studied in each experiment was generally small and different investigators used different species. Also, measurements were taken at differing stages of hepatic encephalopathy by varying means. Not surprising, contradictory conclusions result.

A. WHY CONSIDER ACUTE AND CHRONIC FORMS OF HEPATIC ENCEPHALOPATHY SEPARATELY?

Hepatic encephalopathy can be simply defined as the neuropsychiatric syndrome which occurs in the presence of hepatic failure. Most authors do not differentiate chronic and acute liver failure, assuming that the mechanisms underlying the associated encephalopathies are the same, and that only the rapidity of onset accounts for the differences seen.

Certainly the encephalopathies seen in acute and chronic forms of hepatic failure share many common clinical features. Patients with either acute or chronic forms demonstrate a disturbed mental status with a progressive depression of consciousness, asterixis, pyramidal and extrapyramidal signs and, frequently, fetor hepaticus. There are characteristic electro-encephalograms and evoked potential changes associated with both.[25-27]

However, there are also striking differences which would not be expected if the disturbance in cerebral function were simply a consequence of some essential hepatic process which is lacking in liver failure. Patients with FHF usually present abruptly with delirium and seizures, features rarely seen in chronic liver failure. The prominent pathologic finding is cerebral edema, frequently of sufficient severity to cause intracranial shifts and death. Cerebral edema is almost never seen in chronic hepatic encephalopathy, even in the presence of deep coma.[28,29] Pathologically, the brains of patients or animals with chronic portal-systemic shunting of blood demonstrate changes in protoplasmic astrocytes (referred to as Alzheimer's type I and II astrocytes) to the extent that it has been called a glial syndrome.[30] These changes are not present in FHF.

Consequently, acute and chronic hepatic failure will be considered separately in this chapter. Concepts will be developed from studies which utilize experimental models or patients representative of the type of liver failure being considered. Since much of the experimental work in hepatic encephalopathy has employed models of acute liver failure, FHF will be considered first.

B. FULMINANT HEPATIC FAILURE (FHF)

Fulminant hepatic failure can be defined as a rapidly developing impairment of liver function, complicated by hepatic encephalopathy. The interval of time between the appearance of jaundice and encephalopathy is, by definition, less than two weeks, depending on the investigator.[31] The commonest cause of FHF is acute viral hepatitis, but many other etiologies including drugs, toxins, fatty liver of pregnancy, and hepatic ischemia, have been implicated. The common pathological substrate for FHF is rapid massive hepatocellular necrosis. The course of these patients is frequently complicated by sepsis, renal failure, and pancreatitis, so that other factors may have a role in the development of encephalopathy.

Whatever the cause, the encephalopathy progresses rapidly to coma. The process can be completed reversed, if liver function is restored early. Late in the illness the brain becomes irreversibly damaged from massive cerebral edema. Ware and colleagues reviewed 32 autopsies of patients dying with FHF and found that 16 had evidence of cerebral edema and 4 had evidence of cerebellar tonsillar and/or uncal herniation.[32] The Liver Unit at King's College Hospital reported cerebral edema at necropsy in 13 of 16 consecutive patients, with secondary brain stem compression being responsible for death in 6 patients.[28] The development of cerebral edema is thus clearly implicated as the terminal event in FHF, and any theory on the pathogenesis of FHF must explain the development of cerebral edema.

C. CHANGES IN CEREBRAL BLOOD FLOW AND METABOLISM IN FHF

Although decreased CBF and $CMRO_2$ were first documented in patients with cirrhosis and encephalopathy, many subsequent studies have confirmed similar changes in FHF.[33-37] As the encephalopathy worsens, CBF and $CMRO_2$ progressively decline. Since the encephalopathy of FHF usually ensues rapidly, little is known about CBF and metabolism in the early stages of acute liver failure, before brain function is disturbed. Studies have concentrated on the relationship between pO_2, pCO_2, ICP, and metabolism. In a sense, the measurement of $CMRO_2$ is being exploited as a sensitive and quantitative index of the severity of the hepatic encephalopathy.

Trewby and co-workers examined the integrity of autoregulation in liver failure by measuring hemispheric CBF with a ^{133}Xe clearance method after complete liver devascularization and the creation of a side-to-side portacaval shunt.[33] Signs of liver failure and encephalopathy rapidly appeared and ICP began to rise steadily within 2 h of completion of the surgery. There was a significant correlation between the cerebral perfusion pressure (BP − ICP) and CBF, suggesting that autoregulation had failed. Similar degrees of hypotension in control animals did not affect CBF.

The synergistic effect of hypoxia in aggravating the encephalopathy of FHF has been shown experimentally. Stanley and Cherniack have demonstrated that goats with acute liver failure induced by CCl_4 are more sensitive to the deleterious effects of hypoxia than are controls.[34] Hypoxia failed to produce the expected increased CBF and resulted in decreased $CMRO_2$ at higher levels of pO_2 when compared with baseline studies in the same animals. The fall in CBF appears appropriate to the degree of additional metabolic depression induced by the hypoxia. Strikingly, the level of hypoxia producing this further reduction of metabolism was harmless to healthy animals. It is uncertain whether the brain is more vulnerable to hypoxia, or whether the accompanying liver hypoxia worsens liver function, which is reflected in the observed fall in cerebral metabolism.

Respiratory alkalosis is a constant finding in all forms of hepatic encephalopathy. Hyperventilation, perhaps centrally driven, leads to a progressive fall in the pCO_2. Attempts to correct the relative hypocarbia by having cirrhotic patients inhale CO_2 or by administering acetazolamide result in worse encephalopathy and a further depressed $CMRO_2$.[38] A study using the model of goats with CCl_4-induced acute hepatic failure has shown that the normal response of CBF to CO_2 is blunted, and moreover, that $CMRO_2$ fell in response to hypercarbia that was innocuous to normal animals.[35]

These three studies emphasize that hypotension, hypoxia, and hypercarbia are poorly tolerated by patients with liver failure. In the clinical setting, such disturbances should be promptly and aggressively corrected to avoid further neurological deterioration. It is unclear how such small changes in these factors, inconsequential to healthy patients, deleteriously affect $CMRO_2$ in liver disease. Simplistically it seems that, when neuronal function is already compromised, normal compensatory mechanisms are no longer operating.

Finally in the realm of treatment for FHF, metabolic measurements can show the efficacy of a given therapy. In pigs with totally devascularized livers, cross-circulation with a normal sibling pig resulted in a return to normal CBF and $CMRO_2$, and in prolonged survival.[36]

D. THE BLOOD BRAIN BARRIER IN FHF

There is increasing evidence that the BBB has an important role in the pathogenesis of hepatic encephalopathy and that a disturbance of the BBB is essential to the development of cerebral edema in FHF. Animal models have been used to show an increased permeability of the BBB in acute liver failure.[28] Moreover, the toxic substances that are known to accumulate in liver failure (e.g., ammonia, methyl octanoate, mercaptans, and phenolic acids) are able to disrupt the BBB in rats,[39] suggesting that the cerebral edema seen in FHF is vasogenic (extracellular, secondary to leaky capillaries), as well as cytotoxic (intracellular, secondary to cell membrane failure).[40] Cytotoxic edema results from the failure of the Na^+,K^+-ATPase pump to maintain the intra- to extra-cellular ionic gradients, and the toxins that are found to be elevated in hepatic failure are known to inhibit Na^+,K^+-ATPase.[41] Specifically, sera, from patients with FHF, inhibit Na^+,K^+-ATPase activity in normal rat brain,[41] and the severity of the encephalopathy correlated well with the inhibition of ATPase activity, and not with the serum concentration of hepatic enzymes or bilirubin.

Potvin and colleagues, examining the brains of hepatectomized rats exhibiting acute hepatic coma, found markedly increased brain water content, indicative of cerebral edema.[42] Astrocytic foot processes were swollen and, macroscopically, most of the edema was confined to the grey matter. Capillary endothelial tight junctions were intact but the pinocytotic vesicles were greatly increased in number. Horowitz and co-worker's study, using the galactosamine model of acute liver failure, suggests that the increased permeability of the BBB precedes the onset of encephalopathy.[43]

Failure of the BBB is clearly implicated in the pathogenesis of the cerebral edema present in FHF. It is becoming increasingly apparent that loss of the BBB's integrity may allow entry of substances which are normally excluded, such as GABA, which is known to cause suppressed neuronal function and, ultimately, coma. The coma induced by GABA is "functional" and therefore reversible, whereas, when failure of the BBB leads to cerebral edema, "structural" changes soon appear. When cerebral edema is sufficiently severe to cause intracranial shifts, the resulting secondary brain stem compression produces irreversible coma.

Perhaps an integrated theory on the pathogenesis of FHF would include opening of the BBB by circulating neurotoxins, the influx of substances like GABA which are capable of producing encephalopathy and, finally, the further disruption of the BBB to cause increasing cerebral edema, irreversible coma and death.

V. CHRONIC PORTAL-SYSTEMIC ENCEPHALOPATHY (PSE)

This hepatic encephalopathic syndrome is associated with chronic parenchymal liver disease. It can occur also in the presence of normal liver function if there is sufficient portal-systemic shunting, but usually hepatocellular dysfunction coexists with pathological or surgical (portacaval) shunts. The syndrome is characterized by episodes of encephalopathy precipitated by specific factors such as gastrointestinal bleeding, sedative drugs, excess dietary protein, infection, or constipation. The encephalopathy begins insidiously, with subtle changes in cognitive function or behavior. Seizures occur only rarely, clinically significant cerebral edema does not develop, and the encephalopathy usually clears when the precipitating factor is corrected.

A. CHANGES IN CBF AND METABOLISM IN PSE

In 1956, Fazekas and colleagues used the Kety-Schmidt method to measure CBF and $CMRO_2$ in 20 patients with cirrhosis.[4] They found that CBF and $CMRO_2$ were reduced when compared with age-matched controls. Moreover, patients with clinically apparent encephalopathy had significant further reductions in their $CMRO_2$, while CBF remained unchanged. This reduction in $CMRO_2$ correlated well with the degree of the cerebral disturbance, and was most severe in the comatose patients.

Posner and Plum later repeated these studies in 17 cirrhotic patients whose encephalopathy they assigned a clinical grade.[38] They found that patients without definite encephalopathy had normal $CMRO_2$, and that $CMRO_2$ fell proportionately in patients with increasing degrees of encephalopathy. CBF tended to be higher in patients without encephalopathy, and lower in patients with signs of severe encephalopathy, including coma, when compared to normal subjects. This principle has been confirmed by subsequent studies.[44,45]

These results are consistent with the basic principle that depressed cerebral function, regardless of its cause, is associated with decreased cerebral metabolism. There may be a local reduction in CMR with focal disturbances of cerebral function however, a generalized reduction is expected with diffuse metabolic encephalopathies. $CMRO_2$ can be used as a measure of severity, since it correlates inversely with the grade of the hepatic encephalopathy. For example, $CMRO_2$ increases in response to giving patients with moderate hepatic encephalopathy a course of lactulose.[44]

Although CMRO$_2$ remains normal until encephalopathy appears in patients with liver failure, changes in the CBF and metabolism are already present. Bianchi Porro and colleagues demonstrated that CBF and CMRgl are elevated in patients with cirrhosis and portacaval shunts.[46,47] Using the Kety-Schmidt method, they studied 20 patients with cirrhosis who were alert and had no evidence of encephalopathy.[47] Seven of eight patients undergoing a portacaval shunt had a significant increase in CBF; the exception was a patient whose CBF was high preoperatively. CMRO$_2$ remained normal in all patients. In contrast, CMRgl increased significantly after surgical shunting. As a corollary, the metabolic ratio (the quotient of oxygen uptake divided by glucose uptake, which is normally fixed) decreased after surgery. Mean arterial blood pressure remained constant pre- and postoperatively, and the pCO$_2$ fell only slightly, suggesting that a primary metabolic disturbance was responsible for the observed elevation in CBF. James and co-workers, using the ^{85}Kr inhalation method, have also shown that cirrhotic patients without encephalopathy have higher CBF and CMRgl.[48]

The disturbed metabolic ratio (CMRO$_2$/CMRgl) in chronic hepatic failure has important implications. The increased consumption of glucose may be a clue to the metabolic pathways which are activated in an attempt to detoxify a circulating toxin. The increased CBF demonstrated with cirrhosis and portacaval shunting may represent increased metabolism of glucose via anaerobic pathways even in the presence of an adequate supply of oxygen. This may represent a compensatory phase when the brain is able to metabolize circulating toxins before they are able to interfere with neuronal function.

Knowledge is lacking about the serial changes in CBF, CMRgl, and CMRO$_2$ that occur in patients with increasing encephalopathy from chronic portal-systemic shunting. Gjedde and colleagues measured CBF and CMRO$_2$ in 27 rats, 4 and 8 weeks after end-to-side portacaval shunts, using a modified Kety-Schmidt technique.[49] CBF was elevated from baseline at 8 weeks, but CMRO$_2$ remained normal. When ammonium acetate was infused postoperatively, CMRO$_2$ remaind unchanged at 4 weeks but fell significantly at 8 weeks. These studies demonstrated that, even though blood levels of ammonia were elevated after portacaval shunting, an infusion of exogenous ammonium acetate was necessary to precipitate encephalopathy. Interestingly, Alzheimer type II astrocytes, a constant neuropathological accompaniment of chronic hepatic failure, were present only at 8 weeks. Since Alzheimer type II changes probably signify activation of astrocytes, there is likely a functional change which takes some time to occur, after systemic shunting of portal blood to the brain commences.[28]

More recently this same model of chronic portal-systemic encephalopathy has been studied using autoradiographic techniques to examine local tissue changes in CBF and CMRgl. Cruz and Duffy measured lCMRgl using the [^{14}C]deoxyglucose method in rats at various intervals after portacaval shunting.[50] They found that local tissue consumption of glucose varied according to the specific brain structure and the length of time from surgery. There were few changes in lCMRgl before 8 weeks, while later measurements showed increased glucose utilization in the majority of regions. Only parietal cortex showed a modest fall in lCMRgl. CBF was elevated at 8 weeks but the change was not statistically significant (n = 7). Arterial-venous differences of ammonia demonstrated a marked uptake of ammonia by the brain at 8 weeks after shunting.

Although serum ammonia levels rise shortly after portacaval shunting, there seems to be a gradual cellular adaptation to the hyperammonemia (or other factors) to account for the late changes in lCMRgl. This adaptive change is probably occurring in the protoplasmic astrocytes which have been shown to be involved in the detoxification of ammonia by the brain and, as already discussed, are the site of the subtle neuropathological changes found after 8 weeks in this rat model and in patients with chronic portal-systemic encephalopathy. While Mans and colleagues have obtained conflicting results by demonstrating a depression of CMRgl after portacaval shunting in rats,[51] the validity of the [^{14}C] glucose method they employed has been questioned on methodological grounds.[49]

Lockwood and co-workers later confirmed the presence of increased lCMRgl in rats 8 weeks after portacaval shunting using the [^{14}C] deoxyglucose method.[52] They also demonstrated that the changes in lCMRgl were highest in the phylogenetically older structures including the thalamus, hypothalamus, and basal ganglia, and greatest in the reticular formation which increased by 74%. This is in comparison to the cerebral cortex which showed only modestly increased glucose utilization, increasing 12 to 18%. None of the 20 brain regions examined showed decreased CMRgl. This pattern of increased lCMRgl may account for some of the clinical features of hepatic encephalopathy, including the altered level of consciousness (dependent on the reticular formation), and the common extrapyramidal findings such as rigidity (dependent on the substantia nigra and basal ganglia).

To summarize, there is evidence from the portacaval rat model and from patients with cirrhosis, with and without surgical portacaval shunts, that there is a disturbance of cerebral metabolism, even before signs of encephalopathy occur. The changes include higher glucose utilization which probably results in the initial higher CBF. When measured regionally, these changes are greatest in the reticular formation and deep grey matter structures. Local CMRO$_2$ remains normal throughout this early stage of hepatic failure. Once encephalopathy is clinically apparent, CMRO$_2$ is decreased and continues to fall as neurological function deteriorates. CBF remains tightly coupled to metabolism and, although it initially rises in response to the early elevation of CMRgl, it falls in response to the decreasing CMRO$_2$, as the encephalopathy worsens.

B. THE BLOOD BRAIN BARRIER IN PSE

Most studies examining the BBB in liver disease have used animal models of acute hepatic failure and are therefore less relevant to patients with chronic hepatic failure and encephalopathy. Hawkins recently used an infusion-autoradiographic method to study the transport of substrates in rats with portacaval shunts, an experimental model of PSE.[53] Glucose transport was unhampered, with decreased glucose influx appropriate to the reduced metabolism. Ketone body transport was reduced by 60%, which may be important to energy production if glucose becomes unavailable. Neutral amino acids showed enhanced transport in association with the high concentrations of the aromatic amino acids present in the plasma, during hepatic encephalopathy, whereas the BBB became almost impermeable to basic amino acids 7 to 8 weeks after portacaval shunting. Brain regions demonstrating the greatest increase in the influx of aromatic amino acids were the limbic structures and the reticular formation, possibly relevant to the mechanism of hepatic coma.

Chronic hepatic encephalopathy, although usually reversible, is associated with subtle neuropathological changes. There is proliferation of protoplasmic astocytes, some showing the specific morphological features of Alzheimer type I or II astrocytes. Microscopic and ultrastructural studies performed by Laursen in rats after chronic portacaval shunting have shown that these reactive astrocytes exhibit cytoplasmic edema, with increased numbers of mitochondria, lysosomes, and glial filaments.[30] Laursen found the BBB to be permeable to horseradish peroxidase, a macromolecule usually excluded by normal cerebral capillary membranes.

To summarize, the BBB is altered during both acute and chronic forms of hepatic encephalopathy. The BBB is less severely compromised in PSE than in FHF, and cerebral edema is clinically not important, but the increased permeability of the BBB may still have a significant role in allowing potentially toxic substances access to the brain.

VI. PATHOGENESIS OF HEPATIC ENCEPHALOPATHY

A complete theory of the pathogenesis of hepatic encephalopathy should explain the exact mechanism by which brain function is disturbed secondary to hepatic failure. Ideally, all aspects of the clinical syndrome and the changes in CBF, metabolism, and the BBB would be integrated into this theory.

Early investigations into the pathogenesis of hepatic encephalopathy sought altered concentrations of substances in the blood to correlate with the severity of the encephalopathy. Unfortunately, the presence of a substance in elevated concentrations does not necessarily imply that it is directly responsible for the observed changes in brain function. Evidence is required that inducing a similar alteration in the level of the substance reproduces the encephalopathy and that correcting the alteration will lead to its resolution.[1] Finally, a mechanism must be provided by which this metabolic change can influence neuronal function. Recent studies have approached the problem in reverse, searching for alterations in substances known to depress neuronal function and then measuring their concentrations in models of hepatic encephalopathy (see GABA hypothesis below).

Currently there are three major hypotheses concerning the pathogenesis of hepatic encephalopathy:

1. The synergistic neurotoxins hypothesis[1] which suggests that the accumulation of ammonia and other toxic substances results in neuronal dysfunction.
2. The false transmitter hypothesis[54,55] in which a plasma amino acid imbalance and glutamine efflux from the brain results in augmented synthesis of serotonin (an inhibitory neurotransmitter) and false neurotransmitters, while reducing the production of excitatory neurotransmitters such as dopamine and norepinephrine.
3. The GABA hypothesis[56] which proposes that increased formation of GABA in the gut, decreased GABA extraction by the liver, and entry of GABA through a damaged blood brain barrier results in increased brain concentrations of this potent inhibitory neurotransmitter.

A. SYNERGISTIC NEUROTOXINS HYPOTHESIS

One of the first metabolic disturbances discovered in hepatic encephalopathy was that of elevated serum ammonia.[1,29,57] Although research has focused on patients with cirrhosis and encephalopathy, hyperammonemia occurs in most cases of seriously impaired liver function. Ammonia is generated in the gut by the action of colonic urease-containing bacteria on nitrogenous material (ingested protein, intestinal blood).[29] Ammonia absorption from the bowel is increased with slow transit of fecal material. It enters the liver via the portal circulation, and is normally metabolized by hepatocytes to urea. With hepatic failure, it is not metabolized and is able to enter the systemic circulation, exposing the brain to usually high concentrations.

The blood concentration of ammonia correlates poorly with the severity of encephalopathy, especially in FHF, whereas CSF ammonia concentrations correlate well.[1] The concentration of CSF glutamine, a metabolite of ammonia degradation, also correlates well.[6,57] Patients with PSE appear to benefit clinically and metabolically from lactulose given to reduce ammonia production in the bowel,[44] although its effect in slowing the progression of encephalopathy in FHF is unproven.[28]

If ammonia is the key to the pathogenesis of hepatic encephalopathy, encephalopathy should result from direct infusions of ammonia into the cerebral circulation. Infusion studies in experimental animals produce a clinical syndrome of headache, irritability, progressive obtundation, and eventual coma. The course is accompanied by asterixis, decerebrate posturing, and seizures.[1,57] This has been described as a hyperkinetic syndrome, unlike the generalized depression of cerebral function seen in PSE. Perhaps this state is more like the clinical picture of FHF in which delirium and seizures are prominent. A similar encephalopathy appears in patients with hyperammonemia due to inherited metabolic defects.[57]

Acute infusions of ammonium acetate have produced variable effects on CBF and

CMRO$_2$, depending on the animal model used.[58] Barzilay and co-workers found that whole brain CBF and CMRO$_2$ remained constant in dogs infused with ammonium acetate when PCO$_2$ was kept fixed.[58] However, lCBF in the pons and the midbrain increased. These regional changes again suggest that the reticular formation is selectively involved in hepatic failure. When James and colleagues gave ammonium salts to dogs who were freely ventilating, CBF and CMRgl both increased.[48] This is similar to the changes seen in patients with cirrhosis and in rats with portacaval shunts without encephalopathy already described. Lockwood and co-workers used the [^{14}C]deoxyglucose method in rats given unilateral subthreshold infusions of ammonium acetate.[52] The resulting autoradiograms were compared to those of rats with encephalopathy produced after portacaval shunting. The pattern of augmented lCMRgl was identical except in the substantia nigra, which showed much greater glucose consumption after shunting.

Understanding the way the brain metabolizes ammonia may be a key to our understanding the pathogenesis of hepatic encephalopathy. Excess ammonia is removed by condensation with alpha-ketoglutarate to form glutamate, which is subsequently transformed into glutamine. As discussed previously, the concentration of CSF glutamine correlates well with the severity of the encephalopathy. Recent studies by Butterworth and Giguere have shown that this glutamine elevation is not uniform throughout the brain, but is confined to the midbrain, hypothalamus, medulla-pons, and the spinal white matter.[59] Glutamine was decreased in the striatum and cerebellum. This distribution is somewhat similar to that seen for CMRgl autoradiographically, suggesting that increased glucose consumption might be linked metabolically to ammonia detoxification.

Thus, there is evidence that cerebral blood flow and metabolism are altered by the infusion of ammonium salts. The disturbance seems to be an uncoupling of glucose and oxygen consumption so that glycolytic pathways are augmented, and CBF is secondarily increased. In the case of chronic hepatic failure with portal-systemic shunting, after a latent period, glial function and morphology change so that the brain becomes more vulnerable to further exposure to ammonia. At this stage, cerebral function declines, reflected by falling CMRO$_2$.

Further evidence for the role of ammonia in hepatic encephalopathy is that hyperammonemia itself induces cytoplasmic edema of protoplasmic astrocytes, and increases the amounts of mitochondria and glial filaments.[30] These may represent the ultrastructural changes associated with activated astrocytes attempting to remove excess ammonia.

Since ammonia levels do not account entirely for the presence and severity of hepatic encephalopathy, other factors have been sought. Mercaptans such as methanethiol, which is produced by the metabolism of methionine by gut bacteria, are neurotoxic. Methanethiol is concentrated in the urine of patients with FHF and is believed responsible for the feto hepaticus.[1] Small amounts of mercaptans can induce reversible coma but, like ammonia, they tend to produce a hyperkinetic encephalopathy. The concentrations of mercaptans found in liver failure are not enough in themselves to produce coma.

In a model of acute ischemic hepatic necrosis in rats, brain methanethiol increased fivefold and brain ammonia increased threefold.[1] Individually, neither is enough to induce the observed coma. In his synergistic theory, Zieve proposes that subcoma levels of multiple neurotoxins are responsible for the coma produced experimentally with liver necrosis.[1] Normal rats infused with subcoma concentrations of ammonia salts, methanethiol, and octanoic acid become comatose.[1] Similarly, Zieve also argues that any metabolic disturbance (hypoxia, hypovolemia, or hypoglycemia) may aggravate the existing encephalopathy or precipitate coma.

Ammonia and other toxins have been shown to disrupt the BBB in FHF.[28,57] This opening of the BBB may simply aggravate the situation, by allowing these toxins freer entry to the central nervous system.

The major criticism of the synergistic theory is its inability to provide a mechanism by which ammonia and other substances interfere with neuronal function.

B. FALSE TRANSMITTER HYPOTHESIS

Hyperammonemia increases the brain concentration of aromatic amino acids by two mechanisms: the brain detoxifies ammonia by producing glutamine in the astrocytic Krebs cycle.[29] The efflux of glutamine from the brain is mediated by the large amino acid carrier system,[55] resulting in an augmented influx of tryptophan, tyrosine and phenylalanine by the same carrier. Second, high levels of serum ammonia result in catabolism of branched-chain amino acids by muscle, resulting in low blood concentrations of branched-chain amino acids and high concentrations of aromatic amino acids. The ratio of aromatic to branched-chain amino acids is also increased with liver disease or decreased protein intake. This pattern of amino acids in the blood further enhances the brain's uptake of aromatic amino acids.

Brain concentrations of the neutral aromatic amino acids, including, tryptophan and tyrosine, are elevated in patients dying from FHF.[1,29] The elevated brain levels of the aromatic amino acids result in increased production of serotonin and other inhibitory neurotransmitters. This has also been confirmed experimentally. The metabolic product of serotonin, 5-hydroxyindolacetic acid (5-HIAA) is increased in the CSF of patients with FHF, and brain serotonin, tryptophan, and 5-HIAA are increased in rats with acute hepatic necrosis.[1]

This theory is unable to account for the profound neuronal dysfunction necessary to induce coma; although serotonin and tryptophan can induce sleep, coma does not occur. For the special situation of FHF, these alterations in neurotransmitters do not, by themselves, cause cerebral edema.

C. THE GABA HYPOTHESIS

Schafer and colleagues discovered increased postsynaptic GABA receptors in rabbits with encephalopathy produced by the acute galactosamine model of acute liver failure. This led to further experiments concerning the GABA hypothesis which have been recently reviewed.[60,61] GABA is produced by enteric bacteria and is removed normally from portal blood by the liver which contains most of the body's GABA-transaminase. In galactosamine-induced FHF in rabbits, serum levels of GABA increase tenfold before encephalopathy appears. Since circulating GABA is normally almost totally excluded from the brain, a defect in the BBB must be supposed. Relatively rapid blood to brain transfer of GABA has been documented and the density of postsynaptic GABA receptors is increased. The latter discovery is interesting in light of the tendency of barbiturates and benzodiazepines to aggravate or precipitate hepatic encephalopathy. These drugs act by augmenting GABA neurotransmission. Increased number of postsynaptic receptors also imply increased sensitivity of the brain to GABA. Finally, instillation of small quantities of GABA directly into the brain can induce profound coma.[61]

Specific binding of GABA to postsynaptic receptors increases chloride ion conductance, hyperpolarizing the membrane, and making excitation less probable. Thus there is a known mechanism by which GABA effects its inhibition of neuronal transmission and consequently, failure of neuronal function. Supporting evidence for this mechanism is that the patterns seen with electroencephalography (EEG) and visual evoked potentials (VEP) are similar in hepatic encephalopathy and GABA-induced coma.[28,61]

Recent studies examining concentrations of GABA in patients and animal models of PSE do not substantiate the GABA hypothesis. GABA is not increased in: the brains of rats following end-to-side portocaval anastomosis,[62] the plasma or CSF of cirrhotic patients with encephalopathy,[63] or the brains of cirrhotics dying in hepatic coma.[64] GABA concentrations are elevated in rats following portal vein ligation (a model of PSE), however, there is no change in the density or affinity of the physiologically important GABA binding sites.[65]

New studies demonstrate an accumulation of endogenous substances that bind and modulate the GABA-benzodiazepine-receptor complex in hepatic encephalopathy, findings which support the GABA hypothesis.[66]

Therefore, although the mechanism by which GABA can produce coma has been determined, the evidence that it plays a seminal role in the pathogenesis of hepatic encephalopathy is still lacking. The role of GABA-ergic neurotransmission may be more important in FHF. How the BBB is altered to allow the influx of GABA and cause the severe cerebral edema seen in FHF remains unexplained.

Perhaps a complete understanding of the pathogenesis of hepatic encephalopathy involves integration of elements of all these hypotheses. The presence or absence of cerebral atrophy in association with age or dementia may also influence an individual patient's susceptibility to developing encephalopathy. Ammonia seems to be essential, perhaps responsible for the activation of astrocytes in PSE which is reflected in the increased CMRgl and CBF before the onset of encephalopathy. Whether similar changes occur transiently, in the early (pre-encephalopathic) stages of FHF, is yet to be determined. Also unknown are the functional changes occurring in the brain to account for the delayed susceptibility to increased ammonia in PSE. Ammonia appears to have a role in disrupting the BBB which, one altered, allows circulating toxins easy access to now unshielded neurons. This could lead to the entry of GABA with its potent neuro-inibiting potential. Whatever the neurochemical defect, this later stage is represented clinically by a declining level of consciousness and metabolically by falling $CMRO_2$.

VII. THE FUTURE OF RESEARCH IN THE CEREBRAL CIRCULATION IN HEPATIC ENCEPHALOPATHY

From the point of view of cerebral blood flow and metabolism, the most exciting technology of the 1980s has been the growth of positron emission tomography (PET). Few studies have yet exploited PET's ability to investigate patients with hepatic encephalopathy. Lockwood and colleagues measured lCMRgl and lCBF in patients with PSE and found them increased in the caudate-putamen area, and decreased in the frontal and visual cortices.[67] They postulated that brain regions vary in their susceptibility to specific toxins. The patterns of the metabolic disturbance correlated well with the patient's clinical findings. Specifically, increased muscle tone, decreased attentiveness, and impaired visual processing correspond to decreased metabolism found in the basal ganglia, frontal cortex, the occipital cortex, respectively. Future studies should investigate further the regional changes in CBF and metabolism which evolve as hepatic encephalopathy progresses.

Patients with acute and chronic forms of hepatic encephalopathy could be studied at different stages of their disease. PET will allow repeated, *in vivo*, noninvasive measurements of lCMRgl, $lCMRO_2$, and lCBF in patients in preencephalopathic states (e.g., before and then after portacaval shunting). As these methods become more widely available, these parameters will be used more often by investigators to quantify the severity of encephalopathy. This is especially necessary to objectively evaluate the efficacy of new therapies.

In addition to local tissue measurements of CBF, CMRgl, and $CMRO_2$, future radiopharmaceutical development will allow direct *in vivo* measurement of neurotransmitter receptors and turnover. Positron-labeled tracers for measuring dopamine, opiate, and benzodiazepine receptors are already available.[16] Samson and Bernuau have recently found increased binding of [^{11}C]Ro, a high-affinity selective antagonist of central benzodiazepine receptors, in patients with chronic hepatic encephalopathy as compared to normal individuals.[68] This suggests increased density or affinity of benzodiazepine receptors in chronic PSE, and may account for these patients' increased sensitivity to benzodiazepines.

Although hepatic encephalopathy does not represent a syndrome of cerebral energy failure, the changes in cerebral blood flow and metabolism are important clues to our understanding of the pathogenesis and serve as objective markers of the severity of the condition.

REFERENCES

1. **Zieve, L.,** The mechanism of hepatic coma, *Hepatology,* 1, 360, 1981.
2. **Astrup, J.,** Energy-requiring cell functions in the ischemic brain: their critical supply and possible inhibition in protective therapy, *J. Neurosurg.,* 56, 482, 1982.
3. **Jones, S. C., Fedora, T., Lear, J., Greenberg, J. H., and Reivich, M.,** The flow-metabolism couple in normal rat brain, *J. Cereb. Blood Flow Metab.,* 1 (Suppl. 1), S488, 1981.
4. **Fazekas, J. F., Ticktin, H. E., Ehrmantraut, W. R., and Alman, R. W.,** Cerebral metabolism in hepatic insufficiency, *Am. J. Med.,* 21, 843, 1956.
5. **Wechsler, R. L., Crum, W., and Roth, J. L. A.,** The blood flow and oxygen consumption of the human brain in hepatic coma, *Clin. Res. Proc.,* 2, 74, 1954.
6. **Duffy, T. E. and Plum, F.,** Alpha-ketoglutaramate in the CSF: Clinical implications in hepatic encephalopathy, in *Brain Work,* Ingvar, D. H. and Lassen, N. A., Eds., Munksgaard, Copenhagen, 1975.
7. **Hawkins, R. A.,** Brain energy metabolism and function during hepatic encephalopathy, *Eur. J. Clin. Invest.,* 14, 313, 1984.
8. **Forbes, H. S., Nason, G. L., and Wortman, R. C.,** Cerebral circulation. XLIV. Vasodilatation in the pia following stimulation of the vagus, aortic and carotid sinus nerves, *Arch. Neurol. Psychol.,* 37, 334, 1937.
9. **Forbes, H. S. and Cobb, S. S.,** Vasomotor control of cerebral circulation, *Brain,* 61, 221, 1938.
10. **Hill, L.,** *The Physiology and Pathology of the Cerebral Circulation,* Churchill Livingstone, London, 1986.
11. **Kety, S. S. and Schmidt, C. F.,** The determination of cerebral blood flow in man by the use of nitrous oxide in low concentrations, *Am. J. Physiol.,* 143, 53, 1945.
12. **Obrist, W. D., Thompson, H. K., Jr., Wang, H. S., and Wilkinson, W. E.,** Regional cerebral blood flow estimated by 133-Xenon inhalation, *Stroke,* 6, 245, 1975.
13. **Sokoloff, L.,** The deoxyglucose method: theory and practice, *Eur. Neurol.,* 20, 137, 1981.14.
14. **Greenberg, J. H. and Reivich, M.,** Autoradiographic determination of local cerebral glucose metabolism: physiological and pathological studies, *Adv. Metab. Disord,* 10, 67, 1983.
15. **Phelps, M. E., Mazziotta, J. C., and Huang, S.,** Study of cerebral function with positron-computed tomography, *J. Cereb. Blood Flow Metab.,* 2, 113, 1982.
16. **Phelps, M. E. and Mazziotta, J. C.,** Positron emission tomography: human brain function and biochemistry, *Science,* 228, 799, 1985.
17. **Mchedlishvili, G.,** Physiological mechanisms controlling cerebral blood flow, *Stroke,* 11, 240, 1980.
18. **Lassen, N. A. and Christensen, M. S.,** Physiology of cerebral blood flow, *Br. J. Anaesth.,* 48, 719, 1976.
19. **Silver, F. L., Chawluk, J. B., and Reivich, M.,** The investigation of cerebrovascular disorders with positron emission tomography, in *Cerebrovascular Disease: Research and Clinical Management,* Vol. 1, Lechner, H., Meyer, J. S., and Ott, E., Eds., Elsevier, Amsterdam, 1986, 37.
20. **Astrup, J., Siesjo, B. K., and Symon, L.,** Thresholds in cerebral ischemia — the ischemic penumbra, *Stroke,* 12, 723, 1981.
21. **Kuhl, D. E., Phelps, M. E., Kowell, A. P. et al.,** Effects of stroke on local cerebral metabolism and perfusion: mapping by emission computed tomography, *Ann. Neurol.,* 8, 47, 1980.
22. **Goldstein, G. W.,** The role of brain capillaries in the pathogenesis of hepatic encephalopathy, *Hepatology,* 4, 565, 1984.
23. **Goldstein, G. W. and Betz, A. L.,** Recent advances in understanding brain capillary function, *Ann. Neurol.,* 14, 389, 1983.
24. **Roberts, E.,** The gama-aminobutyric acid (GABA) system and hepatic encephalopathy, *Hepatology,* 4, 342, 1984.
25. **Pappas, S. C. and Jones, E. A.,** Methods of assessing hepatic encephalopathy, *Semin. Liver Dis.,* 3, 298, 1983.
26. **Yang, S.-S., Chu, N.-S., and Liaw, Y.-F.,** Somatosensory evoked potentials in hepatic encephalopathy, *Gastroenterology,* 89, 625, 1985.
27. **Zeneroli, M. L., Pinelli, G., Gollini, G., Penne, A., Messori, E., Zani, G., and Ventura, E.,** Visual evoked potential: a diagnostic tool for the assessment of hepatic encephalopathy, *Gut,* 25, 291, 1984.

28. **Ede, R. J. and Williams, R.,** Hepatic encephalopathy and cerebral edema, *Semin. Liver. Dis.,* 6, 107, 1986.
29. **Fraser, C. L. and Arieff, A. I.,** Hepatic encephalopathy, *N. Engl. J. Med.,* 313, 865, 1985.
30. **Laursen, H.,** Cerebral vessels and glial cells in liver disease, a morphometric and electron microscopic investigation, *Acta Neurol. Scand.,* 65, 381, 1982.
31. **Bernuau, J., Rueff, B., and Benhamou, J.-P.,** Fulminant and subfulminant liver failure: definitions and causes, *Semin. Liver Dis.,* 6, 97, 1986.
32. **Ware, A. J., D'Agostino, A. N., and Combes, B.,** Cerebral edema: a major complication of massive hepatic necrosis, *Gastroenterology,* 61, 877, 1971.
33. **Trewby, P. N., Hanid, M. A., MacKenzie, R. L., Mellon, P. J., and Williams, R.,** Effects of cerebral edema and arterial hypotension on cerebral blood flow in an animal model of hepatic failure, *Gut,* 19, 999, 1978.
34. **Stanley, N. N. and Cherniack, N. S.,** Effect of liver failure on the cerebral circulatory and metabolic responses to hypoxia in the goat, *Clin. Sci. Mol. Med.,* 50, 15, 1976.
35. **Stanley, N. N., Salisbury, B. G., McHenry, L. C., Jr., and Cherniack, N. S.,** Effect of liver failure on the response of ventilation and cerebral circulation to carbon dioxide in man and in the goat, *Clin. Sci. Mol. Med.,* 49, 157, 1975.
36. **Tonnesen, K.,** Cerebral metabolism during cross-circulation in experimental hepatic failure in the pig, *Liver,* 6, 268, 1986.
37. **Pluta, R. and Albrecht, J.,** Changes in arterial and cerebral venous blood gases, cerebral blood flow and cerebral oxygen consumption at different stages of thioacetamide-induced hepatogenic encephalopathy in rat, *Resuscitation,* 14, 135, 1986.
38. **Posner, J. B. and Plum, F.,** The toxic effects of carbon dioxide and acetazolamide in hepatic encephalopathy, *J. Clin. Invest.,* 39, 1246, 1960.
39. **Zaki, A. E. O., Ede, R. J., Davis, M., and Williams, R.,** Experimental studies of blood brain barrier permeability in acute hepatic failure, *Hepatology,* 4, 359, 1984.
40. **Fishman, R. A.,** *Cerebrospinal Fluid Diseases of the Nervous System,* W. B. Saunders, Philadelphia, 1980.
41. **Seda, H. W. M., Hughes, R. D., Gove, C. D., and Williams, R.,** Inhibition of rat brain Na^+,K^+-ATPase activity by serum from patients with fulminant hepatic failure, *Hepatology,* 4, 74, 1984.
42. **Potvin, M., Finlayson, M. H., Hinchey, E. J., Lough, O. J., and Goresky, C. A.,** Cerebral abnormalities in hepatectomized rats with acute hepatic coma, *Lab. Invest.,* 50, 560, 1984.
43. **Horowitz, M. E., Schafer, D. F., Molnar, P., Jones, E. A., Blasberg, R. G., Patlak, C. S., Waggoner, J., and Fenstermacher, J. D.,** Increased blood-brain transfer in a rabbit model of acute liver failure, *Hepatology,* 84, 1003, 1983.
44. **James, I. M. and Garassini, M.,** Effect of lactulose on cerebral metabolism in patients with chronic portosystemic encephalopathy, *Gut,* 12, 702, 1971.
45. **Papenberg, J., Lanzinger, G., Kommerell, B., and Hoyer, S.,** Comparative studies of the electroencephalogram and the cerebral oxidative metabolism in patients with liver cirrhosis, *Klin. Wochenschr.,* 53, 1107, 1975.
46. **Bianchi Porro, G., Maiolo, A. T., and Della Porta, P.,** Cerebral blood flow and metabolism in hepatic cirrhosis before and after portacaval shunt operation, *Gut,* 10, 894, 1969.
47. **Bianchi Porro, G. and Maiolo, A. T.,** Cerebral hemodynamics and metabolism in hepatic cirrhosis, *Digestion,* 3, 111, 1970.
48. **James, I. M., Hamlyn, A. N., Brant, P. C., and Hildrew, P.,** Effect of ornithine alpha oxoglutarate on brain metabolism in patients with chronic liver disease, *J. Neurol. Neurosurg. Psychiatry,* 38, 214, 1975.
49. **Gjedde, A., Lockwood, A., Duffy, T. E., and Plum, F.,** Effect of ammonia on cerebral metabolism of rats with portacaval shunts, *Trans. Am. Neurol. Assoc.,* 101, 180, 1976.
50. **Cruz, N. F. and Duffy, T. E.,** Local cerebral glucose metabolism in rats with chronic portacaval shunts, *J. Cereb. Blood Flow Metab.,* 3, 311, 1983.
51. **Mans, A. M., Biebuyck, J. F., Davis, D. W., Bryan, R. M., and Hawkins, R. A.,** Regional cerebral glucose utilization in rats with portacaval anastomosis, *J. Neurochem.,* 40, 986, 1983.
52. **Lockwood, A. H., Ginsberg, M. D., Rhoades, H. M., and Gutierrez, M. T.,** Cerebral glucose metabolism after portacaval shunting in the rat, *J. Clin. Invest.,* 78, 86, 1986.
53. **Hawkins, R. A.,** Transport of essential nutrients across the blood-brain barrier of individual structures, *Fed. Proc.,* 45, 2055, 1986.
54. **Fischer, J. E. and Baldessarini, R. J.,** False neurotransmitters and hepatic failure, *Lancet,* 2, 75, 1971.
55. **James, J. H., Ziparo, V., Jeppsson, B., and Fischer, J. E.,** Hyperammonaemia, plasma aminoacid imbalance, and blood-brain aminoacid transport: a unified theory of portal-systemic encephalopathy, *Lancet,* 2, 772, 1979.
56. **Schafer, D. E., Thakur, A. K., and Jones, E. A.,** Increased gamma-aminobutyric acid receptors associated with acute hepatic encephalopathy, *Clin. Res.,* 28, 485, 1980.

57. **Flannery, D. B., Hsia, Y. E., and Wolf, B.,** Current status of hyperammonemic syndromes, *Hepatology,* 2, 495, 1982.
58. **Barzilay, Z., Britten, A. G., Koehler, R. C., Dean, J. M., and Traystman, R. J.,** Interaction of CO_2 and ammonia on cerebral blood flow and O_2 consumption in dogs, *Am. J. Physiol.,* 248, H500, 1985.
59. **Butterworth, R. F. and Giguere, J.-F.,** Region-selective glutamine changes in the CNS in relation to function in experimental subacute hepatic encephalopathy, in *Advances in Hepatic Encephalopathy and Urea Cycle Diseases,* S. Karger, Basel, 1984, 394.
60. **Jones, E. A., Schafer, D. F., Ferenci, P., and Pappas, S. C.,** The neurobiology of hepatic encephalopathy, *Hepatology,* 4, 1235, 1984.
61. **Jones, E. A. and Schafer, D. F.,** Hepatic encephalopathy, in *Progress in Liver Disease,* Propper, H. and Schaffner, F., Eds., Grune & Stratton, New York, 1986, 525.
62. **Butterworth, R. F. and Giguere, J.-F.,** Cerebral aminoacids in portal-systemic encephalopathy: lack of evidence for gamma-aminobutyric acid (GABA), *Metab. Brain Dis.,* 1, 221, 1986.
63. **Butterworth, R. F., Lavoie, J., Giguere, J.-F., Layrargues, G. P., and Bergeron, M.,** Cerebral GABA-ergic and glutamatergic function in hepatic encephalopathy, *Neurochem. Pathol.,* 6, 131, 1987.
64. **Moroni, F., Riggio, O., Carla, V., Festuccia, V., Ghinelli, F., Marino, I. R., Merli, M., Natali, L., Pedretti, G., Fiaccadori, F., and Capocaccia, L.,** Hepatic encephalopathy: lack of changes of gamma-aminobutyric acid content in plasma cerebrospinal fluid, *Hepatology,* 7, 816, 1987.
65. **Maddison, J. E., Dodd, P. R., Morrison, M., Johnston, G. A. R., and Farrel, G. C.,** Plasma GABA, GABA-like activity and the brain GABA-benzodiazepine receptor complex in rats with chronic hepatic encephalopathy, *Hepatology,* 7, 621, 1987.
66. **Butterworth, R. F. and Pomier Layrargues, G.,** Benzodiazepine receptors and hepatic encephalopathy, *Hepatology,* 11, 499, 1990.
67. **Lockwood, A. H., Marani, S., Yap, E., Bogue, L., Mullani, N., and Tewson, T. J.,** Cerebral blood flow and glucose metabolism in hepatic encephalopathy, *Ann. Neurol.,* 20, 145, 1986.
68. **Samson, Y. and Bernuau, J.,** Cerebral uptake of benzodiazepine measured by positron emission tomography in hepatic encephalopathy, *N. Engl. J. Med.,* 316, 414-415, 1987.

Chapter 13

DERANGED VOLUME HOMEOSTASIS IN LIVER DISEASE*

Murray Epstein

TABLE OF CONTENTS

* Portions of this review are adapted from: Epstein, M., Renal sodium handling in liver disease, in *The Kidney in Liver Disease*, 3rd ed., Epstein, M., Ed., copyright © by Williams & Wilkins, Baltimore, 1988. With permission.

"When the liver is full of fluid and this overflows into the peritoneal cavity, so that the belly becomes full of water, death follows."

Hippocrates, ca. 400 B.C.[1]

I. INTRODUCTION

The clinical course of patients with decompensated Laennec's cirrhosis is complicated frequently by derangements of renal function varying from progressive impairment of renal sodium and water handling to the hepatorenal syndrome.[2-5] The mechanisms mediating these derangements are exceedingly complex. In this chapter, I will consider the "afferent" events including the major hemodynamic derangements which appear to underlie the renal functional abnormalities. The efferent mechanisms are considered in detail elsewhere in this volume.

A discussion of "afferent" events usually includes consideration of the detector element responsible for the recognition of the degree of volume alterations, as well as a consideration of the extracellular fluid translocations or sequestration into serous spaces or interstitial fluid compartments that characterize advanced liver disease.

In considering the "afferent" events, it is worthwhile to consider two concepts that have been frequently cited in any synthesis of the pathogenesis of the abnormal sodium retention of liver disease: (a) the role of a diminished "effective" volume, and (b) the "overflow" theory of ascites formation. A third hypothesis, the "peripheral arterial vasodilation hypothesis", has recently been proposed.

II. AFFERENT EVENTS

A. ROLE OF DIMINISHED "EFFECTIVE" VOLUME (i.e., "UNDERFILL THEORY")

Traditionally, ascites formation in cirrhotic patients is considered to begin when a critical imbalance of Starling forces develops in the hepatic sinusoids and splanchnic capillaries. This causes an excessive amount of lymph formation, which exceeds the capacity of the thoracic duct to return it to the circulation.[6,7] Consequently, lymph accumulates in the peritoneal space as ascites, with a subsequent contraction of circulating plasma volume. Thus, as ascites develops, there is a progressive redistribution of plasma volume.

Regardless of cause, the diminution of effective plasma volume is believed to constitute an afferent signal to the renal tubule to augment salt and water reabsorption. Thus, the traditional "underfill" formulation suggests that the renal retention of sodium is a secondary rather than a primary event (Figure 1).

B. PERIPHERAL ARTERIAL VASODILATION HYPOTHESIS

Recently an alternative hypothesis, termed "the peripheral arterial vasodilation hypothesis", has been proposed to explain the sodium and water retention of cirrhosis.[8] One may regard this theory as a revision of underfill theory. The principal distinguishing feature of this newly proposed theory is that the decrease in effective blood volume is attributable primarily to an early occurring increase in vascular capacitance. Thus, peripheral vasodilation is the initial determinant of intravascular underfilling, and an imbalance between the expanded capacitance and available volume constitutes a diminished effective volume (Figure 1). This concept brings the hypothesis into accord with some experimental observations that were not consistent with the original postulate. For example, careful balance studies in animals with experimental cirrhosis have clearly shown that sodium retention precedes ascites formation.[9]

Primary systemic hemodynamic changes characterized by peripheral vasodilation with a secondary increase in cardiac output occur very early in experimental cirrhosis and in

THEORIES OF ASCITES FORMATION IN CIRRHOSIS

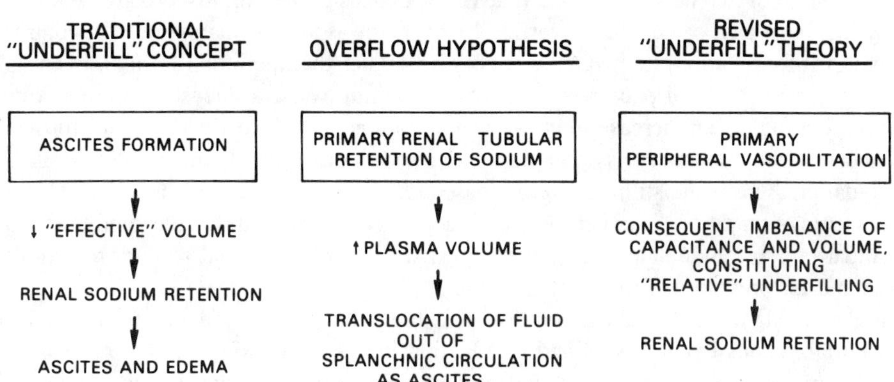

FIGURE 1. Schematic representation of the presumed sequence of events eventuating in ascites formation according to three alternative theories: the traditional "underfill" theory; the "overflow" hypothesis; and the revised "underfill" theory referred to as "the peripheral arterial vasodilation hypothesis". The primary events are shown within the rectangular boxes. According to the traditional underfill concept, the primary event is a diminution in effective volume attributable to the development of abnormal Starling forces in the portal circulation with a maldistribution of circulating volume. This diminished "effective" volume constitutes an afferent signal to the renal tubule to augment renal salt and water reabsorption. In contrast, the overflow theory of ascites formation holds that retention of excessive sodium by the kidneys is the primary event. In the setting of abnormal Starling forces in the portal venous bed, the expanded plasma volume is sequestered preferentially in the peritoneal sac with ascites formation. The most recent hypothesis, which has been termed the "peripheral arterial vasodilation hypothesis" holds that the diminished effective volume is attributable to primary peripheral vasodilation with a consequent imbalance of capacitance and volume. (From Epstein, M., *The Kidney in Liver Disease,* 3rd ed., copyright © by Williams & Wilkins, Baltimore, 1988, 7. With permission.)

humans with compensated cirrhosis.[9-12] The decrease in effective volume induced by these hemodynamic alterations is compounded further by an impaired pressor response to vasoactive agents including exogenous angiotensin II and noradrenaline.[13] Even in those patients who eventually develop an increase in total plasma volume, the relative "fullness" of the arteriovenous tree is decreased.

Total peripheral resistance is diminished significantly in most edematous cirrhotic patients and in animals with toxic cirrhosis[2,9,11] or with bile duct ligation.[12] There is no doubt that the diminution of total peripheral resistance observed in cirrhotic patients is partially related to the above-mentioned vasodilation and consequent increase in vascular capacity. Indeed, when widely developed, these vascular changes may assume the proportion of arteriovenous shunts.[10,11]

The cause of the peripheral vasodilation of liver disease has not been established and is undoubtedly complex. It may be due, at least in part, to vasodilatory hormones secreted by the intestines, such as glucagon, vasoactive intestinal peptide, and substance P, or some other undefined vasodilator. If these hormones bypass the hepatic circulation or are inadequately degraded by the diseased liver, they may exert a vasodilatory effect in the systemic circulation.

Both underfill theories provide a possible explanation of why fluid retention may fail to attenuate the stimulus for continuing sodium and water retention. Despite a progressive increase in total extracellular fluid volume, fluid is sequestered into one or more of the other fluid compartments without succeeding in normalizing effective blood volume. Only correction of the disturbance in the forces governing fluid distribution will permit a reexpansion of effective blood volume to normal.

C. "OVERFILL" THEORY

Over the past two decades, an alternative hypothesis to the diminished effective volume theory has been advocated: the "overflow" theory of ascites formation.[14-16] In contrast to the underfill formulation, the overflow theory postulates that the initial primary event is the inappropriate retention of excessive amounts of sodium by the kidneys. Sodium avidity by the kidney results in an increase in intravascular volume and "overflow" ascites formation.

According to this theory as applied to patients with cirrhosis, an increase in intrahepatic sinusoidal pressure is the stimulus for increased renal sympathetic nerve activity. This view derives from observations in experimental biliary cirrhosis: that relief of elevated intrahepatic sinusoidal pressure by a side-to-side portacaval shunt abolishes renal sodium retention and ascites and restores normal mineralocorticoid escape.

In the setting of abnormal Starling forces in the portal venous bed and hepatic sinusoids (both portal venous hypertension and a reduction in plasma colloid osmotic pressure), the expanded plasma volume is sequestered preferentially in the peritoneal space, with ascites formation. Thus, renal sodium retention and plasma volume expansion *precede rather than follow* the formation of ascites.

The promulgation of the overflow theory of ascites formation has engendered much controversy. The demonstration that plasma volume is increased in cirrhosis with ascites, and that a spontaneous diuresis and natriuresis have been found to occur, independent of measurable changes in the volume of the nonsplanchnic vascular compartment, has been cited as evidence in support of the overflow hypothesis. Additional support derives from a series of elegant investigations carried out by Levy[16,17] on dogs with portal cirrhosis produced by the feeding of dimethylnitrosamine. He demonstrated in sequential studies that renal sodium retention is the initial event that precedes ascites formation. Also, elimination of ascites in these cirrhotic dogs with the LeVeen shunt did not prevent sodium retention during liberal sodium intake.[17] Taken together, therefore, these studies support the view that the initiating event in the renal sodium retention of cirrhosis is not related to "underfilling".

Of interest, in a recent study of cirrhotic patients, Decaux et al.[18] observed a significant increase in the clearance of urea and uric acid, which they attributed to an increase in effective vascular volume.

Although the above observations collectively support the overflow theory of ascites formation, a number of clinical observations in humans are inconsistent with such a formulation.[8,19] Thus, rapid volume expansion with exogenous solutions including saline, mannitol, and albumin and ascitic fluid, frequently result in a transient improvement in renal sodium and water handling.[10,20,21] Similarly, infusion of metaraminol to conteract the peripheral vasodilatation induces a natriuresis.[22] Finally, normalization of Starling forces by surgical decompression of the portal bed in certain patients with cirrhosis may be associated with mobilization of ascites, improvement in renal function, and natriuresis.[23] Of note, all these maneuvers may overcome the circulatory disturbance without improving the function of the cirrhotic liver.

Nevertheless, the fact that several of the utilized maneuvers nonspecifically increase the volume of all fluid compartments and the presumed concomitant alterations in plasma composition have precluded definitive statements regarding the etiologic role of a diminished effective plasma volume. Thus the results of many earlier studies must be considered inconclusive because of the confounding effects of the experimental designs.

D. STUDIES UTILIZING THE WATER IMMERSION MODEL

Studies from our laboratory over the past 20 years have circumvented many of the experimental problems by applying a unique investigative tool, the water immersion model to the assessment of renal function and volume hormonal relationships in diverse edematous disorders.[24-26] Before proceeding to enumerate these findings, it may be useful to describe

TABLE 1
Salient Features of the Model of Head-out Water Immersion

1. Immersion produces a prompt redistribution of circulating blood volume with a relative central hypervolemia.
2. Cardiac output is increased by 25—33% and central blood volume by approximately 700 ml.
3. The alterations in central hemodynamics are sustained throughout a 4 h immersion period and are promptly reversible following cessation of immersion.
4. Immersion-induced central hypervolemia is associated with a profound and progressive natriuresis and diuresis. These alterations are promptly reversible following cessation of immersion.
5. The central hemodynamic and renal effects of immersion are equal in magnitude to those induced by acute saline administration (2 l saline/2 h).
6. The alterations in renal sodium, potassium, and water handling in the sodium-replete state (the only condition as yet studied) occur in the absence of changes in renal plasma flow and GFR.
7. Immersion is associated with a prompt and profound (approximately two thirds) suppression of PRA and plasma aldosterone. Cessation of immersion is associated with a prompt return of both PRA and PA to prestudy levels.
8. Immersion induces a prompt, marked and sustained augmentation of atrial natriuretic factor (ANF). Cessation of immersion is associated with a prompt return of ANF to prestudy levels.
9. The above alterations in renal function, renin-aldosterone, and ANF responsiveness occur in the absence of changes in plasma composition.

briefly the salient features of the model (Table 1) and to underscore the differences between water immersion and the more traditional attempts to achieve ECVE, such as saline administration.

Head-out water immersion of a patient in the seated posture results in a prompt redistribution of blood volume with a sustained increase in central blood volume.[24-27] Furthermore, studies of the "efferent" limb of immersion have demonstrated a marked natriuretic and kaliuretic response during immersion. It has also been demonstrated that the natriuretic and kaliuretic response is indistinguishable from that of saline administration (2 l/120 min) in normal subjects, assuming an identical seated posture.[25] Although water immersion constitutes a potent means of inducing central volume expansion comparable with that induced by the infusion of isotonic saline, it is capable of circumventing many of the problems associated with the infusion of exogenous volume expanders.

In contrast to saline administration, (a) water immersion is associated with a decrease in body weight, rather than the increase that attends saline infusion; (b) the "volume stimulus" of immersion is promptly reversible after cessation of immersion in contrast to the relatively sustained hypervolemia that follows saline administration, and thus constitutes an important attribute in minimizing any risk to the patient; and (c) in contrast to saline administration, the "volume stimulus" of immersion occurs in the absence of changes in plasma composition.[24-26]

The delineation of the immersion model and the demonstration that it constitutes a potent "central volume stimulus", without the necessity of infusing exogenous volume expanders, commended its use in assessing the role of alterations of "effective" plasma volume in the derangements of sodium homeostasis in cirrhosis.

Studies in 32 patients with decompensated cirrhosis demonstrated a striking "normalization" of renal sodium handling, following water immersion. As shown in Figure 2, immersion resulted in marked natriuresis and kaliuresis in the majority of these patients. During the final hour of immersion, $U_{Na}V$ was 20-fold greater than it was during the prestudy hour. Thus, the marked antinatriuresis of cirrhosis was promptly reversed by a manipulation that merely altered the distribution of plasma volume without increasing (and often decreas-

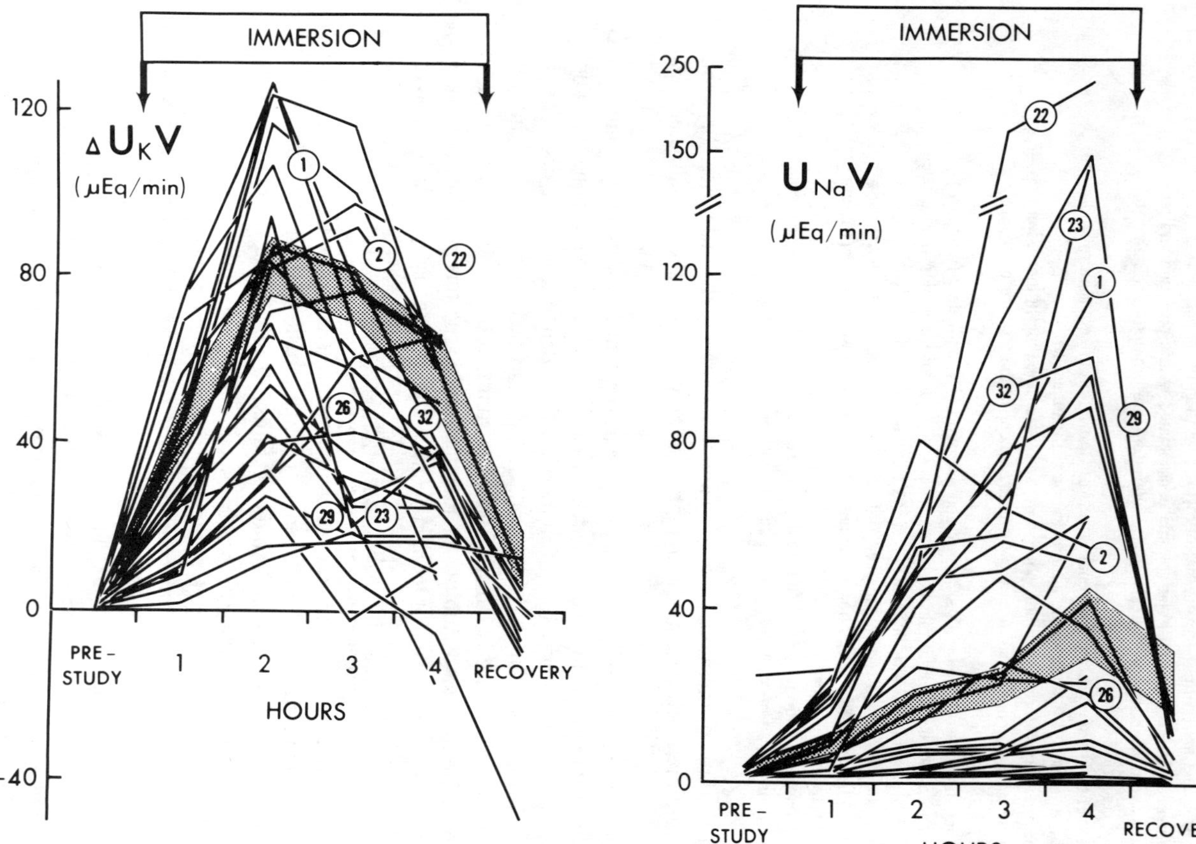

FIGURE 2.   Effects of water immersion following 1 hour of quiet sitting (prestudy) on rate of sodium excretion ($U_{Na}V$) and potassium excretion (U_KV) in a large group of patients with alcoholic liver disease. The circled numbers represent individual patients. Data for U_KV are expressed in terms of absolute changes from prestudy hour (ΔU_KV). The shaded area represents the mean $\pm$ SE for 14 normal control subjects undergoing an identical immersion study while ingesting an identical 10 mEq Na/100 mEq K/day diet. Over half of the cirrhotic patients manifested an appropriate or "exaggerated" natriuretic response. In general, the increase in $U_{Na}V$ was associated with a concomitant increase in ΔU_KV . (From Epstein, M., *The Kidney in Liver Disease,* 3rd ed., copyright © by Williams & Wilkins, Baltimore, 1988, 11. With permission.)

ing) total plasma volume. Indeed in many instances, the natriuresis of such patients exceeded markedly the response manifested by normal subjects to the same procedure. Taken together, these studies lend strong support to the concept that a diminished effective intravascular volume is a major determinant of the enhanced tubular reabsorption of sodium in patients with established cirrhosis.

Further evidence that the immersion-induced natriuretic response is indeed supportive of a role for diminished effective volume and not merely an appropriate response comparable to that of normal subjects can be adduced from the concomitant changes in C_{Cr} during immersion.[2,27] In marked contrast to the findings in normals,[24] immersion was associated with significant increments in C_{Cr} in a majority of cirrhotic patients.[2] Two thirds of the cirrhotic patients manifested increments in C_{Cr} (three- to fivefold) that exceeded markedly the increments observed in sodium-depleted normal subjects. These observations suggest that immersion tends to "normalize" the diminished effective volume of cirrhotic humans with a resultant normalization of renal vascular tone.

Although I believe that the presently available evidence favors a prominent role for diminished effective volume in mediating the avid sodium retention of many cirrhotic patients, it should be emphasized that these two formulations (i.e., diminished effective volume vs. overflow) are not mutually exclusive. As noted elsewhere,[2] cirrhosis is not a static disease, but rather a constantly evolving clinical disorder. Yet, virtually all the available clinical studies of deranged sodium homeostasis were carried out at a single stage of the disease, a time when decompensation was well established, with little information available during the incipient stage of sodium retention. In contrast, the studies with the canine cirrhosis model deal with the relatively early stage of sodium retention. Any formulation that suggests that the same antinatriuretic forces are operative throughout the evolution of sodium retention in cirrhotic humans is probably a marked oversimplification. Rather, one should adopt a more global view of the pathogenesis of abnormal sodium retention in cirrhosis in which differing forces participate in varying degrees as the derangement in sodium homeostasis evolves.

III. SYSTEMIC HEMODYNAMICS

An understanding of the possible causes of the renal functional derangements in cirrhosis requires an appreciation of the alterations in systemic circulatory regulation. A large body of evidence has delineated the florid derangements in systemic hemodynamics that afflict patients with decompensated cirrhosis. The majority of cirrhotic patients with ascites are usually hypotensive,[28,29] despite a high normal to increased plasma volume and an elevated cardiac index.

A. CARDIAC OUTPUT

A large body of evidence have demonstrated that the cardiac output in alcoholic liver disease often is considerably elevated.[30-32] Indeed, this elevated cardiac output has been cited to exonerate the heart as an etiologic factor in the renal hypoperfusion. Cohn has reviewed his findings in a large series of 87 patients with severe alcoholic liver disease.[11] They reported that mean cardiac output was higher than normal and on some occasions was extremely elevated. The peripheral distribution of this high cardiac output in cirrhosis has never been fully delineated. Renal blood flow usually is reduced, and the renal fraction of cardiac output is slow. Skeletal muscle and skin blood flow are at most only slightly increased, and cerebral and coronary blood flow are not likely to be much altered. The splanchnic bed therefore remains as the most likely site of low vascular resistance in this hyperdynamic state.

A minority of patients with decompensated cirrhosis manifest a decrease in cardiac output.[11,19,33] Diminished venous return due to tense ascites,[34] alcohol myopathy, and malnutrition all can interfere with myocardial performance. It is clear, however, that the renal functional derangements of cirrhosis do not merely constitute "cardiorenal syndromes".

Epstein and colleagues[33] studied the relationship of systemic and intrarenal hemodynamics in 20 patients with advanced alcoholic cirrhosis. Among this population, 10 had increased cardiac output (7 to 14 l/min), 7 had normal cardiac output (5 to 7 l/min), and 3 had depressed values (3.7 to 4.1 l/min). Of interest was the observation that renal blood flow did not correlate with the level of cardiac output (Figure 3). Comparable reductions in total renal blood flow, as well as cortical flow, were observed in the low- and high-output groups. This contrasts with the situation in congestive heart failure, where it has been demonstrated that cardiac output directly correlates with cortical flow (as determined by ^{133}Xe washout techniques).[35] These findings suggest that local renal vasoconstrictor influences are extremely important as a final determinant for intrarenal vascular resistance.

B. ROLE OF INCREASED ABDOMINAL AND RENAL VENOUS PRESSURE

Mullane and Gliedman[36] have suggested that pressure on the renal venous system, because of the presence of ascites, will interfere with the renal circulation and cause renal ischemia. Indeed, they have suggested that such increments in renal venous pressure may occur in the absence of ascites. Direct measurements of renal venous pressure in cirrhotic patients do not support this hypothesis. In any event, many patients with tense ascites, where the pressure exerted on the renal veins is in excess of that attributable to the column of fluid because of muscular elasticity, manifest normal renal function.[37,38]

Whether or not removal of ascites by paracentesis improves renal function is unsettled. Gordon[39] observed a transient improvement in renal function in patients with HRS following removal of ascites by paracentesis.

In contrast to the above findings, several other observations militate against a major etiological role for increased renal venous pressure. Relieving the pressure on the renal veins in ascitic patients by placing them in the prone position on a Stryker frame has produced only transient improvement in renal function. Perhaps more to the point is the fact that the pressures that are required to impair renal function in patients with HRS far exceed those that are observed even in patients with the most tense ascites. In summary, it would appear that increased renal venous pressure as a cause of intense renal vasoconstriction is not a major determinant of the renal ischemia or renal functional abnormalities of cirrhosis including HRS.

C. SYNTHESIS OF THE HEMODYNAMIC AND RENAL DERANGEMENTS IN CIRRHOSIS

As detailed above, patients with decompensated cirrhosis present with a unique constellation of findings — hypotension despite expanded plasma volumes and elevated cardiac indices. It is evident that the low arterial pressure manifested by most of these patients is a consequence of a reduced peripheral arteriolar vascular resistance. Given this scenario, it is possible to contemplate how these hemodynamic derangements interact with the known derangements of a number of hormonal and neural systems that supervene in cirrhosis. It is well established that decompensated cirrhosis is associated with activation of the renin-angiotensin and sympathetic nervous systems and elevated vasopressin levels.[40-42]

Studies with antagonists of these hormonal systems suggest that the activation of these vasoconstrictor systems including the renin-angiotensin system, vasopressin, and the sympathetic nervous system constitute an adaptive response to maintain and defend systemic hemodynamics at appropriate levels. As an example, pharmacologic interruption of one of these adaptive mechanisms by the acute administration of inhibitors of the renin-angiotensin system, including saralasin and captopril, produces a marked decrease of arterial pressure in cirrhotic patients with ascites.[43] Unfortunately, there is a tradeoff, and the price the patient

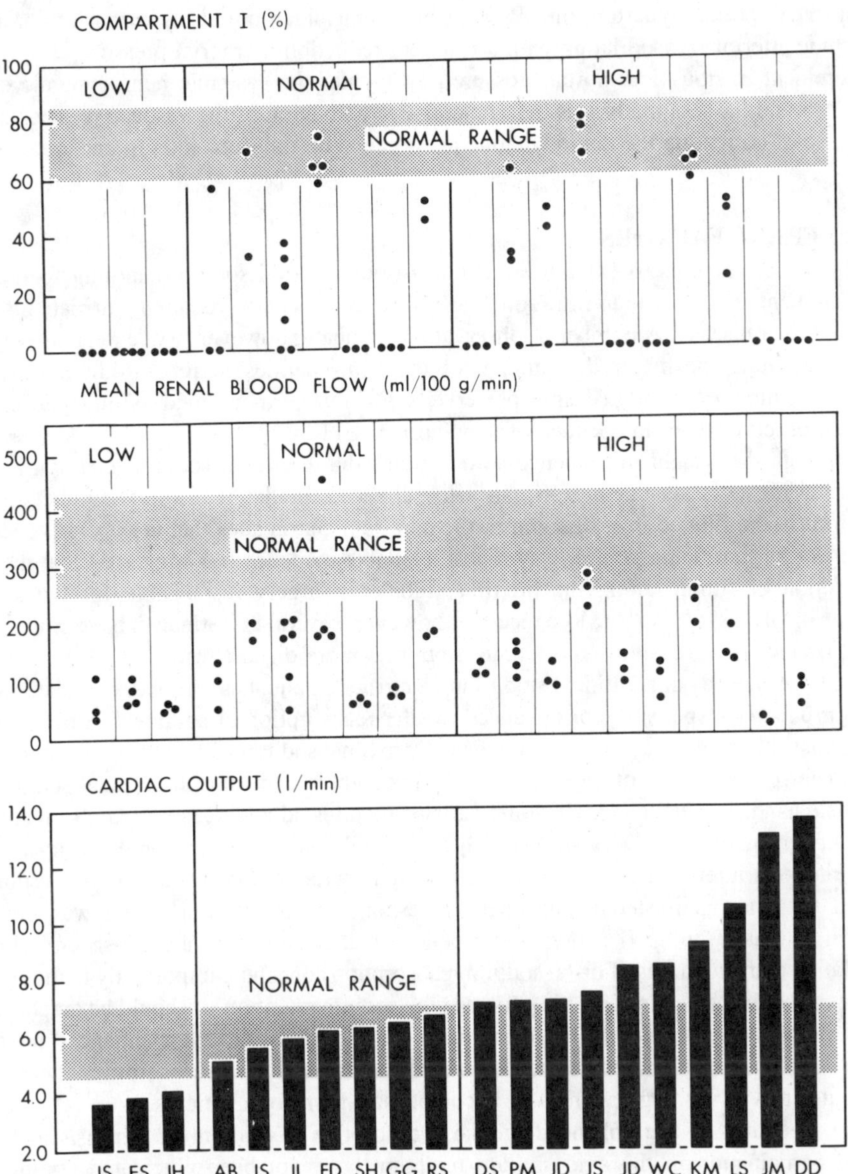

FIGURE 3. Relationship of cardiac output and renal hemodynamics in 20 patients with cirrhosis. The upper panel depicts the percent flow to the rapid flow components (C_1%). The middle panel depicts mean renal blood flow, and the lower panel depicts cardiac output. Each point represents a single xenon washout study. The shaded areas in the upper and middle panels represent mean ± SE of seven normal subjects. The shaded area in the lower panel represents the normal range for cardiac output in this laboratory. The degree of renal hypoperfusion and cortical ischemia was independent of cardiac output. (From Epstein, M., Schneider, N., and Befeler, B., *J. Lab. Clin. Med.*, 89, 1175, 1977. With permission.)

pays for this homeostatic response is avid sodium and water retention. The activity of these neurohumoral vasoactive systems remains increased in an attempt to maintain arterial pressure, thereby perpetuating the retention of sodium and water.

With these events in mind, one may inquire what the initiating events might be. As detailed elsewhere in this book (see Chapter 7), it has been proposed that the initial event is sinusoidal portal hypertension. Presumably, sinusoidal portal hypertension produces splanchnic arteriolar vasodilation with a resultant reduction in arterial pressure. The greater the increment in sinusoidal portal pressure, the greater the systemic hemodynamic disturbance,[44,45] and the less likely it is that the adaptive activation of the vasoactive mechanisms is capable of correcting the hemodynamic disturbance by transient sodium and water retention.

D. EFFERENT FACTORS

The initial attempts to explain the abnormalities of renal sodium handling focused on the decrement in glomerular filtration rate (GFR) that occurs frequently in patients with advanced liver disease. A number of observations indicate, however, that a decrease in GFR cannot constitute the major determinant of the abnormalities in renal sodium handling. Sodium retention occurs often despite preserved GFR. Furthermore, avid sodium reabsorption has been observed even in the face of supranormal GFR.[2,46,47]

Although the weight of evidence demonstrates that the renal sodium retention accompanying cirrhosis is attributable primarily to enhanced tubular reabsorption rather than to alterations in the filtered load of sodium, the precise nephron sites that are operative remain the subject of continuing controversy. Most available evidence has suggested that the avid reabsorption of filtrate along the proximal tubule is largely responsible for the sodium retention of cirrhosis.[20,21,46,48] More recently, however, several investigators have emphasized the importance of excessive sodium reabsorption at more distal sites.[47,49]

We have carried out additional studies in 18 cirrhotic patients in order to elucidate further the nephron sites responsible for enhanced tubular reabsorption of sodium.[49] Since changes in phosphate clearance may provide an index of proximal sodium reabsorption, we undertook to characterize the effects of an immersion-induced volume expansion on renal sodium and phosphate handling (Figure 4). Cirrhotic patients manifested a wide continuum of responses characterized by either a sluggish or barely discernible natriuretic response (group I) or an appropriate natriuretic response (group II). Despite widely varying natriuretic responses, group I patients manifested a phosphaturic response to immersion which was virtually identical to that of group II patients. We believe that our findings are consistent with the formulation that alterations of distal sodium reabsorption contribute importantly to the sodium content of the final urine in cirrhotic patients with sodium retention. It should be emphasized, however, that our observations do not militate against a major role for enhanced proximal tubular reabsorption of sodium; rather, they suggest that enhanced reabsorption at both sites contributes to varying degrees in most decompensated cirrhotic patients.

The mediators of the enhanced tubular reabsorption of sodium in cirrhosis and their relative participation in the avid sodium retention have not been elucidated completely. Several hormonal, neural, and hemodynamic mechanism(s) have been suggested and are enumerated in Table 2. Those mechanism(s) for which there is some evidence and their interrelationships are summarized schematically in Figure 5. The major mechanisms are considered elsewhere in this book.

ACKNOWLEDGMENTS

I am indebted to Audrey Kincaid for her expert preparation of the manuscript.

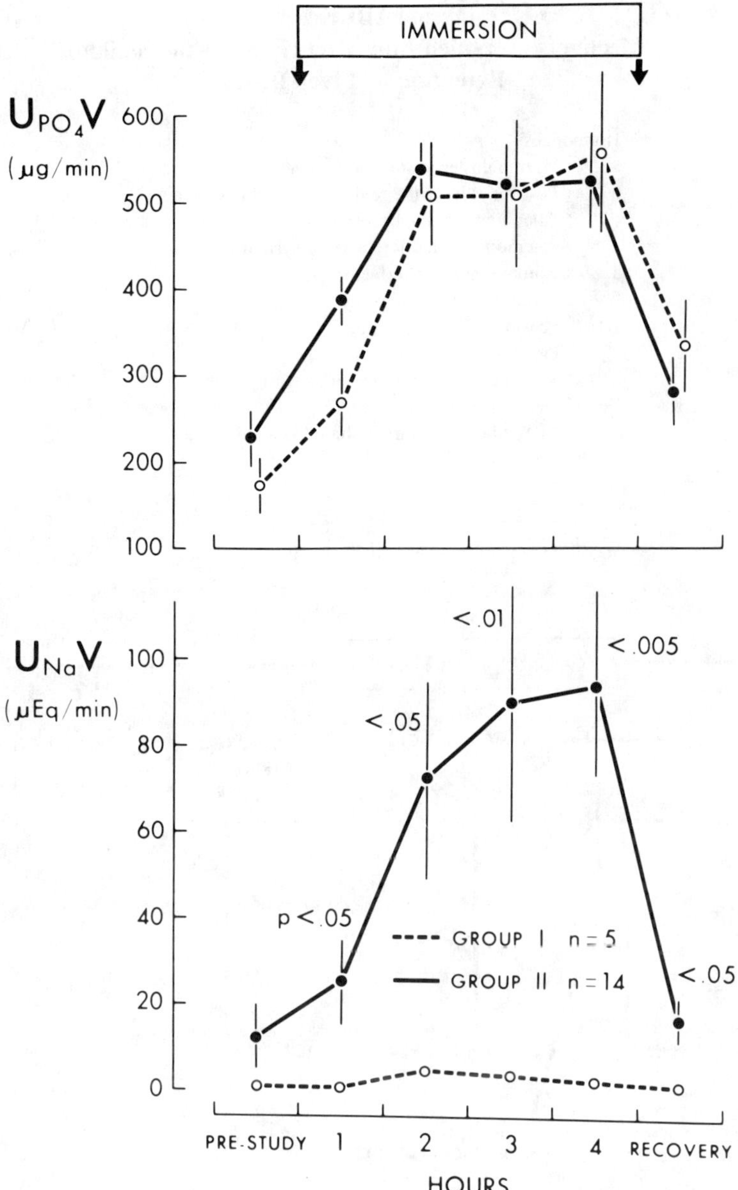

FIGURE 4.   Effect of water immersion on the rate of phosphate excretion ($U_{PO_4}V$, upper panel) and sodium excretion ($U_{Na}V$, lower panel) in 18 cirrhotic patients. Immersion resulted in a marked and progressive phosphaturia in group I patients that was virtually identical with that manifested by group II patients. In contrast to the identical phosphaturic responses, groups I and II manifested marked differences in renal sodium handling. Group I patients manifested a sluggish and barely discernible natriuretic response, whereas group II patients manifested a profound natriuretic response that exceeded that of normal control subjects undergoing an identical immersion study. Results are mean ± SE. (From Epstein, M., Ramachandran, M., and DeNunzio, A. G., *Miner. Electrolyte Metab.*, 7, 311, 1982. With permission of S. Karger, Basel.)

TABLE 2
Mechanisms Which May Participate in the Sodium
Retention of Liver Disease

I.   Hormonal
    a.   Hyperaldosteronism
    b.   Possible role of the renin-angiotensin system
    c.   Alterations in renal prostaglandins
    d.   Alterations in kallikrein-kinin system
    e.   Humoral natriuretic factor
    f.   Atrial natriuretic peptides
    g.   Possible effects of estrogens
    h.   Prolactin
    i.   Vasoactive intestinal peptide
II.   Neural and hemodynamic
    a.   Alterations in intrarenal blood flow distribution
    b.   An increase in sympathetic nervous system activity

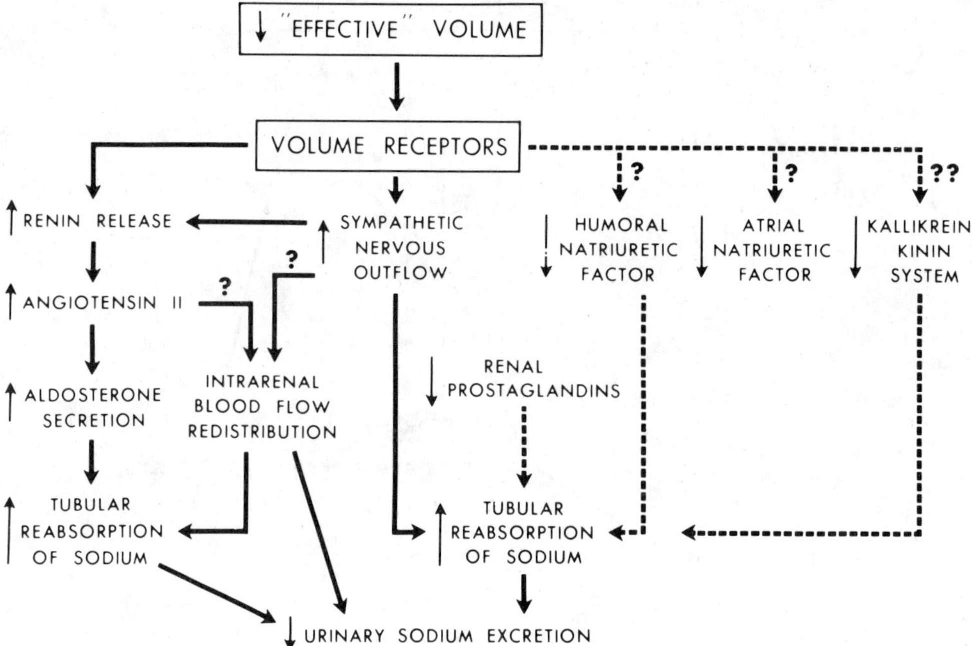

FIGURE 5.   Schematic drawing of possible mechanisms whereby a diminished "effective" volume results in sodium retention. The solid arrows indicate pathways for which evidence is available. The dashed lines represent proposed pathways, the existence of which remains to be established. (From Epstein, M., *The Kidney in Liver Disease,* 3rd ed., copyright © by Williams & Wilkins, Baltimore, 1988, 13. With permission.)

REFERENCES

1. **Hippocrates, Cited in Atkinson, M.,** Ascites in liver disease, *Postgrad. Med. J.,* 32, 482, 1956.
2. **Epstein, M.,** Renal sodium handling in liver disease, in *The Kidney in Liver Disease,* 3rd ed., Epstein, M., Ed., Williams & Wilkins, Baltimore, 1988, 3.
3. **Vaamonde, C. A.,** Renal water handling in liver disease, in *The Kidney in Liver Disease,* 3rd ed., Epstein, M., Ed., Williams & Wilkins, Baltimore, 1988, 31.
4. **Epstein, M.,** Deranged sodium homeostasis in cirrhosis, *Gastroenterology,* 76, 622, 1979.

5. **Epstein, M.,** Hepatorenal syndrome, in *The Kidney in Liver Disease,* 3rd ed., Epstein, M., Ed., Williams & Wilkins, Baltimore, 1988, 89.

6. **Conn, H. O.,** The rational management of ascites, in *Progress in Liver Disease,* Vol. 4, Popper, H., Schaffner, F., Eds., Grune & Stratton, New York, 1972, 269.

7. **Witte, M. H., Witte, C. L., and Dumont, A. E.,** Progress in liver disease: physiological factors involved in the causation of cirrhotic ascites, *Gastroenterology,* 61, 742, 1971.

8. **Schrier, R. W., Arroyo, V., Bernardi, M., Epstein, M., Henriksen, J. H., and Rodés, J.,** Peripheral arterial vasodilation hypothesis: A proposal for the initiation of renal sodium and water retention in cirrhosis, *Hepatology,* 8, 1151, 1988.

9. **Levy, M.,** Sodium retention in dogs with cirrhosis and ascites: Efferent mechanisms, *Am. J. Physiol.,* 233, F586, 1977.

10. **Tristani, F. E. and Cohn, J. N.,** Systemic and renal hemodynamics in oliguric hepatic failure: effect on volume expansion, *J. Clin. Invest.,* 46, 1894, 1967.

11. **Cohn, J. N.,** Renal hemodynamic alterations in liver disease, in *The Kidney in Systemic Disease,* 2nd ed., Suki, W. N. and Eknoyan, G., Eds., John Wiley & Sons, New York, 1981, 509.

12. **Shasha, S. M., Better, O. S., Chaimovitz, C., Doman, J., and Kishon, Y.,** Haemodynamic studies in dogs with chronic bile duct ligation, *Clin. Sci.,* 50, 533, 1976.

13. **Ames, R. P., Borkowski, A. J., Sicinski, A. M., and Laragh, J. H.,** Prolonged infusions of angiotensin II and norepinephrine and blood pressure, electrolyte balance, and aldosterone and cortisol secretion in normal man and in cirrhosis with ascites, *J. Clin. Invest.,* 44, 1171, 1965.

14. **Lieberman, F. L., Denison, E. K., and Reynolds, T. B.,** The relationship of plasma volume, portal hypertension, ascites and renal sodium retention in cirrhosis. The overflow theory of ascites and renal sodium retention in cirrhosis. The overflow theory of ascites formation, *Ann. N.Y. Acad. Sci.,* 170, 202, 1970.

15. **Lieberman, F. L., Ito, S., and Reynolds, T. B.,** Effective plasma volume in cirrhosis with ascites. Evidence that a decreased value does not account for renal sodium retention, a spontaneous reduction in glomerular filtration rate (GFR) and a fall in GFR during drug-induced diuresis, *J. Clin. Invest.,* 48, 975, 1969.

16. **Levy, M.,** Pathophysiology of ascites formation, in *The Kidney in Liver Disease,* 3rd ed., Epstein, M., Ed., Williams & Wilkins, Baltimore, 1988, 209.

17. **Levy, M., Wexler, M. J., and McCaffrey, C.,** Sodium retention in dogs with experimental cirrhosis following removal of ascites by continuous peritoneovenous shunting, *J. Lab. Clin. Med.,* 94, 933, 1979.

18. **Decaux, G., Dumont, I., Naeije, N., Mols, P., Melot, C., and Mockel, J.,** High uric acid and urea clearance in cirrhosis secondary to increased "effective vascular volume", *Am. J. Med.,* 73, 328, 1982.

19. **Better, O. S. and Schrier, R. W.,** Disturbed volume homeostasis in patients with cirrhosis of the liver. *Kidney Int.,* 23, 3031, 1983.

20. **Schedl, H. P. and Bartter, F. C.,** An explanation for and experimental correction of the abnormal water diuresis in cirrhosis, *J. Clin. Invest.,* 39, 248, 1960.

21. **Vlahcevic, Z. R., Adam, N. F., Jick, H., Moore, E. W., and Chalmers, T. C.,** Renal effects of acute expansion of plasma volume in cirrhosis, *N. Engl. J. Med.,* 272, 387, 1965.

22. **Gornel, D. L., Lancestremere, R. G., Papper, S., and Lowenstein, L. M.,** Acute changes in renal excretion of water and solute in patients with Laennec's cirrhosis induced by the administration of the pressor amine, metaraminol, *J. Clin. Invest.,* 41, 594, 1962.

23. **Schroeder, E. T., Anderson, G. H., and Smulyan, H.,** Effect of peritoneovenous shunt on renin in the hepatorenal syndrome, *Kidney Int.,* 15, 54, 1979.

24. **Epstein, M.,** Renal effects of head-out water immersion in man: implications for an understanding of volume homeostasis, *Physiol. Rev.,* 58, 529, 1978.

25. **Epstein, M., Pins, D. S., Arrington, R., DeNunzio, A. G., and Engstrom, R.,** Comparison of water immersion and saline infusion as a means of inducing volume expansion in man, *J. Appl. Physiol.,* 39, 66, 1975.

26. **Epstein, M., Re, R., Preston, S., and Haber, E.,** Comparison of the suppressive effects of water immersion and saline administration on renin-aldosterone in normal man, *J. Clin. Endocrinol. Metab.,* 49, 358, 1979.

27. **Epstein, M., Levinson, R., Sancho, J., Haber, E., and Re, R.,** Characterization on the renin-aldosterone system in decompensated cirrhosis, *Circ. Res.,* 41, 818, 1977.

28. **Nicholis, K. M., Shapiro, M. D., VanPutten, V. J., Kluge, R., Chung, H. M., Bichet, D. G., and Schrier, R. W.,** Elevated plasma norepinephrine concentrations in decompensated cirrhosis: association with increased secretion rate, normal clearance rate and suppressibility by central blood volume expansion, *Circ. Res.,* 56, 457, 1985.

29. **Shapiro, M. D., Nichols, K. M., Groves, B. M., Kluge, R., Chung, H. M., Bichet, D. G., and Schrier, R. W.,** Interrelationship between cardiac output and vascular resistance as determinants of effective arterial blood volume in cirrhotic patients, *Kidney Int.,* 28, 206, 1985.

30. **Murray, F., Dawson, A. M., and Sherlock, S.,** Circulatory changes in chronic liver disease, *Am. J. Med.,* 24, 358, 1958.
31. **Kowalski, H. J. and Abelmann, W. H.,** The cardiac output at rest in Laennec's cirrhosis, *J. Clin. Invest.,* 32, 1025, 1953.
32. **Cohn, J. M., Khatri, I. M., Groszmann, R. J., and Kotelanski, B.,** Hepatic blood flow in alcoholic liver disease measured by an indicator dilution technique, *Am. J. Med.,* 53, 704, 1972.
33. **Epstein, M., Schneider, N., and Befeler, F.,** Relationship of systemic and intrarenal hemodynamics in cirrhosis, *J. Lab. Clin. Med.,* 89, 1175, 1977.
34. **Guazzi, M., Polese, A., Magrini, F., Fiorentini, C., and Olivari, M. T.,** Negative influences of ascites on cardiac function in cirrhotic patients, *Am. J. Med.,* 59, 165, 1975.
35. **Fluck, D. C., Evans, T. R., Siggers, D. C., Crawley, J., and Srivongse, S. A.,** Distribution of blood flow in patients with heart disease, *Clin. Sci.,* 42, 627, 1972.
36. **Mullane, J. R., Gliedman, M. L.,** Elevation of the pressure of the abdominal inferior vena cava as a cause for hepatorenal syndrome in cirrhosis, *Surgery,* 59, 1135, 1966.
37. **Baldus, W. P.,** Etiology and management of renal failure in cirrhosis and portal hypertension, *Ann. N.Y. Acad. Sci.,* 170, 267, 1969.
38. **Maxwell, M. H., Breed, E. S., and Schwartz, I. L.,** Renal venous pressure in chronic congestive heart failure, *J. Clin. Invest.,* 29, 342, 1950.
39. **Gordon, M. E.,** The acute effects of abdominal paracentesis in Laennec cirrhosis upon exchanges of electrolytes and water, renal function and hemodynamics, *Am. J. Gastroenterol.,* 33, 15, 1960.
40. **Epstein, M. and Norsk, P.,** Renin-angiotensin system in liver disease, in *The Kidney in Liver Disease,* 3rd ed., Epstein, M., Ed., Williams & Wilkins, Baltimore, 1988, 331.
41. **Zambraski, E. J. and DiBona, G. F.,** Sympathetic nervous system in hepatic cirrhosis, in *The Kidney in Liver Disease,* 3rd ed., Epstein, M., Ed., Williams & Wilkins, Baltimore, 1988, 469.
42. **Henriksen, J. H., Ring-Larsen, H., Kanstrup, I. L., and Christensen, N. J.,** Sympathetic nervous activity and renal and systematic hemodynamics in cirrhosis: plasma norepinephrine concentration, hepatic extraction and renal release, *Hepatology,* 2, 304, 1982.
43. **Hollenberg, N. K.,** Renin, angiotensin, and the kidney: assessment by pharmacological interruption of the renin-angiotensin system, in *The Kidney in Liver Disease,* 3rd ed., Epstein, M., Ed., WIlliams & Wilkins, Baltimore, 1988, 374.
44. **Bosch, J., Arroyo, V., Betriu, A., Mas, A., Carrilho, F., Rivera, F., Navarro, F., and Rodés, J.,** Hepatic hemodynamics and the renin-angiotensin-aldosterone system in cirrhosis, *Gastroenterology,* 78, 92, 1980.
45. **Bosch, J., Gines, P., Arroyo, V., Navasa, M., and Rodés, J.,** Hepatic and systemic hemodynamics and the neurohumoral systems in cirrhosis, in *The Kidney in Liver Disease,* 3rd ed., Epstein, M., Ed., Williams & Wilkins, Baltimore, 1988, 286.
46. **Klingler, E. L., Jr., Vaamonde, C. A., Vaamonde, L. S., Lancestremere, R. G., Morosi, H. J., Frisch, E., and Papper, S.,** Renal function changes in cirrhosis of the liver, *Arch. Intern. Med.,* 125, 1010, 1970.
47. **Chaimovitz, C., Szylman, P., Alroy, G., and Better, O. S.,** Mechanism of increased renal tubular sodium reabsorption in cirrhosis, *Am. J. Med.,* 52, 198, 1972.
48. **Chiandusi, L., Bartoli, E., and Arras, S.,** Reabsorption of sodium in the proximal renal tubule in cirrhosis of the liver, *Gut,* 19, 497, 1978.
49. **Epstein, M., Ramachandran, M., and DeNunzio, A. G.,** Interrelationship of renal sodium and phosphate handling in cirrhosis, *Miner. Electrolyte Metab.,* 7, 305, 1982.

Chapter 14

EFFECTS OF JAUNDICE ON BODY FLUID VOLUME

Herbert J. Kramer

TABLE OF CONTENTS

I. INTRODUCTION

Acute or chronic jaundice due to bile duct obstruction is often associated with the risks of hypotension, circulatory shock, and acute renal failure. Hypotension and shock may result from impaired cardiac muscle contractility, decreased arterial and venous vascular tone resulting from impaired response of the vascular smooth muscle cell to endogenous vaso-constrictors or to decreased intravascular filling, i.e., decreased effective plasma volume. The effects of jaundice on cardiac performance and on vascular smooth muscle contractility are discussed elsewhere in this volume. The present discussion will therefore be confined to the *effects of jaundice on body fluid volume*, one of the factors possibly related to the hemodynamic risks often encountered in patients with extra- or intrahepatic bile duct obstruction.

Jaundice, in this context, is defined as retention of bile and bile components under conditions of experimental bile duct ligation or in human extra- or intrahepatic bile duct obstruction. Since end-stage hepatic failure, generally due to advanced liver cirrhosis with ascites, is associated with additional impact on systemic and renal hemodynamics eventually leading to the hepatorenal syndrome, the effects of jaundice in this condition will not be discussed in this chapter.

Body fluid volume is maintained essentially by the kidney. Therefore, the discussion will center on the effects of jaundice and related factors on renal handling of fluid and sodium.

II. SODIUM BALANCE AND EXTRACELLULAR FLUID VOLUME IN OBSTRUCTIVE JAUNDICE

In man, acute obstructive jaundice has been shown to be associated with hypovolemia, whereas chronic biliary obstruction with impairment of liver function usually results in renal fluid and sodium retention. Experimental studies to investigate the effects of jaundice on renal handling of fluid and sodium were generally performed in dogs and rats by acute (ABDL) or short-term and long-term chronic bile duct ligation (CBDL).

III. EFFECTS OF JAUNDICE ON RENAL SODIUM EXCRETION

In analogy to acute biliary obstruction in man, *acute* bile duct ligation (ABDL) in the dog, i.e., studies performed after 4 h of bile duct obstruction, has been shown to be associated with a rise in renal blood flow, glomerular filtration rate (GFR), and fractional urinary sodium and water excretion which resulted in a small but insignificant reduction in plasma volume.[1] Dogs with 1-h bile duct ligation showed a normal renal hemodynamic and excretory response to administration of acetylcholine into the renal artery or to acute ECFV expansion with hypotonic saline.[1a] In contrast, experiments with CBDL have led to different and in part conflicting results which may have depended on species-specific effects or differences in the experimental design, e.g., studies in anesthetized vs. conscious animals, or differences in the time of investigation after ligation of the common bile duct. In most studies, CBDL has been found to be associated with renal fluid and sodium retention eventually leading to ascites formation.

Thus, in *short-term chronic* bile duct ligation (CBDL) experiments Bank and Aynedjian[2] observed a positive sodium balance with ascites formation 10 to 14 d after bile duct ligation in rats. In the absence of systemic hemodynamic changes, they demonstrated in micro-puncture studies in anesthetized rats an enhanced sodium reabsorption in superficial cortical nephrons. This may have been due to changes in renal blood flow and intrarenal blood flow distribution with a decrease in outer cortical perfusion. These animals had already developed ascites, which may present an additional important factor for renal hemodynamic alterations. In their experiments, total renal blood flow was normal, but superficial single nephron blood flow was significantly reduced. This finding would suggest intrarenal blood flow distribution towards deep cortical nephrons with increased medullary blood flow. Nevertheless, superficial single nephron filtration rate was normal, suggesting that the increased filtration fraction was a result of efferent arteriolar vasoconstriction. This effect by itself could enhance proximal tubular reabsorption of fluid and sodium by altering peritubular physical forces, i.e., decreased peritubular hydrostatic pressure and increased peritubular oncotic pressure.

Yarger[3] also investigated the effects of bile duct ligation in rats at the time of an initial positive sodium balance and formation of ascites, i.e., 4 to 7 d of CBDL. Despite the positive sodium balance associated with decreased absolute renal sodium excretion at the time of the study, the animals revealed a decrease in plasma fluid volume with a small rise in hematocrit. The author observed a decrease in total renal plasma flow to 57% and in GFR to 59% of control values. A redistribution of intrarenal plasma flow towards the renal medullary tissue may have resulted in differences in fractional sodium reabsorption between superficial, intermediary, and juxtamedullary nephrons, in which blood flow was reduced to 49, 59, and 73% of control values, respectively. Fractional sodium reabsorption was increased in superficial nephrons, which revealed the least decrease in glomerular filtration.

In contrast to the forementioned studies, Better et al.[4] observed no changes in GFR or in proximal tubular sodium reabsorption in CBDL rats, 8 to 10 d after bile duct ligation when they showed normal blood pressure, cardiac output, and systemic vascular resistance, but a twofold rise in renal vascular resistance and a more than 40% decrease in total renal blood flow. In these animals, plasma volume was increased but total blood volume was unaltered. No retention of sodium and a normal natriuretic response to an acute saline load were found by Hishida et al.[4a] in rabbits 10 d after bile duct ligation.

Our studies in conscious rats after 6 d of CBDL revealed a significant decrease in GFR and in absolute renal sodium and chloride excretion.[5] However, fractional sodium and phosphate excretion rates were increased, suggesting a decrease in proximal tubular reabsorption despite a presumed contraction of the extracellular fluid volume which normally results in enhanced proximal tubular absorption.

Equivocal results were also obtained in *long-term* studies of *chronic* bile duct ligation. Whereas Allison et al.[5b] found no sodium retention in CBDL rats 3 weeks after bile duct obstruction, Better and Massry[6] also reported enhanced sodium reabsorption in proximal and distal tubular segments of the CBDL dog 6 weeks after bile duct ligation. These animals, in addition, showed a blunted response to saline loading which may be related partly to a lack of renal vasodilation[1a] and which may be reversed by 5 days oral administration of propranolol.[6a]

IV. EFFECTS OF JAUNDICE ON RENAL CONCENTRATING AND DILUTING ABILITY

Better et al.[4] observed in CBDL rats a defect in the maximal urinary diluting capacity of the kidney which depended on the presence of antidiuretic hormone (ADH). In our studies[5] in conscious CBDL rats, the animals, which had a significantly reduced body weight, were polyuric, with a significantly lower urinary osmolarity than sham-operated rats and revealed a slight reduction in serum sodium concentration. Although we did not measure plasma ADH concentration, which was presumably elevated, nor did we perform a renal concentrating test in these animals, it may be assumed that the collecting tubule in these animals was at least partially resistant to the action of ADH.

V. BILE CONSTITUENTS WHICH MAY AFFECT RENAL FUNCTION IN OBSTRUCTIVE JAUNDICE

Under the conditions of extra- or intrahepatic bile duct obstruction, jaundice is associated with the retention of bile of which bilirubin and bile salts constitute major components besides cholesterol and other lipids. Circulating cholesterol in concentrations observed under these conditions appears to have no major effects on epithelial transport or on renal function, whereas high concentrations of bilirubin may have an effect on renal function and also may contribute to the precipitation of acute renal failure by formation of renal tubular casts leading to tubular obstruction.

Infusion of bile in the dog was shown to result in a rise in urine volume.[7] This was confirmed by Alon et al.[8] when they found that infusion of 1:10 and 1:20 diluted bile into the dog renal artery caused a dose-dependent rise in urinary flow and excretion of sodium and potassium. The rise in urinary flow rate was associated with an increased urinary prostaglandin E_2 and $F_{2\alpha}$ excretion. Pretreatment with a cyclooxygenase inhibitor blunted the rise in urinary prostaglandin excretion and abolished the diuretic, natriuretic, and kaliuretic effects of bile infusion.

VI. EFFECTS OF BILIRUBIN ON RENAL FUNCTION

Hyperbilirubinemia has been shown to potentially affect renal function. Thus, chronic unconjugated hyperbilirubinemia in the GUNN strain of rat results in crystal deposits of bilirubin in the renal papilla and is associated with a urinary concentrating defect, decreased maximal free-water clearance and increased fractional sodium excretion, as well as a decrease in renal medullary urea and sodium concentrations.[9-11] (See Figure 1.) It was also shown in infants that hyperbilirubinemia results in a relative decrease in GFR and in increased fractional excretion of sodium in response to salt and water loading.[12] Since high concentrations of unconjugated bilirubin promotes the secretion of sodium and water in the isolated perfused intestine of the hamster,[13] bilirubin may interfere with epithelial cell transport function (Figure 1). Thus, in the toad bladder it was shown that short-term exposure to bilirubin results in an impaired vasopressin-stimulated active sodium transport without effects on the hydroosmotic response to vasopressin.[14] This is in agreement with previous findings showing that bilirubin has cytotoxic effects[15] and inhibits Na, K-ATPase[16] of human red blood cells in vitro.

Mor et al.,[17] however, found no diuresis in CBDL dogs, despite a significant rise in plasma bilirubin concentration. In contrast, dogs with choledochocaval anastomosis and a somewhat higher bilirubinemia revealed a moderate but significant diuresis, despite an unchanged GFR which suggests that this diuresis was induced by some biliary constituents other than bilirubin. Studies by Alon et al.,[18] in addition, support the notion that bile salts may be the causative factor which induces a diuresis, since direct infusion of sodium taurocholate into the kidney resulted in a significant diuresis, whereas bilirubin infusion was without effect.

VII. EFFECTS OF BILE SALTS ON RENAL FUNCTION

It has long been known that bile acids, which usually undergo enterohepatic recirculation to an extent of 99%, can affect intestinal water and electrolyte transport (Figure 1).

All bile salts formed and excreted by the liver are normally conjugated with the amino acids glycine and taurine prior to their delivery into the biliary canaliculus. The two primary bile acids, cholic acid and chenodeoxycholic acid, are dehydrolyzed to the secondary bile acids, deoxycholic acid and lithocholic acid. Primary bile acids comprise 94, 70, and 64%

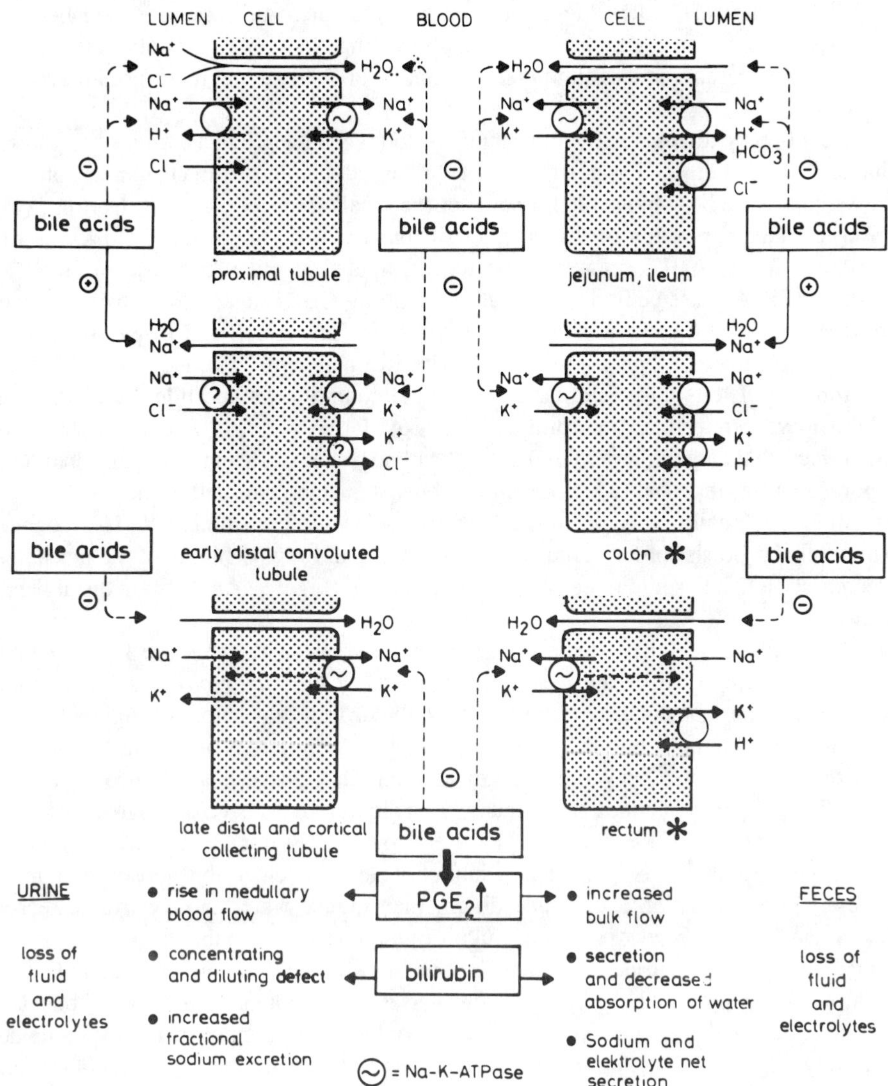

FIGURE 1. Potential effects of bilirubin and bile acids on renal and intestinal handling of fluid and electrolytes. + = stimulation; − = inhibition; (* applies only to superficial epithelial cells).

of total bile acids in the bile, serum, and urine, respectively. In decreasing order of concentrations, total nonesterified bile acids in human plasma comprise chenodeoxycholic acid, deoxycholic acid, cholic acid, and lithocholic acid. Whereas in the bile only small amounts of bile acids are sulfated, in the serum this fraction may rise up to 50% and in the urine up to 72%. Urinary bile acids are mostly polar derivatives and are excreted as sulfates or glucuronides. Bile acid concentrations will rise significantly with partial or complete obstruction of the bile duct and thus may reach the kidney in high concentrations where they are filtered and secreted into the tubular lumen. With cholestasis, urinary bile acid excretion may increase 40- to 100-fold.[19,20]

A. EFFECTS OF BILE SALTS ON RENAL SODIUM EXCRETION AND UNDERLYING MECHANISMS

Infusion of bile salts in dogs has been shown to increase urine output, without a rise in GFR,[18,21] and clinical studies suggest diminished tubular sodium reabsorption before the diluting segment.[22] Thus, Better et al. have shown that sodium taurocholate (0.1 mmol/l) in the tubular perfusate reduces fluid reabsorption by 30% in the microperfused rat proximal tubule *in situ*.[23]

Bile acids may affect renal synthesis of cyclooxygenase products which are known to modulate renal sodium and water excretion by hemodynamic or direct tubular actions[24,25] and are supposed to be responsible for some of the renal effects of bile duct ligation.[26] Thus, the rise in urinary excretion of the potent vasoconstrictor thromboxane B_2 (TXB_2), which we observed in our CBDL rats, may be related to the observed decrease in GFR.[6] The unaltered Na, K-ATPase activities in renal tissue of our CBDL rats[6] do not exclude changes in enzyme activities in specific nephron segments. In fact, Israeli and Bogin demonstrated a significant decrease in Na, K-ATPase activity in microsomal fractions of whole kidney tissue from CBDL rats under similar experimental conditions,[27] and bile acids were found to inhibit in vitro intestinal[28] and brain[29] Na, K-ATPase. We also observed a decrease in renal cortical ATP content in our CBDL rats.[6] Although not sufficient to impair renal tubular transport function, it probably reflects altered energy metabolism within the renal cortex of these animals.[6] Finally, it was shown that bile acids directly inhibit Na-H-exchange in proximal tubular brush border vesicles,[30] which also could represent one of the mechanisms for decreased fluid and sodium reabsorption in proximal (Figure 1) and also in distal nephron segments.

Since no further detailed studies on these issues exist with reference to renal tubular transport we might consider the well-studied *effects of bile acids on intestinal transport*, which shares important features with the renal tubular transport systems (Figure 1).

The human jejunum is normally exposed to high concentrations of conjugated bile acids, and bacterial overgrowth may produce, in addition, large amounts of unconjugated bile acids. In the rat, high concentrations of taurocholate inhibit intestinal electrolyte reabsorption, possibly by inhibition of the Na, K-ATPase enzyme.[31,32] In dogs and in man, conjugated and unconjugated dihydroxy bile acids inhibit water and electrolyte absorption at high concentrations in the colon[33] and, in addition, may induce water and electrolyte secretion in the human colon.[34] *In vivo* perfusion studies in man have shown that unconjugated cholic acid or its glycine and taurine conjugates had no significant effect on water and electrolyte absorption in the proximal jejunum.[35] However, the unconjugated dihydroxy bile acids, deoxycholic acid and chenodeoxycholic acid, as well as their glycine and taurine conjugates, respectively, significantly inhibited water and electrolyte absorption at 3 mM concentration and induced net secretion at 2- to 3-fold higher concentrations.[35] Unconjugated bile acids were also found to inhibit water absorption in the rat jejunum,[36] probably due to changes in epithelial permeability.[37] This was confirmed in human jejunum, ileum, and colon, in which glycine-conjugated dihydroxy bile acids induced net fluid flow. In these studies, bulk flow of fluid was assumed to be intercellular, i.e., by extracellular route, and thus was dissociated from ion exchange which takes place across the luminal surface of the mucosal cell.[38] Additional studies have shown that deoxycholate does not interfere with active transport mechanisms but increases the permeability of the colonic epithelium to sodium ions (Figure 1).[39]

B. EFFECTS OF BILE SALTS ON RENAL WATER EXCRETION

As mentioned earlier, experimental obstructive jaundice in rats is associated with a decrease in renal concentrating ability,[5] and this decrease in maximal concentrating ability was also observed in CBDL dogs by Better and Massry.[6]

With respect to bile salts, on the one hand, studies from Dillingham et al.[40] have shown that sodium taurocholate in the bathing solution increases tubular hydraulic conductivity by a cAMP-independent mechanism in isolated perfused rabbit cortical collecting tubules and induces a dose-dependent leak from tubular lumen to the bathing fluid. With regard to the underlying mechanism, sodium taurocholate was found to be capable of changing the composition and permeability of artificial liposomes.[41] It can alter plasma membrane phospholipid content and regulate sodium and hydrogen ion flux across isolated rat hepatocyte membrane vesicles.[42] It may also stimulate guanylate cyclase activity and cGMP formation.[43]

On the other hand, PGE_2 is known to antagonize the action of ADH by means of a short-loop feedback mechanism through suppression of ADH-induced stimulation of adenylate cyclase activity.[24,44] Since in our studies in CBDL rats urinary PGE_2 excretion, which may reflect renal synthesis of PGE_2 under conditions of endogenous stimulation,[45] was normal, such an antagonistic effect seems unlikely in this *in vivo* experimental condition. The partial resistance of the collecting tubule to ADH under the conditions of obstructive jaundice may simply result from medullary washout[24] due to an increase in medullary blood flow in the presence of normal total renal and reduced outer cortical blood flow.[2]

VIII. SUMMARY

When considering the effects of obstructive jaundice on body fluid volume, the effects of acute bile retention itself on renal function must be strictly separated from biliary obstruction associated with liver damage and formation of ascites. Thus, experimental acute bile duct ligation (ABDL) results in urinary loss of sodium and water, and a reduction in plasma volume similar to the hypovolemia observed in patients with acute obstructive jaundice. In contrast, in animals and in patients with biliary cirrhosis, increased proximal tubular sodium absorption is usually observed in the presence of ascites formation, but fractional sodium absorption may be decreased and extracellular fluid volume be diminished due to preceding urinary fluid loss and a continuous inability of the kidney to concentrate the urine. The major components of bile, which accumulate with bile duct obstruction and impair renal function, are bilirubin and bile salts, both affecting epithelial transport of fluid and sodium.

Bilirubin inhibits the Na, K-ATPase enzyme *in vitro* and results in an increased fractional sodium excretion *in vivo*. Bilirubin also reduces urinary concentrating ability, which is probably due to impaired active sodium transport indirectly stimulated by vasopressin, since it does not affect the hydroosmotic response to vasopressin. A decrease in the medullary osmotic gradient, in addition, may contribute to the resulting urinary concentrating defect.

Bile salts also inhibit renal proximal (and distal) tubular fluid and sodium absorption possibly by inhibiting active sodium transport and the Na, H-exchange mechanism. But, moreover, bile salts may predominantly raise epithelial permeability with increased intercellular, i.e., extracellular, bulk flow as demonstrated for colonic epithelium. Bile acids were shown to increase tubular hydraulic conductivity by a cAMP-independent mechanism, and increased renal prostaglandin E_2 production observed with intrarenal bile infusion may be accompanied by a rise in renal medullary blood flow. Hence, resistance to ADH may primarily result from medullary washout and thereby explain in part the urinary concentrating defect observed under these experimental conditions.

Thus, in addition to the cardiac and vascular impairment which occurs with obstructive jaundice, hypovolemia due to renal fluid and sodium loss with its subsequent contraction of the extracellular fluid volume may contribute to the risks of hypotension and circulatory shock in patients with extra- or intrahepatic bile duct obstruction. In addition to renal hypoperfusion, renal tubular obstruction due to bilirubin cast formation may predispose the jaundiced kidney to acute renal failure.

REFERENCES

1. **Levy, M. and Finestone, H.,** Renal response to four hours of biliary obstruction in the dog, *Am. J. Physiol.,* 244, F516, 1983.

1a. **Melman, A. and Massry, S. G.,** Role of renal vasodilation in the blunted natriuresis of saline infusion in dogs with chronic bile duct obstruction, *J. Lab. Clin. Med.,* 89, 1053,, 1977.

2. **Bank, N. and Aynedjian, H. S.,** A micropuncture study of renal salt and water retention in chronic bile duct obstruction, *J. Clin. Invest.,* 55, 493, 1975.

3. **Yarger, W. E.,** Intrarenal mechanisms of salt retention after bile duct ligation in rats, *J. Clin. Invest.,* 57, 408, 1976.

4. **Better, O. S., Aisenbrey, G. A., Berl, T., Anderson, R. J., Handelman, W. A., Linas, S. L., Guggenheim, S. J., and Schrier, R. W.,** Role of antidiuretic hormone in impaired urinary dilution associated with chronic bile-duct ligation, *Clin. Sci.,* 58, 493, 1980.

4a. **Hishida, A., Honda, N., Sudo, M., Kimura, M., Nagase, M.,** Renal handling of salt and water in the early stage of obstructive jaundice in rabbits, *Nephron,* 30, 368, 1982.

5. **Heidenreich, S., Brinkema, E., Martin, A., Düsing, R., Kipnowski, J., and Kramer, H. J.,** The kidney and cardiovascular system in obstructive jaundice: functional and metabolic studies in conscious rats, *Clin. Sci.,* 73, 593, 1987.

5a. **Allison, M. E. M., Moss, N. G., Fraser, M. M., Dobbie, J. W., Ryan, C. J., Kennedy, A. C., and Blumgart, L. H.,** Renal function in chronic obstructive jaundice: a micropuncture study in rats, *Clin. Sci. Mol. Med.,* 54, 649, 1978.

6. **Better, O. S. and Massry, S. G.,** Effect of chronic bile duct obstruction on renal handling of salt and water, *J. Clin. Invest.,* 51, 402, 1972.

6a. **Winaver, J., Chaimovitz, C., and Better, O. S.,** Natriuretic effect of propranolol on dogs with chronic bile-duct ligation, *Clin. Sci. Mol. Med.,* 54, 603, 1978.

7. **Topuzlu, C. and Stahl, W. M.,** Effect of bile infusion on the dog kidney, *N. Engl. J. Med.,* 52, 760, 1966.

8. **Alon, V., Berant, M., Mordechovitz, D., and Better, O. S.,** The effect of intrarenal infusion of bile on kidney function in the dog, *Clin. Sci.,* 62, 431, 1982.

9. **Call, N. B. and Tisher, C. C.,** The urinary concentrating defect in the Gunn strain of rat, *J. Clin. Invest.,* 55, 319, 1975.

10. **Martinez-Maldonado, M., Suki, W. N., and Schenker, S.,** Nature of the urinary concentrating defect in the Gunn strain of rat, *Am. J. Physiol.,* 216, 1386, 1969.

11. **Odell, G. B., Natzschka, J. C., and Storey, G. N. B.,** Bilirubin nephropathy in the Gunn strain of rat, *Am. J. Physiol.,* 212, 931, 1967.

12. **Broberger, U. and Aperia, A.,** Renal function in infants with hyperbilirubinemia, *Acta Paediatr. Scand.,* 68, 75, 1979.

13. **Whitington, P. F., Olsen, W. A., and Odell, G. B.,** The effect of bilirubin on the function of hamster small intestine, *Pediatr. Res.,* 15, 1009, 1981.

14. **Brem, A. S., Cashore, W. J., Pacholski, M., Tetreault, J., and Lawler, R. G.,** Effects of bilirubin on transepithelial transport of sodium, water, and urea, *Kidney Int.,* 27, 51, 1985.

15. **Kaul, R., Bajpai, V. K., Shipstone, A. C., Kaul, H. K., and Krishna, C. R. M.,** Bilirubin-induced erythrocyte membrane cytotoxicity, *Exp. Mol. Pathol.,* 34, 290, 1981.

16. **Kawai, K. and Cowger, M. L.,** Effect of bilirubin on ATPase activity of human erythrocyte membranes, *Res. Comm. Chem. Pathol. Pharmacol.,* 32, 123, 1981.

17. **Mor, L., Bomzon, A., Mordechovich, D., Blendis, L. M., and Better, O. S.,** Renal bilirubin excretion in canine models of jaundice, *Biochem. Med. Metabol. Biol.,* 36, 252, 1986.

18. **Alon, U., Berant, M., Mordechovitz, D., Hashmonai, M., and Better, O. S.,** Effect of isolated cholaemia on systemic haemodynamics and kidney function in conscious dogs, *Clin. Sci.,* 63, 59, 1982.

19. **Black, P., Spaczynski, K., and Gerok, W.,** Bile-salt glucuronides in urine, *Hoppe-Seyler's Z. Physiol. Chem.,* 355, 749, 1974.

20. **Stiehl, A.,** Bile salt sulphates in cholestasis, *Eur. J. Clin. Invest.,* 4, 59, 1974.

21. **Finestone, H., Fechner, C., and Levy, M.,** Effects of bile and bile salt infusions on renal function in dogs, *Can. J. Physiol. Pharmacol.,* 62, 762, 1984.

22. **Chaimovitz, C., Rochman, J., Eidelman, S., and Better, O. S.,** Exaggerated natriuretic response to volume expansion in patients with primary biliary cirrhosis, *Am. J. Med. Sci.,* 274, 173, 1977.

23. **Better, O. S., Guckian, V., Giebisch, G., and Green, R.,** The effect of sodium taurocholate on proximal tubular reabsorption in the rat kidney, *Clin. Sci.,* 72, 139, 141, 1987.

24. **Kramer, H. J., Glänzer, K., and Düsing, R.,** Role of prostaglandins in the regulation of renal water excretion, *Kidney Int.,* 19, 851, 1981.

25. **Kramer, H. J., Kipnowski, J., and Düsing, R.,** The role of renal prostaglandins in the regulation of renal sodium excretion, *Agents Actions* (Suppl.), 22, 61, 1987.

26. **Alon, V., Davidal, G., Berant, M., and Better, O. S.,** Sodium diclofenac inhibits the natriuretic effect of bile (Abstr.), *Kidney Int., 29,* 328, 1986.
27. **Israeli, B. A. and Bogin, E.,** Biochemical changes in liver, kidney and blood associated with common bile duct ligation, *Clin. Chim. Acta,* 160, 211, 1986.
28. **Parkinson, T. M. and Olson, J. A.,** Inhibitory effects of bile acids on adenosine triphosphatase, oxygen consumption and the transport and diffusion of water-soluble substances in the small intestine of the rat, *Life Sci.,* 3, 107, 1964.
29. **Seda, H. W. M., Grove, C. D., Hughes, R. D., and Williams, R.,** Inhibition of partially purified rat brain Na^+, K^+-dependent ATPase by bile acids, phenolic acids and endotoxin, *Clin. Sci.,* 66, 415, 1984.
30. **Sellinger, M., Haag, K., Mielke, G., Gerok, W., and Knauf, H.,** Hemmung des Na^+/H^+ Antiporters der Bürstensaummembran der menschlichen Niere durch Sulfochenodesoxycholsäure als möglicher Pathomechanismus beim postoperativen Nierenversagen nach Verschlussikterus (Abstr.), *Kidney Int.,* 29, 1257, 1986.
31. **Harries, J. T. and Sladen, G. E.,** Effect of bile acids on small intestinal absorption of glucose, water and sodium, *Gut,* 12, 885, 1971.
32. **Sladen, G. E. and Harries, J. T.,** Studies on the effects of unconjugated dihydroxy bile salts on rat small intestinal function in vivo, *Biochim. Biophys. Acta,* 288, 443, 1972.
33. **Mekhjian, H. S. and Phillips, S. F.,** Perfusion of the canine colon with unconjugated bile acids: effect on water and electrolyte transport, morphology and bile acid absorption, *Gastroenterology,* 59, 120, 1970.
34. **Mekhjian, H. E., Phillips, S. F., and Hofmann, A. F.,** Colonic secretion of water and electrolytes induced by bile acids: perfusion studies in man, *J. Clin. Invest.,* 50, 1569, 1971.
35. **Russell, R. I., Allan, J. G., Gerskowitch, V. P., and Cochran, K. M.,** The effect of conjugated and unconjugated bile acids on water and electrolyte absorption in the human jejunum, *Clin. Sci. Mol. Med.,* 45, 301, 1973.
36. **Forth, W., Rummel, W., and Glasner, H.,** Zur resorptionshemmenden Wirkung von Gallensäuren, *Naunyn-Schmiedebergs Arch. Pharmakol. Exp. Pathol.,* 254, 364, 1966.
37. **Feldman, S. and Gibaldi, M.,** Physiologic surface-active agents and drug absorption. I. Effect of sodium taurodeoxycholate on salicylate transfer across the everted rat intestine, *J. Pharmaceut. Sci.,* 58, 425, 1969.
38. **Wingate, D. L., Krag, E., Mekhjian, H. S., and Phillips, S. F.,** Relationships between ion and water movement in the human jejunum, ileum and colon during perfusion with bile acids, *Clin. Sci. Mol. Med.,* 45, 593, 1973.
39 **Wanitschke, R., Nell, G., Rummel, W., and Specht, W.,** Transfer of sodium and water through isolated rat colonic mucosa under the influence of deoxycholate and oxyphenisatin, *Naunyn-Schmiedebergs Arch. Pharmacol.,* 297, 185, 1977.
40. **Dillingham, M. A., Better, O. S., and Anderson, R. J.,** Sodium taurocholate increases hydraulic conductivity in rabbit collecting tubule, *Kidney Int.,* 33, 782, 1988.
41. **Schubert, R., Jaroni, H., Schoelmerich, J., and Schmidt, K. H.,** Studies on the mechanism of bile-salt induced liposomal membrane damage, *Digestion,* 28, 181, 1983.
42. **Bear, C. E., Petrunka, C. N., and Strasberg, S. M.,** Effect of sodium taurocholate on amiloride-inhibitable sodium uptake and on intracellular pH of isolated rat hepatocytes, *J. Lab. Clin. Med.,* 108, 109, 1981.
43. **Ichihara, K., Larner, J., Kimura, H., Murad, F.,** Activation of liver guanylate cyclase by bile salts and contaminants in crude secretin and pancreozymin preparations, *Biochim. Biophys. Acta,* 481, 734, 1977.
44. **Kramer, H. J., Bäcker, A., Hinzen, S., and Düsing, R.,** Effects of inhibition of prostaglandin-synthesis on renal electrolyte excretion and concentrating ability in healthy man, *Prostaglandins Medicine,* 1, 341, 1978.
45. **Kramer, H. J., Mattern, H., Bäcker, A., Fricke, G., Glänzer, K., Kipnowski, J., and Düsing, R.,** Renal synthesis of prostaglandin E_2 in human subjects with normal renal function, in *Prostaglandins and Other Eicosanoids in the Cardiovascular System,* Schrör, K., Ed., Karger, Basel, 1985, 124.

Chapter 15

ANF AND ITS ROLE IN SODIUM RETENTION IN CIRRHOSIS

P. J. Campbell, Karl Skorecki, and Laurence M. Blendis

TABLE OF CONTENTS

I. INTRODUCTION

It has now been conclusively shown that the atria are a peptide-secreting endocrine gland. The state of molecular biology in the 1980s has permitted rapid progress in the purification, sequencing, and synthesis of the hormone termed atrial natriuretic factor (ANF). Indeed, the endogenous biosynthesis of this peptide and the structural properties of the gene encoding it have been delineated. Autoradiography has revealed specific receptors for this peptide in many organs in the body. Despite these impressive technical advances, the precise role of atrial natriuretic factor in both normal physiological functions and pathophysiological states remains to be elucidated.

In this chapter, we will review the known actions of atrial natriuretic factor, and then discuss the potential role of this peptide in the cardiovascular and renal derangements that occur in chronic liver disease.

II. BACKGROUND

The discovery by deBold and his colleagues that injection of atrial extract from rats could induce a natriuresis, diuresis, and fall in blood pressure[1] represents a culmination of two separate previous lines of investigation that had suggested the atria contained a hormone capable of influencing volume regulation (Table 1).

III. RELEASE OF ATRIAL NATRIURETIC FACTOR

The exact *in vivo* regulation release of ANF is still not clear. Direct atrial distension in animals has been shown to release immunoreactive peptides with ANF activity. In rat heart-lung preparations, increasing the atrial perfusion pressure and distending the atria resulted in the release of an agent that produced a natriuresis and diuresis when infused into bioassay rats,[12] and in the perfusates of distended atria from isolated perfused rat hearts, an increase in immunoreactive ANF-like material was demonstrated.[13] In conscious dogs, distension of either right or left atria by partial obstruction of the mitral or tricuspid valve produced an increase in the concentration of ANF in plasma, and circulating levels of the peptide reverted to control values shortly after return of atrial pressure to normal.[14] In the dog, a 1 mmHg rise in atrial pressure results in an increase of 10 to 15 pmol/l rise in plasma (p) ANF levels. The response is unaffected by cardiac denervation.[14]

In man[15-17] acute volume expansion with intravenous saline results in the releases of ANF. Other maneuvers in man known to elevate atrial pressure, namely, head-out water immersion (HWI),[18-20] assumption of the supine posture,[21,22] and exercise[23] also result in increased plasma levels of ANF. In response to an increase in sodium in the diet, plasma levels of ANF in normal volunteers rise.[21] These accumulated data are consistent with the release of ANF in response to either ECF volume expansion or central redistribution.

Other mechanisms of stimulation of atrial ANF release include increase in sodium concentration.[24] *In vitro* incubation of rat atria with α- and β-adrenergic agonists[25-26] and vasopressin resulted in a marked increase in natriuretic activity,[27,28] with depletion of the natriuretic activity of the atrial tissue. These effects were inhibited by the specific antagonists, atropine and phentolamine. Since these substances activate the phosphoinositol system, inositol triphosphate was suggested as the second messenger of the stimulus to secretion in atrial cells.[27,28]

The above evidence would then implicate at least two separate mechanisms for ANF release: first, stretch itself, and second, neurohormonal stimulation of specific receptors.

TABLE 1
The Background History of ANF

Year	Author	Comment	Ref.
1956	Kersch	Identification of atrial granules	2
1964	Jamieson and Palade	Granules distinguished from lysozymes	3
1974	Huet and Cantin	Further characterization of atrial granules	4
1979	deBold	Relationship between presence of granules and salt and water balance established	5
1981	deBold et al.	Injection of atrial extract causes natriuresis	1
1982—1983	Garcia et al.	Identification of natriuretic	6
	deBold et al.	Properties of atrial granules	7
1982—1983	deBold	Purification and identification of atrial peptides, including the circulating active 28-amino acid form, ANF	9
	Thibault et al.		8
	Trippodo et al.		10
	deBold and Flynn		11

IV. ACTIONS OF ANF

A. CELLULAR LEVEL; ANF RECEPTORS AND CYCLIC GMP (cGMP) PRODUCTION

The topic of ANF receptors has previously been reviewed in detail.[28-32] Although the precise details concerning the mechanism of action of ANF at a cellular level are not known, cyclic GMP (cGMP) is considered to be a potential intracellular, second messenger.[33] It has subsequently been demonstrated that ANF activates particulate guanylate cyclase in target tissues,[34-38] and that the increase in cGMP by ANF correlates with the distribution of particulate guanylate cyclase.[37] The rise in cGMP appears to be the result of direct stimulation, rather than inhibition of cGMP degradation.[37] In man, bolus injection of 50 mg of ANF,[39] volume expansion with saline,[40] or HWI[20] produce rises in both urinary and plasma cGMP.[39-40]

Cyclic GMP is eliminated from the circulation largely by renal excretion, the plasma half life being approximately 15 min.[41] Therefore, utilizing cGMP as a biological marker, investigators have studied the effects of ANF on various target organs. In the kidney, ANF has been demonstrated to stimulate cGMP accumulation in the glomeruli,[42] primary cultures of inner medullary collecting ducts,[43] and renal epithelial cell lines.[44] In microdissected nephron segments, synthetic ANF (1 mM) markedly increased cGMP content only in rat glomeruli and inner medullary collecting ducts.[43]

However, there is an apparent discrepancy between the dose required to bind to receptors and stimulate end organ biological activity and the higher dose that is required to stimulate cGMP.[45-47] This discrepancy can be explained in part by the identification of at least two distinct ANF receptors characterized from cultured canine kidney tubular (MDCK) cells and rat thoracic aortic smooth muscle (RTASM) cells.[48] These receptor subtypes include a disulfide-linked 140-kDa protein found in RTASM cells which is probably analogous to the guanylate cyclase-uncoupled vascular receptor. A second subtype is a disulfide-unlinked 120-kDa protein which is analogous to the guanylate cyclase-coupled renal receptor. A third subtype, nonreducible 68- to 70-kDa protein was found in both MDCK and RTASM cells, which with the reducible 140-kDa protein showed a strong affinity for the full length ANF peptide. Thus, the concept of two types of receptor has been developed, one linked to guanylate cyclase for metabolic effect of ANF, the other unlinked for clearance of ANF from plasma. Indeed, it has been more recently shown that the resolution of ANF receptor density with varying salt intake pertained specifically to the clearance type, but not to guanylate cyclase-linked receptor.

TABLE 2
Systemic Hemodynamic Effects of ANF

Study	Results	Ref.
Large dose bolus infusion in animals	Fall in BP and PVR	57, 58
	No change in PVR	59, 60
	Transient hypotension	61, 62
Low dose continuous infusion	Fall in CO, secondary fall in BP	57, 59
High dose infusion into coronary arteries	Coronary vasoconstriction	63

There is conflicting evidence as to the effect of ANF on cyclic AMP (cAMP) production. It was suggested that ANF does not directly compete with hormone receptors stimulating adenylate cyclase,[49] but may stimulate inhibitory receptors coupled to the adenylate cyclase.[44]

B. PHYSIOLOGICAL/PHARMACOLOGICAL ACTIONS
1. Vascular Actions

Original experiments with crude atrial extracts from rats and human atrial tissue demonstrated relaxation of preconstricted rabbit aorta and chick rectal smooth muscle preparations.[50] With the preparation of synthetic ANF, the vasodilator profile of ANF has been further studied. ANF appears to have some degree of selectivity in terms of its effects on specific vascular beds. Renal artery and aorta appear highly sensitive, but mesenteric, carotid, femoral, and vertebral arteries have been found to be relatively unresponsive.[51-52] The vasodilator profile of ANF has been compared to that of nitroprusside, both in *in vitro* experiments,[53] and appears to be endothelial independent.[54,55]

2. Systemic Hemodynamics (Table 2)

The effect of ANF on systemic hemodynamics in various animal models has been previously extensively reviewed.[56] In summary, mean arterial blood pressure (MAP) usually but not always falls.

3. Regional Blood Flow Studies

Blood flow to splanchnic organs has been reported to decrease,[63-65] whereas flow to skeletal muscle has been documented to either increase[64] or decrease.[57,59] In intact animals, ANF administration has been reported to produce a selective increase in renal blood flow with a fall[49,65,67] or a rise in renal vascular resistance in conscious rats.[59] The precise reasons for these conflicting reports are not immediately obvious. However, in the functioning isolated rat kidney, perfused without vasoconstrictors, ANF has been reported to cause a gradual consistent rise in renal vascular resistance.[71] However, in preparations perfused by vasoconstrictors (angiotensin II, norepinephrine, vasopressin), infusion of ANF results in a decrease of renal vascular resistance towards prevasoconstrictor levels.[71] These results suggest that ANF may under some circumstances have a mild renal vasoconstrictor effect which competes with more powerful vasoconstrictors when present, resulting in vasodilatation.

4. Renal Effects
a. Glomerular Filtration Rate (Table 3)

An increase in glomerular filtration rate (GFR) has been reported in rats with a continuous infusion of atrial extract[72] or synthetic ANF.[73,68] The increase in GFR and filtration fraction is accompanied by a small but significant rise in renal vascular resistance. This has led to the suggestion that ANF is a preferential efferent vasoconstrictor in the glomerular vasculature, thereby elevating glomerular capillary pressure and hence GFR.[76] Similar work by Burnett et al.[77] noted that there was an increase in filtration fraction with no change in renal

TABLE 3
The Renal Effects of ANF

Preferential Efferent (Weak) Vasoconstrictor

Glomerular filtration rate — no change
Renal plasma flow — no change or increased
Renal medullary blood flow — no change or increased
Filtration fraction — increased
Peritubular capillary pressure — increased
Renal vascular resistance — increased

Tubular Sodium Transport Inhibitor

Generalized proximal tubular reabsorption — normal or decreased
Juxta medullary tubular reabsorption — decreased

Medullary Collecting Duct — Inhibition

Direct via blockage of amiloride-sensitive sodium channels
Indirect via increased peritubular capillary, pressure with backflux of sodium, rich interstitial fluid

blood flow, which led to the suggestion that the increase in GFR may be mediated by a balanced action on segmental renal vascular resistances, i.e., preglomerular resistance is decreased and postglomerular resistance is increased. Direct study of glomeruli has not fully resolved this.[78-84]

b. Changes in Tubular Function

There is considerable disagreement on the presence or absence of ANF receptors in the proximal tubule and on whether ANF affects sodium reabsorption.[69,70,85-87] Furthermore, micropuncture studies showed no increase in solute concentration at end superficial proximal tubules, indicating no increased proximal tubule reabsorption.[70] In addition, no effects of ANF were found on isolated perfused segments of Henle's loop,[88] and inhibition of sodium transport was described with microcatheterization of papillary collecting ducts.[89]

c. Medullary "Washout"

Evidence that there is a redistribution of blood flow to "deeper" nephrons is controversial.[75] Yet, the natriuresis following ANF administration is secondary to a rise in GFR, and if glomerulotubular balance is maintained, then the increased filtered load should be reabsorbed. It has therefore been proposed that accompanying the rise in GFR there is a rise in medullary plasma flow, leading to a medullary "washout".[75,76] Such a medullary "washout" has previously been proposed to inhibit sodium reabsorption from the ascending limb, leading to increased delivery to the distal nephron and then to a natriuresis.[79] In support of this concept, Maack et al. note that a synthetic ANF in dogs leads to a decrease in urine osmolality without a change in free water clearance.[75] Furthermore, there is an increase in papillary blood flow in rats following administration of atrial extract, as measured by the albumin distribution method and a decreased papillary urea concentration due to a direct ability of ANF to alter urea permeability.[74]

More substantial evidence exists for an effect on more distal sites, i.e., the medullary collecting duct, the main site, apart from the glomerulus for the presence of ANF receptors.[43,44] Sodium transport in the inner medullary collecting duct of anesthetized rats was characterized by microcatheterization before and during intravenous infusion of atrial extract[89] and synthetic ANF.[90] During ANF infusion there was not only increased delivery of sodium, but also reduced fractional reabsorption of sodium. This was contrasted with KCl infusion, which also induced enhanced sodium delivery to the duct, but had no effect on absorption. However, the precise mechanism of this inhibition was not clear from this study. Furthermore, prevention of the medullary washout effect of infused ANF by clamping of the renal artery also prevented the natriuresis seen in the contralateral kidney.[91] The effect also occurred even in the presence of a drop in GFR in young rats.[92] More recent studies with more exact methodology have confirmed the association with increased medullary blood flow.[93,94]

Initial studies demonstrated that ANF did not inhibit Na^+,K-ATPase. However, there is now evidence that ANF inhibits sodium entry in inner medullary collecting duct cells, prepared from rabbit kidney outer medulla via blockage of amiloride-sensitive sodium channels.[95] The possibility also exists that ANF induces rises in peritubular capillary pressure in the renal medulla resulting in back flux of sodium-rich interstitial fluid into the collecting duct lumen.

Although there is little doubt the ANF can increase glomerular filtration rate, it is highly questionable that this is primarily responsible for the resultant natriuresis and diuresis — particularly as, in many reports, this occurs only at relatively high plasma levels. There would also seem to be an important contribution to the natriuresis by primary tubular inhibition of sodium reabsorption in the collecting duct system as well as secondary to changes in it, and the current evidence favors the inner medullary collecting duct as the predominant site of action.

V. ANF IN CIRRHOSIS

Certain cirrhotic patients demonstrate progressive impairment of renal sodium and water excretion. Despite extensive investigation, the primary effector mechanism(s) responsible leading to salt and water retention remain unclear. Furthermore, the volume status of such individuals, i.e., the nature of the stimulus to salt and water retention is also controversial.

The discovery of ANF has led naturally to an investigation into its possible contribution to the salt and water retention in cirrhosis. It has been the opinion of some investigators that the failure to excrete salt and water is secondary to a deficiency of a natriuretic hormone(s). It is possible in the context of ANF to extend that hypothesis to a deficiency in either synthesis/release or a deficiency in end organ action, i.e., to raise the possibility of end organ resistance.

In an effort to investigate these possibilities, several types of study have been undertaken:

1.   Static measurements: the determination of plasma levels or atrial content of ANF in cirrhotics compared to normal controls.
2.   Dynamic measurements: manipulation of the volume status of cirrhotics, to study the response of the ANF system, to changes in intravascular volume.
3.   Direct infusion of ANF: to study the direct effects of the hormone.

A. STATIC MEASUREMENTS

Jimenez et al., in 1986, studied the atrial content of carbon tetrachloride-induced cirrhotic rats compared to normal controls, by assaying the atrial content in anesthetized normovolemic rats.[96] Atrial extracts from cirrhotic and control rats were injected with normal animals and the rise in urine volume following cirrhotic extracts was 40% and sodium excretion 20% of that of controls. It was therefore concluded that the atrial content of ANF is reduced in cirrhotic rats, due to either a deficiency in synthesis, or to chronic depletion of ANF in the storage form due to excessive release.

Measurement of plasma levels in man has produced conflicting results. Several investigators have noted the plasma levels of ANF in cirrhotics are elevated compared to normal volunteers.[97-101] However, other investigators have found relatively normal levels.[102-103]

The precise reason for the disparity in the results is not clear. Certainly, differences in technique as regards the radioimmunoassay and extraction do occur. However, it is quite clear that in many of the studies reported, there has been no reported attempt to control one very important study variable, that is the sodium content of the diet. It has been quite clearly documented in normal volunteers that the plasma levels of ANF vary with sodium intake.[104] In studies, therefore, the purpose of which is to compare static levels, it is important that the sodium content of the diet is rigorously controlled. Studies from our own institution, which have been performed under strict metabolic conditions, have clearly demonstrated that ANF levels in cirrhotics with and without documented sodium retention are elevated, compared to normal volunteers consuming the same sodium diet.[105] With the present controversy in plasma ANF levels in cirrhosis, any corroborative evidence is welcome. The increased activation of particulate guanylate cyclase activity by elevated circulating ANF levels should lead to both elevated plasma cGMP levels and urinary cGMP excretion. With this in mind, we have recently compared and found a significant correlation between plasma ANF levels and both these parameters.[20,105]

This criticism of previous studies is of course only valid, if it can be shown that the sodium content of the diet has an influence on plasma levels of ANF in cirrhotics. Such a study would also document the responsiveness of the ANF system to changes in dietary sodium load. We have performed a simple balance study to examine this question.

1. Influence of Dietary Sodium on Plasma ANF in Cirrhosis

Six biopsy-proven cirrhotics without (group 1) and five with previously documented ascites (group 2) were admitted to our metabolic unit and placed sequentially on first a constant 20-mM sodium and then a constant 100-mM sodium diet. Each diet lasted 7 days. Diuretic therapy was discontinued prior to admission to the unit. While on the respective diets, after a 5 d equilibration period, two serial 24 h urine collections were obtained for measurement of creatinine clearance and sodium excretion. Fasting recumbent overnight blood samples were drawn for measurement of ANF, creatinine, and aldosterone. ANF was assayed as previously described.[100] Differences in the parameters measured between diets were analyzed by paired t-testing. Results are presented as the mean ± SE.

2. Results

Cirrhotic patients in group 1 tended to be in slight positive sodium balance on both 20 and 100 mM sodium diets associated with nonsignificant rises in pANF and pcGMP levels and suppression of plasma renin activity (PRA) and serum aldosterone levels. In contrast, in patient in group 2, mean 24 h urine sodium excretion on the 20 mmol sodium diet was 8.7 ± 2.8 mM/d, this was significantly less than on the 100 mM diet; 33 ± 12 mM/d ($p < 0.05$). Mean serum aldosterone on the 20 mM sodium diet was 1593 ± 460 pmol/l, this decreased significantly to 235 ± 49 pmol/l ($p < 0.05$) on the 100 mM diet. Mean plasma ANF on the 20 mM diet was 29 ± 4 pg/ml, this increased significantly to 62 ± 9 pg/ml ($p < 0.05$) on the 100 mM diet. There was a significant correlation between pcGMP and pANF levels, supporting the contentions both that pANF levels were indeed elevated and biologically active.

In conclusion, this study documents that it is essential to control sodium intake in cirrhotics as well as normal subjects, when comparing ''baseline'' levels of ANF. In addition, it provides evidence that the ANF system in cirrhotics is responsive to a rise in sodium intake. However, despite the increase in ANF, the patients in group 2 remained in positive sodium balance, excreting only one third of the ingested sodium.

B. DYNAMIC STUDIES

As stated previously, the precise volume status of cirrhotics with salt and water retention is unclear.[95] By alteration of the volume status of such patients, we can document the responsiveness of hormonal systems involved in salt and water retention.

We have therefore employed two models to study volume redistribution in cirrhotics with sodium retention; (1) the response to peritoneovenous shunting (PVS); and (2) the response to head-out water immersion (HWI), and compared them to ANF infusion.

1. PVS

PVS is widely used for the management of ascites refractory to standard medical therapy.[106] Although, the effectiveness of this relatively simple procedure is well known, the precise reason for the partial reversal of salt and water retention is still not clear. Both the immediate and long term physiological consequences of PVS in cirrhotics has been well documented. In the immediate postinsertion period, there is an acute volume load as demonstrated by a rise in cardiac output and a fall in the hematocrit of approximately 15% without a change in overall red cell mass.[107] Accompanying the dramatic increase in cardiac output effect renal plasma flow and creatinine clearance usually rise significantly, accompanied by a diuresis and natriuresis, even in the absence of diuretics. Diuretics which previously had been ineffective are usually effective in the immediate postoperative period even in small doses. In the absence of shunt failure, most patients postdischarge, have little or no ascites, however, they must still limit their sodium intake, and or use a small dose of diuretic, because sodium retention can be induced by dietary salt loading.[108] As regards hormonal changes, although there is an eventual decline in elevated levels of plasma renin activity PRA, serum aldosterone,[107] plasma catecholamines,[109] and arginine vasopressin,[110] there is little or no immediate change in these parameters in the first few hours following shunting. We therefore studied the acute response to PVS of plasma ANF and urinary cGMP, in six cirrhotics with massive refractory ascites.[99] The cirrhotics were studied under strict metabolic conditions prior to and for the first 8 h immediately post PVS.

Five out of the six cirrhotics experienced an immediate significant natriuresis and diuresis. In the 5 immediate responders, there was an immediate and progressive fall in hematocrit, a rise in cardiac output, without a significant fall in mean arterial blood pressure, i. e., systemic vasodilatation occurred. Mean right atrial pressure rose from a baseline value of 6.3 ± 1.1 mmHg to a peak at 2 h of 11.6 ± 1.4 mmHg ($p < 0.05$). ANF rose immediately from a mean preoperative value of 72.7 ± 15 pg/ml, to a peak value at 2 h of 303.4 ± 21.9 pg/ml ($p < 0.01$) (Figure 1). There was a subsequent decline in both right atrial pressure and ANF, but the mean ANF value at 8 h post PVS was still significantly elevated; 186.5 ± 19.2 pg/ml ($p < 0.01$). In these 5 subjects, urinary cGMP excretion increased from a preoperative mean value of 311 ± 108 pmol/min to peak at 4 h at 1829 ± 840 pmol/min ($p < 0.05$). It remained elevated compared to baseline throughout the 8 h of observation (Figure 1).

PRA in the 5 immediate responders fell progressively from a mean preoperative level of 10.68 ± 2.85 ng/l/S to a nadir at 6 h of 2.88 ± 1.15 ng/l/S ($p < 0.05$). Mean aldosterone fell gradually and was significantly below preshunt values only at 8 h postshunt (Figure 1).

The most important observation that derived from this study was the finding that levels of ANF rose significantly in response to an acute volume load, in cirrhotics. This would indicate that even in cirrhotics with massive refractory ascites, there is no failure of release of ANF, in response to a volume stimulus, and thus no evidence of atrial depletion of ANF, as seen in experimental animals.[96] Furthermore, we documented a rise in urinary cyclic GMP levels, indicating that the ANF release is biologically active. It is of course tempting to propose that the acute response to PVS in terms of a natriuresis and diuresis is secondary to this massive rise in ANF, especially as previous studies have demonstrated no change in plasma catecholamines and AVP and only a gradual fall in aldosterone, resulting in persistent hyperaldosteronism during the first 4 postoperative hours. For example, despite the fact that

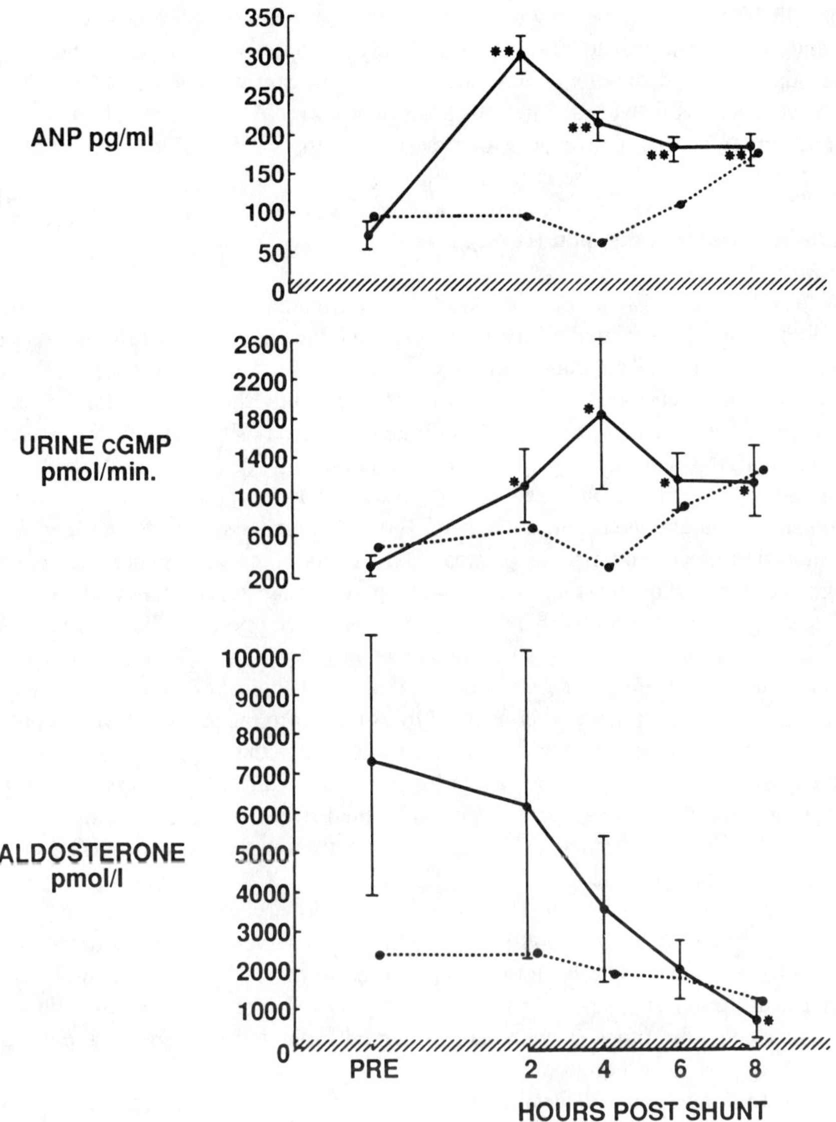

FIGURE 1. Acute changes in plasma ANP, urine cyclic guanosine monophosphate (cGMP) and serum aldosterone levels from preoperative baseline values. Dotted line indicates a delayed response in one patient.

AVP levels do not fall in the immediate postshunt period,[110] there was a prompt fall in urine osmolality, which could be secondary to a direct antagonism of the action of AVP by ANF at the level of the collecting duct. As regards the natriuresis, there was also a rise in creatinine clearance; however, we found no correlation between the mean rise in creatinine clearance and the mean rise in urinary sodium excretion. Furthermore, it has been previously documented that in the acute post PVS period, although there is an increase in C_{PAH} there is no change in mean filtration fraction.[109] These results provide indirect evidence that the natriuresis is not simply a consequence of the rise in GFR or changes in proximal peritubular capillary forces and are more consistent with a tubular rejection of sodium, i.e., would be consistent with a direct tubular action of ANF.

Since this report, there has been a subsequent study reported with almost identical results.[111] In 10 cirrhotic patients with ascites, mean preoperative plasma ANF levels were 82 ng/l and rose significantly to 308 ng/l immediately postoperative. The levels then gradually fell over the next 7 d at which they were still significantly elevated (140 ng/l) above preoperative levels. However, at 3 months postshunt plasma ANF levels had fallen to within the normal range (75 ng/l). However, in contrast these authors did not find a direct relationship between changes in ANF and sodium excretion.

2. Head-Out Water Immersion (HWI)
a. The Study
HWI results in a redistribution of blood volume, increasing central, i.e., intrathoracic blood volume, and is associated with a natriuresis and diuresis.[112] Although the exact mechanism responsible for the resultant natriuresis and diuresis even in normal subjects is still unclear, this method has been used by investigators to study the pathogenesis of renal salt and water retention in cirrhotics.[113,114] In normal subjects, HWI results in a moderate rise in both plasma ANF and urinary cyclic GMP excretion.[20] We have therefore studied the response to HWI in cirrhotic patients without a history of ascites and a group of 12 cirrhotics, in documented sodium retention, to 3 h of HWI. Patients without ascites had both an exaggerated natriuresis and rise in plasma ANF levels compared to normal controls.[115] Although the explanation for this is unclear, it may be due to an increased extracellular volume and great expansion of the intravascular volume. Support for this was provided by a more significant fall in the peripheral hematocrit in the patients compared to controls.

Twelve cirrhotics were admitted to our metabolic unit, diuretics were discontinued, and a constant 20 mM sodium diet was consumed for 8 d prior to the study.[116] All patients were in positive sodium balance on this diet. Prior to the study, the patients were further characterized by their ability to excrete a standard water load; 20 ml/kg of IV D5W, administered over 15 to 20 min, the urine response being measured over 5 h. Each patient was studied on both a control and an immersion day. Details of the immersion and control day have been previously reported.[115]

Of the 12 cirrhotics, only 6 had a marked rise in urinary sodium excretion, sufficient for them to enter into a negative sodium balance, i.e., achieve an hourly sodium excretion in excess of 0.83 mmol. The cirrhotics were therefore divided into 2 groups, depending upon their natriuretic response to HWI. The 6 that achieved a negative sodium balance were termed responders, the other 6, who had a markedly blunted natriuretic response, were termed nonresponders. Although all the cirrhotics were in positive sodium balance, only 2 out of the 6 responders had detectable ascites, whereas all 6 nonresponders had obvious ascites. Furthermore, none of the nonresponders were able to excrete 50% of the standard water load in 5 h, but 5 out of the 6 responders did excrete more than 50% of the water load. When baseline levels of PRA and aldosterone were compared, the responder group had levels within our laboratory normal range, for a 20 mM sodium diet. However, all the nonresponders were above the normal range for PRA and aldosterone and the mean values of these parameters in the nonresponders were significantly elevated compared to the responders. The baseline mean pANF level in the nonresponders was 33.4 $\pm$ 4.6 pg/ml, which was not significantly different to the responders mean value of 25.7 $\pm$ 2.4 pg/ml. Similarly mean baseline urinary cGMP excretion was equivalent in both groups.

When the response of plasma ANF to HWI was compared in both groups, there was a significant and comparable rise (Figure 2). Although the plasma ANF responses to water immersion was not different and therefore did not correlate with the absence or presence of a natriuresis, we considered the possibility of biochemical resistance to the action of ANF. Urinary cGMP was used as a marker of the biochemical activity of ANF. Both groups of patients again showed a significant and comparable rise in this parameter during HWI (Figure 2).

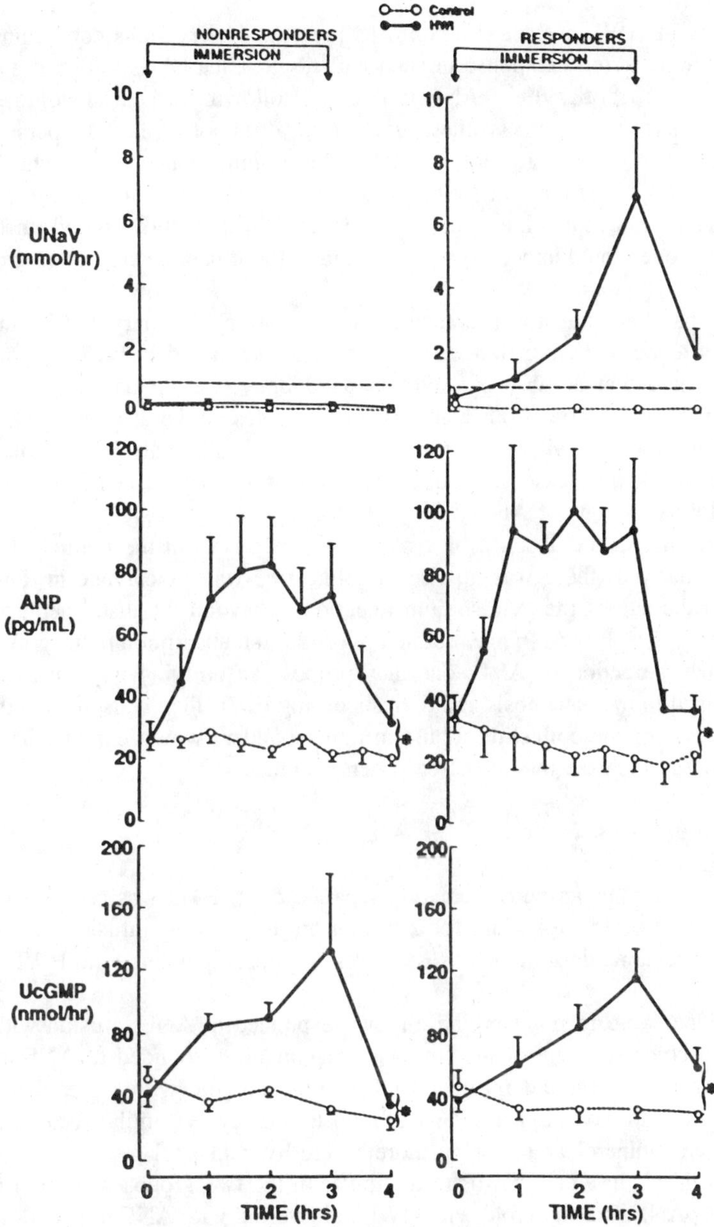

FIGURE 2. Effect of head-out water immersion (HWI) on urine sodium (UNaV) plasma ANP and urinary cGMP excretion.

As regards the effect of water immersion on other urinary parameters, there was no effect on creatinine clearance, but of interest, urinary potassium excretion rose in a comparable fashion in both groups. Similarly there was an increase in urine volume in both groups; however, when this was separated into osmolar and solute free water clearance, it was apparent that only the responders had a significant increase in solute free water clearance. Therefore, the increase in the urinary volume during HWI in the nonresponders was a result of an increase in osmolar clearance.

b. Comments

This study of HWI in cirrhotics confirms previous observations concerning the heterogeneity of the natriuretic response in such patients.[117] Clearly, as with the data observed in the post PVS cirrhotics,[100,112] ANF is released following a central volume challenge. Therefore a deficiency of ANF synthesis and release does not explain the persistent sodium retention present in certain cirrhotic subjects. These nonresponders were characterized by higher PRA and aldosterone values, obvious ascites, and failure to excrete a water load. Although plasma catecholamines were not measured in this study, based on the work of Nicholls et al., one would expect to see elevation in these parameters in this group as well, compared to the responders.[114]

The fact that there was no difference in the generation of urinary cGMP, indicates that there appears to be a dissociation between the end organ biochemical response and the proposed physiological activity of ANF on the kidney, i.e., a natriuresis and diuresis. Presumably it is secondary to other antinatriuretic forces active at a site separate to ANF receptor coupling and cGMP generation. Unfortunately, although cGMP does serve as a useful marker for ANF release, it is not known for certain whether cGMP is responsible for the observed renal actions of ANF.

The kaliuresis, in the absence of a natriuresis, observed in the nonresponders was of interest particularly as there was no rise in solute free water clearance in these subjects, implying that the site of the avid sodium retention is beyond the distal nephron. As there is evidence to suggest that ANF may both inhibit sodium reabsorption in the collecting duct[89] and antagonize the action of AVP, one may propose an unifying hypothesis. Namely, if ANF is involved in the natriuresis and diuresis during HWI, then resistance to the action of ANF at the level of the collecting tubule in nonresponders would explain the failure of a natriuresis and an increase in solute free water clearance.

3. Infusion Studies vs. HWI

a. The Study

In 12 cirrhotic patients with ascites on separate days, HWI was compared to infusion of ANF in a dose of 15 ng/kg/min for 2 h after an initial bolus infusion of 35 ng/kg/min for 5 min.[118] The same definition for responders and nonresponders with HWI was used as previously.

Five patients were responders and all five responded to ANF infusion with a marked natriuresis. In contrast, none of the seven nonresponders responded to ANF infusion. As found previously, nonresponders tended to be hyponatremic with lower daily urine and sodium excretion, to have higher PRA and aldosterone levels, similar mean arterial blood pressure and creatinine clearances, but more severe liver disease.

Increases in pANF and UcGMP were similar in the two groups with both maneuvers. In responders pANF rose threefold with HWI and fivefold with ANF infusion. Yet, sodium excretion increased to 6 mmol/hr with HWI compared to 4.2 mmol/hr with ANF infusion. There was no change in creatinine clearance in either group, in either maneuver. Of interest, kaliuresis once again occurred with HWI in both groups, but in neither group with ANF infusion. HWI induced a significantly greater suppression of PRA and aldosterone compared to ANF infusion.

b. Comments

The pANF levels achieved with low dose infusion were comparable to levels following PVS. Yet, whereas the latter invariably results in a natriuresis, in this study the majority of patients did not respond. This indicates that the response to PVS is not due to sixfold elevation in pANF levels alone, but requires additional changes to overcome final renal resistance to ANF resulting, for example, from acute expansion of the intravascular volume.

This is suggested by the greater natriuresis with HWI despite lower peak pANF levels. This in turn will result in both changes in physical factors within the kidney and suppression of antinatriuretic factors which combined with further elevation in pANF levels results in a natriuresis even in the nonresponders.

Brabant et al.[119] reported the effect of a single large bolus dose (30 mg) of ANF in ten cirrhotics with ascites. No subjective or objective side effects were noted apart from a slight fall in mean arterial blood pressure of approximately 10 mmHg. All the subjects had an apparent, but variable natriuresis and diuresis with an inverse correlation between percent increase in sodium excretion and ANF levels. However, the levels of ANF in plasma, required to induce the natriuresis and diuresis were not reported.

Salerno et al.[120] also reported the effect of a single bolus injection of ANF, administered in large dose, i.e., 1 mg/kg, to 14 cirrhotics (9 with and 5 without ascites) on a 35 to 40 mmol sodium diet for 7 d with all diuretics discontinued, compared to 6 controls. The resulting natriuretic and diuretic response was highly variable. Post study, the cirrhotics were divided into 2 groups based on their basal urine sodium excretion, those with either moderate or avid sodium retention, i.e., less than 5 mEq sodium per day. The first group had a significant diuresis and natriuresis which was blunted compared to controls. The avid sodium-retaining cirrhotics experienced a blunted diuresis, but no natriuresis. In the cirrhotics, as a whole, the decline in blood pressure -18 ± 2.5 mmHg was greater than controls, -9 ± 2 mmHg. It was not stated whether or not this decline in blood pressure was equal in both groups of cirrhotics. Glomerular filtration rate as measured by creatinine clearance was unchanged in both cirrhotics and controls. Neither baseline nor increases in plasma ANF achieved by the bolus administration were reported.

More recently Laffi et al.[121] used a smaller dose of 50 mcg bolus of ANF, followed by 0.1 mcg/min/kg for 45 min in 15 cirrhotics with ascites. Five patients had a natriuretic response which was related to the increase in effective renal plasma flow and GFR. Both responders and nonresponders had a similar reduction in blood pressure, similar fourfold rise in pANF levels and a sixfold rise in pcGMP levels. The lack of rise in renal plasma flow in nonresponders might be due to overwhelming renal vasoconstriction due to increased renal sympathetic nerve activity.

VI. SUMMARY

Have the plethora of physiological studies on ANF and the few studies of ANF in cirrhosis helped us to understand its role in the pathogenesis of salt and water retention in these patients? It now appears that at some stage in the natural history of the disease, some cirrhotic patients develop increasing resistance to ANF. The major site of action of ANF appears to be at the medullary collecting duct. Then failure to deliver sodium to that site for any reason or failure of the medullary circulation to respond to ANF would prevent its action. An attractive unifying hypothesis would then involve a gradual reduction in renal blood flow and GFR increased salt and water absorption along the nephron in relation to that and sodium retaining hormones and renal vasoconstriction affecting medullary blood flow. It is possible that only by reversing all three abnormalities will the patient again become responsive to ANF and once again obtain sodium homeostasis.

REFERENCES

1. **deBold, A. J., Borenstein, H. B., Veress, A. T., and Sonnenberg, H.,** A rapid and potent natriuretic response to intravenous injection of atrial myocardial extract in rats, *Life Sci.*, 28, 89, 1981.
2. **Kersch, B.,** Electron microscopy of the atrium of the heart. I. Guinea Pig, *Exp. Med. Surg.*, 14, 99, 1956.

3. **Jamieson, J. D. and Palade, G. E.,** Specific granules in atrial muscle cell, *J. Cell. Biol.,* 23, 151, 1964.
4. **Huet, M. and Cantin, M.,** Ultrastructural cytochemistry of atrial muscle cells. II. Characterization of the protein content of specific granules, *Lab. Invest.,* 30, 525, 1974.
5. **deBold, A. J.,** Heart atria granularity. Effects of changes in water and electrolyte balance, *Proc. Soc. Exp. Biol. Med.,* 161, 508, 1979.
6. **Garcia, R. and Cantin, M., Thibault, G., and Genest, J.,** Relationship of specific granules to the natriuretic and diuretic activity of rat atria, *Experientia,* 38, 1071, 1982.
7. **deBold, A. J.,** Tissue fractionation studies on the relationship between an atrial natriuretic factor and specific atrial granules, *Can. J. Physiol. Pharmacol.,* 60, 324, 1982.
8. **Thibault, G., Garcia, R., Cantin, M., and Genest, J.,** Atrial natriuretic factor. Characterization and partial purification, *Hypertension,* 5 (Suppl. 1), 75, 1983.
9. **deBold, A. J.,** Atrial natriuretic factor of the rat heart. Studies on isolation and properties, *Proc. Soc. Exp. Biol. Med.,* 170, 133, 1982.
10. **Trippodo, N. C., MacPhee, A. A., and Cole, F. E.,** Partially purified human and rat atrial natriuretic factor, *Hypertension,* 5, (Suppl. 1), 181, 1983.
11. **deBold, A. J. and Flynn, T. G.,** Cardionatrin I-A novel heart peptide with potent diuretic and natriuretic properties, *Life Sci.,* 33, 297, 1983.
12. **Dietz, J. R.,** Release of natriuretic factor from rat heart-lung preparation by atrial distension, *Am. J. Physiol.,* 247, R1093, 1984.
13. **Lang, R. E., Tholken, H., Ganten, D., Luft, F. C., Ruskoaho, H., and Unger, T. H.,** Atrial natriuretic factor a circulating hormone stimulated by volume loading, *Nature,* 314, 264, 1985.
14. **Goetz, K. L., Wang, B. C., Geer, P. G., Leadley, R. J., Jr., and Reinhardt, H. W.,** Atrial stretch increases sodium excretion independently of release of atrial peptides, *Am. J. Physiol.,* 250, R946, 1986.
15. **Yamaji, T., Ishibashi, M., and Takafu, F.,** Atrial natriuretic factor in human blood, *J. Clin. Invest.,* 76, 1705, 1985.
16. **Anderson, J. V., Donckier, J., McKenna, W. J., and Bloom, S. R.,** The plasma release of atrial natriuretic peptide in man, *Clin. Sci.,* 71, 151, 1986.
17. **Schenker, Y., Sider, R. S., Ostafin, E. A., and Grekin, R. J.,** Plasma levels of immunoreactive atrial natriuretic factor in healthy subjects and in patients with edema, *J. Clin. Invest.,* 76, 1684, 1985.
18. **Epstein, M., Loutzenheiser, R. D., Friedland, E., Aceto, R. M., Carmargo, M. J. F., and Atlas, S. A.,** Increases in circulating atrial natriuretic factor during immersion-induced central hypervolaemia in normal humans, *J. Hypertens.,* 4, 593, 1986.
19. **Ogihara, T., Shima, J., and Hara, H. et al.,** Significant increase in plasma immunoreactive atrial natriuretic polypeptide concentration during head out water immersion, *Life Sci.,* 38, 2413, 1986.
20. **Leung, W. M., Skorecki, K. L., Campbell, P. J., Debowski, T. E., Bull, S. B., Wong, P. Y., Blendis, L. M., and Logan, A. G.,** Urinary cyclic GMP as a marker of the renal response to atrial peptide during water immersion, *Can. J. Physiol. Pharmacol.,* 65, 2076, 1987.
21. **Soloman, L. R., Atherton, J. C., Bobinski, H., and Green, R.,** Effect of dietary sodium chloride and posture on plasma immunoreactive atrial natriuretic pepetide concentrations in man, *Clin. Sci.,* 72, 201, 1987.
22. **Hollister, A. S., Tanaka, I., and Imada, T. et al.,** Sodium loading and posture modulate human atrial natriuretic factor plasma levels, *Hypertension,* 8 (Suppl. 2), 2, 106, 1986.
23. **Richards, A. M., Tonolo, G., and Cleland, J. G. F., et al.,** Plasma atrial natriuretic peptide concentrations during exercise in sodium replete and deplete normal man, *Clin. Sci.,* 72, 159, 1987.
24. **Arjamaa, O. and Vuolteenaho, O.,** Sodium ion stimulates the release of atrial natriuretic polypeptides (ANP) from rat atria, *Biochem. Biophy. Res. Commun.,* 132, 375, 1985.
25. **Currie, M. G., Newman, W. H.,** Evidence for alpha 1 adrenergic receptor regulation of atriopeptin release from the isolated rat heart, *Biochem. Biophys. Res. Commun.,* 137, 94, 1986.
26. **Schiebinger, R. J., Baker, M. Z., and Linden, J.,** Effect of adrenergic and muscarinic cholinergic agonists on atrial natriuretic peptide secretion in isolated rat atria, *J. Clin. Invest.,* 80, 1687, 1987.
27. **Sonnenberg, H. and Veress, A. T.,** Cellular mechanism of release of atrial natrial factor, *Biochem. Biophys. Res. Commun.,* 124, 443, 1984.
28. **Sonnenberg, H.,** Mechanisms of release and renal tubular action of atrial natriuretic factor, *Fed. Proc.,* 45, 2106, 1986.
29. **Ballerman, B. J. and Brenner, B. M.,** Biologically active peptides, *J. Clin. Invest.,* 76, 2041, 1985.
30. **Gerzer, R., Weil, J., Strom, J., and Muller, T.,** Mechanisms of action of atrial natriuretic factor: clinical consequences, *Klin. Wochenschr.,* 64 (Suppl. 6), 21, 1986.
31. **Hamet, P., Tremblay, J., and Pang, S. C. et al.,** Cyclic GMP as mediator and biological marker of atrial natriuretic factor, *J. Hypotens.,* 4 (Suppl. 2), S49, 1986.
32. **Ballerman, B. J., Hoover, R. L., Karnovsky, M. J., and Brenner, B. M.,** Physiological regulation of atrial natriuretic peptide receptors in rat renal glomeruli, *J. Clin. Invest.,* 76, 2049, 1985.

33. **Hamet, P., Tremblay, J., and Pang, S. C. et al.,** Effect of native and synthetic atrial natriuretic factor on cyclic GMP, *Biochem. Biophys. Res. Commun.,* 123, 515, 1984.
34. **Gerzer, R., Tremblay, J., Pang, S., Vinay, P., DeLean, A., and Hamet, P.,** Atrial natriuretic factor activates mammalian particulate guanylate cyclase, *Fed. Proc.,* 44, 698, 1985.
35. **Waldman, S. A., Rapoport, R. M., and Murad, F.,** Atrial natriuretic factor selectively activates particulate guanylate cyclase and elevates cyclic GMP in rat tissues, *J. Biol. Chem.,* 259, 14332, 1984.
36. **Winquist, R. J., Faison, E. P., Waldman, S. A., Schwartz, K., Murad, F., Rapoport, R. M.,** Atrial natriuretic factor elicits an endothelium independent relaxation and activates particulate guanylate cyclase in vascular smooth muscle, *Proc. Natl. Acad. Sci. U.S.A.,* 81, 7661, 1984.
37. **Tremblay, J., Gerzer, R., Vinary, P., Pang, S., Beliveau, R., and Hamet, P.,** The increase of cGMP by atrial natriuretic factor correlates with the distribution of particulate guanylate cyclase, *FEBS Lett.,* 181, 17, 1985.
38. **Kremer, S., Troyer, D., Kreisberg, J., Skorecki, K.,** Interaction of atrial natriuretic peptide-stimulated guanylate cyclase and vasopressin-stimulated calcium signaling pathways in the glomerular mesangial cell, *Arch. Biochem. Biophys.,* 260, 763, 1988.
39. **Gerzer, R., Witzgall, H., Tremblay, J., Gutowska, J., and Hamet, P.,** Rapid increase in plasma and urinary cGMP after bolus injection of atrial natriuretic factor in man, *J. Clin. Endocr. Metab.,* 61, 1217, 1985.
40. **Weil, J., Lang, R. E. Suttman, H., Rampf, U., Bidlingmeier, F., Gerzer, R.,** Concimitant increase in plasma atrial natriuretic peptide and cyclic GMP in man during volume loading, *Klin. Wochenschr.,* 63, 1265, 1985.
41. **Blonde, L., Wehmann, R. E., Steiner, A. L.,** Plasma clearance rates and renal clearance of 3H-labeled cyclic AMP, and 3H-labeled cyclic GMP in the dog, *J. Clin. Invest.,* 53, 163, 1974.
42. **Stokes, T. J., McCoukey, C. L., Jr., and Martin, K. J.,** Atriopeptin 3 increases cGMP in glomeruli but not in proximal tubules of dog kidney, *Am. J. Physiol.,* 250, F24, 1986.
43. **Nonoguchi, H., Knepper, M. A., and Manganiello, V. C.,** Effects of atrial natriuretic factor on cyclic guanosine monophosphate and cyclic adenosine monophosphate accumulation in microdissected nephron segments from rats, *J. Clin. Invest.,* 80, 500, 1987.
44. **Ishikawa, S., Saito, T., Okada, K., Kuzuya, K., Kangawa, K., and Matuso, H.,** Atrial natriuretic factor increases cyclic GMP and inhibits cyclic AMP in rat renal papillary collecting tubule cells in culture, *Biochem. Biophys. Res. Commun.,* 130, 1147, 1985.
45. **DeLean, A., Gutowska, J., McNicoll, N., Schiller, P. W., Cantin, M., and Genest, J.,** Characterization of specific receptor for atrial natriuretic factor in bovine adrenal zone glomerulosa, *Life Sci.,* 35, 2311, 1984.
46. **Kudo, T., Baird, A.,** Inhibition of aldosterone production in the adrenal glomerulosa by atrial natriuretic factor, *Nature,* 312, 20, 1984.
47. **Schiffrin, E. L., Chartier, L., Thibault, G., St. Louis, J., Cantin, M., and Genest, J.,** Vascular and adrenal receptors for atrial natriuretic factor in the rat, *Circ. Res.,* 56, 801, 1985.
48. **Pandey, K. N., Inagami, T., and Misono, K. S.,** Three distinct forms of ANF receptors; kidney tubuluar epithelium cells and vascular smooth muscle cells contain different types of receptors, *Biochem. Biophys. Res. Commun.,* 147, 1146, 1987.
49. **Anad-Srivastava, M. B., Franks, D. J., Cantin, M., and Genest, J.,** Atrial natriuretic factor inhibits adenylate cyclase activity, *Biochem. Biophys. Res. Commun.,* 121, 855, 1984.
50. **Currie, M. G., Geller, D. M., Cole, B. R., Boylan, J. C., Wu, Y. S., Holmberg, S. W., and Needleman, P.,** Bioactive cardiac substances: potent vasorelaxant activity in mammalian atria, *Science,* 221, 71, 1983.
51. **Garcia, R., Thibault, G., Cantin, M., and Genest, J.,** Effect of a purified atrial natriuretic factor on rat and rabbit vascular strips and vascular beds, *Am. J. Physiol.,* 247, R34, 1984.
52. **Ishihara, T., Aisaka, K., and Hattori, S. et al.,** Vasodilatory and diuretic actions of x-human atrial natriuretic polypeptide (x-hANP), *Life Sci.,* 36, 1205, 1985.
53. **Bolli, P., Muller, F. B., and Linder, L.,** The vasodilator potency of atrial natriuretic peptide in man, *Circulation,* 75, 221, 1987.
54. **Linz, W., Albus, U., Wiemer, G., Schdkens, B. A., and Konig, W.,** Atriopeptin III induces endothelium independent relaxation and increases cGMP levels in rabbit aorta, *Klin. Wochenschr.,* 64 (Suppl. 6), 27, 1986.
55. **Fujita, T., Ito, Y., Noda, H., Sato, Y., Ando, K., Kangawa, K., and Matsuo, H.,** Vasodilatory actions of x-human atrial natriuretic peptide and high calcium effects in normal man, *J. Clin. Invest.,* 80, 832, 1987.
56. **Pegram, B. L., Trippodo, N. C., and Natsume, T. et al.,** Hemodynamic effects of atrial natriuretic hormone, *Fed. Proc.,* 45, 2382, 1986.
57. **Fujioka, S., Tamaki, T., Fukui, K., Okahara, T., Abe, Y.,** Effects of a synthetic human atrial polypeptide on regional blood flow in rats, *Eur. J. Pharmacol.,* 109, 301, 1985.

58. **Pegram, B. L., Kardon, M. B., Trippodo, N. C., Cole, F. E., and MacPhee, A. A.**, Atrial natriuretic factor: haemodynamic effects in conscious Wistar-Kyoto and spontaneously hypertensive rats, *Am. J. Physiol.*, 249, H265, 1985.

59. **Lappe, R. W., Smits, V. F. M., Todt, J. A., Debets, J. J. M., and Wendt, R. L.**, Failure of atriopeptin II to cause arterial vasodilatation in the conscious rat, *Circ. Res.*, 56, 606, 1985.

60. **Marsh, E. A., Seymour, A. A., and Haley, A. B. et al.**, Renal and blood pressure responses to synthetic atrial natriuretic factor in spontaneously hypertensive rats, *Hypertension*, 7, 386, 1985.

61. **Lappe, R. W., Todt, V. A., and Wendt, R.**, Haemodynamic effects of infusion versus bolus administration of atrial natriuretic factor, *Hypertension*, 8, 866, 1986.

62. **Trippodo, N. C., Kardon, M. B., Pegram, B. L., Cole, F. E., MacPhee, A. A.**, Acute haemodynamic effects of the atrial natriuretic hormone in rats, *J. Hypertens.*, 4 (Suppl. 2), S35, 1986.

63. **Wanger, R. D., Brehaus, B. A., Otero, H. O., Hastings, D. A., Holzman, M. D., Sane, H. H., Sparks, H. V., and Chimoskey, J. E.**, Coronary vasoconstrictor effects of atriopeptin II, *Science*, 230, 558, 1985.

64. **Hintze, T. H., Currie, M. G., and Needleman, P.**, Atrial peptins: renal-specific vasodilators in conscious dogs, *Am. J. Physiol.*, 248, 4587, 1985.

65. **Wakitani, K., Cole, B. R., Geller, D. M., Currie, M. G., Adams, S. P., Fok, K. F., and Needleman, P.**, Atriopeptins: correlation between renal vasodilatation and natriuresis, *Am. J. Physiol.*, 249, F49, 1985.

66. **Wakitani, K., Oshina, T., Lowey, A. D., Holmberg, S. W., Cole, B. R., Adams, S. P., Fok, K. F., Currie, M. G., and Needleman, P.**, Comparative vascular pharmacology of the atriopeptins, *Circ. Res.*, 56, 621, 1985.

67. **Caramelo, C., Fernandez-Cruz, A., Villamediana, L. M., Sanz, E., Rodriguez-Puyol, D., Hermando, L., and Lopez-Novok, J. M.**, Systemic and regional haemodynamic effects of a synthetic atrial natriuretic peptide in conscious rats, *Clin. Sci.*, 71, 323, 1986.

68. **Maack, T., Marion, D. N., Camargo, M. J. G., Kleinert, H. D., Laragh, J. H., Vaughan, E. D., and Atlas, S. A.**, Effects of auriculin (atrial natriuretic factor) on blood pressure renal function and the renin-aldosterone system in dogs, *Am. J. Med.*, 77, 1069, 1984.

69. **Burnett, J. C., Jr., Graujer, J. P., and Ongenoth, T. S.**, Effects of synthetic atrial natriuretic factor on renal function and renin release, *Am. J. Physiol.*, 247, F863, 1984.

70. **Huang, C. L., Lewicki, J., Johnson, L. K., and Cogan, M. G.**, Renal mechanism of action of rat atrial natriuretic factor, *J. Clin. Invest.*, 75, 769, 1985.

71. **Camargo, M. J. F., Atlas, S. A., Sealey, J. F., Laragh, J. H., and Maack, T.**, Vascular effects of atrial extract in isolated perfused rat kidney (IK), *Fed. Proc.*, 43, 723, 1984.

72. **Beasley, D. and Malvin, R. L.**, Atrial extract increases glomerular filtration rate *in vivo*, *Am. J. Physiol.*, 248, F24, 1985.

73. **Huang, C. L., Lewicki, J., Johnson, L. K., and Cogan, M.**, Renal mechanisms of action of rat atrial natriuretic factor, *J. Clin. Invest.*, 75, 769, 1985.

74. **Camargo, M. J. F., Kleinert, H. D., Atlas, S. A., Sealey, J. E., Laragh, J. H., and Maack, J.**, Ca-dependant haemodynamic and natriuretic effects of atrial extract in isolated rat kidney, *Am. J. Physiol.*, 246, F447, 1984.

75. **Maack, T., Atlas, S. A., Camargo, M. J. F., and Cogan, M. G.**, Renal haemodynamic and natriuretic effects of atrial natriuretic factor, *Fed. Proc.*, 45, 2128, 1986.

76. **Maack, T., Camargo, M. J. F., Kleinert, H. D., Laragh, J. H., and Atlas, S. A.**, Atrial natriuretic factor: structure and functional properties, *Kidney Int.*, 27, 607, 1985.

77. **Burnett, J. C., Granger, J. P., and Openorth, T. J.**, Effects of synthetic atrial natriuretic factor on renal function and renin release, *Am. J. Physiol.*, 247, F863, 1984.

78. **Fried, T. A., McCog, R. N., Osgood, R. W., Reineck, H. J., and Stein, J. H.**, The effects of atrial natriuretic peptide on glomerular dynamics, *Clin. Res.*, 33, 587A, 1985.

79. **Ichikawa, I., Dunn, B. R., Troy, J. L., Maack, T., and Brenner, B. M.**, Influence of atrial natriuretic peptide on glomerular microcirculation, *in vivo*, *Clin. Res.*, 33, 487A, 1985.

80. **Sonnenberg, H. and Cupples, W. A.**, Intrarenal localization of the natriuretic effect of cardiacs atrial extract, *Can. J. Physiol. Pharmacol.*, 60, 1149, 1982.

81. **Borenstein, A. B.**, The effect of natriuretic atrial extract on renal haemodynamics and urinary excretion in anaesthetized rats, *J. Physiol. (London)*, 334, 133, 1983.

82. **Seymour, A. A., Blaine, E. H., and Whitney, M. A.**, Renal effects of synthetic atrial natriuretic factor, *Life Sci.*, 36, 33, 1985.

83. **Murray, R. D., Itoh, S., Inagarni, T., Misono, K., Seito, S., Scicli, G., and Carretero, O. A.**, Effects of synthetic atrial natriuretic factor in the isolated perfused rat kidney, *Am. J. Physiol.*, 249, F603, 1985.

84. **Yukimura, T., Ho., K., Takenaga, T., Yamamoto, K., Kangawa, K., and Matsuo, H.**, Renal effects of a synthetic x-human atrial natriuretic polypeptide (x-hANP) in anaesthetized dogs, *Eur. J. Pharmacol.*, 103, 363, 1984.

85. **Burnett, J. C., Opgenorth, T. J., and Granger, J. P.,** The renal action of atrial natriuretic peptide during control of glomerular filtration, *Kidney Int.,* 30, 16, 1986.
86. **Hammond, T. G., Yusufi, A. N. K., Knox, F. G., and Dousa, T. P.,** Administration of atrial natriuretic factor inhibits sodium coupled transport in proximal tubules, *J. Clin. Invest.,* 75, 1983, 1985.
87. **Baum, M. and Toto, R. D.,** Lack of a direct effect on atrial natriuretic factor in the rabbit proximal tubule, *Am. J. Physiol.,* 250, F66, 1986.
88. **Kondo, Y., Imai, M., and Kangawa, K.,** Lack of direct action of beta human atrial natriuretic polypeptide on the *in vitro* perfused segments of Henle's loop isolated from rabbit kidney, *Pfluegers Arch.,* 406, 273, 1986.
89. **Borenstein, H. B., Cupples, W. A., Sonnenberg, H., and Veress, A. T.,** The effects of natriuretic atrial extract on renal hemodynamics and urinary excretion in anesthetised rats, *J. Physiol.,* 334, 133, 1983.
90. **Sonnenberg, H., Honrath, U., Chong, C. K., and Wilson, D. R.,** Atrial natriuretic factor inhibits sodium transport in medullary collecting duct, *Am. J. Physiol.,* 250, F963, 1986.
91. **Sosa, R. E., Volpe, M., Marion, D. N., Atlas, S. A., Laragh, J. H., Vaughan, E. D., and Maack, T.,** Relationship between renal hemodynamic and natriuretic effects of atrial natriuretic factor, *Am. J. Physiol.,* 250, F520, 1986.
92. **Roy, D. D.,** Effect of synthetic ANP on renal and loop of Henle functions in the young rat, *Am. J. Physiol.,* 251, F220, 1986.
93. **Takezawa, K., Cowley, A. W., Skelton, M., and Roman, R. J.,** Atriopeptin III, alters renal medullary hemodynamics and the pressure diuresis response in rats, *Am. J. Physiol.,* 80, 1595, 1987.
94. **Kiberd, B. A., Larson, T. S., Robertson, C. R., and Jamieson, R. L.,** Effect of atrial natriuretic peptide on vasa recta blood flow in the rat, *Am. J. Physiol.,* 252, F1112, 1987.
95. **Zeidel, M. L., Seifter, J. L., Lear, S., Brenner, B. M., and Silva, P.,** Atrial peptides inhibit oxygen consumption in kidney medullary collecting duct cells, *Am. J. Physiol.,* 251, F379, 1986.
96. **Jimenez, W., Martinez-Pardo, A., and Arroya, V. et al.,** Atrial natriuretic factor reduced cardiac content in cirrhotic rats with ascites, *Am. J. Physiol.,* 250, F749, 1986.
97. **Fernandez-Cruz, A., Marco, J., and Cvadrado, L. M.,** Plasma levels of atrial natriuretic peptide in cirrhotic patients, *Lancet,* 2, 1439, 1985.
98. **Gines, P., Jimenez, W., Arroyo, V., Navaga, M., Lopez, C., Tito, L., Serra, A., Bosch, J., Sanz, G., Rivera, F., and Rodés, J.,** Atrial natriuretic factor in cirrhosis with ascites. Plasma levels cardiac release and splanchnic extraction, *Hepatology,* 8, 636, 1988.
99. **Campbell, P., Skorecki, K. L., Logan, A. G., Wong, P. Y., Leung, W. M., Greig, P., and Blendis, L. M.,** The acute effects of peritoneovenous shunting (PVS) on plasma atrial natriuretic peptide in cirrhotics with massive refractory ascites, *Am. J. Med.,* 84, 112, 1988.
100. **Juppner, H., Brabant, G., Kapteina, U.,** Direct radioimmunoassay for human atrial natriuretic peptide (hANP) and its clinical evaluation, *Biochem. Biophys. Res. Commun.,* 139, 1215, 1986.
101. **Nischiuchi, T., Santo, H., Yamasaki, Y., and Santo, S.,** Radioimmunoassay for atrial natriuretic peptide method and results in normal subjects and in patients with various diseases, *Clin. Chem. Acta,* 159, 45, 1986.
102. **Shenker, Y., Sider, R. S., Ostafin, E. A., and Grekin, R. J.,** Plasma levels of immunoreactive atrial natriuretic factor in healthy subjects and in patients edema, *J. Clin. Invest.,* 76, 1684, 1985.
103. **Henriksen, J. H., Schutten, H. J., Bendtsen, F., and Warberg, J.,** Circulating atrial natriuretic peptide (ANP) and central blood volume (CBV) in cirrhosis, *Liver,* 6, 361, 1986.
104. **Sagnella, G. A., Markandu, N. D., Shore, A. C., MacGregor, G. A.,** Effects of changes in dietary sodium intake and saline infusion on immunoreactive atrial natriuretic peptide in human plasma, *Lancet,* ii, 1208, 1985.
105. **Warner, L., Campbell, P. J., Logan, A. G., Skorecki, K., and Blendis, L. M.,** The response of atrial natriuretic factor (ANF) and sodium excretion to dietary sodium challenges in cirrhotic patients, *Hepatology,* 8, 1389, 1988.
106. **LeVeen, H. H., Christoudias, G., Moon, I. P., Luft, R., Falk, G., and Grosberg, S.,** Peritoneovenous shunting for ascites, *Ann. Surg.,* 180, 580, 1974.
107. **Blendis, L. M., Greig, P. D., Langer, B., Baigrie, R. S., Ruse, J., and Taylor, B. R.,** The renal and hemodynamic effects of the peritoneovenous shunt for intractable heaptic ascites, *Gastroenterology,* 77, 250, 1979.
108. **Greig, P. D., Blendis, L. M., Langer, B., Taylor, B. R., and Colapinto, R. F.,** The renal and hemodynamic effect of the peritoneovenous shunt. Long term effect, *Gastroenterology,* 80, 119, 1981.
109. **Blendis, L. M., Sole, M. J., Lossing, A. G., Greig, P. D., Taylor, B. R., and Langer, B.,** The effect of peritoneovenous shunting on catecholamine metabolism in patients with hepatic ascites, *Hepatology,* 7, 143, 1987.
110. **Reznick, R. K., Langer, B., Taylor, B. R., Seif, S., and Blendis, L. M.,** Hyponatremia and ADH secretion in patients with refractory hepatic ascites undergoing peritoneovenous shunting, *Gastroenterology,* 87, 713, 1983.

111. **Klepetko, W., Muller, C. H., Hartter, E., Hiholics, J., Schwarz, C. H., Woloszczuk, W., and Woeschl, P.,** Plasma atrial natriuretic factor in cirrhotic patients with ascites, *Gastroenterology*, 95, 764, 1988.
112. **Epstein, M.,** Renal effects of head-out water immersion in man, *Physiol. Rev.*, 58, 529, 1978.
113. **Epstein, M., Levinson, R., Sancho, J., Haber, E., and Re, R.,** Characterization of the renin-aldosterone system in decompensated cirrhosis, *Circ. Res.*, 41, 818, 1977.
114. **Nicholls, K. M., Shapiro, M. D., and Dluge, R. et al.,** Sodium excretion in advanced cirrhosis: effect of expansion on central blood volume and suppression of plasma aldosterone, *Hepatology*, 6, 235, 1986.
115. **Campbell, P. J., Leung, W. M., Logan, A. G., Debowski, T. E., Blendis, L. M., and Skorecki, K. L.,** Hyperresponsiveness to water immersion in sodium retaining cirrhotics. The role of atrial natriuretic factor, *Clin. Invest. Med.*, 11, 392, 1988.
116. **Skorecki, K. L., Leung, W. M., Campbell, P. J., Warner, L. C., Wong, P. Y., Bull, S., Logan, A., and Blendis, L. M.,** Role of atrial natriuretic peptide in natriuretic response to central volume expansion induced by head-out water immersion in sodium retaining cirrhotic subjects, *Am. J. Med.*, 85, 375, 1988.
117. **Bichet, D. G., Van Putten, V. J., and Schrier, R. W.,** Potential role of increased sympathetic activity in impaired sodium and water excretion in cirrhosis, *N. Engl. J. Med.*, 307, 1552, 1982.
118. **Legault, L., Warner, L., Leung, W. M., Logan, A., Skorecki, K., and Blendis, L. M.,** A comparison in natriuretic response between head-out water immersion and infusion of atrionatriuretic factor, in preparation.
119. **Brabant, G., Juppner, H., Kirschner, M., Boker, K., Schmidt, F. W., and Hesch, R. D.,** Human atrial natriuretic peptide (ANP) for the treatment of patients with liver cirrhosis and ascites, *Klin. Wochenschr.*, 64 (Suppl.), 108, 1986.
120. **Salerno, F., Badalamenti, S., Incerti, P., Capozza, L., and Mainardi, L.,** Renal response to atrial natriuretic peptide in patients with advanced liver cirrhosis, *Hepatology*, 8, 21, 1988.
121. **Laffi, G., Pinzani, M., Meacci, E., LaVilla, G., Renzi, D., Baldi, E., Cominelli, F., Marra, F., and Gentilini, P.,** Renal hemodynamic and natriuretic effects in human atrial natriuretic factor infusion in cirrhosis with ascites, *Gastroenterology*, 96, 167, 1989.

Chapter 16

ALCOHOL-INDUCED INCREASE IN PORTAL BLOOD FLOW—MECHANISM, INTERACTION WITH ANESTHETICS, AND CLINICAL IMPLICATIONS

F. J. Carmichael and Hector Orrego

TABLE OF CONTENTS

I. INTRODUCTION

The fact that the liver (1) has a high oxygen requirement, (2) receives 60 to 70% of its blood supply through a vein, and (3) has a perivenular zone of the acinus which is normally in a state of hypoxia relative to the periportal zone, renders this organ highly susceptible to hypoxic cell damage. Preservation of normal liver function and hepatocellular integrity, therefore, requires a fine balance between the consumption and the delivery of oxygen to the liver.

The oxygen tension in the sinusoids supplying the cells in the periportal area (Zone I) is of the order of 65 to 70 mmHg, while in the perivenular area (Zone III), the oxygen tension drops to about 30 mmHg, indicating that oxygen is removed along the sinusoidal length.[1] This latter value constitutes an average oxygen tension resulting from a mixture of blood flowing through sinusoids of different lengths that can have oxygen tensions as low as 2 mmHg (approximately 0.1 mM).[2,3] This level may be critical for maintaining cellular function since the K_m for cytochrome oxidase is approximately 0.2 mM.[4] These factors explain why several studies that have measured the redox potential of liver cells have found that the perivenular area of the liver acinus is normally in a state of partial hypoxia.[5] If conditions of increased oxygen demand are not accompanied by a corresponding increase in oxygen delivery, the low oxygen tensions in the perivenular area could result in a critical focal hypoxic state and liver cell damage. Thus, situations that increase the requirements of the liver for oxygen, such as fever,[6] hyperthyroidism,[7,8] ethanol,[9] or reduced oxygen deliver, such as anemia,[10] congestive heart failure,[11] and anesthesia,[12] can potentially result in hepatocellular necrosis.[13]

Ethanol has been found to increase oxygen consumption by the liver,[3,13,15-18] an effect that, as stated above, accentuates the state of relative hypoxia that normally exists in Zone III of the liver acinus,[17,19-23] rendering these areas more susceptible to hypoxic damage. Nevertheless, the degree of perivenular hypoxia induced by ethanol per se is obviously not sufficient to produce liver damage because hepatocellular necrosis is not observed during acute or chronic alcohol intake in most animal models, despite the presence of an increased oxygen consumption by the liver.[24-27] The same is probably also true in most human beings since alcoholic hepatitis and cirrhosis occur in only a small fraction of persons abusing alcohol.[28]

To account for this observation, the hypoxic theory of alcohol-induced liver damage postulates that, in order for necrosis to occur, two factors must be present simultaneously: (1) an increase in oxygen demand by the liver, which is a constant effect of alcohol consumption, and (2) a decrease in oxygen delivery to the liver. This second effect occurs at random, only in certain individuals. Conditions that would decrease oxygen delivery to the liver such as anemia, respiratory depression, smoking, chronic lung diseases, or sleep apnea, etc., are frequent in chronic alcoholics.[29-33]

This hypothesis has been tested in experiments conducted in rats given alcohol chronically. These animals were found to develop hepatocellular necrosis in Zone III of the liver acinus when the delivery of oxygen to the liver was reduced, under conditions such as low atmospheric oxygen tension, induction of experimental anemia, or ligation of the hepatic artery.[13,16,34-37] The hypoxic theory of liver cell damage can account for three of the characteristics of alcohol-induced hepatocellular necrosis: (1) it affects only certain individuals, (2) it is focal in nature, and (3) it is localized mainly to the perivenular zone of the liver acinus.

An important factor that could account for the resistance of most species, including man, to alcohol-induced liver damage is the existence of a compensatory increase in blood flow through the liver in the presence of ethanol. In studies where alcohol was administered either acutely or chronically, the increase in blood flow delivered to the liver was sufficient to compensate for the alcohol-induced increase in oxygen consumption.[14,18,38,39]

II. ALCOHOL AND LIVER BLOOD FLOW

Studies of the effects of ethanol on the splanchnic circulation have produced contradictory results.[9,14,15,38-53,109] This is probably due in part to methodological difficulties derived from the use of dyes such as indocyanine green,[16,38,43,44,47,52] and especially sulfobromophthalein.[39,42,48,50,51] The latter has the problem of extrahepatic uptake and excretion[54] and of enterohepatic circulation:[55] both can introduce pitfalls in the measurements of liver blood flow. In addition, some workers used anesthetic agents[9,14,15,42-46,48,39] that, as discussed below, can interfere with the effect of alcohol on liver blood flow.[41] Further, the dose of ethanol used in some of the studies, resulted in blood alcohol concentrations below 3 mM (see below).[9,42,47,48,51] It is of interest that since 1981 all workers have found, in a number of animal species from rats to humans, an increase in liver blood flow following alcohol administration (Table 1).

In our laboratory over a period of about 2 years, in twelve different studies, we have found a consistent increase in portal blood flow from 42.2 ± 3.5 ml/kg/min in 83 controls to 63.4 ± 6.5 ml/kg/min in 87 rats given oral ethanol.

In experiments using radiolabeled microspheres, which allow for the separate determination of portal vein and liver arterial blood flows, the increase in liver blood flow has been shown to be the result of an increase in flow through the portal vein, with little or no effect on the hepatic artery (Figure 1). The increase in portal blood flow results from a vasodilation at the level of the splanchnic organs that drain into the portal vein, as shown by a sharp decrease in preportal vascular resistance. This effect results in an increase in the percentage of cardiac output flowing through the portal circulation from 20.4 ± 0.8 in controls to 26.8 ± 1.1 (p <0.05) in rats receiving 2g/kg ethanol orally.

III. MECHANISM OF THE ALCOHOL-INDUCED INCREASE IN PORTAL BLOOD FLOW

Three mechanisms could explain the alcohol-induced increase in portal blood flow: (1) an effect of vasoactive hormones released by ethanol, (2) a direct effect of ethanol on the splanchnic vasculature, or (3) an effect dependent on the metabolism of alcohol to acetaldehyde or to acetate.

Among the hormones possibly involved in the response to ethanol, glucagon appeared to be the most attractive candidate for the following reasons: (1) alcohol has been reported to increase circulating glucagon levels;[45,56,57] (2) glucagon is known to increase splanchnic blood flow (Figure 2);[56,58,59] and (3) glucagon increases oxygen consumption by the liver.[59,60] Therefore, glucagon might explain both the increase in portal blood flow and the increase in liver oxygen consumption that follows alcohol administration. However, a role of glucagon in the hemodynamic effects of alcohol can be excluded based upon two findings:

1. The ethanol-induced increase in portal blood flow occurs without a concomitant increase in circulating glucagon concentration;[49]
2. Neither the infusion of glucose, which decreased arterial glucagon concentration by 40%,[59] nor somatostatin, at doses that markedly reduced the release in glucagon by the pancreas,[61] interferes with the effect of ethanol on portal blood flow (Figure 3).

Two features of the ethanol-induced increase in portal blood flow are important. First, ethanol maximally increases portal blood flow at a blood concentration of 3.5 mM (Figure 4), a concentration at which the alcohol dehydrogenase pathway is saturated. Second, ethanol, when given at doses that result in blood concentrations up to 27 mM, continues to increase portal blood flow until it is metabolized to blood levels of less than 4 mM.[41] These experiments

TABLE 1
Studies Showing Increased Liver Blood Flow Following Ethanol

Author	Model/Method	Ethanol dose (blood conc.)	Condition	Increase (%)	Ref.
Mendeloff 1954	Man/BSP	(9.9 mM)	Awake	45	50
Stein et al. 1963	Man/ICG	0.5—0.8 g/min i.v.	Awake	21	51
Abrams and Cooper 1976	Rat/Lipid colloid	0.7 g/kg i.p. (10 mM)	Awake	49	40
Shaw et al. 1977	Baboon/BSP	1.75 g/kg (6 mM)	Ketamine, nembutal	80	39
Villeneuve 1981	Dog/^{99}Tc-albumin	2.0 g/kg p.o.	Awake	89	18
Jauhonen et al. 1982	Baboon/ICG	1.1 g/kg (26 mM)	Ketamine	54	38
Israel et al. 1983	Rats/microsphere	4 g/kg p.o.	Ketamine	50	43
Bredfeldt et al. 1985	Rats/microsphere	Liquid diets (34 mM)	Ketamine	33	14
Yoshihara et al. 1985	Man/Doppler	25 g p.o. (13 mM)	Awake	24	53
McKaigney et al. 1986	Rats/microsphere	0.5—4.0 g/kg p.o. (3.5—27 mM)	Awake	65	49
Jenkins et al. 1986	Rat/Xe-133 colloid	.03—.12 mg/g/min (14 mM)	Pentobarbital	46	46
Carmichael et al. 1987	Rat/microsphere	0.5—4.0 g/kg p.o.	Awake	60	41

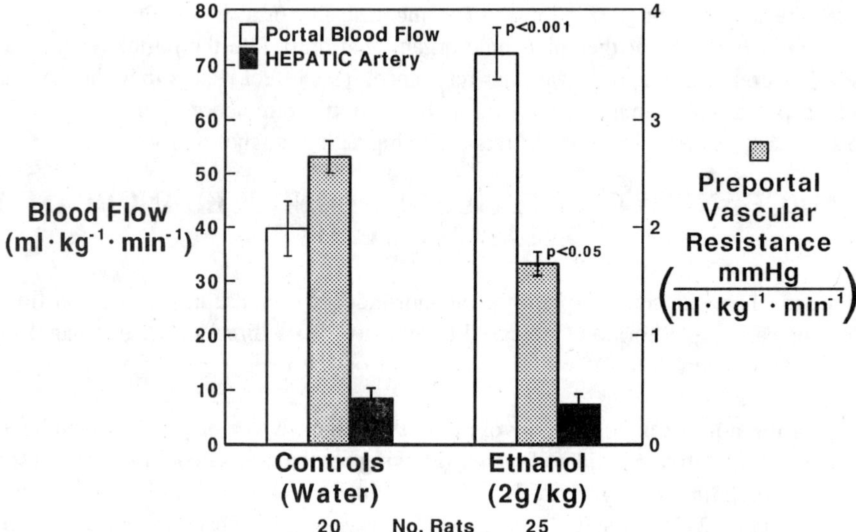

FIGURE 1.   Effect of ethanol (2 g/kg) orally on portal blood flow, hepatic artery blood flow, and preportal vascular resistance in rats. Control rats received an equivalent volume of water orally. Cardiac output and blood flows were measured using the labeled, 15 μm, microsphere technique as described previously.[49]

suggest an involvement of the alcohol dehydrogenase pathway in the hemodynamic response to ethanol. Further support of a role of this pathway is the demonstration that the administration of 4-methylpyrazole, a powerful inhibitor of alcohol dehydrogenase,[62] blocks completely the effect of ethanol on portal blood flow while resulting in higher blood ethanol levels (Figure 4). These observations also demonstrate that the increase in portal blood flow is not the result of a direct effect of ethanol on the splanchnic blood vessels but, rather, this increased flow is mediated by factors resulting from the metabolism of alcohol.

When metabolized by the liver, alcohol is converted sequentially into acetaldehyde and then into acetate. These two substances are possible mediators of the hemodynamic effects of ethanol since both have been reported to have vasoactive properties.[63-70]

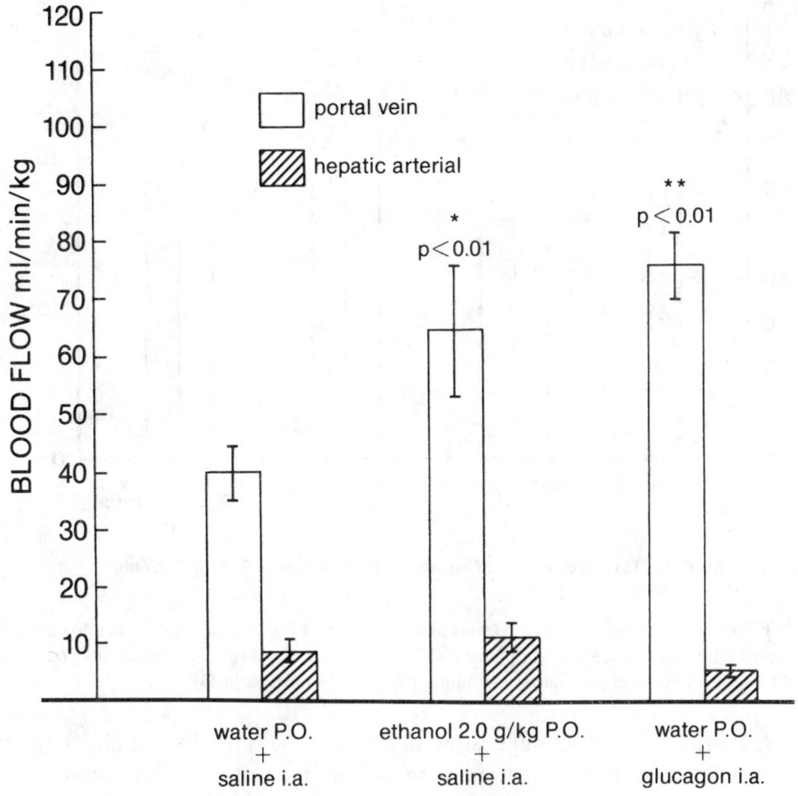

FIGURE 2.   Effects of oral ethanol (2 g/kg) and intra-arterial glucagon (20 μg/kg/min) on portal blood flow and hepatic artery blood flow in rats. Control rats received an equivalent volume of water orally and of saline intra-arterially. Cardiac output and blood flows were determined as in Figure 1.

Cyanamide is an inhibitor of aldehyde dehydrogenase which when combined with alcohol, produces a marked increase in circulating acetaldehyde concentration.[71] The concomitant administration of cyanamide with ethanol (2 g/kg) results in an increase in arterial acetaldehyde concentrations from 4 ± 3 μM in rats receiving ethanol alone to 293 ± 40 μM in the animals treated with cyanamide plus ethanol.[72] Under these conditions, the addition of cyanamide produces a significant reduction of the ethanol-induced increase in portal blood flow, rather than an increase as would have been expected had acetaldehyde been the mediator (Figure 5). Moreover, the infusion of acetaldehyde directly into the arterial circulation or into the portal vein has no effect on basal portal blood flow, nor on the ethanol-induced increase in portal blood flow, despite attaining arterial concentrations of acetaldehyde greater than 200 μM. It would, therefore, appear that circulating acetaldehyde does not play a role in the effect of ethanol on the splanchnic circulation. It is likely that the inhibitory effect of cyanamide could be the result of two actions of this drug (1) a decrease in the production of acetate from acetaldehyde, and (2) a decrease in the rate of metabolism of ethanol.[72]

From the above-experiments, acetate appeared as a likely mediator of the effects of ethanol on portal blood flow. In fact, *in vivo* acetate per se, at concentrations comparable to those resulting from alcohol metabolism, produces an increase in portal blood flow. In the rat, the intra-arterial infusion of acetate (0.023 mM/kg/min) results in an increase in portal blood flow from 38.0 ± 2.3 ml/kg/min in the controls to 50.5 ± 2.8 ml/kg/min ($p < 0.05$).[42]

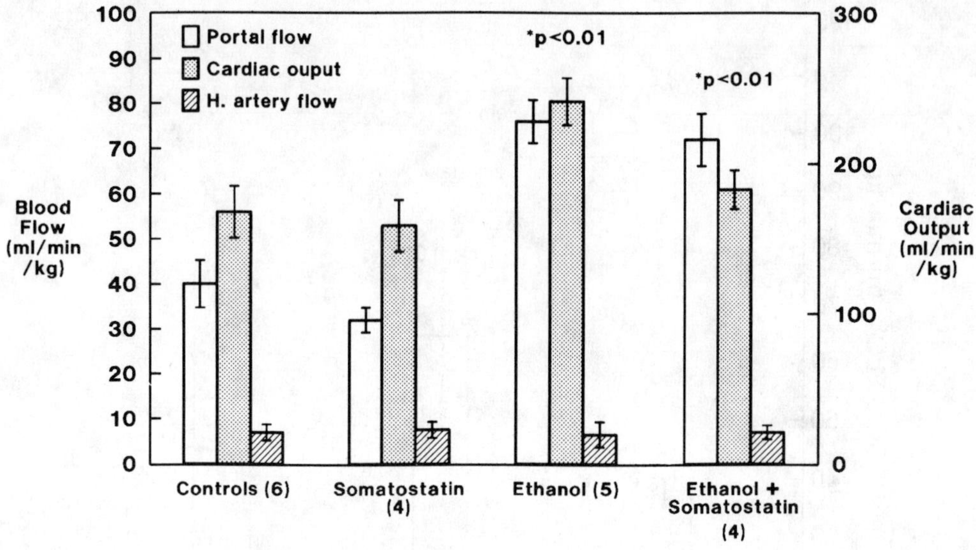

FIGURE 3.   Effects of somatostatin (1 μg/kg bolus plus infusion of 7.5 μg/kg/min for 5 min into the left ventricle) prior to measurement of cardiac output and portal and hepatic artery blood flow in control rats and in rats treated with ethanol (2 g/kg orally). Cardiac output and blood flows determined as in Figure 1.

There is, however, evidence suggesting that acetate does not have a direct effect per se on the splanchnic vasculature. First, *in vitro* acetate induces vasoconstriction in isolated mesenteric arterioles and venules, which would reduce portal blood flow.[66] Second, in *in vivo* studies using fluoroacetate, which inhibits the metabolism of acetate, the hemodynamic effects of acetate are abolished.[69] Although these experiments, either *in vitro* or using a powerful metabolic poison, must be viewed with caution, they suggest that the vascular effects of acetate might be caused not by acetate itself but by a substance that is associated with its metabolism.

Several studies have shown that acetate increases the concentration of adenosine in tissues.[73-75] Adenosine has been shown to be a powerful vasodilator,[76-81] and may, at least in part, be the mediator for the vascular effects of acetate.[69,73-75] The increased adenosine concentration following acetate administration results from the metabolism of acetate to acetyl CoA with the formation of 5′-AMP from ATP. 5′-AMP is metabolized to adenosine by the membrane-bound enzyme 5′-nucleotidase.[69,82] It is of interest that the activity of 5′-nucleotidase is especially high in the smooth muscle of the small intestine.[77] This could result in higher levels of adenosine in the splanchnic vasculature, explaining a selective increase in blood flow in the splanchnic territory. Although 5′-nucleotidase is primarily an ectoenzyme, it has been shown that the synthesis of adenosine occurs intracellularly as a result of the small fraction of this enzyme that exists within the cell.[83] This would mean that the synthesized adenosine would likely have to be transported out of the cell before exerting its effects on adenosine receptors.

Adenosine is a powerful vasodilator in the splanchnic circulation, increasing portal blood flow from 41.3 ± 2.3 ml/kg/min in the controls (n = 19) to 81.7 ± 8.0 ml/kg/min (n = 6) ($p < 0.05$) in animals receiving an intra-arterial infusion of adenosine (0.17 mg/kg/min) (Figure 6). As with ethanol, adenosine decreases the preportal vascular resistance by 62% and, as expected, also increases the percentage of the cardiac output flowing through the portal vein from $19.1 \pm 0.9\%$ in the controls to $26.7 \pm 2.3\%$ in the animals infused with adenosine ($p < 0.05$).

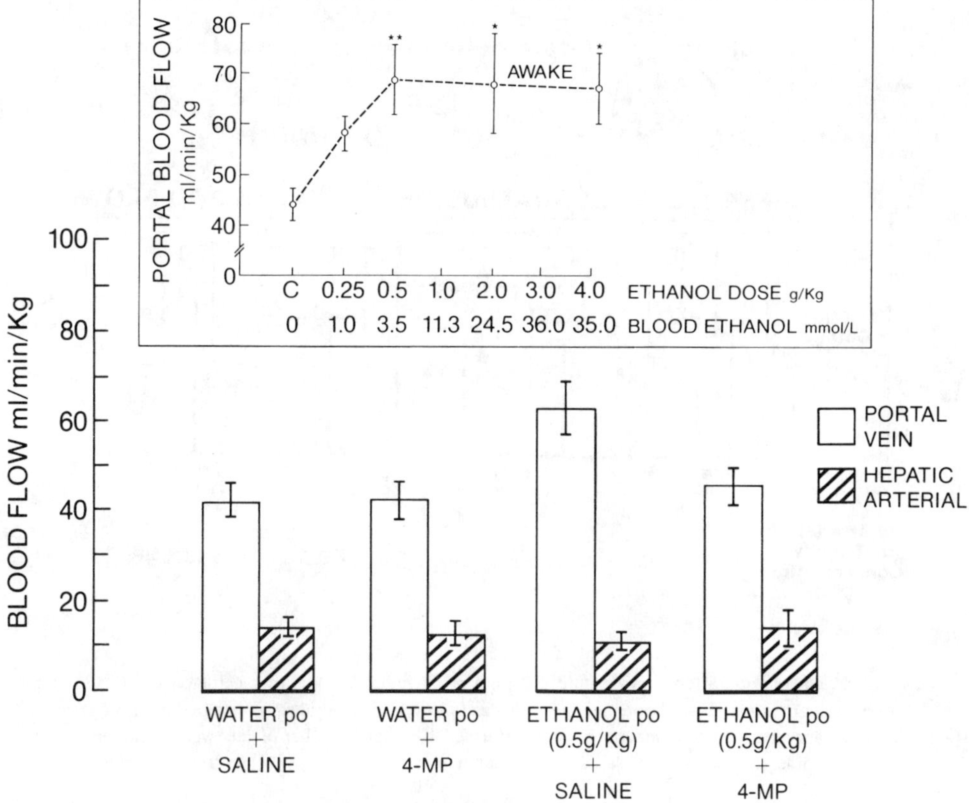

FIGURE 4. Top: Effect of increasing doses of oral ethanol (0.25 to 4.0 g/kg) on portal blood flow and blood ethanol concentrations. Bottom: Effect of 4-methylpyrazole (4 MP) (1.0 mmol/kg intra-arterially) on portal vein and hepatic artery blood flow in rats. Controls received an equivalent oral volume of water or of intra-arterial saline. Blood flows determined as in Figure 1. (Reprinted with permission of the *Canadian Journal of Physiology and Pharmacology.*)

A specific inhibitor of adenosine receptors, 8-phenyltheophylline,[82] that blocks the effects of adenosine on the splanchnic vasculature (Figure 6), was found to also suppress the portal blood flow responses and the fall in preportal vascular resistance, induced both by ethanol (Figure 7) and by acetate.[42] It should be noted that 8-phenyltheophylline does not block the increase in portal blood flow that follows the administration of isoproterenol[58,111] or of glucagon.[96] These results suggest that the vascular effects of ethanol and of acetate are, at least in part, mediated through adenosine.

The administration of ethanol to animals results in a marked increase in hepatic 5′-AMP,[84] an effect that is also expected to occur in tissues outside the liver, since the bulk of the acetate generated in the metabolism of ethanol leaves the liver and is oxidized in the periphery.[48,85] It is of interest that this increase in 5′-AMP induced by ethanol has been proposed to constitute an important mechanism in the increased production of uric acid, the final metabolite of the purine nucleotides, and in the production of gout following alcohol consumption.[25,74,86,87]

Also in keeping with the idea of acetate playing an important role in the hemodynamic effects of ethanol is the finding, already discussed, that the effect of ethanol on portal blood flow is maximal at blood concentrations of ethanol above 3 mM, that saturate the alcohol dehydrogenase pathway. At this concentration, the rate of production of acetate has been shown to be maximal and remains increased while the blood concentration of ethanol is above 3 mM.[85]

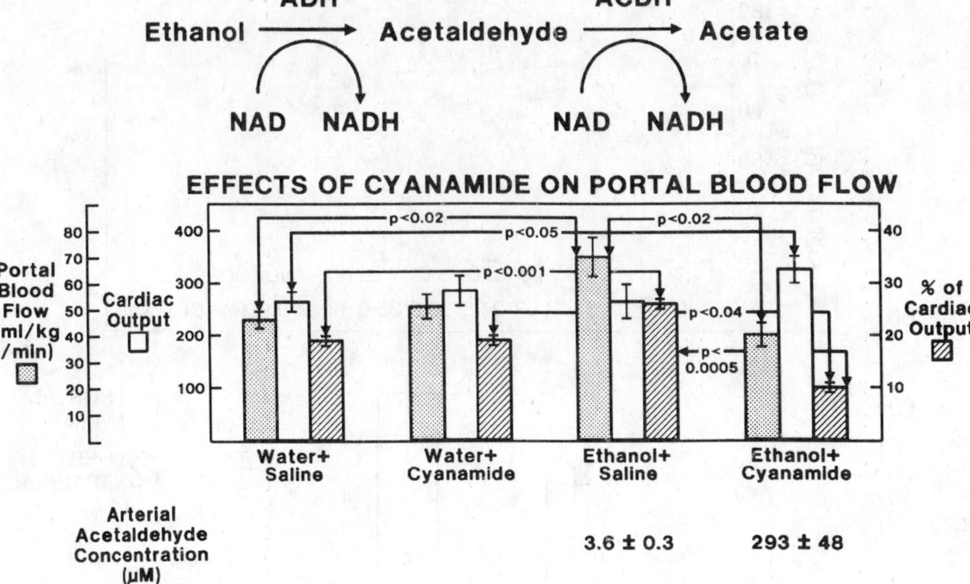

FIGURE 5.   Effect of intra-arterial cyanamide (10 mg/kg) on portal blood flow, cardiac output, and arterial acetaldehyde concentration in rats. Cyanamide infusion was followed by the oral administration of 1g/kg of ethanol. Blood flows and acetaldehyde determinations were performed 1 h later. Number of rats were: water + saline = 7; water + cyanamide = 7; ethanol + saline = 8; ethanol + cyanamide = 8. (Data from Reference 72).

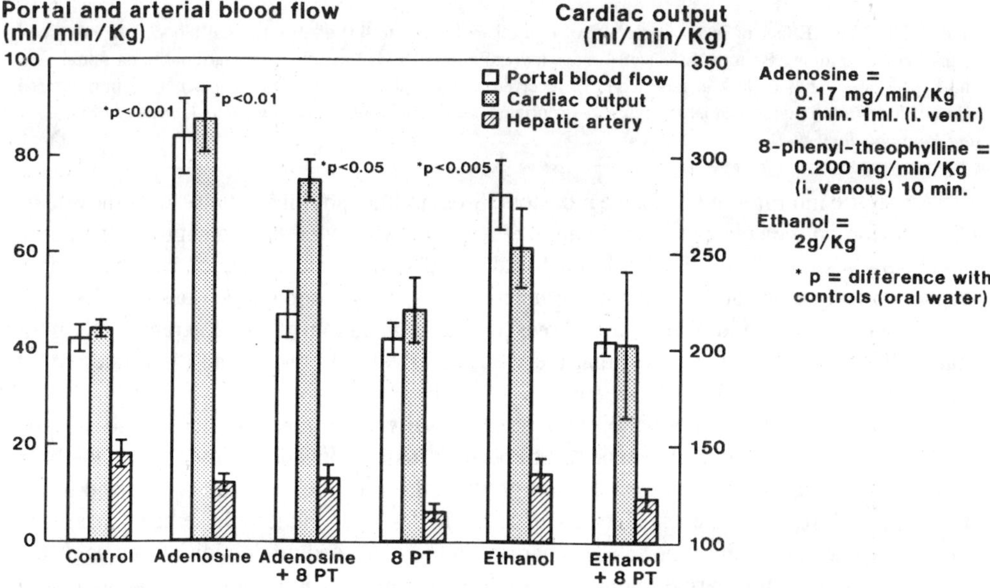

FIGURE 6.   Effect of adenosine (0.17 mg/min/kg intra-arterially), ethanol (2 g/kg orally), and 8-phenyltheophylline (0.2 mg/min/kg intravenously) on cardiac output, portal and hepatic artery blood flow in rats. Controls received equivalent volumes of water orally and saline either intra-arterially or intravenously. Cardiac output and blood flows determined as in Figure 1. (Data from Orrego, H., Carmichael, F. J., Saldivia, V., Giles, H. G., Meggiorini, S., and Israel, Y., *Am. J. Physiol.*, 254, 495, 1988. With permission.)

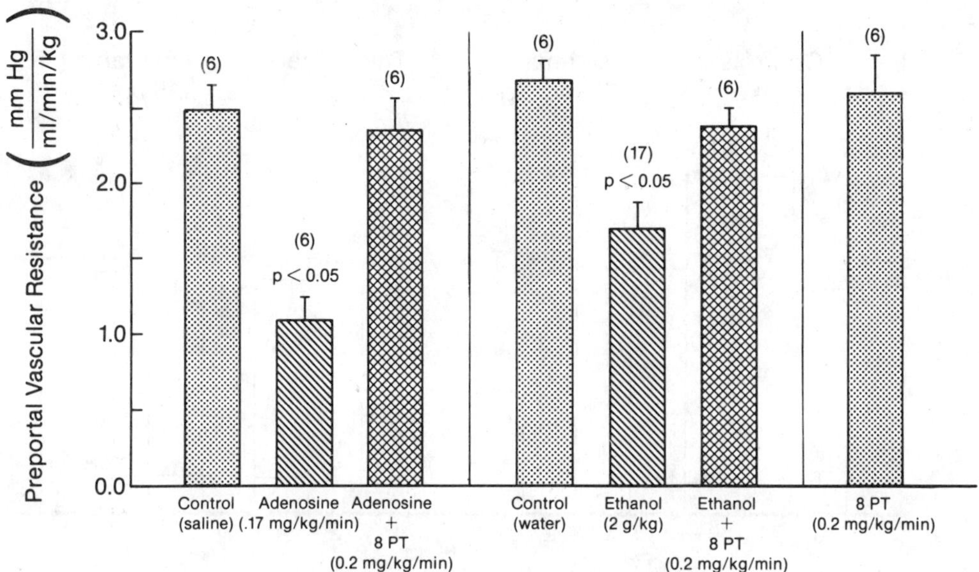

FIGURE 7. Effect of 8-phenyltheophylline (0.2 mg/min/kg intravenously) on the adenosine (0.17 mg/min/kg intra-arterially) and ethanol (2 g/kg orally) induced changes in preportal vascular resistance. (Data from Orrego, H., Carmichael, F. J., Saldivia, V., Giles, H. G., Meggiorini, S., and Israel, Y., *Am. J. Physiol.*, 254, 495, 1988. With permission.)

It is important to note that theoretically, other factors besides acetate may be involved in the increase in adenosine following ethanol consumption. Hypoxia could also contribute to an increase in circulating adenosine following ethanol administration. It is known that hypoxia releases adenosine from several tissues.[76] This increase results from a reduced production of ATP from ADP in the presence of hypoxia. Since ADP is in equilibrium through the adenylate kinase reaction with 5'-AMP (2 ADP $\rightarrow$ AMP + ATP), the tissue concentration of 5'-AMP will increase. The increased production of adenosine under hypoxic conditions is, in fact, known to constitute a most powerful stimulus, increasing blood flow in a number of tissues including the myocardium,[88,89] skeletal muscle,[90] the brain,[76] and the gastrointestinal tract.[91]

As indicated earlier, ethanol increases the degree of relative hypoxia in the perivenular zone of the liver acinus (Zone III). This effect may contribute to the increased production of adenosine, since it has been shown that even mild degrees of hypoxia markedly increase the release of adenosine from perfused livers and isolated hepatocytes.[92,93] Moreover, it has been proposed that the liver is a major exporter of adenosine for use in other tissues with poor capability for *de novo* synthesis of purines such as erythrocytes and the intestinal mucosa.[92-94]

Confirming this idea in the rat, we have found an increase in arterial adenosine concentration 60 min after the oral administration of ethanol (2 g/kg). Arterial adenosine concentration increased from 0.04 $\pm$ 0.02 μM (before ethanol) to 0.17 $\pm$ 0.02 μM ($p < 0.01$), an increase of 400%. It should be noted, however, that circulating levels of adenosine do not necessarily reflect interstitial adenosine concentrations at A_1 and A_2 receptors due to an active metabolism of adenosine by endothelial cells.[95]

It is clear that by itself the release of adenosine from the liver does not provide a complete explanation for the vasodilatory effects of ethanol, since the adenosine levels were below those that have been shown to be effective locally in inducing vasodilation.[91] Furthermore,

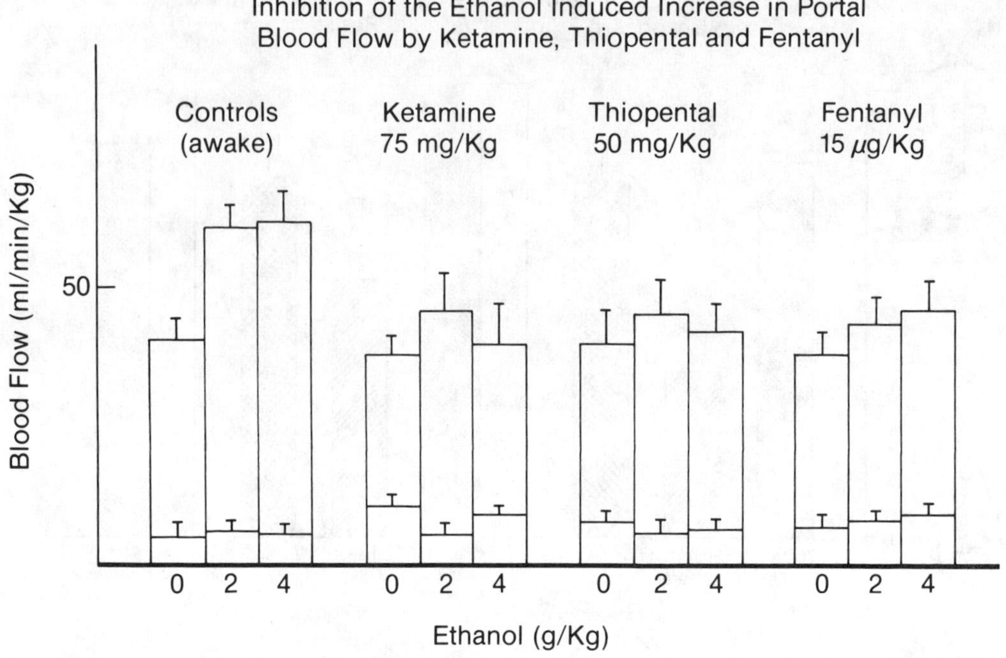

FIGURE 8.   Effect of intramuscular ketamine (75 mg/kg), thiopental (50 mg/kg), and fentanyl (15 μg/kg) on the ethanol (2 or 4 g/kg orally) induced changes in portal and hepatic artery blood flow. Blood flows determined as in Figure 1. (From Carmichael, F. J., Saldivia, V., Israel, Y., McKaigney, J. P., and Orrego, H., *Hepatology*, 7, 89—94, 1987. © by the American Association for the Study of Liver Diseases. With permission.)

ethanol did not lead to an increase in hepatic arterial or coronary flows (controls = 11.8 ± 0.9; ethanol (2 g/kg) = 12.5 ± 1.9 ml/kg/min),[96] which would have been expected if the effects of ethanol were mediated solely by a release of adenosine from the liver resulting in a general increase in systemic circulating adenosine. These differences in flow between systemically administered adenosine and oral ethanol can easily be explained by factors that control the local concentration of adenosine resulting from acetate metabolism in tissues: (1) differences in the rate of acetate metabolism in various organs, (2) activity of 5′-nucleotidase in tissues, and (3) of activity of adenosine deaminase.

IV. INTERACTION BETWEEN ANESTHETIC AGENTS AND ALCOHOL ON PORTAL BLOOD FLOW

The possibility of an interaction between anesthetic agents and alcohol has implications both from the experimental and from the clinical point of view. Experimentally, animals are often studied under conditions of anesthesia, while in humans, the use of anesthetics during emergency surgery in alcoholic or intoxicated patients may render these patients more susceptible to hypoxic liver damage. Therefore, it would appear important to define whether an interaction exists, and to determine the potency of anesthetic agents in this interaction.

Three intravenous anesthetic drugs in current clinical use (ketamine, thiopental, fentanyl) and three inhalational anesthetics (ether, halothane, or isoflurane) have been shown to interact with ethanol on portal blood flow. When administered by intramuscular injection to awake rats, ketamine (75 mg/kg), thiopental (50 mg/kg) or fentanyl (15 μg/kg) do not modify basal liver blood flow through the hepatic artery or portal vein. Each of these anesthetics, when given 15 min before blood flow determinations, however, completely blocked the increase in portal vein blood flow induced by ethanol (Figure 8). This suppression of the ethanol-induced increase in portal blood flow was found to be dose-dependent and time-dependent.[41]

The two inhalational anesthetics, halothane and isoflurane, on the other hand, were found to modify basal blood flow through the liver. Portal vein flows were decreased only slightly, while the hepatic arterial flows were increased by 40% and 60%, respectively. This is similar to previous findings in pigs[97] and rats.[98] As was found with the intravenous anesthetics, both halothane and isoflurane attenuated the ethanol-induced increase in portal blood flow, however, halothane resulted in a complete block while isoflurane only partially blocked this increase in flow.[112] These data suggest that halothane, by reducing the supply of oxygen to the liver under conditions of increased oxygen requirements, may be more hepatotoxic than isoflurane. This increased hepatotoxic potential for halothane is in agreement with some reported experimental studies, which show increased liver damage with halothane compared to isoflurane.[99] Ether, an agent commonly used in experimental studies, also blocked the ethanol-induced increase in portal blood flow.

These six anesthetic agents, therefore, can markedly interfere with the effect of ethanol on liver blood flow. The fact that all of these agents with different molecular structures and chemical characteristics inhibit the effects of ethanol on the blood flow, points to a general consequence of anesthesia per se. In general, anesthetics are known to reduce autonomic tone[100] which might mediate part of these effects. Alternatively, the lipid soluble property of general anesthetic would result in an interaction with hydrophobic environments which may play a role in the effects observed. Alcohol dehydrogenase is known to contain hydrophobic pockets to which molecules such as ethanol, propanol, and butanol can bind.[101] Anesthetics might also interact at these domains, reducing ethanol metabolism which is required for the hemodynamic response to ethanol. This interaction between anesthetics and alcohol may be linked to the previous observation that the hemodynamic effects of ethanol are dependent upon alcohol metabolism by the alcohol dehydrogenase pathway. It is of interest that ether has been found to reduce the rate of ethanol metabolism and that this effect has been attributed to a direct inhibition of the alcohol dehydrogenase enzyme.[102] An effect of this type would also result in a decrease in oxygen consumption by the liver and in acetate production, and therefore, in a decrease in adenosine concentrations at the A_1 and A_2 receptors. Whether the interaction between ethanol and the other anesthetic agents is a result of the same mechanism has yet to be determined.

It is of great importance that, when these agents are used experimentally, the lack of an effect on basal blood flow should not be taken as a guarantee that these drugs will not affect other physiological or pharmacological responses. In this respect, it is of interest that other authors who have studied the effect of ethanol on splanchnic blood flow under anesthesia have failed to comment upon the possibility of an interaction between ethanol and the anesthetic agent used. Our data suggest that caution must be used in interpreting data obtained from anesthetized animals. As well, these findings may help explain some of the discrepancies that exist in the literature with regard to the effect of ethanol on liver blood flow.[49] It would appear that the intravenous anesthetic, ketamine, which has the shortest duration of action, or the inhalational anesthetic, isoflurane, may be the anesthetics of choice for blood flow experiments while still providing a period of good anesthesia.

V. PATHOGENIC IMPLICATIONS

In the presence of alcohol-induced liver disease, several factors could operate to make this compensatory increase in liver blood flow less effective. Among these would be:

1. The presence of portosystemic shunts that would result in most of the increased portal blood flow bypassing the liver;
2. The presence of enlarged hepatocytes compressing the sinusoids and decreasing sinusoidal blood flow;[103] and

3.   Abnormalities in the space of Disse, such as the accumulation of collagen[104] and the capillarization of the sinusoids[105] that might introduce new barriers for oxygen diffusion.[104]

These factors could constitute a vicious-cycle type of mechanism that would contribute to the increasing sensitivity of the liver to damage by alcohol in patients with liver disease who continue to drink even moderate amounts of ethanol.[106]

Portal hypertension and its complications are determined by the combined effects of an increase in intrahepatic resistance and of portal blood flow. In a situation where portal blood flow would be increased, such as in the presence of ethanol, portal hypertension would increase with the possible consequence of bleeding from esophageal varices. It has been reported that alcohol consumption is related to an increased incidence of variceal bleeding.[107]

On the other hand, it is likely that a reduction in portal pressure would be of help in the treatment of esophageal variceal bleeding. In fact, the most common medical treatments of this condition (e.g., vasopressin and somatostatin) act by decreasing portal blood flow and therefore, intravariceal pressure. In patients bleeding from esophageal varices in the presence of ethanol, methylxanthines such as 8-phenyltheophylline that block adenosine receptors may be beneficial, since they would reduce the ethanol-induced increase in portal blood flow. It is of interest that this situation is opposite to that following ethanol intake in individuals with normal livers, where the increase in portal blood flow would be beneficial, since it would prevent hypoxic liver damage by compensating for the increase in oxygen requirements resulting from ethanol metabolism.

VI. CONCLUSIONS

Evidence has accumulated in the recent years which would support the concept of alcohol-induced liver necrosis being of a hypoxic nature. It has furthermore been shown that necrosis is the most important determinant of prognosis in alcoholic liver disease.[31] Therefore, an efficient balance between the increase in oxygen consumption produced by alcohol and the delivery of oxygen to the liver could be an essential determinant in the production, as well as the prognosis, of alcohol-induced liver disease.

Of the mechanisms that increase oxygen delivery to the liver, the most important is an increase in liver blood flow in the presence of ethanol. This increase in liver blood flow requires the metabolism of alcohol by the liver, which results in both hypoxia in the perivenular zone of the liver acinus, and in the production and export of acetate into the systemic circulation. Adenosine, a powerful splanchnic vasodilator, could play an important role in the alcohol-induced increase in portal blood flow. Adenosine would be released as a result of the metabolism of acetate in peripheral tissues, and perhaps by the alcohol-induced liver hypoxia. Failure of this adenosine-mediated increase in portal blood flow in response to ethanol could result in hypoxic liver cell necrosis.

These findings may well have clinical implications. It is possible that other xanthines, found in coffee, tea, cola drinks, and chocolate,[108] could compete for adenosine receptors in the splanchnic vasculature and might have the detrimental effect of suppressing the compensatory increase in portal blood flow. This response could potentiate the hypoxic effects of ethanol resulting in liver cell necrosis. Alcoholics are also heavy consumers of coffee. The interference by anesthetic agents in the compensatory changes in liver blood flow may also be detrimental to liver cells under certain conditions. Indeed, the hepatocellular necrosis found in ethanol-treated rats given halothane in an environment of reduced oxygen tension[109] may be related to a reduction in oxygen delivery to the liver in the presence of these agents.

REFERENCES

1. **Nauck, M., Wolfle, D., Katz, N., and Jungermann, K.,** Modulation of the glucagon dependent induction of phosphoenolpyruvate carboxykinase and tyrosine aminotransferase by arterial and venous oxygen concentration in hepatocyte cultures, *Eur. J. Biochem.,* 119, 657, 1981.
2. **Eguchi, H., Sato, N., Matsumura, T., Kawano, S., and Kamada, T.,** *In vivo* estimation of oxygen saturation of hemoglobin in hepatic lobules in rats, in *Oxygen Transport to Tissue, Advances in Biology and Medicine,* Vol. 10, in press.
3. **Kessler, M.,** Normal and critical O_2 supply of the liver, in *Oxygen Transport in Blood and Tissue,* Lubbers, D. W., Luft, V. C., Theivs, E., and Witzleb, E., Eds., Theime Verlag, Stuttgart, 1968, 242.
4. **Chance, B.,** Molecular basis of oxygen affinity for cytochrome oxidase, in *Oxygen and Physiological Function,* Jobsis, F. F., Ed., Professional Information Library, Dallas, 14.
5. **Israel, Y. and Orrego, H.,** Hypermetabolic state and hypoxic liver damage, in *Recent Developments in Alcoholism,* Galanter, M., Ed., Plenum Press, New York, 1984, 119.
6. **Gore, I., Isaacson, N. H.,** The pathology of hyperpyrexia. Observations at autopsy in 17 cases of fever therapy, *Am. J. Pathol.,* 25, 1029, 1948.
7. **McIver, M. A. and Winter, E. A.,** Deleterious effects of anoxia on the liver of the hyperthyroid animal, *Arch. Surg.,* 46, 171, 1943.
8. **Myers, J. D., Brannon, E. S., and Holland, B. C.,** A correlative study of the cardiac output and the hepatic circulation in hyperthyroidism, *J. Clin. Invest.,* 29, 1069, 1950.
9. **Bravo, I. R., Acevedo, C. G., and Gallardo, V.,** Acute effects of ethanol on liver blood circulation in the anesthetized dog, *Alcoholism: Clin. Exp. Res.,* 4, 248, 1980.
10. **Hines, J. D. and Cowan, D. J.,** Anemia and alcoholism, in *Drugs and Hematological Reactions,* Dimitrov, N. V. and Nodene, J. H., Eds., Grune & Stratton, New York, 1974, 141.
11. **Myers, J. D. and Hickam, J. B.,** An estimation of the hepatic blood flow and splanchnic oxygen consumption in heart failure, *J. Clin. Invest.,* 27, 620, 1948.
12. **Gelman, S.,** Disturbances in hepatic blood flow during anesthesia and surgery, *Arch. Surg.,* 111, 881, 1976.
13. **Israel, Y., Kalant, H., Orrego, H., Khanna, J. M., Videla, L., and Phillips, J. M.,** Experimental alcohol-induced hepatic necrosis: suppression by propylthiouracil, *Proc. Nat. Acad. Sci. U.S.A.,* 72, 1137, 1975.
14. **Bredfeldt, J. E., Riley, E. M., and Groszmann, R. J.,** Compensatory mechanisms in response to an elevated hepatic oxygen consumption in chronically ethanol-fed rats, *Am. J. Physiol.,* 248, 507, 1985.
15. **Israel, Y. and Orrego, H.,** Hypermetabolic state, hepatocyte expansion and liver blood flow: an interaction triad in alcoholic liver injury, *Ann. N.Y. Acad. Sci.,* 492, 303—323, 1987.
16. **Israel, Y., Orrego, H., Khanna, J. M., Stewart, D. J., Phillips, M. J., and Kalant, H.,** Alcohol induced susceptibility to hypoxic liver damage: possible role in the pathogenesis of alcoholic liver disease?, in *Alcohol and the Liver,* Fisher, M. M. and Rankin, J. G., Eds., Plenum Press, New York, 1977, 323.
17. **Ji, S., Lemasters, J. J., Christenson, V., and Thurman, R. G.,** Periportal and pericentral pyridine nucleotide fluorescence from the surface of the perfused liver: evaluation of the hypothesis that chronic treatment with ethanol produces pericentral hypoxia, *Proc. Natl. Acad. Sci. U.S.A.,* 79, 5415, 1982.
18. **Villeneuve, J. P., Pomier, G., and Huet, P. M.,** Effect of ethanol on hepatic blood flow in unanesthetized dogs with chronic portal and hepatic vein catheterization, *Can. J. Physiol. Pharmacol.,* 59, 598, 1981.
19. **Jungermann, K. and Katz, N.,** Functional hepatocellular heterogeneity, *Hepatology,* 2, 385, 1982.
20. **Miyamoto, K. and French, S. W.,** Role of hypoxia in pathogenesis of alcohol-induced liver injury in rats, *Hepatology,* 6, 1124(A), 1986.
21. **Orrego, H., Blake, J. E., Medline, A., and Israel, Y.,** Interrelation of the hypermetabolic state, necrosis, anemia and cell enlargement as determinants of severity in alcoholic liver disease, *Acta Med. Scand.,* 703, 81, 1985.
22. **Quistorff, B., Chance, B., and Takeda, H.,** Two- and three-dimensional redox heterogeneity of rat liver. Effects of anoxia and alcohol on the lobular redox pattern, in *Frontiers of Biological Energetics,* Vol. 2, Academic Press, New York, 1978, 1487.
23. **Sato, N., Kamada, T., Kawano, S., Hayashi, N., Kishida, Y., Meren, H., Yoshihara, H., and Abe, H.,** Effect of acute and chronic ethanol consumption on hepatic tissue oxygen tension in rats, *Pharmacol. Biochem. Behav.,* 18, 443, 1983.
24. **French, S. W., Ruebner, B. H., Mezey, E., Tamura, T., and Halsted, C. H.,** Effect of chronic ethanol feeding on hepatic mitochondria in the monkey, *Hepatology,* 3, 34, 1983.
25. **Lieber, C. S. and De Carli, L. M.,** Animal models of ethanol dependence and liver injury in rats and baboons, *Fed. Proc.,* 35, 1232, 1976.
26. **Popper, H. and Lieber, C. S.,** Histogenesis of alcoholic fibrosis and cirrhosis in the baboon, *Am. J. Pathol.,* 98, 695, 1980.

27. **Rogers, A. E., Fox, J. G., and Gottlieb, L. S.,** Effects of ethanol and malnutrition on non-human primate liver, in *Frontiers of Liver Disease,* Berk, P. D. and Chalmers, T. C., Eds., Thieme-Stratton, New York, 1981, 167.

28. **Orrego, H., Israel, Y., and Blendis, L. M.,** Alcoholic liver disease: information in search of knowledge?, *Hepatology,* 1, 267, 1981.

29. **Emirgil, C., Sobol, B. J., Heymann, B., and Shibutani, K.,** Pulmonary function in alcoholics, *Am. J. Med.,* 57, 69, 1974.

30. **Maletzky, R. M. and Klotter, J.,** Smoking and Alcoholism, *Am. J. Psychiat.,* 131, 445, 1974.

31. **Orrego, H., Blake, J. E., Blendis, L. M., and Medline, A.,** Prognosis of alcoholic cirrhosis in the presence and absence of alcoholic hepatitis, *Gastroenterology,* 92, 208, 1987.

32. **Rankin, J. G. and Wilkinson, P.,** Alcohol and tobacco smoking, in *The Health of a Metropolis,* Krupinski, J. and Stoller, A., Eds., Heineman Educational Australia, 1971, 61.

33. **Taasan, V. C., Block, A. J., Boysen, P. G., Wynne, J. W., White, C., and Lindsey, S.,** Alcohol increases sleep apnea and oxygen desaturation in asymptomatic man, *Am. J. Med.,* 71, 240, 1981.

34. **French, S. W., Benson, N. C., and Sun, P. S.,** Centrilobular liver necrosis induced by hypoxia in chronic ethanol-fed rats, *Hepatology,* 4, 912, 1984.

35. **French, S. W., Miyamoto, K., and Tsukamoto, H.,** Ethanol-induced hepatic fibrosis in the rat: role of the amount of dietary fat, *Alcoholism: Clin. Exp. Res.,* 10(S), 13, 1986.

36. **Kalant, H., Israel, Y., Phillips, M. J., Woo, N., Kanna, J. M., and Orrego, H.,** Necrosis produced by hepatic arterial ligation in alcohol-fed rats, *Fed. Proc.,* 34, 719(A), 1975.

37. **Perrissoud, D., Maignan, M. F., and Dumont, J. M.,** Antinecrotic effect of 3-palmitoy(+)-catechin against liver damage induced by galactosamine-ethanol in the rat, *Liver,* 5, 55, 1985.

38. **Jauhonen, P., Baraona, E., Miyakawa, H., and Lieber, C. S.,** Mechanism for selective perivenular hepatotoxicity of ethanol, *Alcoholism: Clin. Exp. Res.,* 6, 350, 1982.

39. **Shaw, S., Heller, E. A., Friedman, H. S., Baraona, E., and Lieber, Ch. S.,** Increased hepatic oxygenation following ethanol administration in the baboon, *Proc. Soc. Exp. Biol. Med.,* 156, 509, 1977.

40. **Abrams, M. A. and Cooper, C.,** Mechanisms of increased hepatic uptake of unesterified fatty acid from serum of ethanol-treated rats, *Biochem. J.,* 156, 47, 1976.

41. **Carmichael, F. J., Saldivia, V., Israel, Y., McKaigney, J. P., and Orrego, H.,** Ethanol-induced increase in portal hepatic blood flow: interference by anesthetic agents, *Hepatology,* 7, 89, 1987.

42. **Carmichael, F. J., Saldivia, V., Israel, Y., Orrego, H.,** The effect of acetate on splanchnic hemodynamics, *Hepatology,* 7, 1987.

43. **Israel, Y., Macdonald, A., and Orrego, H.,** Contribution of portal and arterial flow to the increase in liver blood flow induced by acute ethanol administration, *Gastroenterology,* 84, 1377, 1983.

44. **Iturriaga, H., Bunout, D., Peterman, M., Ugarte, G., and Israel, Y.,** Effects of ethanol on hepatic blood flow in the rat, *Alcoholism: Clin. Exp. Res.,* 5, 221, 1981.

45. **Jauhonen, V. P.,** Effect of acute ethanol load on plasma immunoreactive insulin and glucagon, *Horm. Metab. Res.,* 10, 214, 1978.

46. **Jenkins, S. A., Baxter, J. N., Devitt, P., Taylor, I., and Shields, R.,** Effects of alcohol on hepatic haemodynamics in the rat, *Digestion,* 34, 236, 1986.

47. **Jorfeldt, L. and Juhlin-Dannfeldt, A.,** The influence of ethanol on splanchnic and skeletal muscle metabolism in man, *Metabolism,* 27, 97, 1976.

48. **Lundquist, F., Tygstrup, N., Winkler, K., Mellemgaard, K., and Manck-Petersen, S.,** Ethanol metabolism and production of free acetate in the human liver, *J. Clin. Invest.,* 41, 955, 1962.

49. **McKaigney, J. P., Carmichael, F. J., Saldivia, V., Israel, Y., and Orrego, H.,** Role of ethanol metabolism in the ethanol-induced increase in splanchnic circulation, *Am. J. Physiol.,* 250, 518, 1986.

50. **Mendeloff, A. I.,** Effect of intravenous infusions of ethanol upon estimated hepatic blood flow in man, *J. Clin. Invest.,* 33, 1298, 1954.

51. **Smythe, C. McC., Heinemann, H. O., and Bradley, S. E.,** Estimated hepatic blood flow in the dog. Effect of ethyl alcohol on it, renal blood flow, cardiac output and arterial pressure, *Am. J. Physiol.,* 172, 737, 1953.

52. **Stein, S. W., Lieber, C. S., Leevy, C. M., Cherrick, G. R., and Abelman, W. H.,** The effect of ethanol upon systemic and hepatic blood flow in man, *Am. J. Clin. Nutr.,* 13, 68, 1963.

53. **Yoshihara, H., Sato, N., Sasaki, Y., Uchima, E., Inoue, A., Matsumura, T., Hayashi, N., Kawano, S., Kamada, T., and Abe, H.,** Effect of alcohol ingestion on portal venous blood flow in healthy volunteers: comparison between the subjects with and without ALDH isoenzyme, *Alcohol,* 2, 463, 1985.

54. **Leevy, C. M., Silverberg, M., and Naylor, J.,** Physiology of dye extraction by the liver: comparative studies of sulfobromophthalein and indocyanine green, *Ann. N.Y. Acad. Sci.,* 111, 161, 1963.

55. **Lorber, S. H., Oppenheimer, M. J., Shay, H., Lynch, P., and Siplet, H.,** Enterohepatic circulation of bromsulphalein: intraduodenal, intraportal and intravenous dye administration in dogs, *Am. J. Physiol.,* 173, 259, 1953.

56. **Kock, N. G., Roding, P., Hahnloser, P., Tibblin, S., and Schenk, W. G.,** The effect of glucagon on hepatic blood flow, An experimental study in the dog, *Arch. Surg.*, 100, 147, 1970.

57. **Tiengo, A., Fedele, D., Frasson, P., Muggeo, M., and Crepaldi, G.,** Ethanol effect on glucagon secretion in the pig, *Horm. Metab. Res.*, 6, 245, 1974.

58. **Krarup, N. and Larsen, J. A.,** The effect of glucagon on hepatosplanchnic hemodynamics, functional capacity, and metabolism in the liver in cats, *Acta Physiol. Scand.*, 91, 42, 1974.

59. **McKaigney, J. P., Carmichael, F. J., Saldivia, V., Israel, Y., and Orrego, H.,** Is glucagon a mediator of ethanol-induced increase in splanchnic blood flow, *Hepatology* 5, 978(A), 1985.

60. **Balaban, R. S. and Blum, J. J.,** Hormone-induced changes in NADH fluorescence and O_2 consumption of rat hepatocytes, *Am. J. Physiol.*, 242, 172, 1982.

61. **Limburg, B. and Kommerell, B.,** Correction of altered plasma amino acid pattern in cirrhosis of the liver by somatostatin, *Gut* 25, 1291, 1984.

62. **Li, T. K. and Theorell, H.,** Human liver alcohol dehydrogenase: inhibition by pyrazole and pyrazole analogs, *Acta Chem. Scand.*, 23, 892, 1969.

63. **Aizawa, Y., Ohmori, T., Imai, Y., Nara, M., Matsuoka, M., and Hirasawa, Y.,** Depressant action of acetate upon the human cardiovascular system, *Clin. Nephrol.*, 8, 477, 1977.

64. **Altura, B. M., and Altura, B. T.,** Microvascular and vascular smooth muscle actions of ethanol, acetaldehyde and acetate, *Fed. Proc.*, 41, 2447, 1982.

65. **Altura, B. M., Carella, A., and Altura, B. T.,** Acetaldehyde on vascular smooth muscle: possible role in vasodilator action of ethanol, *Eur. J. Pharmacol.*, 52, 73, 1978.

66. **Altura, B. M. and Gebrewold, A.,** Failure of acetaldehyde or acetate to mimic the splanchnic arteriolar or venular dilator actions of ethanol: direct in situ studies on the microcirculation, *Br. J. Pharmacol.*, 73, 580, 1981.

67. **Gailis, L.,** Cardiovascular effects of acetaldehyde: evidence for the involvement of tissue SH groups, in *The Role of Acetaldehyde in the Actions of Ethanol*, Lindros, K. O. and Eriksson, C. J. P., Eds., Kauppakirjapaino, Helsinki, 1975, 135.

68. **Kirkendol, P. L., Devia, C. J., Bower, J. D., and Holbert, R. D.,** A comparison of the cardiovascular effect of sodium acetate, sodium bicarbonate and other potential sources of fixed base in hemodialysate solutions, *Trans. Am. Soc. Artif. Int. Organs*, 23, 399, 1977.

69. **Liang, C. S. and Lowenstein, J. M.,** Metabolic control of the circulation. Effects of acetate and pyruvate, *J. Clin. Inv.*, 62, 1029, 1978.

70. **Rix, K. J. B.,** *Alcohol and Alcoholism*, Montreal Eden Press, Montreal, 1977.

71. **Cederbaum, A. I.,** The effect of cyanamide on acetaldehyde oxidation by isolated rat liver mitochondria and on the inhibition of pyruvate oxidation by acetaldehyde, *Alcoholism: Clin. Exp. Res.*, 5, 38, 1981.

72. **Carmichael, F. J., Israel, Y., Saldivia, V., Giles, H. G., Meggiorini, S., and Orrego, H.,** Blood acetaldehyde and the ethanol-induced increase in splanchnic circulation, *Biochem. Pharmacol.*, 36, 2673, 1987.

73. **Molnar, J. I., Scott, J. B., Frohlich, E. D., and Haddy, F. J.,** Local effects of various anions and H^+ on dog limb and coronary vascular resistances, *Am. J. Physiol.*, 203, 125, 1962.

74. **Puig, J. G. and Fox, I. H.,** Ethanol-induced activation of adenosine nucleotide turnover. Evidence for a role of acetate, *J. Clin. Inv.*, 74, 936, 1984.

75. **Steffen, R. P., McKenzie, J. E., Bockman, E. L., and Haddy, F. J.,** Changes in dog gracilis muscle adenosine during exercise and acetate infusion, *Am. J. Physiol.*, 244, 387, 1983.

76. **Berne, R. M., Winn, H. R., Knabb, R. M., Ely, S. W., and Rubio, R.,** Bloodflow regulation by adenosine in heart, brain and skeletal muscle, in *Regulatory Function of Adenosine*, Berne, R. M., Rall, T. W., and Rubio, R., Eds., Martinius Nijhoff, The Hague, 1983, 293.

77. **Burger, R. M. and Lowenstein, J. M.,** Preparation and properties of 5'nucleotidase from smooth muscle of small intestine, *J. Biol. Chem.*, 245, 6274, 1970.

78. **Dobson, J. G., Ordway, R. N., and Fenton, R. A.,** Endogenous adenosine inhibits catecholamine contractile responses in normoxic hearts, *Am. J. Physiol.*, 251, 455, 1986.

79. **Eintrei, C. and Carlsson, C.,** Effects of hypotension induced by adenosine on brain surface oxygen pressure and cortical cerebral blood flow in the pig, *Acta Physiol. Scand.*, 126, 463, 1986.

80. **Haddy, F. J., Chou, C. C., Scott, J. B., and Dabney, J. M.,** Intestinal vascular responses to naturally occurring vasoactive substances, *Gastroenterology*, 54, 444, 1967.

81. **Lautt, W. W. and Legare, D. J.,** The use of 8-phenyltheophylline as a competitive antagonist of adenosine and an inhibitor of the intrinsic regulatory mechanism of the hepatic artery, *Can. J. Physiol. Pharmacol.*, 63, 717, 1985.

82. **Daly, J. W.,** Adenosine receptors: targets for future drugs, *J. Med. Chem.*, 25, 197, 1982.

83. **Schutz, W., Schrader, J., and Gerlach, E.,** Different sites of adenosine formation in the heart, *Am. J. Physiol.*, 240, 963, 1981.

84. **Lindros, K. O., Kivikataja, R. L., and Soukas, A.,** Elevation by ethanol and its metabolites of liver adenosine monophosphate, *Alcohol*, 3, 63, 1986.

85. **Soukas, A., Forsander, O., and Lindros, K.,** Distribution and utilization of alcohol-derived acetate in the rat, *J. Stud. Alcohol,* 45, 381, 1984.

86. **Faller, J. and Fox, I. H.,** Ethanol-induced hyperuricemia. Evidence for increased urate production by activation of adenine nucleotide turnover, *N. Engl. J. Med.,* 307, 1598, 1982.

87. **Wyngaarden, J. B. and Kelley, W. N.,** Drug-induced hyperuricemia and gout, in *Gout and Hyperuricemia,* Grune & Stratton, New York, 1976, 369.

88. **McKenzie, J. E., Steffen, R. P., and Haddy, F. J.,** Relationships between adenosine and coronary resistance in conscious exercising dogs, *Am. J. Physiol.,* 242, 24, 1982.

89. **Schrader, J., Haddy, F. J., and Gerlach, E.,** Release of adenosine, inosine and hypoxanthine from the isolated guinea pig heart during hypoxia, flow-autoregulation and reactive hyperemia, *Pfluegers Arch.,* 369, 1, 1977.

90. **Thompson, L. P., Gorman, M. W., and Sparks, H. V.,** Aminophylline and interstitial adenosine during sustained exercise hyperemia, *Am. J. Physiol.,* 251, 1232, 1986.

91. **Granger, D. N., Valleau, J. D., Parker, R. E., Lane, R. S., and Taylor, A. E.,** Effects of adenosine on intestinal hemodynamics, oxygen delivery, and capillary fluid exchange, *Am. J. Physiol.,* 235, H707, 1978.

92. **Arnold, S. T. and Cysyk, R. L.,** Adenosine export from the liver: oxygen dependency, *Am. J. Physiol.,* 251, 34, 1986.

93. **Belloni, F. L., Elkin, P. L., and Giannotto, B.,** The mechanism of adenosine release from hypoxic rat liver cells, *Brit. J. Pharmacol.,* 85, 441, 1985.

94. **Pritchard, J. B., O'Connor, B., Oliver, J. M., and Berlin, R. D.,** Uptake and supply of purine compounds by the liver, *Am. J. Physiol.,* 229, 967, 1975.

95. **Sparks, H. V., Dewitt, D. F., Wangler, R. D., Gorman, M. W., and Bassigthwaighte, J. B.,** Capillary transport of adenosine, *Fed. Proc.,* 44, 2620, 1985.

96. **Orrego, H., Carmichael, F. J., Saldivia, V., Giles, H. G., Meggiorini, S., and Israel, Y.,** Ethanol-induced increases in portal blood flow: role of adenosine, *Am. J. Physiol.,* 254, 495, 1988.

97. **Lundeen, G., Manohav, M., and Parke, C.,** Systemic distribution of blood flow in swine while awake and during 1.0 and 1.5 MAC isoflurane anesthesia with or without 50% nitrous oxide, *Anesth. Analg.,* 62, 499, 1983.

98. **Miller, E. D., Kistner, J. R., and Epstein, R. M.,** Whole body distribution of radioactively labelled microspheres in the rat during anesthesia with halothane, enflurane, or ketamine, *Anesthesiology,* 52, 296, 1980.

99. **VanDyke, R. A.,** Hepatic centrilobular necrosis in rats after exposure to halothane, enflurane, or isoflurane, *Anesth. Analg.,* 61, 812, 1982.

100. **Marshall, B. E. and Wollman, H.,** General anesthetics, in *Goodman and Gilman's, the Pharmacological Basis of Therapeutics,* 6th ed., Gilman, A. G., Goodman, L. S., Rall, T. W., and Murad, F., Eds., Macmillan, New York, 1985, 276.

101. **Cornell, N. W., Hansch, C., Kim, K. H.,** The inhibition of alcohol dehydrogenase *in vitro* and in isolated hepatocytes by 4-substituted pyrazoles, *Arch. Biochem. Biophys.,* 227, 81, 1983.

102. **Normann, P. T., Ripel, A., and Morland, J.,** Diethyl ether inhibits ethanol metabolism *in vivo* by interaction with alcohol dehydrogenase, *Alcoholism: Clin. Exp. Res.,* 11, 163, 1987.

103. **Vidins, E. I., Britton, R. S., Medline, A., Blendis, L. M., Israel, Y., and Orrego, H.,** Sinusoidal caliber in alcohol and nonalcoholic liver disease: diagnostic and pathogenic implications, *Hepatology,* 5, 408, 1985.

104. **Orrego, H., Medline, A., Blendis, L. M., Rankin, J. G., and Kreaden, D. A.,** Collagenisation of the Disse space in alcoholic liver disease, *Gut,* 20, 673, 1979.

105. **Schaffner, F. and Popper, H.,** Capillarization of hepatic sinusoids in man, *Gastroenterology,* 44, 239, 1963.

106. **Orrego, H., Blake, J., Blendis, L., Compton, K., and Israel, Y.,** Long-term propylthiouracil in the treatment of alcoholic liver disease, *N. Engl. J. Med.,* 317, 1421, 1987.

107. **Garcia-Tsao, Groszmann, R. J., Fisher, R. L., Conn, H. O., Atterbury, C. E., and Glickman, M.,** Portal pressure, presence of gastroesophageal varices and variceal bleeding, *Hepatology,* 5, 419, 1985.

108. **Fredholm, B. B.,** Are methylxanthine effects due to antagonism of endogenous adenosine?, *Trends Pharmacol. Sci.,* 1, 129, 1980.

109. **Tagaki, T., Ishii, H., Takahashi, H., Kato, S., Okuno, F., Ebihara, Y., Yamauchi, H., Nagata, S., Tashiro, M., and Tsuchiya, M.,** Potentiation of halothane hepatoxicity by chronic ethanol administration in rat: an animal model of halothane hepatitis, *Pharmacol. Biochem. Behav.,* 18, (Suppl. 1), 461, 1983.

110. **Castenfors, H., Hultman, E., and Josephson, B.,** Effect of intravenous infusions of ethyl alcohol on stimulated hepatic blood flow in man, *J. Clin. Invest.,* 39, 776, 1960.

111. **Lautt, W. W.,** Autoregulation of superior mesenteric artery is blocked by adenosine antagonism, *Can. J. Physiol. Pharmacol.,* 64, 1291, 1986.

112. **Roldan et al.,** unpublished results.

Chapter 17

EFFECTS OF VASOACTIVE DRUGS ON THE SYSTEMIC AND SPLANCHNIC CIRCULATION

Didier Lebrec and Samuel S. Lee*

TABLE OF CONTENTS

*   Dr. Lee held a fellowship from the Medical Research Council of Canada.

I. INTRODUCTION

Patients with liver disease are known to have alterations in sympathetic nervous system activity, so it is not surprising that much clinical and experimental research has focused on the hemodynamic effects of sympathomimetic and sympatholytic agents and other vasoactive drugs. Research with these drugs has two major goals: first, to better understand the pathophysiological mechanisms responsible for the deranged sympathetic function in liver disease, and second, as a natural outgrowth of the first, to suggest possible new treatments for the complications of portal hypertension. This chapter will briefly review the methodology for circulatory studies and then focus on the hemodynamic effects of pharmacological agonists and antagonists of the α- and β-adrenergic and serotonergic systems as well as the effects of nitrates.

II. METHODS AND MODELS FOR STUDYING THE CIRCULATION

In humans, the systemic circulation is accessible to study by many methods. Cardiac output is measured readily by the Fick principle, using either thermodilution with a pulmonary artery catheter, or dye dilution with simultaneous arterial and venous catheterization. Systemic vascular resistance can then be calculated from the arterial pressure and cardiac output.

By contrast, the splanchnic circulation is much more difficult to study. In normal subjects, no valid method yet exists to quantify portal tributary blood flow. In patients with chronic liver disease, because of the portosystemic collaterals, even total splanchnic blood flows cannot be approximated by measuring hepatic blood flow. At present, we can only obtain indirect information about the splanchnic circulation in cirrhosis. Portal pressure can be measured directly by either the percutaneous or umbilical vein approach. However, these techniques may be hazardous in patients with ascites or coagulopathy, so less invasive techniques have become more popular. In particular, the wedged hepatic venous pressure and the hepatic venous pressure gradient (the wedged minus the free hepatic venous pressure) can easily be measured, and closely reflect the portal pressure and the sinusoidal contribution to the portal pressure, respectively.[1] One disadvantage is that these pressures underestimate true portal pressure in presinusoidal causes of portal hypertension. In addition, the hepatic venous pressure gradient may not adequately reflect the magnitude of change in portal pressure after vasoactive drug administration.[2] However, the direction of change in pressures will be the same.

Hepatic blood flow can also be measured by hepatic dye clearance techniques. In patients with abnormal liver architecture, accurate measurement of hepatic extraction is essential; otherwise estimates of flow based on plasma clearance alone lead to large errors.

Blood flow in the portal vein trunk and the splenic and superior mesenteric veins has been estimated by measuring flow velocity by Doppler scanning and simultaneously, vessel size by ultrasound sector scans.[3-5] While very promising as a completely noninvasive method of quantifying deep abdominal venous responses, this technique remains to be fully validated.[6] In particular, questions have been raised about its reproducibility.

Since the portosystemic collaterals are so important, attempts have been made to measure a part of this circulation. Following up the original report by Bosch and Groszmann,[7] the Barcelona unit and our unit have validated the use of the azygos venous blood flow as an index of superior portocollateral flow (Figure 1).[8,9] Neither the size of esophageal varices nor the risk of bleeding correlate with azygos flow. However, good correlations with hepatic venous pressure gradient and cardiac output provide circumstantial evidence that the azygos reflects portocollateral flow.[8,9] More recently, the estimate of oxygen and bile salt content of the azygos venous blood clearly established that at least part of this blood is derived from a splanchnic source.[10]

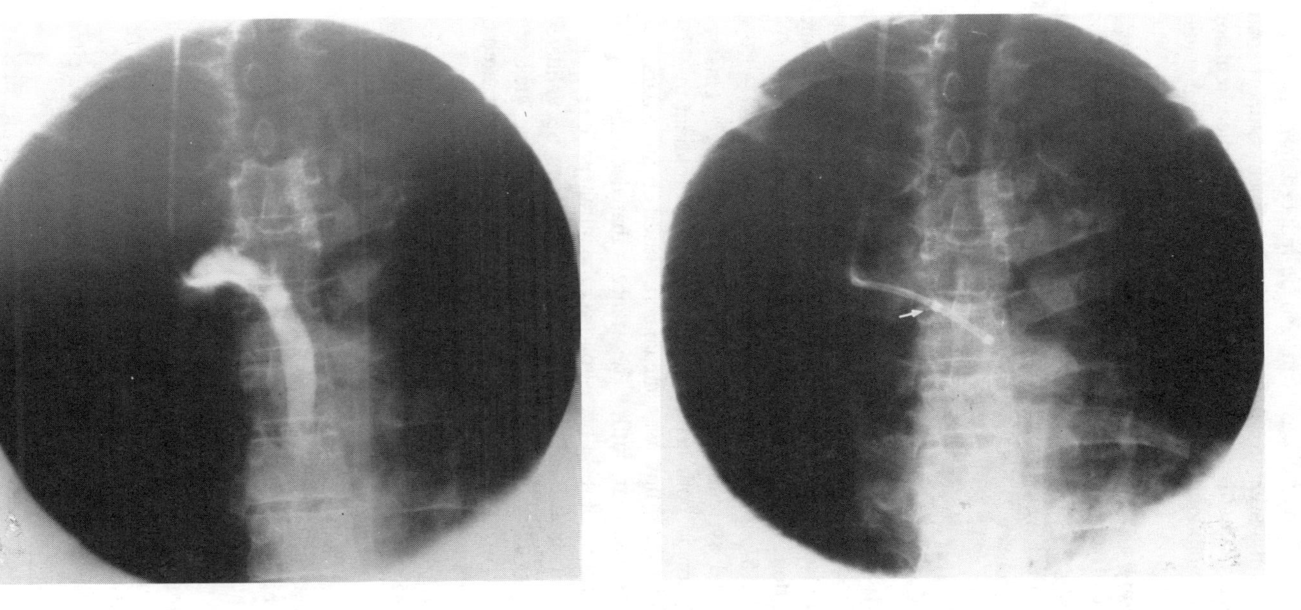

FIGURE 1.   (A) Opacification of the arch of the azygos vein in a patient with cirrhosis. (B) The continuous thermodilution catheter has been introduced and advanced in the azygos vein. The arrow indicates the proximal thermoresistance.

Since splanchnic hemodynamics are so difficult to measure directly in man, animal models of liver disease have been developed. Much research in pathophysiological mechanisms has used the portal vein-stenosed rat, a model of prehepatic portal hypertension.[11] Cirrhosis can be induced in rats by either chronic administration of carbon tetrachloride[12] or chronic bile duct ligation.[13] Chronic liver disease can also be induced in dogs by bile duct ligation[14] or administration of dimethylnitrosamine;[15] however, since canine hepatic veins have powerful sphincters, many investigators have abandoned splanchnic circulatory work in this species. Other species, including pigs, rabbits, and cats have also been studied sporadically, but good models of chronic liver disease in these animals are lacking. When interpreting animal studies, it should be kept in mind that: (a) models with prehepatic portal hypertension have essentially normal livers, and (b) anesthesia may markedly change hemodynamics, as shown recently for dogs[16] and rats[17] undergoing controlled hemorrhage, the portal vein-stenosed rats[18] and bile duct-ligated rats.[19] The models are discussed in greater detail elsewhere in this book (see Chapter 2).

III. DRUGS ACTING ON α-ADRENOCEPTORS

A. α-ADRENOCEPTOR AGONISTS

Clonidine is a centrally active α_2-agonist. This presynaptic α_2-stimulation decreases total sympathetic nervous overflow, as reflected in diminished catecholamine levels. Two studies in patients with cirrhosis have been done and the results show generally good agreement.[20,21] In the Australian study, a dose of 2.5 μg/kg led to decreases in cardiac output (-13%), mean arterial pressure (-23%), and systemic vascular resistance (-15%).[20] This was associated with a significant reduction in both hepatic venous pressure gradient (-27%) and portal pressure (-19%). Hepatic blood flow was unchanged. Based on these data, they calculated a "postsinusoidal hepatic vascular outflow resistance" that decreased significantly, suggesting that the principal action of this drug is to lower the intrahepatic resistance. However, their concept of "postsinusoidal outflow resistance" remains to be validated. Therefore, at present their hypothesis must remain conjectural. An alternative idea, that clonidine causes splanchnic vasoconstriction, perhaps mediated by baroreflexes triggered by the fall in arterial pressure, also remains speculative.

Our study used a dose of 150 μg in Pugh class B and C patients with severe ascites.[21] We also found reductions in cardiac output (-17%) and mean arterial pressure (-12%), but systemic vascular resistance did not change. Splanchnic findings included decreases in hepatic venous pressure gradient (-20%) and azygos blood flow (-27%), with unchanged hepatic blood flow. Although peripheral and renal vein noradrenaline levels decreased markedly, peripheral renin activity and aldosterone remained unaffected.

From these studies, several conclusions can be drawn:

1. Clonidine is an effective sympatholytic agent in cirrhosis. All patients in the two studies showed diminished serum noradrenaline levels or a noradrenaline spillover index.
2. As expected, this sympatholysis led to decreases in the hyperkinetic systemic circulation.
3. Decreased sympathetic tone also was associated with decreases in portal pressure and probably portocollateral flow.
4. The sympathetic nervous system is activated in patients with advanced cirrhosis and is at least partially responsible for mediating some of the systemic and splanchnic hyperkineticism.
5. Although this short-term amelioration in the hyperkinetic circulation is promising, any potential therapeutic use may be hampered by the hypotensive action.

Mastai et al. recently reported the effects of peripheral α-adrenergic stimulation with methoxamine, a predominant α_1-agonist.[22] This resulted in a slight but significant 10% decrease in hepatic venous pressure gradient, reductions in cardiac output, and increased arterial pressure. This study is discussed in further detail below (see Section B).

B. α-ADRENOCEPTOR ANTAGONISTS

Only two clinical studies using peripheral α-adrenergic antagonists have been reported.[23,24] Ikeda measured portal pressure intraoperatively in six patients with portal hypertension, before and after phenoxybenzamine administration, and found a 22% decrease.[23] However, firm conclusions cannot be drawn from these promising results due to the small sample size and possibly confounding intraoperative factors: measurements were done during major abdominal surgery, under general anesthesia, with blood being transfused.

Mills et al. tested the long-term effects of prazosin, an α_1-antagonist, after 3 and 8 weeks of administration.[24] The hepatic venous pressure gradient decrease significantly by 18% at 8 weeks, while systemic vascular resistance and cardiac output did not change significantly. Although mean arterial pressure remained unchanged, considerable orthostatic diastolic hypotension occurred.

No studies of α-blockade or α-stimulation in animal models of liver disease have yet been reported.

How is one to reconcile the results of all these studies on α-adrenergic agents? It seems that no matter what the α-adrenoreceptor stimulus, portal pressure decreases. First, central α-stimulation with clonidine is radically different from peripheral α-adrenoreceptor effects, since it results in decreases in both α- and β-adrenergic tone. Second, it is possible that the effects of short- and long-term α-stimulation differ considerably. Such discrepancy has already been described with prazosin, in hypertensive patients, and is presumed to be due to long-term compensatory mechanisms such as resetting of baroreflexes.[25] It is clear that much work, especially in animal models, still needs to be done.

III. DRUGS ACTING ON β-ADRENOCEPTORS

A. β-ADRENOCEPTOR AGONISTS

There is a paucity of information on this topic, insofar as liver disease is concerned, probably because most interest has been diverted to the therapeutic possibilities of β-blockade. In patients and animal models with liver disease, there seems to be attenuated circulatory response to β-adrenergic stimulation. Ramond et al. documented that the dose of isoprenaline required to raise the heart rate by 25 beats per min was significantly greater in cirrhotic patients than in controls.[26] This blunted chronotropic response to isoprenaline has also been demonstrated in anesthetized portal hypertensive rats.[27]

Dobutamine, a relatively selective β_1-agonist at low doses, was administered to patients with cirrhosis by Mikulic et al.[28] This resulted in increased cardiac output and decreased systemic vascular resistance, but no change in hepatic venous pressures or blood flow. A similar hyporesponsiveness in dobutamine-induced splanchnic hyperemia has been noted in anesthetized portal hypertensive rats.[29] The reasons for this hyposensitivity to β-stimulation are unclear, but β-adrenoceptor desensitization by downregulation has been suggested, since serum catecholamines are elevated in cirrhosis.[30] The only study to examine this issue found significant differences in lymphocyte β_2-receptor density only in a subgroup of patients with severe ascites.[31]

B. β-ADRENOCEPTOR ANTAGONISTS

Although β-adrenergic antagonists have been in therapeutic use for over a quarter-century and known to affect the splanchnic circulation for two decades, it remained for Lebrec and his colleagues, in 1980, to show that propranolol lowered the hepatic venous pressure gradient and to suggest that this may be useful as a medical treatment for portal hypertension.[32] Subsequently, further research by this unit and many others have detailed the systemic and splanchnic circulatory effects, side effects, and finally, a number of controlled trials of prophylaxis of variceal bleeding. All these topics except the last will now be reviewed.

1. Circulatory Effects in Humans

Thirteen major hemodynamic studies have elucidated the short-term and long-term effects of β-blockade on the systemic and splanchnic circulation (Table 1).[8,22,24,33-42] From these results some issues are now clear. As far as systemic parameters are concerned, patients with cirrhosis react in much the same manner as normals and differently from arterial hypertensives subjects: propranolol increases systemic vascular resistance and has no effect on arterial pressure. It also universally decreases cardiac output and heart rate.

Splanchnic circulatory effects are less uniform. There now seems no doubt that propranolol reduces portal pressure in the majority of patients — every study has found a significant decrease in either portal pressure or hepatic venous pressure gradient ranging from 13% to 31%. This effect is independent of the type of cirrhosis, since patients with posthepatitic and cryptogenic cirrhosis also seem to respond. Age is not a factor; one study has documented a portal hypotensive action even in children.[43] Furthermore, it is also clear that the short-term (within the first 1 to 2 h) and long-term actions of β-blockers are essentially identical. None of the studies have found any evidence of tachyphylaxis during long-term administration up to 2 years.

Most studies also find a certain percentage of nonresponders, i.e., patients in whom portal pressure either increases or does not change, ranging from 0 to 41% (see Table 1). The reasons for this uneven response are unknown. It might be hypothesized that, since sympathetic nervous activity tends to be correlated with the degree of liver failure,[30] patients with more advanced disease would not respond as well as those in good condition. This issue was examined in two studies and both concurred that the degree of liver failure as assessed by Child-Turcotte and Pugh criteria, did not correlate with hemodynamic response.[41,44] No identifiable clinical, laboratory, or hemodynamic criteria can predict which patient will respond. Nor do other tests, such as plasma propranolol levels[45] or isoprenaline infusion test, identify responders (unpublished observations). Although these two tests are useful in determining if systemic β-blockade is sufficient, this may not necessarily indicate that parallel splanchnic circulatory changes are occurring.

One factor in the variable response is undoubtedly inadequate propranolol dose. This was found in the New England study wherein half the original 40% of "nonresponders" subsequently responded to increased doses.[41] In several of these secondary responders, the additional doses were able to effectively decrease hepatic venous pressure gradient without further affecting heart rate.

In contrast to the variable portal pressure results, azygos blood flow decreases remarkably consistently: in the four studies that include azygos measurement, reductions after propranolol range from 30 to 35%, despite concomitantly uneven hepatic venous pressure responses (nonresponder rate varied from 13 to 35% [Table 1]). Indeed, the preoccupation with changes in portal pressure may be irrelevant; it is possible that the consistent action of propranolol on superior portocollateral flow is much more important in diminishing variceal bleeding risk. In this debate, there is much "logical" supposition and little hard evidence. For example, consensus opinion holds that above a certain level (somewhere around 8 to 12 mmHg), the absolute height of portal pressure does not affect bleeding risk. Yet much hemodynamic work is based on the premise that decreasing the portal pressure in any individual patient also decreases bleeding risk. One prospective study that has examined this issue failed to demonstrate a relation between degree of portal hypotensive response

TABLE 1
Hemodynamic Effects of Propranolol in Patients with Liver Disease

First author	Number of patients	Dose (mg)	Reduction (%)				Nonresponders (%)	Ref.
			Cardiac output	Hepatic venous pressure gradient	Hepatic blood flow	Azygos blood flow		
Lebrec	12	40 p.o. (40—400 p.o./d)	31 (32)	23 (23)	12 (16)		0	33
Burroughs	20	(40—400 p.o./d)		(36)			Not available	34
Mills	8	(120—160 p.o./d)	(31)	(25)			Not available	24
Westaby	9	2 i.v.	13	31	21		0	35
Calès	15	15 i.v.	24	15	19	34	13	8
Bosch	23	40—120 p.o.	22	12	13	35	35	36
Ohnishi	10	5 i.v.	25	18	27		11	37
Okumura	20	5 i.v.	24	23	13		Not available	38
Rector	27	(320—960 p.o./d)		14[a]			41	39
Kanazawa	7	0.2/kg i.v.	18	24	18	33	Not available	40
Garcia-Tsao	50	40 p.o.		14			40	41
Kong	9	5 i.v.	15	24			11	42
Mastai	12	10 i.v.	17	10	7	31	Not available	22

Note: Numbers in brackets are percentages found during continuous administration of propranolol.

[a] Portal pressure.

TABLE 2
Hemodynamic Effects of Nonselective and Selective β-Blockers in Patients with Liver Disease

First author	β-Blocker	No. of patients	Dose (mg)		Cardiac output		Hepatic venous pressure gradient		Ref.
Gatta	Nadolol[a]	12		(40—160 p.o./d)		(19)		(20)	48
Wink	Mepindolol[a]	6	0.65 i.v.		9	(21)	36	(52)	49
Braillon	Mepindolol	8	0.6 i.v.		22		18		50
Hillon	Atenolol[b]	14	100 p.o.		32		16		51
Mills	Atenolol	8		(100 p.o./d)		(12)		(18)	24
Zoli	Atenolol	10	100 p.o.	(100 p.o./d)	9	(23)	6	(34)	52
Bützow	Metoprolol[b]	10		(180 p.o./d)		(10)		(17)	53
Westaby	Metoprolol	9	2 i.v.		17		18		35
Bihari	ICI 118551[c]	17	10—100 p.o.		3—14		11—9		54

Note: Numbers in brackets are percentages found during continuous administration of β-blockers.

[a] Nonselective β-blocker.
[b] Cardioselective β-blocker.
[c] β_2-blocker.

and subsequent bleeding.[46] On the other hand, correlations between azygos response to propranolol and bleeding risk have not yet been examined. As more experience is gained with the azygos technique, these important issues will be clarified.

Although hepatic blood flow decreased significantly in only three of the 13 studies (Table 1), it is very likely that propranolol slightly reduces this flow. This conjecture remains to be proven, and indeed in the largest series of patients wherein in this phenomenon was studied, no significant change was detected.[47] However, estimated hepatic blood flow decreased in every study, ranging from 7 to 27%, a clearly suggestive trend. Failure to demonstrate statistical significance in most studies may be due to the large interindividual variability in response, coupled with relatively small sample sizes. On the other hand, it is extremely unlikely that this slight decrease in hepatic blood flow is clinically significant. This matter is discussed further in "side effects".

A few studies of nonselective β-blockers other than propranolol, such as nadolol and mepindolol,[48-50] show hemodynamic effects similar to propranolol (Table 2). Since nadolol has a longer half-life, it can be administered once daily, thus possibly improving compliance. The disadvantage is that there is much less experience with this drug compared to propranolol. Mepindolol, because of its intrinsic sympathomimetic activity, was the object of two small studies:[49,50] although both found significant reductions in hepatic venous pressure gradient, one found an unchanged cardiac output whereas the other, in a formal comparison with propranolol, found equivalent reductions in cardiac output and heart rate. The advantage of intrinsic sympathomimetic activity in β-blockade thus remains to be established.

Selective β_1- or β_2-blockade has also been investigated, in order to determine which subtype is important in mediating the major effects and also to perhaps avoid some selective side effects (Table 2). With reasoning analogous to therapy for arterial hypertension, in which β_1-selective drugs are used to avoid possible bronchospastic effects of β_2-blockade, several studies have shown mild portal hypotensive effects with the former class of drugs.[24,35,51-53] However, the consensus seems to be that these drugs reduce portal pressure to a lesser extent than nonselective β-blockers. This is not surprising, given that splanchnic vessels are devoid of β_1 receptors. Thus these agents act solely by decreasing cardiac output. This was borne out in a study by Hillon et al.[51] wherein the decrease in portal pressure correlated with the decrease in cardiac output after the β_1-blocker atenolol. In the same

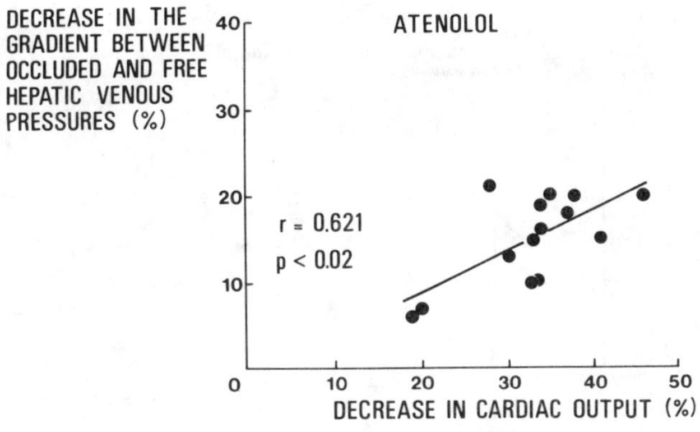

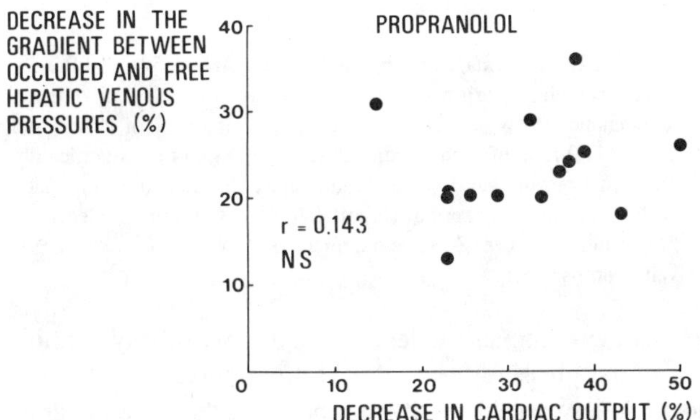

FIGURE 2. Correlation between the decrease in the gradient between occluded and free hepatic venous pressures and the decrease in cardiac output after oral administration of atenolol or propranolol in patients with cirrhosis. (From Hillon, P., Lebrec, D., Munoz, C., Jungers, M., Goldfarb, G., and Benhamou, J.-P., *Hepatology*, 2, 528—531, 1982, copyright © by the American Association for the Study of Liver Diseases. With permission.)

patients, a comparable dose of propranolol induced a greater fall in portal pressure, which was not correlated with the decrease in cardiac output (Figure 2).

The other possibility, β_2-blockade, was theoretically attractive since it would avoid some of the possible cardiodepressant side effects of β_1-blockade. This had been tested in one study in cirrhotic patients, and found to cause mild but significant decreases in hepatic venous pressure gradient associated with modest reduction in cardiac output.[54] This study is interesting for several reasons:

1. The slight but significant reductions in cardiac output and heart rate suggest that β_2 cardiac receptors also subserve both chronotropic and inotropic function, even in cirrhosis.
2. Analogous to ketanserin action (see Section V), there was discrepant timing of the systemic and splanchnic responses — systemic effects were more marked at 30 min, while the portal hypotensive actions were uncorrelated with cardiac output changes, and were more marked at 60 min, when cardiac output tended to return to baseline.

Unfortunately, hepatic blood flow and azygos blood flow were not measured in this study, so further characterization of the circulatory response to β_2-blockade in cirrhosis awaits future research.

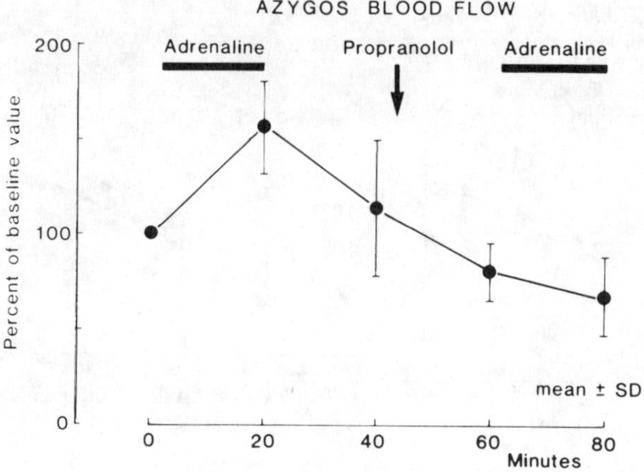

FIGURE 3.   Percentages from baseline value in azygos blood flow in
6 patients with cirrhosis receiving in successive order a 20-min infusion
of adrenaline (50 ng/kg min), propranolol (i.v. injection of 15 mg) and
a second 20-min infusion of adrenaline (50 ng/kg min). *Significantly
different from the basal value. Significantly different from the value
of the previous study period. (From Valla, D., Gaudin, C., Geoffroy,
P., Braillon, A., Lee, S. S., and Lebrec, D., *J. Hepatol.*, 4, 86, 1987.
With permission.)

Based only on all these human studies, one could reasonably surmise that nonselective
β-blockade lowers portal pressure by a marked diminution in portal tributary blood flow.
The decreased portal inflow would result from both the decrease in cardiac output and also
a direct or reflexively mediated splanchnic vasoconstriction. Selective β_2-blockers may
decrease portal inflow by a direct splanchnic vasoconstriction.

Various human studies have been done in an effort to sort out these hypotheses and to
delineate exact mechanisms. It has been widely speculated that β-blockade allows unopposed
vasoconstrictive α-adrenergic action. In a laudable attempt to test this idea, Mastai et al.[22]
administered methoxamine, an α_1-adrenergic agonist, propranolol, and in a third group of
patients, both drugs, and then compared the responses in each group. α-Adrenergic stimulation produced reductions in cardiac output and hepatic venous pressure gradient, thus
mimicking β-blockade, but there the resemblance stopped: mean arterial pressure increased,
hepatic blood flow decreased and azygos blood flow was not affected. Administering methoxamine to patients already β-blocked resulted in a slight but significant increase, however,
still did not return azygos blood flow to the prepropranolol baseline. In addition hepatic
blood flow again significantly decreased. Although these results do demonstrate that α_1-
adrenergic stimulation produces different hemodynamic patterns than β-blockade, this does
not necessarily disprove that the latter phenomenon acts by unopposed α_1-adrenergic stimulation. The crucial weakness in the protocol is that absent β-tone with unopposed tonic α_1-
adrenergic activity (propranolol) is not the same as basal β-adrenergic tone plus increased
α_1-adrenergic tone (methonamine), or absent β-tone with increased α_1-tone (the combination). However, a workable alternative protocol to test this question is difficult to imagine.

The mechanism of propranolol effect on azygos blood flow was investigated recently
in our unit. Successive infusions of adrenaline, then propranolol, then the combination,
revealed that adrenaline increased azygos blood flow, propranolol decreased this flow, and
the combination further decreased flow (Figure 3).[55] In other words, the normal incremental
effect of adrenaline on azygos blood flow was reversed after propranolol. This may explain
the postulated efficacy of propranolol in reducing superior portosystemic (variceal) flow.

2. Circulatory Effects in Animals

Due to the previously discussed limitations in measuring splanchnic circulatory phenomena in humans, animal studies have been used to define exact mechanisms of β-blocker action. The postulated reduction in portal tributary blood flow was indeed found in the portal vein-stenosed rat model by several laboratories.[56-58] Comparable results in cirrhotic rats with portal vein and hepatic arterial flows measured by electromagnetic flowmeters, have also been reported.[59] In particular, these 20 to 30% decreases in portal tributary blood flow associated with only modest 10 to 20% reductions in portal pressure due to large increases in portocollateral resistance, seemed to coincide well with the hemodynamic studies in patients, especially explaining the marked changes in azygos blood flow, and variable and lesser changes in portal pressure. Unfortunately, most of these studies were done in a rat model with no liver disease and all were done in anesthetized rats, thus immensely complicating their interpretation.

Indeed preliminary results from our unit suggest that anesthesia markedly changes the circulatory response to both β_1-blockade and nonselective β-blockade.[60, 61] In conscious animals, only extremely high doses of β-blockers seem capable of overcoming autoregulatory mechanisms in the mesenteric circulation.[60,61]   All things considered, it may very well be that the conclusions from the earlier studies in anesthetized rats are correct. However, verification is needed by studies in conscious models, preferably with liver disease.

3. Side Effects

β-Blockers have many potential side effects of which bronchospasm and cardiac conduction blocks are the best known. Of course, patients with liver disease are not immune to any of these, but several real or hypothetical side effects are particularly relevant in these patients.

Portosystemic encephalopathy precipitated by a postulated decrease in liver perfusion was initially thought to be a risk. Indeed, there were sporadic reports of acute encephalopathy,[62,63] and increases in serum NH_3 levels[64] associated with propranolol. Two studies with objective measures of encephalopathy such as the Reitan trail test, however, failed to detect any increased risk.[65,66] In the large-scale clinical trials, of 157 patients receiving propranolol, only one had encephalopathy.[34,67-69] We suspect that the rare patient with encephalopathy after β-blockade may represent an idiosyncratic reaction similar to that seen in patients without hepatopathy. The possibility of propranolol-induced decrease in cerebral blood flow as a cause for encephalopathy also appears unlikely, as a preliminary study found cerebral flow to be completely unaffected by this drug.[70] Other measures of standard liver function remained unchanged after β-blockade.[34,67-69]

Renal hemodynamics and thus, function, might be affected by β-blockade. This was demonstrated in two studies not to be a factor: despite the decrease in cardiac output, renal perfusion was autoregulated and renal function did not change.[48,71] Indeed, the known hyporeninemic effect of β-blockade was postulated to be beneficial in the management of patients with ascites. One short-term study (1 to 4 h) showed no beneficial effect on sodium or urine output.[72] Another long-term study (1 to 12 months) showed a decrease in total body sodium levels compared to controls taking placebo.[73]

The vasoconstrictive action of propranolol can also affect the pulmonary circulation. The intriguing discovery that propranolol could augment arterial pO_2 tension in patients with chronic obstructive lung disease, was reported recently.[74] In a preliminary report,[75] although propranolol did not change pO_2, the drug-induced decrease in systemic oxygen delivery (by decreasing cardiac output) was compensated by increased O_2 extraction so that oxygen uptake did not change.

The negative inotropic action of propranolol led to worries about difficulty in resuscitating bleeding patients on chronic therapy. In practice, experience from several centers has shown that sufficient doses of isoprenaline, dopamine and glucagon, among other drugs, can overcome the β-blockade successfully.[76]

Finally, the demonstration of upregulation in β-adrenergic receptors in asthmatic and arterial hypertensive patients on long-term β-blockade, along with the known cardiovascular complications of sudden withdrawal (precipitation of unstable angina, arrhythmias, myocardial infarction and sudden death) in patients with cardiac disease led to worries about similar splanchnic circulatory events occurring in cirrhotic patients. Indeed, several sporadic reports[77,78] and analysis of a larger series[79] suggested that abrupt termination of chronic therapy is followed by recurrence of variceal bleeding. We tried to experimentally reproduce this situation and showed the existence of a transient β-adrenergic hypersensitivity 2 days after abruptly stopping chronic propranolol therapy in the portal vein-stenosed rats.[27] One could speculate that similar phenomena occur in patients, and we advise graded withdrawal of long-term β-blocker therapy.

4. Clinical Trials

The logical consequence of the promising hemodynamic results was the testing of β-blockade as a prophylactic treatment to prevent variceal bleeding. To date the results of these randomized controlled trials are discrepant. Further analysis of these trials and possible reasons for this variability will not be discussed here but the reader is referred to recent reviews of this topic.[80,81]

V. SEROTONIN (5-HYDROXYTRYPTAMINE)

This vasoactive amine, despite its ubiquity in body tissues, remains almost as enigmatic today as when it was first discovered four decades ago. This is largely because its effects vary markedly, depending on dose, route of administration, vascular bed studied, species and coexisting sympathetic tone. In 1979 Peroutka and Snyder[82] proposed two subtypes of serotonin receptors, labeled S_1 and S_2. Further research has now led to the subclassification of the S_1 receptor into the S_{1A} and S_{1B} subtypes.[83] The situation is far from settled, as there is even evidence of yet more types of serotonin receptors, not conforming to S_1 and S_2 patterns.[84] Older serotonin antagonists such as methysergide and cyproheptadine, are nonselective, while newer agents such as ketanserin are highly selective for S_2.[85] Unfortunately, pharmacological studies are complicated by the fact that ketanserin, for example, also has weak α_1-blocking effects[85] and perhaps even some dopaminergic D_2 effects.[85]

In the early 1960s there was some interest in the role of serotonin in portal hypertension. However, serotonin infusion at 30 μ/kg min failed to produce any effects on arterial pressure, cardiac output, hepatic blood flow, and wedged hepatic or intrasplenic pressures, in patients with cirrhosis.[86]

Interest in serotonin then remained dormant for two decades until the development of elective serotonin antagonists. In 1985, Gasic et al. found that ketanserin decreased the pressor effects of phenylephrine on wedged hepatic pressure in normal subjects.[87]

We have investigated the systemic and splanchnic circulatory effects of ketanserin in patients with cirrhosis.[88] A 10 mg slow intravenous bolus caused significant reduction in mean arterial pressure, but unchanged cardiac output and systemic vascular resistance. Splanchnic parameters affected were decreased hepatic venous pressure gradient, primarily due to a decrease in wedged hepatic venous pressure, and azygos blood flow. Hepatic blood flow did not change. Interestingly, there seemed to be a dissociated response between splanchnic and systemic changes, since the azygos flow decrease was gradual and progressive over the 1 h period while mean arterial pressure fell within 5 to 10 min and then gradually returned toward baseline (Figure 4). The short-term hypotensive effects were correlated with the Pugh score; in other words, patients with more severe liver disease were more sensitive

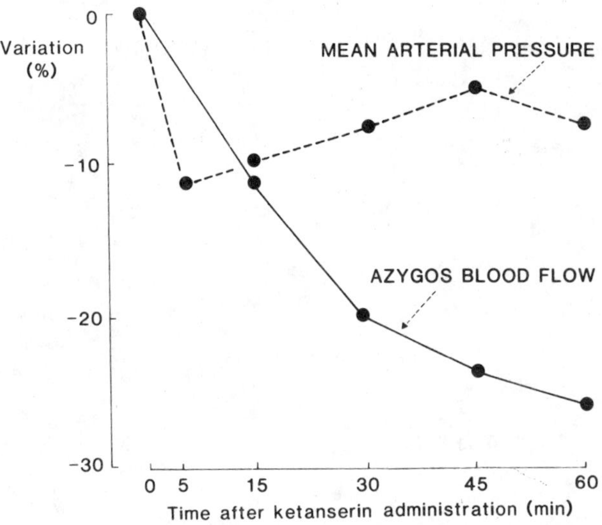

FIGURE 4.   Effects of intravenous administration of 10 mg of ketanserin on mean arterial pressure and azygos blood flow in patients with alcoholic cirrhosis. (From Hadengue, A., Lee, S. S., Moreau, R., Braillon, A., and Lebrec, D., *Hepatology*, 7, 644—647, 1987, copyright © by the American Association for the Study of Liver Diseases. With permission.)

to ketanserin hypotensive action. The azygos blood flow showed no such correlation. The reasons for this divergent sensitivity in systemic and splanchnic circulation are unclear. However, since Gasic and colleagues also found a similar divergent response with this drug to α_1-stimulation in normals, it may be an intrinsic effect of ketanserin itself, rather than differential regional sensitivity of serotonin receptors.

The exact mechanism of ketanserin splanchnic effects remain conjectural. In this regard, some illuminating results are provided by Cummings et al.[89] In ketamine-anesthetized portal hypertensive rats, ketanserin decreased cardiac output, mean arterial pressure, portal pressure, and portal venous inflow. These results suggest that S_2-blockade decreased portal pressure directly by splanchnic venous dilatation and also by decreasing portal venous inflow. This latter phenomenon was thought to be due to the reduced cardiac output (due to splanchnic venous pooling) and reflexly mediated splanchnic vasoconstriction due to decreased arterial pressure.

These human and experimental results suggest that serotonin plays a role in the initiation or maintenance of portal hypertension, but further clarification awaits the arrival of "purer" specific serotonin antagonists.

VI. ORGANIC NITRATES

The troublesome complications of vasopressin led several investigators during the 1970s to research various drugs to counterbalance the hypertensive and cardiodepressant effects; and although Gelman and Ernst first demonstrated that nitroprusside prevented the adverse effects of vasopressin in normal dogs,[90] it remained for Groszmann et al.[91] to show a beneficial effect of this combination in patients and dogs with portal hypertension. Naturally, since their results showed yet further diminutions in portal pressure when intravenous nitroglycerin was added to vasopressin, interest was stimulated on possible beneficial effects of nitrates alone. To date, seven studies have examined systemic or splanchnic circulatory effects of nitrates alone in humans (Table 3).[75,92-97] Several trends are evident:

TABLE 3
Hemodynamic Effects of Nitrates in Patients with Cirrhosis

First author	Nitrate	Dose (mg)	Number of patients	Reduction (%)				
				Cardiac output	Mean arterial pressure	Hepatic venous pressure gradient	Hepatic blood flow	Ref.
Hallemans	Isosorbide dinitrate	5 sl	10	14	20	21		92
Dawson	Isosorbide dinitrate	5 p.o.	8		42[a]	< 5		93
Freeman	Isosorbide dinitrate	10 i.v.	10			35		94
		80 p.o./d	6			44		
Gibson	Nitroglycerin	0.6—2.4 p.o.	7		15[a]	22[b]		95
Zoli	Isosorbide dinitrate	5 sl	8				28[c]	96
Merkel	Isosorbide dinitrate	5 sl	13	17	30	34	2	97
Moreau	Nitroglycerin	25—75 i.v./mean	21	23	22			75

[a] Systolic arterial pressure.
[b] Portal pressure.
[c] Portal blood flow.

1. Nitrates in these therapeutic doses cause marked decreases in arterial pressure. The Birmingham study reported a mean 42 mmHg fall in systolic pressure! Examination of the data from others shows that several individual subjects had precipitous drops in blood pressure.
2. Cardiac output is also reduced, likely as a result of a decrease in preload due to the known venodilator action.
3. Portal pressure is very likely reduced at these doses — only one study did not find a decrease in hepatic venous pressure gradient or portal pressure.[93]
4. There is suggestive evidence from the Belgian study and our study, of a detrimental effect on tissue oxygenation.[75,92] In the Belgian study, oxygen delivery significantly decreased by 13%, but oxygen uptake did not change. Therefore tissue oxygen extraction must have increased, as evidenced by a slight but significant decrease in mixed venous PO_2. Their conclusion that this decrease in venous pO_2 is evidence of tissue hypoxia is thus debatable. However, while we dispute their reasoning, we agree with their conclusion. Our study found significant decreases in oxygen delivery and uptake. Thus, despite an 18% increase in the oxygen extraction ratio, this compensatory effect was insufficient to prevent significant decrease in oxygen uptake. Further evidence of this deterioration in tissue oxygenation was the 31% increase in arterial lactate levels.

Hepatic blood flow, measured only in one study, appears not to be affected.[96] Data on azygos blood flow response to nitrate, so far only in preliminary form, shows variable results.[98,99]

Work in animal models suggests that nitrates decrease splanchnic inflow by a predominant effect on arterial pressure. At low doses, as demonstrated in the conscious normal dog[100] and anesthetized portal hypertensive rat,[101] modest falls in arterial pressure are associated with splanchnic arteriolar constriction. Since it is difficult to imagine a selective direct constrictor effect in the splanchnic territory, a much more plausible explanation is that reflex splanchnic vasoconstriction reduces portal venous inflow. Blei and Gottstein recently tried to identify different factors that modify the response to nitrates.[101] They observed that at low doses this reflex splanchnic vasoconstriction did not lead to decrease in portal pressure, due to a rise in portal vascular resistance. At higher doses, cardiac output and mean arterial pressure decreased markedly, while portal venous inflow remained unchanged, and portal pressure diminished only modestly, thus indicating decrease in portal vascular resistance. These divergent dose-responses must be considered in interpreting circulatory studies with this drug. However, in humans with cirrhosis, it appears that doses of nitrates in the low-to-moderate therapeutic range produce relatively uniform responses.

Our conclusion is that organic nitrates alone have no therapeutic interest because of their clear marked hypotensive effects associated with evidence of detrimental tissue oxygenation. Further clinical research on this drug should only be done in the carefully monitored confines of a hemodynamic laboratory.

REFERENCES

1. **Boyer, T. D., Triger, D. R., Horisawa, M., Redeker, A. G., and Reynolds, T. B.,** Direct transhepatic measurement of portal vein pressure using a thin needle. Comparison with wedged hepatic vein pressure, *Gastroenterology*, 72, 584, 1977.
2. **Valla, D., Bercoff, E., Menu, Y., Bataille, C., and Lebrec, D.,** Discrepancy between wedged hepatic venous pressure and portal venous pressure after acute propranolol administration in patients with alcoholic cirrhosis, *Gastroenterology*, 86, 1400, 1984.
3. **Ohnishi, K., Saito, M., Sato, S., Sugita, S., Tanaka, H., and Okuda, K.,** Clinical utility of pulsed doppler flowmetry in patients with portal hypertension, *Am. J. Gastroenterol.*, 81, 1, 1986.

4. **Moriyasu, F., Ban, N., Nishida, O., Nakamura, T., Miyake, T., Uchino, H., Kanematsu, Y., and Koizumi, S.,** Clinical applicatioon of an ultrasonic duplex system in the quantitative measurement of portal blood flow, *J. Clin. Ultrasound,* 14, 579, 1986.

5. **Zoli, M., Marchesini, G., Cordiani, M. R., Pisi, P., Brunori, A., Trono, A., and Pisi, E.,** Echo-doppler measurement of splanchnic blood flow in control and cirrhotic subjects, *J. Clin. Ultrasound,* 14, 429, 1986.

6. **Burns, P., Taylor, K., and Blei, A. T.,** Doppler flowmetry and portal hypertension, *Gastroenterology,* 92, 824, 1987 (Editorial).

7. **Bosch, J. and Groszmann, R. J.,** Measurement of azygos venous blood flow by a continuous thermal dilution technique: an index of blood flow through gastroesophageal collaterals in cirrhosis, *Hepatology,* 4, 424, 1984.

8. **Calès, P., Braillon, A., Jiron, M. I., and Lebrec, D.,** Superior portosystemic collateral circulation estimated by azygos blood flow in patients with cirrhosis. Lack of correlation with esophageal varices and gastrointestinal bleeding. Effect of propranolol, *J. Hepatol.,* 1, 37, 1984.

9. **Bosch, J., Mastai, R., Kravetz, D., Bruix, J., Rigau, J., and Rodés, J.,** Measurement of azygos venous blood flow in the evaluation of portal hypertension in patients with cirrhosis. Clinical hemodynamic correlations in 100 patients, *J. Hepatol.,* 1, 125, 1985.

10. **Hadengue, A., Lee, S. S., Moreau, R., and Lebrec, D.,** Oxygen and bile acid content in the azygos blood. Clues to the azygos derivation in patients with portal hypertension, *J. Hepatol.,* 5, 98, 1987.

11. **Halvorsen, J. F. and Myking, A. O.,** Prehepatic portal hypertension in the rat. Immediate and long-term effects on portal vein and aortic pressure of a graded portal vein stenosis, followed by occlusion of the portal vein and spleno-renal collaterals, *Eur. Surg. Res.,* 11, 89, 1979.

12. **Cameron, G. R. and Karunaratne, W. A. E.,** Carbon tetrachloride cirrhosis in relation to liver regeneration, *J. Pathol and Bacteriol.,* 42, 1, 1936.

13. **Cameron, G. R. and Oakley, C. L.,** Ligation of the common bile duct, *J. Pathol. Bacteriol.,* 35, 769, 1932.

14. **Ohlsson, E. G., Rutherford, R. B., Haalebos, M. M. P., Wagner, H. N., and Zuidema, G. D.,** The effect of biliary obstruction on hepatosplanchnic blood flow in dogs, *J. Surg. Res.,* 10, 201, 1970.

15. **Madden, J. W., Gertman, P. M., and Peacock, E. E., Jr.,** Dimethylnitrosamine-induced hepatic cirrhosis: a new canine model of an ancient human disease, *Surgery,* 68, 260, 1970.

16. **Zimpfer, M. W., Manders, T., Barger, A. C., and Vatner, S. F.,** Pentobarbital alters compensatory neural and humoral mechanisms in response to hemorrhage, *Am. J. Physiol.,* 243, H713, 1982.

17. **Seyde, W. C., McGowan, L., Lund, N., Duling, B., and Longnecker, D. E.,** Effects of anesthetics on regional hemodynamics in normovolemic and hemorrhaged rats, *Am. J. Physiol.,* 249, H164, 1985.

18. **Lee, S. S., Girod, C., Valla, D., Geoffroy, P., and Lebrec, D.,** Effects of pentobarbital sodium anesthesia on splanchnic hemodynamics of normal and portal-hypertensive rats, *Am. J. Physiol.,* 249, G528, 1985.

19. **Lee, S. S., Girod, C., Braillon, A., Hadengue, A., and Lebrec, D.,** Hemodynamic characterization of chronic bile duct-ligated rats: effect of pentobarbital sodium, *Am. J. Physiol.,* 251, G176, 1986.

20. **Willett, I. R., Esler, M., Jennings, G., and Dudley, F. J.,** Sympathetic tone modulates portal venous pressure in alcoholic cirrhosis, *Lancet,* 2, 939, 1986.

21. **Moreau, R., Lee, S. S., Hadengue, A., Braillon, A., and Lebrec, D.,** Hemodynamic effects of a clonidine-induced decrease in sympathetic tone in patients with cirrhosis, *Hepatology,* 7, 149, 1987.

22. **Mastai, R., Bosch, J., Navasa, M., Kravetz, D., Bruix, J., Viola, C., and Rodés, J.,** Effects of alpha-adrenergic stimulation and beta-adrenergic blockade on azygos blood flow and splanchnic haemodynamics in patients with cirrhosis, *J. Hepatol.,* 4, 71, 1987.

23. **Ikeda, M.,** Effect of phenoxybenzamine (POB) on portal venous pressure in patients with portal hypertension, *Am. J. Gastroenterol.,* 71, 389, 1979.

24. **Mills, P. R., Rae, A. P., Farah, D. A., Russell, R. I., Lorimer, A. R., and Carter, D. C.,** Comparison of three adrenoreceptor blocking agents in patients with cirrhosis and portal hypertension, *Gut,* 25, 73, 1984.

25. **Colucci, W. S.,** Alpha-adrenergic receptor blockade with prazosin. Consideration of hypertension, heart failure, and potential new applications, *Ann. Intern. Med.,* 97, 67, 1982.

26. **Ramond, M.-J., Comoy, E., and Lebrec, D.,** Alterations in isoprenaline sensitivity in patients with cirrhosis: evidence of abnormality of the sympathetic nervous activity, *Br. J. Clin. Pharmacol.,* 21, 191, 1986.

27. **Lee, S. S., Braillon, A., Girod, C., Geoffrey, P., and Lebrec, D.,** Haemodynamic rebound phenomena after abrupt cessation of propranolol therapy in portal hypertensive rats, *J. Hepatol.,* 3, 38, 1986.

28. **Mikulic, E., Munoz, C., Puntoni, L. E., and Lebrec, D.,** Hemodynamic effects of dobutamine in patients with alcoholic cirrhosis, *Clin. Pharmacol. Ther.,* 34, 56, 1983.

29. **Braillon, A., Calès, P., Girod, C., and Lebrec, D.,** Alteration in response of the portal tributary vascular bed to the β-agonist dobutamine in rats with extrahepatic portal hypertension, *J. Hepatol.,* 2, 267, 1986.

30. **Henriksen, J. H., Ring-Larsen, H., and Christensen, N. J.,** Sympathetic nervous activity in cirrhosis. A survey of plasma catecholamine studies, *J. Hepatol.,* 1, 55, 1984.
31. **Gerbes, A. L., Remien, J., Jüngst, D., Sauerbruch, T., and Paumgartner, G.,** Evidence for down-regulation of β_2-adrenoceptors in cirrhotic patients with severe ascites, *Lancet,* 1, 1409, 1986.
32. **Lebrec, D., Nouel, O., Corbic, M., and Benhamou, J.-P.,** Propranolol — a medical treatment for portal hypertension?, *Lancet,* 2, 180, 1980.
33. **Lebrec, D., Hillon, P., Munoz, C., Goldfarb, G., Nouel, O., Benhamou, J.-P.,** The effect of propranolol on portal hypertension in patients with cirrhosis: a hemodynamic study, *Hepatology,* 2, 523, 1982.
34. **Burroughs, A. K., Jenkins, W. J., Sherlock, S., Dunk, A., Walt, R. P., Osuafor, T. O. K., Mackie, S., and Dick, R.,** Controlled trial of propranolol for the prevention of recurrent variceal hemorrhage in patients with cirrhosis, *N. Engl. J. Med.,* 309, 1539, 1983.
35. **Westaby, D., Bihari, D. J., Gimson, A. E. S., Crossley, I. R., and Williams, R.,** Selective and nonselective β-receptor blockade in the reduction portal pressure in patients with cirrhosis and portal hypertension, *Gut,* 25, 121, 1984.
36. **Bosch, J., Masti, R., Kravetz, D., Bruix, J., Gaya, J., Rigau, J., and Rodés, J.,** Effects of propranolol on azygos venous blood flow and hepatic and systemic hemodynamics in cirrhosis, *Hepatology,* 4, 1200, 1984.
37. **Ohnishi, K., Nakayama, T., Saito, M., Hatano, H., Tsukamoto, T., Terabayashi, H., Sugita, S., Wada, K., Nomura, F., Koen, H., and Okuda, K.,** Effects of propranolol on portal hemodynamics in patients with chronic liver disease, *Am. J. Gastroenterol.,* 80, 132, 1985.
38. **Okumura, H., Sekiyama, T., Katsuta, Y., Akaike, M., Sekino, M., Terada, H., Satomura, K., Aramaki, T., Sesoko, M., and Honda, M.,** Effective oral doses of propranolol and endoscopic findings on the effects of propranolol on esophageal varices, *Jpn. J. Gastroenterol.,* 82, 621, 1985.
39. **Rector, W. G.,** Propranolol for portal hypertension. Evaluation of therapeutic response by direct measurement of portal vein pressure, *Arch. Intern. Med.,* 145, 648, 1985.
40. **Kanazawa, H., Matsusaka, S., Tada, N., Kuroda, H., and Kobayashi, M.,** Measurement of azygos blood flow by a continuous thermodilution method in liver disease, *Acta Hepatol. Jpn.,* 27, 1132, 1986.
41. **Garcia-Tsao, G., Grace, N. D., Groszmann, R. J., Conn, H. O., Bermann, M. M., Patrick, J. C., Morse, S. S., and Algerts, J. L.,** Short-term effects of propranolol on portal venous pressure, *Hepatology,* 6, 101, 1986.
42. **Kong, C.-W., Lay, C.-S., Tsai, Y.-T., Lee, S.-D., Lai, K.-H., Lo, K.-J., and Chiang, B. N.,** Hemodynamic effect of propranolol on portal hypertension in patients with Hb_sAg positive cirrhosis, *Dig. Dis. Sci.,* 31, 1303, 1986.
43. **Ozsoylu, S., Kocak, N., and Yuce, A.,** Propranolol therapy for portal hypertension in children, *J. Ped.,* 106, 317, 1985.
44. **Braillon, A., Calès, P., Valla, D., Gaudy, D., Geoffroy, P., and Lebrec, D.,** Influence of the degree of liver failure on systemic and splanchnic haemodynamics and on response to propranolol in patients with cirrhosis, *Gut,* 27, 1204, 1986.
45. **Jiron, M. I., Delhotal, B., Lebrec, D.,** Relationship between dose, blood level and hemodynamic response in patients with cirrhosis receiving propranolol, *Eur. J. Clin. Pharmacol.,* 28, 353, 1985.
46. **Valla, D., Jiron, M. I., Poynard, T., Braillon, A., and Lebrec, D.,** Failure of haemodynamic measurement to predict recurrent gastrointestinal bleeding in cirrhotic patients receiving propranolol, *J. Hepatol.,* 5, 144, 1987.
47. **Braillon, A., Lee, S. S., Girod, C., Peignoux-Martinot, M., Valla, D., and Lebrec, D.,** Role of portasystemic shunts in the hyperkinetic circulation of the portal hypertensive rat, *J. Lab. Clin. Med.,* 108, 543, 1986.
48. **Gatta, A., Sacerdoti, D., Merkel, C., Milani, L., Battaglia, G., and Zuin, R.,** Effects of nadolol treatment on renal and hepatic hemodynamics and function in cirrhotic patients with portal hypertension, *Am. Heart J.,* 108, 1167, 1984.
49. **Wink, K.,** Acute and chronic effects of the beta-receptor blocker mepindolol on hemodynamics and the portal circulation, *Int. J. Clin. Pharmacol. Ther. Toxicol.,* 22, 447, 1984.
50. **Braillon, A., Calès, P., and Lebrec, D.,** Comparison of the short-term effects of mepindolol and propranolol on splanchnic and systemic haemodynamics in patients with cirrhosis, *Int. J. Clin. Pharmacol. Ther. Toxicol.,* 4, 223, 1985.
51. **Hillon, P., Lebrec, D., Munoz, C., Jungers, M., Goldfarb, G., and Benhamou, J.-P.,** Comparison of the effects of a cardioselective and a nonselective β-blocker on portal hypertension in patients with cirrhosis, *Hepatology,* 2, 528, 1982.
52. **Zoli, M., Marzocchi, A., Marchesini, G., Marrozzini, C., Dondi, C., and Pisi, E.,** Atenolol in portal hypertension: a haemodynamic study, *Ital. J. Gastroenterol.,* 17, 252, 1985.
53. **Bützow, G. J., Remmecker, J., and Bräuer, A.,** Metoprolol in portal hypertension. A controlled study, *Klin. Wochenschr.,* 60, 1311, 1982.

54. **Bihari, D., Westaby, D., Gimson, A., Crossley, I., Harry, J., and Williams, R.,** Reductions in portal pressure by selective β_2-adrenoceptor blockade in patients with cirrhosis and portal hypertension, *Br. J. Clin. Pharmacol.,* 17, 753, 1984.

55. **Valla, D., Gaudin, C., Geoffroy, P., Braillon, A., Lee, S. S., and Lebrec, D.,** Reversal of adrenaline-induced increase in azygos blood flow in patients with cirrhosis receiving propranolol, *J. Hepatol.,* 4, 86, 1987.

56. **Calès, P., Braillon, A., Girod, C., and Lebrec, D.,** Acute effect of propranolol on splanchnic circulation in normal and portal hypertensive rats, *J. Hepatol.,* 1, 349, 1985.

57. **Kroeger, R. J. and Groszmann, R. J.,** Increased portal venous resistance hinders portal pressure reduction during the administration of β-adrenergic blocking agents in a portal hypertensive model, *Hepatology,* 5, 97, 1985.

58. **Spina, G. P., Galeotti, F., Opocher, E., Santambrogio, R., Merlo, L., Paro, M., Cucchiaro, G., and Marchetti, G.,** The effect of levomoprolol on portal hemodynamics in rats: comparison with propranolol, *Curr. Ther. Clin. Exp. Res.,* 36, 211, 1984.

59. **Jenkins, S. A., Baxter, J. N., Johnson, J. N., Devitt, P., and Shields, R.,** Effects of propranolol on hepatic hemodynamics in the cirrhotic and noncirrhotic rat, *Br. J. Surg.,* 72, 354, 1985.

60. **Lebrec, D., Girod, C., Hadengue, A., Lee, S. S., Koshy, A., and Cerini, R.,** Hemodynamic dose response curves of propranolol in conscious portal hypertensive rats, *Hepatology,* 6 (Abstr.), 1127, 1986.

61. **Lee, S. S., Hadengue, A., Girod, C., Braillon, A., and Lebrec, D.,** Discrepant responses to betaxolol in conscious and anesthetized portal hypertensive rats, *Hepatology,* 6 (Abstr.), 1127, 1986.

62. **Traver, D., Walt, R. P., Dunk, A. A., Jenkins, W. J., and Sherlock, S.,** Precipitation of hepatic encephalopathy by propranolol in cirrhosis, *Br. Med. J.,* 287, 585, 1983.

63. **Wiesner, R. H.,** Does propranolol precipitate hepatic encephalopathy?, *J. Clin. Gastroenterol.,* 8, 74, 1986.

64. **Van Buuren, H. R., Van Der Velden, P. C., Koorevaar, G., and Silberbusch, J.,** Propranolol increases arterial ammonia in liver cirrhosis, *Lancet,* 2, 30, 1982 (correspondence).

65. **Arthur, M. J. P., Tanner, A. R., Patel, C., George, C. F., and Wright, R.,** Portal hypertension, propranolol, and hepatic encephalopathy, *Lancet,* 2, 879, 1982 (correspondence).

66. **Watson, P. P. and Hayes, J. R.,** Cirrhosis, hepatic encephalopathy, and propranolol, *Br. Med. J.,* 287, 1067, 1983.

67. **Lebrec, D., Poynard, T., Hillon, P., and Benhamou, J.-P.,** Propranol for prevention of recurrent gastrointestinal bleeding in patients with cirrhosis, *N. Engl. J. Med.,* 305, 1371, 1981.

68. **Villeneuve, J.-P., Pomier-Layrargues, G., Infante-Rivard, C., Willems, B., Huet, P.-M., Marleau, D., and Viallet, A.,** Propranolol for the prevention of recurrent variceal hemorrhage: a controlled trial, *Hepatology,* 6, 1239, 1986.

69. **Queuniet, A. M., Czernichow, P., Lerebours, E., Durcotte, P., Tranvouez, J. L., and Colin, R.,** Étude contrôlée du propranolol dans la prévention des récidives hémorragiques chez les patients cirrhotiques, *Gastroentérol. Clin. Biol.,* 11, 41, 1987.

70. **Calès, P., Pierre-Nicolas, M., Guell, A., Caucanas, J. P., Vinel, J. P., and Pascal, J. P.,** Effects du propranolol sur le débit sanguin cérébral au cours de la cirrhose, *Gastroentérol. Clin. Biol.,* 11 (Abstr.), 159A, 1987.

71. **Bataille, C., Bercoff, E., Pariente, E. A., Valla, D., and Lebrec, D.,** Effects of propranolol on renal blood flow and renal function in patients with cirrhosis, *Gastroenterology,* 86, 129, 1984.

72. **Rector, W. G., Jr. and Reynolds, T. B.,** Propranolol in the treatment of cirrhotic ascites, *Arch. Int. Med.,* 144, 1761, 1984.

73. **Hayes, P. C., Stewart, W. W., and Bouchier, I. A. D.,** Influence of propranolol on weight and salt and water homoeostasis in chronic liver disease, *Lancet,* 2, 1064, 1984.

74. **Vincent, J.-L., Lignian, H., Gillet, J.-B., Berre, J., and Contu, E.,** Increase in PaO_2 following intravenous administration of propranolol in acutely hypoxemic patients, *Chest,* 88, 558, 1985.

75. **Moreau, R., Lee, S. S., Hadengue, A., Ozier, Y., Sicot, C., and Lebrec, D.,** Effects of vasoactive drugs on O_2 utilization in patients with cirrhosis: evidence for a subclinical tissue hypoxia, *J. Hepatol.,* 5 (Abstr.) (Suppl. 2), S171, 1987.

76. **Opie, L. H.,** Drugs and the heart. I. β-blocking agents, *Lancet,* 1, 693, 1980.

77. **Lebrec, D., Bernuau, J., Rueff, B., and Benhamou, J.-P.,** Gastrointestinal bleeding after abrupt cessation of propranolol administration in cirrhosis, *N. Engl. J. Med.,* 307, 560, 1982 (correspondence).

78. **Maringhini, A., Simonetti, R. M., Marceno, M. P., and Pagliaro, L.,** Propranolol for gastrointestinal bleeding in cirrhosis, *N. Engl. J. Med.,* 307, 1710, 1982 (correspondence).

79. **Poynard, T., Lebrec, D., Hillon, P., Sayegh, R., Bernuau, J., Naveau, S., Chaput, J. C., Klepping, C., Rueff, B., and Benhamou, J.-P.,** Propranolol for prevention of recurrent gastrointestinal bleeding in patients with cirrhosis: a prospective study of factors associated with rebleeding, *Hepatology,* 7, 447, 1987.

80. **Schalm, S. W. and Van Buuren, H. R.,** Prevention of recurrent variceal bleeding: nonsurgical procedures, *Clin. Gastroenterol.,* 14, 209, 1985.

81. **Lebrec, D.,** β-bloquants et hémorragies digestive, *Gastroentérol. Clin. Biol.,* 11, 37, 1987 (editorial).
82. **Peroutka, S. J. and Synder, S. H.,** Multiple serotonin receptors: differential binding of (^{3}H)5-hydroxytryptamine, (^{3}H)lysergic acid diethylamide and (^{3}H)spiroperidol, *Mol. Pharmacol.,* 16, 687, 1979.
83. **Pedigo, N. W., Yamamura, H. I., and Nelson, D. L.,** Discrimination of multiple [^{3}H]5-hydroxytryptamine binding sites by the neuroleptic spiperone in rat brain, *J. Neurochem.,* 36, 220, 1981.
84. **Kaumann, A. J.,** Two classes of myocardial 5-hydroxytryptamine receptors that are neither 5-HT$_1$ nor 5-HT$_2$, *J. Cardiovasc. Pharmacol.,* 7 (Suppl. 7), S76, 1985.
85. **Janssen, P. A. J.,** Pharmacology of potent and selective S$_2$-serotonergic antagonists, *J. Cardiovasc. Pharmacol.,* 7 (Suppl. 7), S2, 1985.
86. **Chiandussi, L., Greco, F., Indovina, D., Cesano, L., Vacarrino, A., and Muratori, F.,** Effect of drug infusion on splanchnic circulation. II. Serotonin infusion in normal and cirrhosis subjects, *Proc. Soc. Exp. Biol. Med.,* 112, 326, 1963.
87. **Gasic, S., Eichler, H. G., and Korn, A.,** Effect of ketanserin on phenylephrine-dependent changes in splanchnic hemodynamics and systemic blood pressure in healthy subjects, *J. Cardiovasc. Pharmacol.,* 7, 219, 1985.
88. **Hadengue, A., Lee, S. S., Moreau, R., Braillon, A., and Lebrec, D.,** Beneficial hemodynamic effects of ketanserin in patients with cirrhosis: possible role of serotonergic mechanisms in portal hypertension, *Hepatology,* 7, 644, 1987.
89. **Cummings, S. E., Groszmann, R. J., and Kaumann, A. J.,** Hypersensitivity of mesenteric veins to 5-hydroxytryptamine- and ketanserin-induced reduction of portal pressure in portal hypertensive rats, *Br. J. Pharmacol.,* 89, 501, 1986.
90. **Gelman, S. and Ernst, E. A.,** Nitroprusside prevents adverse hemodynamic of vasopressin, *Arch. Surg.,* 113, 1465, 1978.
91. **Groszmann, R. J., Kravetz, D., Bosch, J., Glickman, M., Bruix, J., Bredfeldt, J., Conn, H. O., Rodés, J., and Strorer, E. H.,** Nitroglycerin improves the hemodynamic response to vasopressin in portal hypertension, *Hepatology,* 2, 757, 1982.
92. **Hallemans, R., Naeije, R., Mols, P., Melot, C., and Reding, P.,** Treatment of portal hypertension with isosorbide dinitrate alone and in combination with vasopressin, *Crit. Care Med.,* 11, 536, 1983.
93. **Dawson, J., Gertsch, P., Mosimann, F., West, R., and Elias, E.,** Endoscopic variceal pressure measurements: response to isosorbide dinitrate, *Gut,* 26, 843, 1985.
94. **Freeman, J. G., Barton, J. R., and Record, C. O.,** Effect of isosorbide dinitrate, verapamil, and labetalol on portal pressure in cirrhosis, *Br. Med. J.,* 291, 561, 1985.
95. **Gibson, P. R., Mclean, A. J., and Dudley, F. J.,** The hypotensive effect of oral nitroglycerin on portal venous pressure in patients with cirrhotic portal hypertension, *J. Gastroenterol. Hepatol.,* 1, 201, 1986.
96. **Zoli, M., Marchesini, G., Brunori, A., Cordiani, M. R., and Pisi, E.,** Portal venous flow in response to acute β-blocker and vasodilatatory treatment in patients with liver cirrhosis, *Hepatology,* 6, 1248, 1986.
97. **Merkel, C., Finucci, G., Zuin, R., Bazzerla, G., Bolognesi, M., Sacerdoti, D., and Gatta, A.,** Effects of isosorbide dinitrate on portal hypertension in alcoholic cirrhosis, *J. Hepatol.,* 4, 174, 1987.
98. **Garcia-Tsao, G., Hanson, J. S., and Groszmann, R. J.,** Splanchnic hemodynamics in portal hypertensive patients during nitroglycerin administration, *Gastroenterology,* 88 (Abstr.), 1659, 1985.
99. **Notsumata, K.,** The effects of propranolol or nitroglycerin on azygos blood flow of patients with portal hypertension, *Jpn. J. Gastroenterol.,* 83, 1489, 1986.
100. **Vatner, S. F., Pagani, M., Rutherford, J. D., Millard, R. W., and Manders, W. T.,** Effects of nitroglycerin on cardiac function and regional blood flow distribution in conscious dogs, *Am. J. Physiol.,* 234, H244, 1978.
101. **Blei, A. T. and Gottstein, J.,** Isosorbide dinitrate in experimental portal hypertension: a study of factors that modulate the hemodynamic response, *Hepatology,* 6, 107, 1986.

Chapter 18

DRUGS ACTING ON THE RENIN-ANGIOTENSIN-ALDOSTERONE SYSTEM

Mauro Bernardi, Franco Trevisani, and Giovanni Gasbarrini

TABLE OF CONTENTS

I. INTRODUCTION

Several drugs can modulate the activity of the renin-angiotensin system, by either direct or indirect influence. In this chapter, only those drugs which have been employed in cirrhosis to specifically counteract the activated renin-aldosterone axis will be briefly discussed. Among them, antimineralocorticoids are the only drugs currently used in clinical practice. Adrenergic β-receptor blocking drugs are also widely employed, but their clinical use is directed to lower portal hypertension through mechanisms other than renin release inhibition. However, the knowledge of the effects of these drugs has been and is very useful in understanding the pathophysiology of this system in cirrhosis.

The pharmacological inhibition of the renin-angiotensin system can occur at different sites: (1) release of renin from the juxtaglomerular apparatus; (2) inhibition of angiotensin-converting enzyme activity; (3) blockade of receptors for angiotensin II. Other means are represented by renin antibodies, inhibitors of renin, and substrate analogues.[1] To the best of our knowledge, none of the latter have been used in cirrhotics.

Aldosterone biological activity can be counteracted by the inhibition of its secretion or by the selective antagonism at mineralocorticoid receptors.

II. BETA-ADRENERGIC ANTAGONISTS

Most of the available information on the effect of β-adrenergic receptor blockade in patients with cirrhosis is based on the results obtained by propranolol administration. Therefore, the present discussion will focus on this drug, recalling variant effects by other β-adrenergic antagonists when relevant.

Propranolol is a competitive antagonist at both β_1- and β_2-adrenoreceptors. Thus, it reduces renin release from the juxtaglomerular apparatus by blunting sympathoadrenergic afferents to it.

Pharmacological effects of propranolol are dose related. After oral administration to normal subjects, it is almost completely absorbed, but its bioavailability is low because of extensive presystemic metabolism by the liver.[2] It circulates heavily (up to $\approx 90\%$) bound to plasma proteins, mainly α_1-glycoprotein and albumin.[3] The free fraction is pharmacologically active. The clearance of the drug is related to the hepatic blood flow[4] and the half-life ranges from 3 to 5 h after a single dose and is slightly prolonged by repeated administration.[5]

Due to these characteristics, it is not surprising that propranolol pharmacokinetics are grossly deranged in patients with cirrhosis. After an intravenous administration of 40 mg of propranolol, the half-life was prolonged, distribution volume increased, and drug clearance reduced. The latter fall was proportional to that of indocyanine green clearance, thus suggesting that hepatic blood flow was a limiting factor. The most prominent abnormalities were found in patients with severe hypoalbuminemia (<3 g/dl).[6] Two h after an oral dose of 20 mg, which rarely leads to detectable plasma levels in the normal man, from 9 to 81 ng/ml of propranolol were measured.[7] Moreover, in patients with severely impaired residual liver function (plasma albumin <3 g/dl), propranolol was still present 24 h after dosing. Protein binding was only moderately reduced.[7] Similar results were obtained in a further study, which also showed that atenolol pharmacodynamics in cirrhosis did not differ from that in healthy subjects.[8] Since the reduction in heart rate was proportional to the plasma propranolol concentrations,[7] a message of caution should originate from the above studies. Propranolol administration to cirrhotic patients should preferably be initiated in hospital, with low (20 mg) starting doses.

Initial interest on the effects of β-blockade in cirrhosis was focused on the renin-angiotensin-aldosterone system, in order to unravel its complex pathophysiology. We shall not discuss any further either this aspect, which has been widely commented upon in the chapter dealing with the renin-angiotensin-aldosterone system in liver disease (Chapter 3, Section II. A.2.e and f; B.2.b; C.1), or the impact of β-blockade on portal pressure, which is beyond the scope of the present review. We shall rather try to evaluate the clinical effects of propranolol administration, as far as systemic hemodynamics and renal function are concerned. This is of interest, since the drug, which succeeds in lowering portal pressure,[9] is currently used to prevent rebleeding from esophageal varices and hemorrhagic gastritis in cirrhosis.[10-12]

Effective β-blockade by propranolol, evaluated as reduction of resting (>15 to 20%[13-15]) or postexercise (>10%[16]) pulse rate, does not significantly affect blood pressure of cirrhotic patients, either without[13] or with[14-16] ascites. This may be surprising, particularly in patients with advanced cirrhosis and ascites. In fact, the drug lowers cardiac output,[13,14] mainly by reducing heart rate, and depresses PRA.[13,15,16] As discussed elsewhere in this book (Chapter 3, Section II.A.2.d), blood pressure maintenance in decomposed cirrhotics is strictly dependent on the activation of the renin-angiotensin system. However, unlike the other drugs inhibiting the renin-angiotensin system activity (such as captopril and saralasin, see below), β-adrenergic antagonists also influence the final adrenergic afference by leaving an unopposed α-receptor-mediated stimulation of vascular contractility. In fact, systemic vascular resistances are significantly increased by propranolol in cirrhotics both with[14] and without[13,17] ascites. Thus, it appears a safer agent in this respect.

Greater concern may derive from the possible effects of propranolol on the renal function, since it has been shown to reduce renal perfusion in patients without liver disease.[18-20] In contrast, total renal blood flow, blood flow distribution within the renal cortex, glomerular filtration rate, and renal vascular resistance were not affected in patients without[13,17] and with[14-16] ascites. In some studies, the changes in renal sodium excretion were not statistically significant. However, by analyzing individual changes, when reported, renal sodium excretion increased in a number of cases: 7/10 cases,[13] 5/11 (unchanged in two further cases).[16] In a further series, after 1 week of propranolol administration, patients without ascites increased significantly their natriuresis, which returned towards baseline level 2 weeks later.[17] In our experience,[15] 15 out of 17 cirrhotics with ascites taking oral propranolol for 1 week increased renal salt excretion, so that the mean change, although mild, was statistically significant.

The mechanisms underlying propranolol influence on renal function of cirrhotic patients are not completely understood. The maintenance of renal perfusion has been attributed to the suppression of the renin-angiotensin system and/or activation of vasodilating substances, such as prostaglandins or bradykinin.[13] The latter mechanism, however, has not been substantiated in cirrhotics without ascites.[17] As far as patients with ascites are concerned, our data may help in clarifying this matter. The activity of sympathoadrenergic system may be increased in patients with ascites.[21] Taking into account that sympathoadrenergic tone can influence vascular responsiveness to propranolol, we divided our patients[15] according to their baseline plasma norepinephrine concentration, as an index of sympathetic nervous system activity. Once an effective β-blockade was reached, patients with high baseline plasma norepinephrine and, presumably, reduced systemic vascular resistances, showed a significant increase in glomerular filtration rate, whereas cirrhotics with normal baseline plasma norepinephrine did not show significant changes (Figure 1). The former finding may be explained through an increase in effective blood volume secondary to an improvement in vascular resistances. This assumption was indirectly supported by a significant reduction of formerly elevated plasma norepinephrine levels, a feature found only in such a subset of cirrhotics. Interestingly, the increase in renal sodium excretion reported above was confined to these patients and largely related to the increase in the filtered sodium load. As previously reported in a study where urine aldosterone excretion was measured,[16] the changes in renal

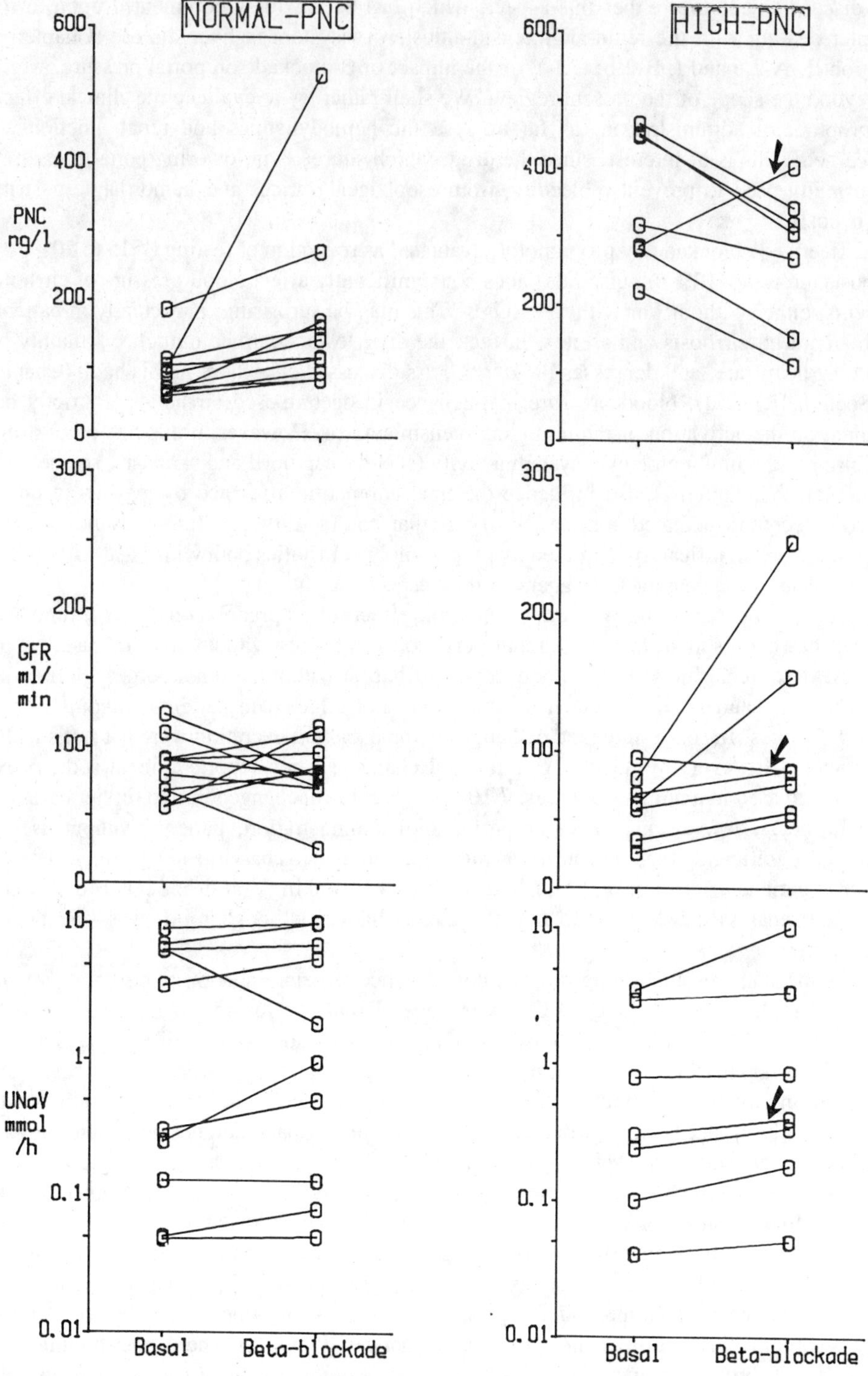

FIGURE 1.   Plasma norepinephrine concentration (PNC), glomerular filtration rate (GFR) and renal sodium excretion ($U_{Na}V$) under basal conditions and after effective β-blockade in 17 patients with cirrhosis and ascites. The patients were divided according to the baseline plasma norepinephrine concentration (normal-PNC and high-PNC). Please note that GFR did not improve in the only "high-PNC" patient whose PNC was not reduced after β-blockade (arrows). (From Bernardi, M., de Palma, R., Trevasani, F., Tamé, M. R., Ciancaglini, G. C., Pesa, O., Ligabue, A., Baraldini, M., and Gasbarrini, G., *J. Hepatal.*, 8, 279, 1989. With permission.)

sodium excretion also appeared to be strictly related to those of plasma aldosterone concentration, which underwent a significant reduction. Thus, the changes in aldosterone secretion played a permissive, if not determinant, role.

Results similar to those seen after propranolol were also observed after β-blockade achieved in 12 cirrhotics (3 with mild ascites) by nadolol administration.[22] In this study, the unimpaired renal perfusion could also be explained by the fact that nadolol may possess a direct renal vasodilatatory effect.[23]

Coming back to propranolol, the study by Rector and Reynolds[24] is somewhat at variance with those cited above. In fact, by comparing the effect of diuretic and diuretic plus propranolol in patients with ascites, these authors found that the combined regimen led to a lower sodium excretion. Apart from the obvious differences in the study protocol and the higher propranolol dosage (160 to 640 mg/d vs. ≤ 160 mg/d,[16] 186 ± 106 [S.D.] mg/d,[13] 40 to 120 mg/d,[14] 40 to 80 mg/d,[15] such a result remains intriguing. In fact, glomerular filtration rate during propranolol plus diuretic administration was not lower than during the diuretic alone administration and systolic blood pressure (mean blood pressure was not reported) declined by a mean value of 12 mmHg.

As a whole, these results would imply that propranolol should not induce detrimental effects on renal function even in advanced cirrhosis, but a close monitoring is advisable in such patients. In any case, propranolol does not have a place in the treatment of renin-aldosterone axis abnormalities and their consequences in cirrhosis.

An exception to this statement may be diuretic-induced uremia without blood volume depletion. Diuretics readily induce renal impairment and this is usually due to over-diuresis with too rapid a contraction of the plasma volume. Occasionally, however, it has been observed in the absence of a negative fluid balance. Renal function impairment was associated with a striking increase in PRA[25,26] and both subsided when therapy was discontinued.[26] This would suggest that diuretics activated the renin-angiotensin system via a mechanism other than volume depletion and such activation played a role in inducing renal failure, possibly through intrarenal vasoconstriction. The simultaneous administration of β-adrenergic antagonists seems to protect the kidney from such an adverse effect.[26]

III. ANGIOTENSIN I-CONVERTING ENZYME INHIBITORS

Captopril was the first available orally effective inhibitor of the angiotensin -converting enzyme. Therefore, most information on the effects of converting enzyme inhibition in cirrhosis come from the administration of this drug.

In normal man, after oral administration, it is rapidly absorbed with peak blood levels reached in 30 to 90 min. Food in the gastrointestinal tract can reduce absorption by 30 to 40%. Captopril is protein bound in blood by 30% and promptly distributed to most tissues, except in the central nervous system. Its metabolism is rapid, so that the half-life of unchanged captopril is probably less than 2 h. Within 4 h of administration, ≈50% of the drug appears in the urine, rising to 66% within 24 h. The elimination of captopril and its metabolites is closely correlated with endogenous creatinine clearance.[27]

Captopril is a specific inhibitor of the angiotensin -converting enzyme. However, the enzyme is also involved in the degradation of the vasodilator bradykinin (Chapter 3, Section I. A. 2). Therefore, its effects are the integrate result of the action on both renin-angiotensin and kinin systems. The relative contribution of these actions can vary according to the pathophysiological background of different clinical settings. It has also been reported that captopril decreases hepatic extraction of renin by the isolated perfused rat liver.[28]

The blockade of angiotensin I conversion in cirrhosis has been devoted to evaluate the effect of renin-angiotensin system inhibition on portal hypertension,[29] aldosterone secretion,[30-34] and renal[31,35] and systemic[35,36] hemodynamics. The pathophysiological mechanisms of such effects have already been discussed in Chapter 3 (Section II.A.2.c and e; B.2.c). Here, we shall attempt to present a clinically relevant, integrated overview.

A main target for captopril administration to cirrhotics with "refractory" ascites would be the inhibition of angiotensin II (III)-induced secondary hyperaldosteronism. Natriuresis should therefore ensue. The administered captopril dose was extremely variable, ranging from 18.75 to 450 mg daily. Furthermore, in most studies diuretics were simultaneously given,[31,37] while in another, no mention was made about diuretic treatment.[32] As a matter of fact, elevated plasma concentration or urine excretion of aldosterone fell in all studies,[30-33,37] but one.[34] A reduction in plasma aldosterone concentration was also observed by Eriksson et al.,[29] who gave 12.5 to 50 mg of captopril to patients without and with ascites (diuretic therapy not stated) to evaluate the effect of the drug on portal hemodynamics. Despite the favorable effect on hyperaldosteronemia, an enhanced natriuresis was not usually achieved. In fact, apart from one case described by Jorgensen et al.[37] (who was also treated with furosemide [240 mg.daily] and spironolactone [100 mg/daily], and two cases described by Mantero et al.,[33] the only report of a captopril-induced natriuresis comes from Saruta et al.[30] A lack of natriuretic effect of captopril was also found by Pariente et al.[35] in a well-designed study which, unfortunately, did not include plasma aldosterone measurement. The kind of hyperbolic relationship linking aldosterone with renal sodium excretion explains in part such a failure (see Chapter 3, Section II.C.1). Indeed, renal sodium excretion fell in the 4 patients of Wood's et al.[31] report (in spite of simultaneous furosemide administration (40 to 120 mg/daily) and in two out of six patients of Pariente et al.[35] study. The antinatriuretic effect of captopril, which also led to a blunted effect of furosemide, has been further confirmed by Daskalopoulos et al. in patients with cirrhosis and ascites.[38]

The variance of these results may be somehow confusing. However, in addition to the differences in both experimental conditions, in some cases not being rigorously controlled, and the kind of patient investigated, a possible explanation may originate from taking into account the changes in systemic and renal hemodynamics induced by captopril administration to cirrhotics. In fact, it often led to a significant decrease in blood pressure[29,31,32,34-36,38] due to a reduction in arteriolar resistances. Interestingly, such a reduction was mainly attributable to the fall in renal vascular resistances, presumably confined at the postglomerular level.[31,35,38] Thus, it can be explained why glomerular filtration rate declined in the face of a steady or even increased renal blood flow. The role of blood pressure fall in determining the decrease in glomerular filtration rate was clearly supported by the close direct correlation found between these two variables, suggesting an impairment in renal autoregulation.[31,35] The final result was a striking reduction in the filtered load of sodium, which could have obscured any possible favorable effect on the aldosterone-dependent tubular handling of the ion. An indirect confirmation arises from those studies where blood pressure perturbations did not occur.[30,33,37] In fact, an (often moderate) increase in renal sodium excretion was only reported by these authors.

Captopril administration (25 to 50 mg q.i.d.) was also attempted in five patients with hepatorenal syndrome, without improving either renal function or the final outcome of the syndrome.[39]

Summarizing, we are inclined to believe that a clinical role of angiotensin -converting enzyme inhibition is unlikely in the management of renal sodium retention in cirrhosis. This assumption is based on the knowledge of the hemodynamic effects of the drug, which can be expected to be particularly hazardous precisely in those patients in whom a treatment alternative to the classical diuretic regimes would be most tempting. In fact, cirrhotics with refractory ascites usually show a trend to arterial hypotension, renal hypoperfusion, and hence, a strikingly activated renin-angiotensin system which plays an important role in maintaining blood pressure and renal autoregulation.

IV. ANGIOTENSIN II ANALOGUES

Some angiotensin II analogues compete with the hormone for receptor sites, so that their administration allows the attainment of a selective inhibition of the renin-angiotensin system. The best known of the group is saralasin, which derives its name from the replacement of the first two amino acid moieties with sarcosine and alanine (1-sar, 8-ala angiotensin II). 1-sar, 8-ile angiotensin II is another analogue in which the substitution in position 8 is made with isoleucine. Both analogues possess a partial angiotensin II agonistic effect, which is more evident for 1-sar, 8-ile angiotensin II.[40]

Few studies have been carried out by administering angiotensin II analogues to cirrhotic patients and those are mainly confined to the pathophysiological approach.[30,41,42] The results obtained, which have been described in detail in Chapter 3 (Section II.A.2.c, d, and e; B.2.b), makes it possible to formulate some considerations. As found after captopril utilization (see above), in patients with an activated renin-angiotensin system, the angiotensin II analogue infusion led to a reduction in blood pressure.[41,42] This was primarily attributable to the fall in peripheral vascular resistances, although a certain decrease in cardiac index was also observed.[41] Interestingly, the degree of the saralasin-induced fall of arterial pressure was directly correlated with the baseline PRA value[41] and a depressor response to 1-sar, 8-ile angiotensin II was found only in patients with high basal PRA levels.[30,42] Moreover, salt repletion, attained by high oral sodium intake plus saline infusion, succeeded in reducing the sensitivity of the blood pressure to saralasin in cirrhotics with ascites.[42] These features strongly suggest that angiotensin II hyperproduction in cirrhosis, when present, has to be seen as a compensatory mechanism, essential in maintaining a reset cardiovascular homeostasis. Moreover, the relationships between the changes in systemic and splanchnic hemodynamics after saralasin observed by Arroyo et al.,[41] makes it unlikely that the putative contribution of angiotensin II to the development of portal hypertension cannot be attributed to its effects on systemic hemodynamics.

Based on the finding that under certain experimental and clinical conditions, such as sodium restriction and either low or high output heart failure, the blockade of angiotensin II markedly increases the renal blood flow,[43] Arroyo et al.[44] attempted to improve the renal perfusion in three cirrhotics with hepatorenal syndrome by infusing 0.4 μg/kg/min of saralasin for 110 min. Such a treatment failed in increasing renal plasma flow and glomerular filtration rate. In spite of the low dose employed, blood pressure fell in every case. Similar results were obtained by Wilkinson (unpublished results) by infusing saralasin into the renal artery. Therefore, as for captopril, the concomitant changes in systemic hemodynamics did not allow the evaluation of the possible role of angiotensin II in the development/maintenance of the intrarenal vasoconstriction of hepatorenal syndrome.

V. ANTIMINERALOCORTICOIDS

Antimineralocorticoids are the most widely used drugs to counteract the effects of activated renin-aldosterone axis in liver disease. They form a class of substances — spirolactones — which compete with aldosterone by occupying its receptors due to their structural analogy with mineralocorticoid hormones.[45,46] Although aldosterone synthesis inhibition by spironolactone was demonstrated ''in vitro''[47] and in the early phases of treatment of patients with primary hyperaldosteronism,[48] such an effect was not demonstrated in normal man.[49] On the contrary, after prolonged spironolactone administration, secretion rate and plasma levels of aldosterone increased,[49] due to the simultaneous activation of the renin-angiotensin system.

Among antimineralocorticoids, spironolactone has been widely employed for more than 20 y. More recently, the water-soluble derivative canrenoate-K (thus also available for i.v. administration) has been introduced in practice.

After a single oral administration, spironolactone is extensively transformed in a single hepatic passage, so that the unmetabolized drug is not recovered from the urine. Spironolactone metabolism is complex, leading to generation of many compounds, canrenone being the most important.[50] More than 90% of this metabolite is bound to plasma proteins[50] and possesses 10% of the affinity of spironolactone for aldosterone receptors.[46] Investigations measuring plasma canrenone by high-pressure liquid-chromatography[51-53] have shown that its contribution to the antimineralocorticoid effect of acutely administered spironolactone is substantially lower than was assumed from early studies,[50,54] in which not entirely specific assay methods were employed. Other metabolites may therefore play an important pharmacodynamic role. After multiple doses, canrenone accumulates due to its long half-life, thus accounting for 72% of spironolactone pharmacologic activity.[55] Agreement is not general, however, on these results.[51,53]

Canrenoate-K is inactive and rapidly converted to canrenone in the plasma via the canrenoic acid.[50] The elimination of antimineralocorticoid metabolites is mainly renal, biliary with excretion accounting for a very small amount.

Canrenone half-life after a single spironolactone administration to cirrhotic patients is prolonged (healthy subjects: 13.5 to 24 h; cirrhotics: 32 to 105 h).[56] Other authors, however, failed to show this difference.[56] In any case, there is no evidence that the half-life prolongation is accompanied by additional accumulation of canrenone in plasma after repeated dosage.[56,57] The observed prolongation of canrenone half-life has therapeutical implications. In fact, if steady-state levels can be expected after 4 d in normal subjects, 12 d may be necessary in cirrhotics.[56]

The effectiveness of spironolactone administration in counteracting sodium retention in cirrhosis, providing renal impairment is not present, has long been recognized.[58,59] A further demonstration came more recently from a controlled clinical trial by Pérez-Ayuso et al.[60] Moreover, in this study, the administration of 150 to 300 mg/d of spironolactone was more effective than 80 to 160 mg/d of furosemide in promoting natriuresis in cirrhotics with ascites (glomerular filtration rate: 100.5 ± 7.8 ml/min and 95.6 ± 9.9 ml/min, in the two groups studied). Namely, only 1/19 patient did not respond to spironolactone (and did not subsequently to furosemide) whereas 10/21 patients did not respond to furosemide, 9 of them showing subsequently natriuresis on spironolactone. These results seem to be paradoxical when considering only the intrinsic natriuretic potency of the two drugs employed. However, they may easily be explained by taking into account the enhanced activity of aldosterone in cirrhosis, so that any amount of sodium delivered to the distal nephron is taken up by a large amount at this site.

Due to the mechanism of action of antimineralocorticoids, the degree of hyperaldosteronism strongly influences the amount of drug needed to promote a negative sodium balance in the absence of other factors favouring salt retention or ascites compartmentalization. In fact, we found a direct correlation between plasma aldosterone concentration and ''effective'' daily dose of spironolactone in 23 ascitic patients with preserved renal perfusion (glomerular filtration rate: 60 to 132 ml/min.).[61] This implies that in the presence of marked hyperaldosteronism, elevated dosages have to be reached in order to expect a satisfactory diuresis. Indeed, dosages exceeding 300 mg/d had to be reached in 22% of our cases (Figure 2). Accordingly, the 2 patients who did not respond to 300 mg/daily of spironolactone in the trial of Pérez-Ayuso et al.[60] had a very high plasma aldosterone concentration. Moreover, Eggert[58] and Campra and Reynolds[59] demonstrated that some cirrhotics with ascites need up to 1 g/d of aldosterone to attain natriuresis.

On the other hand, it must be remembered that in clinical practice the relationship linking antimineralocorticoid dose and aldosteronaemia may be obscured by factors other than poor renal perfusion, since severe hypoalbuminemia ($\leq$ 3 g/dl) and hyponatremia ($\leq$ 136 mmol/l) may affect such a relationship.[61]

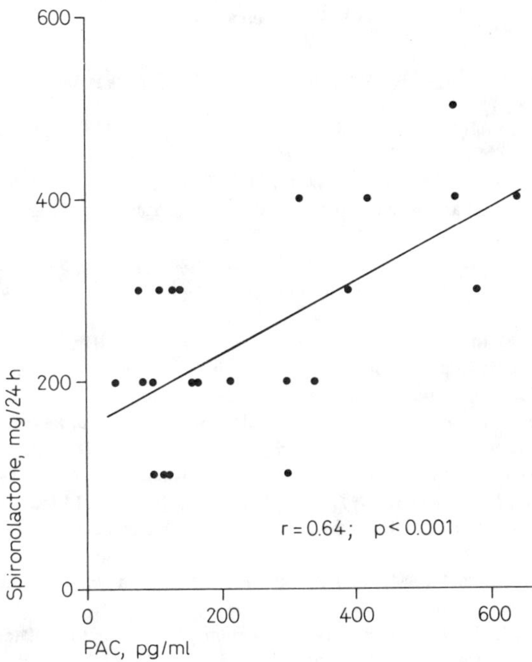

FIGURE 2. Correlation between daily dosage of spironolactone needed to promote a negative sodium balance in 23 patients with cirrhosis and ascites (glomerular filtration rate $\geq$ 60 ml/min) and plasma aldosterone concentration (PAC) measured before the start of therapy (normal range: 32 to 150 pg/ml).

As reported in normal subjects,[49] prolonged administration of spironolactone in cirrhotics can lead to an activation of the renin-angiotensin system, via the depletion of plasma volume.[49] Interestingly, this also occurred in some cases after a relatively short time, without evidence of volume depletion, and it could be involved in renal perfusion impairment.[25,26] Patients with high baseline PRA appeared to be more prone to develop such an effect.[25]

Although free water clearance impairment is an expected effect of loop diuretics,[62] it also occurred in cirrhotics with spironolactone administration.[25] The mechanism of this finding is not clear. However, assuming that the enhanced proximal sodium absorption is a major factor leading to impaired diluting ability in cirrhosis,[63] the aldosterone-dependent distal hyperabsorption may be seen as a partial counterbalance of such a defect.[64] Thus, aldosterone antagonism by spironolactone could further impair free water generation.

In conclusion, spironolactone is a first choice drug to counteract renal sodium retention in cirrhosis. In patients with preserved renal perfusion, not showing hyponatremia and severe hypoalbuminemia, it is effective, provided that a sufficient dosage, related to the degree of hyperaldosteronism, is reached. It must also be employed when loop diuretics are needed, to allow them to fully display their potency and to limit the occurrence of side effects such as excessive kaliuresis and chloruresis.[60,62]

REFERENCES

1. **Haber, E. and Burton, J.,** Inhibitors of renin and their utility in physiologic studies, *Fed. Proc.,* 38, 2768, 1979.
2. **Paterson, J. W., Connolly, M. E., Dollery, C. T., Hayes, A., and Coopre, R. G.,** The pharmacodynamics and metabolism of propranolol in man, *Eur. J. Clin. Pharmacol.,* 2, 127, 1970.
3. **Evans, G. H., Nies, A. S., and Shand, D. G.,** The disposition of propranolol. III. Decreased half-life and volume of distribution as a result of plasma binding in man, monkey, dog and rat, *J. Pharmacol. Exp. Ther.,* 186, 114, 1973.
4. **George, C. F., Orme, M. E., Buranapong, P., Macerlean, D., Breckenridge, A. M., and Dollery, C. T.,** Contribution of the liver to overall elimination of propranolol, *J. Pharmacokinet. Biopharm.,* 4, 17, 1976.
5. **Evans, G. H. and Shand, D. G.,** Disposition of propranolol. V. Drug accumulation and steady state concentrations during chronic oral administration in man, *Clin. Pharmacol. Ther.,* 4, 487, 1973.
6. **Branch, R. A., James, J., and Read, A. E.,** A study of factors influencing drug disposition in chronic liver disease, using the model drug (+)− propranolol, *Br. J. Clin. Pharmacol.,* 3, 243, 1976.
7. **Arthur, M. J. P., Taner, A. R., Patel, C., Wright, R., Renwik, A. G., and George, C.,** Pharmacology of propranolol in patients with cirrhosis and portal hypertension, *Gut,* 26, 14, 1985.
8. **Rocher, I., Decourt, S., Leneveu, A., Lebrec, D., Rosier, S. P., and Flouvat, B.,** Hemodynamics and pharmacokinetic study of propranolol and atenolol in cirrhosis patients, *Clin. Pharmacol. Ther. Toxicol.,* 23, 406, 1985.
9. **Lebrec, D., Nouel, O., Corbic, M., and Benhamou, J. P.,** Propranolol — a medical treatment for portal hypertension?, *Lancet,* 2, 180, 1980.
10. **Lebrec, D., Poynard, T., Hillon, P., and Benhamou, J. P.,** Propranolol for prevention of recurrent gastrointestinal bleeding in patients with cirrhosis, *N. Engl. J. Med.,* 305, 1371, 1982.
11. **Pascal, J. P. and Cales, P.,** Multicenter Study Group: Propranolol in the prevention of first upper gastrointestinal tract hemorrhage in patients with cirrhosis of the liver and esophageal varices, *N. Engl. J. Med.,* 317, 856, 1987.
12. The Italian Multicenter Project for Propranolol in Prevention of Bleeding, Propranolol for prophylaxis of bleeding in cirrhotic patients with large varices: a multicenter randomized clinical trial, *Hepatology,* 8, 1, 1988.
13. **Bataille, C., Bercoff, E., Pariente, E. A., Valla, D., and Lebrec, D.,** Effects of propranolol on renal blood flow and renal function in patients with cirrhosis, *Gastroenterology,* 86, 129, 1984.
14. **Bosch, J., Masti, R., Kravetz, D., Bruix, J., Gaya, J., Rigau, J., and Rodés, J.,** Effects of propranolol on azygos venous blood flow and hepatic and systemic hemodynamics in cirrhosis, *Hepatology,* 4, 1200, 1984.
15. **Bernardi, M., De Palma, R., Trevisani, F., Tamé, M. R., Ciancaglini, G. C., Peas, O., Ligabue, A., Baraldini, M., Gasbarrini, G.,** Renal function and effective β-blockade in cirrhosis with ascites. Relationship with baseline sympathoadrenergic tone, *J. Hepatol.,* 8, 279, 1989.
16. **Wilkinson, S. P., Bernardi, M., Smith, I. K., Jowett, T. P., Slater, J. D. H., and Williams, R.,** Effect of β-adrenergic blocking drugs on the renin-aldosterone system, sodium excretion, and renal hemodynamics in cirrhosis with ascites, *Gastroenterology,* 73, 659, 1977.
17. **Meacci, E., La Villa, G., Laffi, G., Cominelli, F., Di Donato, M., Dabizzi, P., Albani, F., and Gentilini, P.,** Systemic haemodynamics, renal and platelet function during chronic propranolol administration in patients with compensated cirrhosis, *Liver,* 7, 110, 1987.
18. **De Leeuw, P. W. and Birkenhäger, W. H.,** Renal response to propranolol treatment in hypertensive humans, *Hypertension,* 4, 125, 1982.
19. **Wilkinson, R.,** β-blockers and renal function, *Drugs,* 23, 195, 1982.
20. **Epstein, M. and Oster, J. R.,** Beta-blockers and the kidney, *Mineral Electrolyte Metab.,* 8, 237, 1982.
21. **Henriksen, J. H., Ring-Larsen, H., and Christensen, N. J.,** Sympathetic nervous activity in cirrhosis. A survey of plasma catecholamine studies, *J. Hepatol.,* 1, 55, 1984.
22. **Gatta, A., Sacerdoti, D., Merkel, C., Milani, L., Battaglia, G., and Zuin, R.,** Effects of nadolol on renal and hepatic hemodynamics and function in cirrhotic patients with portal hypertension, *Am. Heart J.,* 108, 1167, 1984.
23. **Textor, S. C., Fouad, F. M., Bravo, E. L., Tarazi, R. C., Vidt, D. G., and Gifford, R. W.,** Redistribution of cardiac output to the kidneys during oral nadolol administration, *N. Engl. J. Med.,* 307, 601, 1982.
24. **Rector, W. G. and Reynolds, T. B.,** Propranolol in the treatment of cirrhotic ascites, *Arch. Int. Med.,* 144, 1761, 1984.
25. **Bernardi, M., Trevisani, F., Capelli, M., Bugiardini, G., and Gasbarrini, G.,** Study of renal function, renin-aldosterone axis and plasma electrolytes during diuretic treatment of patients with cirrhosis of the liver, *Ital. J. Gastroenterol.,* 14, 199, 1982.

26. **Wilkinson, S. P., Bernardi, M., Wheeler, P. G., Smith, I. K., and Williams, R.,** Diuretic-induced renal impairment without volume depletion in cirrhosis: changes in the renin-angiotensin system and the effect of β-adrenergic blockade, *Postgrad. Med. J.,* 55, 862, 1979.
27. **Vidt, D. G., Bravo, E. L., and Fouad, F. M.,** Captopril, *N. Engl. J. Med.,* 306, 214, 1982.
28. **Keiser, J. A., Romero, J. C., Kost, L. J., and LaRusso, N. F.,** Hepatic extraction of renin: quantitation and characterization in the isolated perfused rat liver, *Hepatology,* 7, 1254, 1987.
29. **Eriksson, L. S., Kågedal, B., and Wahren, J.,** Effects of captopril on hepatic venous pressure and blood flow in patients with liver cirrhosis, *Am. J. Med.,* 76, 66, 1984.
30. **Saruta, T., Eguchi, T., and Saito, I.,** Angiotensin antagonists in liver disease, in *The Kidney in Liver Disease,* 2nd ed., Epstein, M., Ed., Elsevier, New York, 1983, 441.
31. **Wood, L. J., Goergen, S., Stockigt, J. R., Powell, L. W., and Dudley, F. J.,** Adverse effects of captopril in treatment of resistant ascites, a state of functional bilateral renal artery stenosis, *Lancet,* 2, 1008, 1985 (letter).
32. **Espiner, E. A. and Nicholls, M. G.,** Hormones and fluid retention in cirrhosis, *Lancet,* 2, 501, 1982 (letter).
33. **Mantero, F., Boscolo, R., Zotti, S., Fallo, F., Opocher, G., and Furlanut, M.,** The renin-angiotensin-aldosterone system in liver disease, in *The Endocrines and the Liver,* Langer, M., Chiandussi, L., Chopra, I. J., and Martini, L., Eds., Academic Press, London, 1982, 245.
34. **Schlienger, J. L., Imbs, J. L., Chabrier, G., Doffoel, M., and Imler, M.,** Traitement de l'ascite cirrhotique. Absence d'effet favorable du capropril, *Nouv. Presse Méd.,* 11, 1570, 1982.
35. **Pariente, E. A., Bataille, C., Bercoff, E., and Lebrec, D.,** Acute effects of captopril on systemic and renal hemodynamics and renal function in cirrhotic patients with ascites, *Gastroenterology,* 88, 1255, 1985.
36. **Stanek, B., Renner, F., Sedlmayer, A., and Silberbauer, K.,** Effect of captopril on renin and blood pressure in cirrhosis, *Eur. J. Clin. Pharmacol.,* 33, 249, 1987.
37. **Jorgensen, F., Badskjaer, J., and Nordan, H.,** Captopril and resistant ascites, *Lancet,* 2, 405, 1983 (letter).
38. **Daskalopoulos, G., Pinzani, M., Murray, N., Hirschberg, R., and Zipser, R. D.,** Effects of captopril on renal function in patients with cirrhosis and ascites, *J. Hepatol.,* 4, 330, 1987.
39. **Cobden, I., Shore, A., Wilkinson, R., and Record, C. O.,** Captopril in the hepatorenal syndrome, *J. Clin. Gastroenterol.,* 7, 354, 1985.
40. **Needleman, P., Douglas, J. T., Jr., Jakschik, B. A., Blumberg, A., Isaksin, P. C., and Marshall, G. P.,** Angiotensin antagonists as pharmacological tools, *Fed. Proc.,* 35, 2488, 1976.
41. **Arroyo, V., Bosch, J., Mauri, M., Rivera, F., Navarro-Lopez, F., and Rodés, J.,** Effect of angiotensin II blockade on systemic and hepatic hemodynamics and on the renin-angiotensin-aldosterone system in cirrhosis with ascites, *Eur. J. Clin, Invest.,* 11, 221, 1981.
42. **Schroeder, E. T., Anderson, G. H., Goldman, S. H., and Streeten, D. U. P.,** Effect of blockade of angiotensin II on blood pressure, renin and aldosterone in cirrhosis, *Kidney Int.,* 9, 511, 1976.
43. **Arendshorst, W. J. and Finn, W. F.,** Renal hemodynamics in the rat before and during inhibition of angiotensin II, *Am. J. Physiol.,* 233, F290, 1977.
44. **Arroyo, V., Bosch, J., Rivera, F., and Rodés, J.,** The renin-angiotensin system in cirrhosis: its relation to functional renal failure, in *Hepatorenal Syndrome,* Bartoli, E. and Chiandussi, L., Eds., Piccin Medical Books, Padova, 1979, 201.
45. **Kagawa, C. M.,** Blocking the renal electrolyte effects of mineralocorticoids with an orally active steroidal spironolactone, *Endocrinology,* 67, 125, 1960.
46. **Corvol, P., Claire, M., Oblin, M. E., Geering, K., and Rossier, B.,** Mechanism of the antimineralo-corticoid effects of sprironolactones, *Kidney Int.,* 20, 1, 1981.
47. **Cheng, S. C., Suzuki, K., Sadée, W., and Harding, B. W.,** Effects of spironolactone, canrenone and canrenoate-K on cytochrome P450, and 11β- and 18-hydroxylation in bovine and human adrenal coritcal mitochondria, *Endocrinology,* 99, 1097, 1976.
48. **Conn, J. W. and Hinerman, D. L.,** Spironolactone-induced inhibition of aldosterone biosynthesis in primary aldosteronism: morphological and functional studies, *Metabolism,* 26, 1293, 1977.
49. **Gaillard, R. C., Riondel, A. M., Chambert, P., and Vallotton, M. B.,** Effect of spironolactone on aldosterone regulation in man, *Clin. Sci.,* 58, 227, 1980.
50. **Karim, A., Zagarella, J., Hribar, J., and Dooley, M.,** Spironolactone. I. Disposition and metabolism, *Clin. Pharmacol. Ther.,* 19, 158, 1976.
51. **Abshagen, U., Besenfelder, E., Endele, R., Koch, K., and Neubert, B.,** Kinetics of canrenone after single and multiple doses of spironolactone, *Eur. J. Clin. Pharmacol.,* 16, 255, 1979.
52. **Dahlöf, C. G., Lunborg, P., Persson, B. A., and Regardh, C. G.,** Re-evaluation of the antimineralo-corticoid effect of the spironolactone metabolite, canrenone, from plasma concentrations determined by a new high-pressure liquid-chromatographic method, *Drug Metab. Dispos.,* 7, 103, 1979.
53. **Krause, W., Karras, J., and Seifert, W.,** Pharmacokinetics of canrenone after oral administration on spironolactone and intravenous injection of canrenoate-K in healthy man, *Eur. J. Clin. Pharmacol.,* 25, 449, 1983.

54. **Sadée, W., Dagcioglu, M., and Schöder, R.,** Pharmacokinetics of spironolactone, canrenone and canrenoate-K in humans, *J. Pharmacol. Exp. Ther.,* 185, 686, 1973.

55. **Ramsay, L., Asbury, M., Shelton, J., and Harrison, I.,** Spironolactone and canrenoate-K: relative potency and steady state, *Clin. Pharmacol. Ther.,* 21, 602, 1977.

56. **Jackson, L., Branch, R., Levine, D., and Ramsay, L.,** Elimination of canrenone in congestive heart failure and chronic liver disease, *Eur. J. Clin. Pharmacol.,* 11, 177, 1977.

57. **Abshagen, U., Rennekamp, H., and Luszpinki, G.,** Disposition kinetics of spironolactone in hepatic failure after single doses and prolonged treatment, *Eur. J. Clin. Pharmacol.,* 11, 169, 1977.

58. **Eggert, R. C.,** Spironolactone diuresis in patients with cirrhosis and ascites, *Br. Med. J.,* 4, 401, 1970.

59. **Campra, J. L. and Reynolds, T. B.,** Effectiveness of high-dose spironolactone therapy in patients with chronic liver disease and relatively refractory ascites, *Dig. Dis. Sci.,* 23, 1025, 1978.

60. **Pérez-Ayuso, R. M., Arroyo, V., Planas, R., Gaya, J., Bory, F., Rimola, A., Rivera, F., Rodés, J.,** Randomized comparative study of efficacy of furosemide versus spironolactone in nonazotemic cirrhosis with ascites, *Gastroenterology,* 84, 961, 1983.

61. **Bernardi, M., Servadei, D., Trevisani, F., Rusticali, A. G., and Gasbarrini, G.,** Importance of plasma aldosterone concentration on natriuretic effect of spironolactone in patients with liver cirrhosis and ascites, *Digestion,* 31, 189, 1985.

62. **Bernardi, M., De Palma, R., Trevisani, F., Santini, C., Patrono, D., Motta, R., Servadei, D., and Gasbarrini, G.,** Effects of a new loop diuretic (Muzolimine) in cirrhosis with ascites: comparison with furosemide, *Hepatology,* 6, 400, 1986.

63. **Schedl, H. P. and Bartter, F. C.,** An explanation for and experimental correction of the abnormal water diuresis in cirrhosis, *J. Clin. Invest.,* 39, 248, 1960.

64. **Chiandussi, L., Bartoli, E., and Arras, S.,** Reabsorption of sodium in the proximal renal tubule in cirrhosis of the liver, *Gut,* 19, 497, 1978.

Chapter 19

VASOPRESSIN AND SOMATOSTATIN—HEMODYNAMIC EFFECTS, EFFICACY, AND COMPLICATIONS IN THE TREATMENT OF ACUTE VARICEAL BLEEDING

David Kravetz

TABLE OF CONTENTS

I. INTRODUCTION

Gastrointestinal bleeding from ruptured esophageal varices is one of the main complications of portal hypertension.[1-4] Control of these bleeding episodes is still a difficult problem. The mortality rate from variceal hemorrhage remains extremely high[5,6] despite the efforts to control bleeding by means of a variety of surgical,[7] endoscopic,[8,9] and pharmacological therapies.[10,11]

In recent years, much effort has been focused in the development of new and more effective treatments for bleeding esophageal varices. Specifically, there has been a renewed interest in the use of pharmacological agents that decrease portal pressure by reducing the inflow of blood into the portal venous system through splanchnic vasoconstriction.

The present chapter will discuss the hemodynamic effects, efficacy, and complications of the two more widely used splanchnic vasoconstrictors: vasopressin and somatostatin and its derivatives, in the treatment of variceal bleeding in patients with portal hypertension.

II. VASOPRESSIN

Vasopressin has been the most widely used drug in the treatment of variceal bleeding: Vasopressin in a hormone of the posterior lobe of the pituitary gland. Its potent vasoconstrictor effect was first described by Oliver in 1895.[12] It is also called antidiuretic hormone because of its antidiuretic effect.[13] The elimination half-life of vasopressin in man is short, approximately 24 min,[14] and it is inactivated at multiple sites, including the kidneys, liver, and vasculature.[15] The original vasopressin used in clinical practice was a combination of arginine-8-vasopressin (bovine) and lysine-8-vasopressin (porcine).[11] The preparation of the hormone was standardized by bioassays on the basis of the effect on blood pressure in the dog. One unit is the activity present in 0.5 mg of standard powder of the pituitary gland.[16] Today, synthetic preparations of arginine vasopressin and lysine vasopressin, with a very similar activity, are available for clinical use.

A. HEMODYNAMIC EFFECTS OF VASOPRESSIN

When vasopressin is infused at pharmacological doses, it produces generalized vasoconstrictive effects. Various regional beds exhibit different sensitivity, but it is the splanchnic vasculature where the vasopressin exerts a more pronounced vasoconstrictive action.[10,17-21]

Several experimental studies have been performed in order to assess the relationship between the rate of vasopressin infusion and the decrease in portal blood flow and portal pressure.[21-24] These dose response studies that have not been performed in man,[25] suggest that portal blood flow reduction by vasopressin is more pronounced with increasing doses, with variable sensitivity in the different species studied.[24,26] After achieving maximal effects increasing the dose of vasopressin, infusion is associated with severe toxicity.[25]

Vasopressin is an effective agent in reducing portal pressure in patients with cirrhosis and in portal hypertensive animals.[2,17-20,24-32] Infusion of this drug, regardless of the route of administration, produces a marked vasoconstriction in the mesenteric and splenic arteries.[20,33,34] This vasoconstriction in the main tributaries of the portal vein reduces the inflow of blood into the portal venous system, resulting in a fall in portal pressure. Studies in cirrhotic patients with portal hypertension show that vasopressin infusion (0.2 to 0.4 U/min, i.v.) produces a marked decrease in total hepatic blood flow, ranging between 25 to 40%, and a similar decrease in portal pressure.[27,29,31,32] The results of hemodynamic studies investigating the effects of vasopressin have been questioned recently because they were performed in hemodynamically stable patients or animals, which is quite different from the situation in which vasopressin is clinically used in hypovolemic patients with variceal bleeding receiving blood transfusion. In that regard, recent studies in portal hypertensive rats demonstrated that vasopressin infusion did not decrease the portal bleeding rate.[35] In addition, the dose of vasopressin infusion that decreased portal pressure and blood flow in the stable animal was without effect in the hemorrhaged transfused rat. Only when 10 times larger doses of vasopressin were used, were hemodynamic effects noted.[20]

The effects of vasopressin administration on hepatic artery blood flow are confused. Published studies present divergent results. It has been reported that vasopressin infusion may cause a decrease,[36] an increase,[37] biphasic response,[38] or no change[20,24] in hepatic artery blood flow. The reason for these discrepant results is not known, but it might be related to different routes of administration, dosages, or species studied. Recently, with the introduction of measurements of azygos blood flow,[39,40-42] as an index of blood flow through the gastroesophageal collaterals draining into the azygos venous system, it has become possible to assess the effects of different drugs on the gastroesophageal varices.[40,41] In that regard, it has been shown that in patients with cirrhosis, intravenous vasopressin infusion at 0.4 U/min for 30 min produces a significant decrease of 35% on the azygos blood flow, suggesting that vasopressin administration effectively reduces blood flow through the esophageal varices.[43,44] In addition, it has recently been shown that a bolus injection of 1 IU of vasopressin produces a significant reduction (14%) in variceal pressure, measured by direct puncture of the varices in patients undergoing endoscopic sclerotherapy.[45,46]

Together with these beneficial effects, vasopressin induces frequent and severe side effects, which are due to its potent vasoconstrictive effects on the heart and systemic circulation.[10,11,26,27,29,31,32,47] Vasopressin increases peripheral vascular resistance, with a concomitant increase in arterial pressure and a baroreceptor-mediated bradycardia.[25] These effects, together with a direct impairment of cardiac contractility[47] lead to a fall in cardiac output and coronary blood flow, and are probably the factors responsible for the many cardiovascular complications observed during vasopressin therapy.[48-53]

B. VASOPRESSIN IN THE TREATMENT OF ACUTE VARICEAL BLEEDING

Since the introduction of vasopressin in clinical practice for the treatment of variceal hemorrhage, its dosage and route of administration have varied.[54] At the beginning, vasopressin (pitressin) was administered intravenously as a bolous or as short infusions in a dose of 20 IU.[55,56] However, due to its short action, to the development of tachyphylaxis and considerable side effects, this schedule of vasopressin administration was promptly abandoned. In 1968 Nusbaum et al.[57] suggested that variceal bleeding could be controlled by a continuous, selective infusion of lesser amounts of vasopressin into the superior mesenteric artery. The hypothesis was that the infusion of small amounts of vasopressin directly into the bleeding site was more effective, and caused fewer systemic side effects than via the intravenous route. However, several studies demonstrated that continuous selective infusions of vasopressin into the superior mesenteric artery caused similar systemic effects and complications as continuous intravenous infusions.[26,54,58] Furthermore, intraarterial infusions are associated with additional complications related to the catheterization technique, and result in a delay of several hours in starting therapy.[54] Two clinical controlled trials[54,58] demonstrated that the continuous intravenous infusion of vasopressin is as effective as selective intraarterial infusions in the treatment of variceal bleeding (Table 1).

Based on these studies, the currently preferred route of vasopressin administration is as a continuous intravenous infusion, starting at a dose of 0.4 U/min with a maximum dose up to 0.8 U/min, depending on the effectiveness in controlling variceal hemorrhage and on the development of side effects.

Despite the extensive clinical experience with vasopressin infusion in the treatment of variceal hemorrhage, only three randomized clinical trials comparing vasopressin infusion versus conventional[49,59] or placebo therapy[50] have been reported, and only one was a double-blind investigation[50] (Table 2). The two trials that compared intraarterial vasopressin infusion

TABLE 1
Comparison between Intraarterial and Intravenous Vasopressin Infusions in Controlling Variceal Hemorrhage

	Chojkier et al.[54]	Johnson et al.[58]
Dose (U/min)		
Intraarterial	0.1—0.5	0.4
Intravenous	0.3—0.5	0.4
Control of bleeding		
Intraarterial	6/12 (50%)	7/14 (50%)
Intravenous	5/10 (50%)	7/11 (64%)
Mortality		
Intraarterial	9/12 (75%)	4/14 (29%)
Intravenous	7/10 (70%)	5/11 (46%)

TABLE 2
Controlled Clinical Trials Assessing the Efficacy of Vasopressin Infusion in the Treatment of Variceal Hemorrhage

	Conn et al.[49]	Mallory et al.[59]	Fogel et al.[50]
Route of administration	Intraarterial	Intraarterial	Intravenous
Dose (U/min)	0.04—0.4	0.4	0.4
Control of bleeding			
Vasopressin	12/17 (71%)	2/5 (40%)	4/14 (29%)
Conventional	4/16 (25%)[a]	1/6 (16%)	7/19 (37%)
Mortality			
Vasopressin	9/17 (53%)	2/5 (40%)	7/14 (50%)
Conventional	19/16 (63%)	3/6 (50%)	8/19 (42%)

[a] $p < 0.05$ vs. vasopressin. In the Conn and Mallory studies, conventional therapy include Sengstaken-Blakemore tube and gastric lavage. In the Fogel study, conventional therapy means placebo treatment.

with conventional therapy[49,59] showed that vasopressin was more effective than conventional treatment in controlling variceal hemorrhage. The last study, by Fogel et al.[50] questioned the effectiveness of vasopressin in controlling the hemorrhage. In this trial, intravenous vasopressin infusion was even less effective (29%) than placebo treatment (37%). However, there are some data in this study suggesting that vasopressin could be better than placebo as the first treatment (i.e., the need of surgery in the first 24 hr was greater in the placebo-treated group, and the infusions was stopped more frequently in placebo-treated patients because of persistent bleeding).

Importantly none of the studies have documented an improvement in survival in the vasopressin-treated patients as compared to those receiving placebo or conventional therapy.

All these results indicate that vasopressin therapy is far from an ideal treatment for the control of variceal bleeding. Moreover, vasopressin therapy is associated with frequent (50%) and sometimes severe complications (Table 3), that require cessation of therapy in up to a quarter of the patients.[52]

III. VASOPRESSIN PLUS NITROGLYCERIN

If the toxic effects of vasopressin could be prevented while maintaining the therapeutic benefit of portal pressure reduction, vasopressin might become a more effective and safe

TABLE 3
Complications Associated with Vasopressin Infusion

Minor complications	Major complications[a]
Cardiac arrhythmias	Cardiorespiratory arrest
Arterial hypertension	Mycocardial infarction
Hyponatremia	Pulmonary edema
Bacteremia	Cerebral hemorrhage
Activation of fibrinolysis	Septicemia
Abdominal cramps	Bowel ischemia
Diarrhea	Bowel necrosis
Nausea and vomiting	Local tissue necrosis

[a] Requiring discontinuation of therapy.

therapy for the treatment of variceal bleeding. The administration of nitroglycerin, a potent venous and mild arterial vasodilator, during vasopressin infusion has recently been shown to abolish the deleterious cardiocirculatory effects, while causing a further decrease in portal pressure.[32] The addition of nitroglycerin to vasopressin infusion improves cardiac performance by increasing coronary blood flow and peak dp/dt and decreasing left ventricular end diastolic pressure.[47] Furthermore, the increased arterial and right atrial pressure and the decreased cardiac output and heart rate observed during vasopressin infusion[31,32,47] are normalized after nitroglycerin administration.[32] Similar results had been published with isoproterenol[60] and nitroprusside.[61] Recently, the addition of nitroglycerin infusion at 200 μg/min to intravenous vasopressin further lowered the mean portal pressure in cirrhotic patients from 13.7 to 11.7 mmHg.[61a]

Two controlled clinical trials[62,63] demonstrated that the combined administration of nitroglycerin can prevent or reverse the cardiotoxic systemic side effects of vasopressin infusion during the treatment of acute variceal bleeding (Table 4). In addition, significantly fewer patients given nitroglycerin had to be withdrawn from vasopressin therapy because of complications related to the treatment. However, in these trials, vasopressin plus nitroglycerin also failed to improve the survival rate, suggesting that mortality is more closely related to the severity of the underlying liver disease than to the side effects associated with vasopressin infusion.

IV. VASOPRESSIN ANALOGUES

The serious complication associated with vasopressin therapy, its rapid degradation, the development of tachyphylaxis, and the increase in plasma levels of plasminogen activator promote the investigation of new vasopressin analogues in an attempt to improve its specificity, prolong the biological half-life of a single injection, and reduce the cardiovascular side effects. Triglycyllysine vasopressin (also called glypressin or terlypressin) is a new structural analogue[64] in which in about 5 to 10% of the drug administered the N-terminal triglycyl group of the molecule is cleaved *in vivo*, resulting in a slow release of lysine vasopressin, which is the active principle.[65] The rest is excreted unchanged in the urine.[66] The half-life of this substance is about 10 h.[67] However, the decrease in portal pressure observed after a bolus injection of glypressin of 1 mg/4—6 h lasts on average from 53[68] to 104 min.[19]

Early studies reported that glypressin lowers mesenteric blood flow and portal pressure[19,68] without any significant change in the cardiac output. However, the lack of effects of glypressin on systemic hemodynamics has not been confirmed by other investigators, who found

TABLE 4

**Comparison between Vasopressin (VP) and
Vasopressin Plus Nitroglycerin (VP + NG) in the
Treatment of Variceal Bleeding**

	Gimson et al.[62]	Tsai et al.[63]
Dosis		
VP	0.4 U/min	0.66 U/min
VP + NG	0.4 U/min	0.66 U/min
	+	+
	40 μg/min to	0.6μg
	400 μg/min	
Control of Bleeding		
VP	15/34 (44%)	4/19 (21%)
VP + NG	26/38 (68%)[a]	9/20 (45%)
Major complications		
VP	7/34 (20%)	6/19 (32%)
VP + NG	1/38 (3%)[b]	2/20 (10%)[a]
Mortality		
VP	9/30 (30%)	11/19 (42%)
VP + NG	9/32 (28%)	11/20 (55%)

Note: In the study by Gimson et al., vasopressin and vasopressin plus
nitroglycerin were administered intravenously for 12 h. In the
study by Tsai et al., vasopressin was given intravenously for
24 h, and nitroglycerin sublingualy every 30 min for 6 h.

[a] $p < 0.05$.
[b] $p < 0.02$ vs. vasopressin.

that glypressin administration produced a decrease of cardiac output and heart rate and an
increase of arterial pressure of the same magnitude as that observed with vasopressin infusion.[19,68,69] The only difference between the two vasoconstrictors was a longer duration
of the glypressin effect. Experimental studies in dogs failed to demonstrate any significant
difference on portal pressure reduction between glypressin bolus injection and vasopressin
infusion (39 vs. 38% reduction, respectively), portal venous blood flow (40 vs. 35%,
respectively) and systemic hemodynamics.[19] Glypressin, unlike vasopressin,[53] did not modify
the plasma levels of plasminogen activator.[70] This difference might result in better control
of bleeding. However, the elevation of plasminogen activator observed with vasopressin
infusion did not result in demonstrable fibrinolysis.[65]

The effects of glypressin in controlling variceal bleeding were evaluated in two randomized controlled trials[71,72] (Table 5). Both studies reported that glypressin is more effective
than vasopressin in the control of hemorrhage. However, the results of these studies have
been questioned because of defects in the study design. The study by Freeman et al.[71] had
an unexpectedly low success rate for vasopressin in controlling variceal hemorrhage (9%),
with 85% of the patients Child's A-B, influencing the relatively low mortality (Table 5). In
the trial by Walker et al.[72] it is impossible to assess the efficacy of glypressin because of
the concomitant use of the Sengstaken-Blakemore tube in about 80% of the patients. The
only difference observed between glypressin and vasopressin administration was that sclerotherapy was required more frequently in the vasopressin group (48%) compared to the
glypressin group (20%). No major complication requiring interruption of therapy was reported in these studies.

TABLE 5
Controlled Clinical Trials Comparing Intravenous Terlipressin
(Glypressin) and Vasopressin or Placebo in Acute Variceal
Hemorrhage

	Dose	Control of bleeding	Mortality
Freeman et al.[71]			
Terlipressin	2 mg/6 h	7/10 (70%)	1/10 (10%)
Vasopressin	0.4 U/min	1/11 (9%)[a]	4/11 (37%)
Walker et al.[72]			
Terlipressin	2 mg + 1 mg/4 h	20/25 (80%)	3/25 (12%)
Placebo	—	13/25 (52%)[b]	8/25 (32%)

[a] $p < 0.02$ vs. terlipressin.

[b] $p < 0.05$.

V. SOMATOSTATIN

In 1973, the tetradecapeptide somatostatin was isolated from the sheep hypothalamus.[73] It was later found in a series of other locations including the gastrointestinal tract,[74] pancreas,[75] central and peripheral nervous system,[76,77] and thyroid gland of different species.[78] Its physiological role in man has not been completely elucidated, but it is probably involved in the perception of sensory stimuli, in the short-loop negative feedback control system for regulation of glucagon and insulin. In addition, it has been suggested that somatostatin also participates in the control of the rate at which nutrients enter the circulation by inhibition of all gut secretion, intrinsic as well as extrinsic.[79,80]

The half-life of somatostatin ranges between 1 to 4.5 min in dogs, healthy subjects, and cirrhotic patients.[81-83] This rapid plasma disappearance of somatostatin suggests that the peptide is destroyed in many areas of the body.[84 86] In that regard, Webb et al.[87] recently demonstrated that during somatostatin infusion, the splanchnic extraction of the hormone reached 45%, while the hepatic extraction was 38%. Similar figures was observed in the rat (36%)[88] and in the dog (29%).[86]

A. HEMODYNAMIC EFFECTS OF SOMATOSTATIN

It has been shown that somatostatin infusion reduces splanchnic blood flow in healthy subjects and in experimental animals,[89-93] by approximately 30%. Early studies by Tyden et al.,[94] in a small number of cirrhotic patients, demonstrated that somatostatin infusion reduced portal pressure and suggested that somatostatin might be useful in the treatment of acute variceal hemorrhage.[94,95] Recently, it has been demonstrated in a larger series of patients that somatostatin administration significantly reduced both the portal pressure and hepatic blood flow.[27] In this study, somatostatin administrated as an intravenous bolus injection of 0.5, 1, and 2 μg/kg caused a fall in portal pressure, averaging 28% within 30 sec. Portal pressure returned gradually to control values by 2 min. This short-lasting pressure drop correlates with the half-life of the peptide. When somatostatin was given as a constant intravenous infusion of 7.5 μg/min, smaller (17%), but still significant reductions in portal pressure and hepatic blood flow were observed. Similar results have been found in cirrhotic rats.[96] All this data suggests that somatostatin reduces portal pressure by decreasing splanchnic blood flow, probably due to a selective splanchnic vasoconstriction, since cardiac output remains unchanged. Not all studies agree,[91,97,98] due perhaps to different doses or to the administration of a bolus injection prior to continuous somatostatin infusion.[27]

The effects of somatostatin on the azygos venous blood flow in cirrhotic patients with portal hypertension were recently studied.[40,43,44] Somatostatin caused a significant reduction in azygos blood flow in patients with esophageal varices,[40,43,44] reflecting a decrease in the esophageal collateral blood flow. This beneficial effect was much greater following bolus injections of 1 μg/kg (43%) than after a continuous intravenous infusion of 7.5 μg/min preceded by a bolus injection of 1 μg/kg (21%).[44] These results suggest that bolus injections are of greater therapeutic potential, provided the effects can be sustained. Reduction of azygos blood flow was still evident when the effects of somatostatin on portal pressure were disappearing.[43] In this study, it was found that for a similar reduction in the porto-hepatic gradient, somatostatin induced a greater fall in azygos blood flow than vasopressin, suggesting a greater effect of somatostatin on the gastroesophageal collaterals. In addition to the reduction in azygos blood flow, other investigators recently reported that somatostatin injection in cirrhotic patients produced a significant reduction in variceal pressure measured by direct variceal function.[45]

There are conflicting results in relation to the effects of somatostatin on the hepatic artery blood flow. While hepatic arterial blood flow decreased in normal subject,[89] this effect was not observed in normal dogs[93,99] or in normal rats[100] in which hepatic blood flow increased significantly, but not in portal hypertensive rats, probably because hepatic artery blood flow is already maximally increased in response to the diversion of portal blood through the portocollateral circulation.

The main advantage of somatostatin over vasopressin infusion is the absence of adverse effects on the systemic circulation.[27,92,96,98] Neither the cardiac output, heart rate, systemic vascular resistance and nor arterial pressure are significantly affected by somatostatin infusion.[27]

However, bolus injections are accompanied by a transient reduction in heart rate and cardiac output, and a rise in mean arterial blood pressure.[10,44,96]

Somatostatin infusion reduces portal pressure through a splanchnic arteriolar vasoconstriction,[10,96] the mechanism of which is unclear. It is possible that somatostatin has a direct vasoconstrictor effect on the splanchnic vasculature, as suggested by the very rapid onset of portal pressure reduction following bolus injection.[27,90] Recent *"in vitro"* studies have shown that somatostatin has a direct venoconstrictor effect[101] accounting for the increase in inferior vena cava pressure and portal venous resistance in portal hypertensive rats receiving somatostatin. It is possible that suppression of vasodilating gastrointestinal hormones may play a relevant role contributing to the reduction of splanchnic blood flow and portal pressure. For example, increased circulating levels of glucagon may be one of humoral determinants of the splanchnic vasodilation associated with chronic portal hypertension,[102,103] and portocaval shunt,[104] Removal of circulating pancreatic glucagon by the administration of glucagon antiserum reduced the portal blood flow of portal hypertensive rats by approximately 30%,[103] and somatostatin infusion, in portal hypertensive rats, caused a marked decrease of plasma glucagon concentration (47%) with a concomitant reduction in portal pressure (14%) and portal blood flow (29%).[100]

B. SOMATOSTATIN IN THE TREATMENT OF ACUTE VARICEAL BLEEDING

There are several reports on the use of somatostatin infusion in the treatment of hemorrhage due to esophageal varices[94,95,105] and also for the treatment of gastrointestinal bleeding from other sources.[106,107] However, the use of somatostatin in the treatment of acute variceal bleeding in cirrhotic patients has been assessed in two published controlled randomized trials,[51,108] both comparing the effectiveness and complications of somatostatin and vasopressin intravenous infusions. As shown in Table 6, in both studies somatostatin was associated with increased control of bleeding during the first day of therapy. Although Jenkins et al.[108] found that somatostatin was significantly better than vasopressin, this was not confirmed in the second study.[51] The latter included a much larger number of patients who were given comparable doses of drug infusion (250 μg/h), except for a smaller bolus injection

TABLE 6
Controlled Clinical Trials Comparing the Effects of
Intravenous Infusions of Somatostatin and Vasopressin in the
Treatment of Variceal Bleeding

	Kravetz et al.[51]	Jenkins et al.[108]
Duration of therapy (hours)	48	18—24
Control of bleeding at 24 h		
Somatostatin	26/30 (87%)	10/10 (100%)
Vasopressin	23/31 (74%)	4/12 (33%)[a]
Control of bleeding at 48 h		
Somatostatin	16/30 (53%)	—
Vasopressin	18/31 (58%)	—
Major complications (%)		
Somatostatin	0/30	0/10
Vasopressin	8/31 (26%)[a]	2/12 (17%)
Minor complications		
Somatostatin	3/30 (10%)	—
Vasopressin	15/31 (48%)[a]	—
Mortality		
Somatostatin	14/30 (47%)	2/10 (20%)
Vasopressin	14/31 (45%)	4/12 (33%)

[a] $p < 0.05$ vs somatostatin. In both studies somatostatin and vasopressin were administered as intravenous constant infusions. Requiring discontinuation of therapy.

at the beginning (50 μg vs. 250 μg). Despite this high initial success in controlling variceal bleeding, a relatively large number of patients rebelled during therapy, so that the hemorrhage was completely controlled only in about half of them, a number that does not differ from that observed with vasopressin.[51,49,59]

Unfortunately, there is no study comparing somatostatin infusion to placebo therapy, which is the only way to assess objectively the efficacy of somatostatin in the treatment of acute variceal hemorrhage. This is especially important since a recent study suggested that vasopressin is not superior to a placebo in the treatment of this severe complication.[50] However, as summarized in Table 6, somatostatin appears to be much safer than vasopressin, as evidenced by a significantly lower number of complications related to therapy in both studies.[51,108] Although vasopressin caused major complication in a relatively high number of patients (Table 6), this does not appear to markedly influence the outcome, as suggested by the similar mortality during hospitalization of both treatment groups in the two studies.

VI. SOMATOSTATIN ANALOGUES

During the past few years, several efforts had been made in an attempt to develop new somatostatin analogues with major specificity and longer half-life than the normal tetradecapeptide currently used.[109-111] Recently, a new synthetic compound of long-acting somatostatin (SMS 201—995) was developed with a plasma half-life of 10 min after intravenous injection or 22 min following subcutaneous administration.[111] The analogue is an octapeptide with a more potent inhibitory effect on glucagon, insulin, growth hormone, and gastric acid secretion than somatostatin.[111] The optimal dose of this compound has not been clearly identified. Doses from 5 to 100 μg given intravenously or subcutaneously have been tested, but no clear relationship has been found between the observed effects and the given doses.[112]

It has been shown that these somatostatin analogues produce a similar effect on splanchnic hemodynamics. Hepatic blood flow was reduced in normal subjects by 30 to 35%,[112] and in cirrhotic patients wedged hepatic pressure[28] and hepatic blood flow were reduced to a similar extent by somatostatin and the analogue.[28,112] The only difference observed between them was that while the effects of somatostatin cease immediately after discontinuation of the infusion, the effects of the analogue were present until approximately 1 h after the end of the administration.[112,113] Recently, an experimental study in cirrhotic rats[113] demonstrated that either the intravenous infusion or the subcutaneous administration of this somatostatin analogue produces similar and marked decreases in portal pressure, portal blood flow, and hepatic blood flow. These splanchnic effects started immediately after intravenous infusion (2 to 4 μg/kg bw), but after 18 min with subcutaneous administration (2 μg/kg bw). As happens with somatostatin, the synthetic analogue did not modify systemic hemodynamic parameters.

Clearly, further studies and controlled clinical trials are required to determine the effectiveness of this promising somatostatin analogue both in the control of acute variceal hemorrhage and in the long-term management of portal hypertension in patients with cirrhosis.

ACKNOWLEDGMENTS

The author wishes to thank Dr. Jaime Bosch for his valuable assistance in preparing this chapter, and Mónica Masllorens and Eulàlia Ventura for the careful typing.

REFERENCES

1. **Groszmann, R. J. and Atterbury, C. E.,** The pathophysiology of portal hypertension: A basis for classification, *Semin. Liver Dis.,* 2, 117, 1982.
2. **Bosch, J., Mastai, R., Kravetz, D., Navasa, M., and Rodés, J.,** Hemodynamic evaluation of the patient with portal hypertension, *Semin. Liver Dis.,* 6, 309, 1986.
3. **Boyer, T. D.,** Portal hypertension and its complications: bleeding esophageal varices, ascites and spontaneous bacterial peritonitis, in *Hepatology. A Textbook of Liver Disease,* Zakim, D. and Boyer, T. D., Eds., W. B. Saunders, Philadelphia, 1982, 464.
4. **Sherlock, S.,** *Diseases of the Liver and Biliary System,* 5th ed., Blackwell Scientific, Oxford, 1975, 194 pp.
5. **Graham, D. Y. and Smith, J. L.,** The course of patients after variceal hemorrhage, *Gastroenterology,* 80, 800, 1981.
6. **Conn, H. O.,** Cirrhosis, in *Diseases of the Liver,* 4th ed., Schiff, L., Ed., J. B. Lippincott, Philadelphia, 1975.
7. **Franco, D. and Smadja, C.,** Prevention of recurrent variceal bleeding: surgical procedures, *Clin. Gastroenterol.,* 14, 233, 1985.
8. **Sivak, M. V.,** Sclerotheraphy for esophageal varices, in *Therapeutic Gastrointestinal Endoscopy,* Silvus, S., Ed., Igaru Shoin Medical Publishers, New York, 1985.
9. **Paquet, K. J. and Freussner, H.,** Endoscopic sclerosis and esophageal balloon in acute hemorrhage from esophago gastric varices. A prospective controlled randomized trial, *Hepatology,* 5, 580, 1985.
10. **Bosch, J.,** Effect of pharmacological agents on portal hypertension: a haemodynamic appraisal, *Clin. Gastroenterol.,* 14, 169, 1985.
11. **Groszmann, R. J. and Atterbury, C. E.,** The pharmacological therapy of portal hypertension, *Adv. Intern. Med.,* 31, 341, 1986.
12. **Oliver, G. and Schafer, E. A.,** On the physiological action of the extracts of pituitary body and certain other glandular organs, *J. Physiol.,* 18, 277, 1985.
13. **Goodman, L. S. and Gilman, A.,** *The Pharmacological Basis of Therapeutics,* Macmillan, London, 1970.
14. **Baumann, G. and Dingman, J. F.,** Distribution, blood transport and degradation of anti-diuretic hormone in man, *J. Clin. Invest.,* 57, 1109, 1976.
15. **Blei, A. T.,** Pharmacokinetic-hemodynamic interaction in cirrhosis, *Semin. Liver Dis.,* 6, 299, 1986.
16. **Goth, A.,** *Medical Principles and Concepts,* 6th ed., C. V. Mosby, St. Louis, 1972.

17. **Shaldon, S., Dolle, W., Guevara, L., Iber, F. L., and Sherlock, S.,** Effects of pitressin on the splanchnic circulation in man, *Circulation,* 24, 797, 1961.
18. **Freeman, A. R., Keer, J. C., and Swan, K. G.,** Primate mesenteric blood flow. Effects of vasopressin and its route of delivery, *Gastroenterology,* 74, 875, 1978.
19. **Blei, A. T., Groszmann, R. J., Gusber, R., and Conn, H. O.,** Comparison of vasopressin and triglycil-lysine vasopressin on splanchnic and systemic hemodynamics in dogs, *Dig. Dis. Sci.,* 25, 688, 1980.
20. **Kravetz, D., Cummings, S. A., and Groszmann, R. J.,** Hyposensitivity to vasopressin in a hemorrhaged transfused rat model of portal hypertension, *Gastroenterology,* 93, 170, 1987.
21. **Schmid, P. G., Abboud, F. M., Wendling, M. G., Ramberg, E. S., Mark, A. L., Heistad, D. D., Eckstein, J. W.,** Regional vascular effects of vasopressin: plasma levels and circulatory response, *Am. J. Physiol.,* 227, 998, 1974.
22. **Athanasoulis, C. A., Waltman, A. C., Simmons, J. T., Sheehan, B., and Coggins, C. H.,** Effects of intravenous vasopressin on canine mesenteric arterial blood flow, bowel oxygen consumption and cardiac output, *Am. J. Roentgenol.,* 130, 1033, 1978.
23. **Eriksson, B. F.,** The effects of vasopressin on the distribution of cardiac output and organ blood flow in the anesthetized dog, *Acta Chir. Scand.,* 137, 729, 1971.
24. **Gaskill, H. V., Sirinek, K. R., Barry, A. L.,** Hemodynamic effects of vasopressin. Can large doses be safely given?, *Arch. Surg.,* 118, 434, 1983.
25. **Polio, J. and Groszmann, R. J.,** Hemodynamic factors involved in the development and rupture of esophageal varices: a pathophysiologic approach to treatment, *Semin. Liver Dis.,* 6, 318, 1986.
26. **Barr, J. W., Lakin, R. C., and Rosch, J.,** Similarity of arterial and intravenous vasopressin on portal and systemic hemodynamics, *Gastroenterology,* 69, 13, 1975.
27. **Bosch, J., Kravetz, D., and Rodés, J.,** Effects of somatostatin on hepatic and systemic hemodynamics in patients with cirrhosis of the liver: comparison with vasopressin, *Gastroenterology,* 80, 518, 1981.
28. **Richardson, P. D. I. and Withrington, P. G.,** The effects of intraarterial and intraportal injections of vasopressin on the simultaneously perfused hepatic arterial and portal vascular beds of the dog, *Circ. Res.,* 43, 496, 1978.
29. **Millete, B., Huet, P. M., Lavoie, P., and Viallet, A.,** Portal and systemic effects of selective infusion of vasopressin into the superior mesenteric artery in cirrhotic patients, *Gastroenterology,* 69, 6, 1975.
30. **Groszmann, R. J., Blei, A. T., Storer, E. H., Conn, H. O.,** Pharmacological vs. mechanical reduction in portal pressure: a comparative study, *Surgery,* 84, 679, 1978.
31. **Silva, V. J., Moffart, R. C., and Walt, A. J.,** Vasopressin effect on portal and systemic hemodynamics. Studies in intact, unanesthetized humans, *JAMA,* 210, 1065, 1968.
32. **Groszmann, R. J., Kravetz, D., Bosch, J., Glickman, M., Bruix, J., Bredfeldt, J. E., Conn, H. O., Rodés, J., and Storer, E. H.,** Nytroglycerin improves the hemodynamics response to vasopressin in portal hypertension, *Hepatology,* 2, 757, 1982.
33. **Haddy, F. J. and Scott, J. B.,** Cardiovascular pharmacology, *Annu. Rev. Pharmacol.,* 6, 49, 1966.
34. **Cohen, M. M., Sitar, D. S., McNeill, J. R., and Greenway, C. V.,** Vasopressin and angiotensin on resistance vessels of spleen, intestine and liver, *Am. J. Physiol.,* 218, 1704, 1970.
35. **Valla, D., Geoffroy, P., Girod, C., and Lebrec, D.,** Circulatory actions of vasopressin in anaesthetized rats with portal hypertension subjected to haemorrhage, *J. Hepatol.,* 2, 328, 1986.
36. **Drapanas, T., Crowe, C. P., Shim, W. K. T., and Shenk, W. G.,** The effects of pitressin on cardiac output and coronary, hepatic and intestinal blood flow, *Surg. Gynecol. Obstet.,* 113, 48-, 1961.
37. **Barr, J. W., Lakin, R. C., and Rosch, J.,** Effect of selective celiac infusion of vasopressin on the hepatic artery, *Inv. Radiol.,* 10, 1975.
38. **Bynum, T. E. and Fara, J. W.,** Hepatic artery response to vasopressin, *Am. J. Physiol.,* 239, G378, 1980.
39. **Bosch, J. and Groszmann, R. J.,** Measurement of the azygos venous blood flow through gastroesophageal collaterals in cirrhosis, *Hepatology,* 4, 424, 1984.
40. **Bosch, J., Mastai, R., Kravetz, D., Bruix, J., Rigau, J., and Rodés, J.,** Measurement of azygos venous blood flow in the evaluation of portal hypertension in patients with cirrhosis. Clinical and hemodynamic correlation in 100 patients, *J. Hepatol.,* 1, 125, 1985.
41. **Bosch, J., Mastai, R., Kravetz, D., Bruix, J., Gaya, J., Rigau, J., and Rodés, J.,** Effects of propranolol on gastroesophageal collateral blood flow and on hepatic and systemic hemodynamics in cirrhosis, *Hepatology,* 4, 1200, 1984.
42. **Cales, P., Braillon, J., Jiron, M., Lebrec, D.,** Superior portosystemic collateral circulation estimated by azygos blood flow in patients with cirrhosis, *J. Hepatol.,* 1, 37, 1985.
43. **Bosch, J., Kravetz, D., Mastai, R., Bruix, J., Rigau, J., and Rodés, J.,** Azygos venous blood flow in cirrhosis: effects of balloon tamponade, vasopressin, somatostatin and propranolol, *Hepatology,* 3 (Abstr.), 855, 1983.

44. **Mastai, R., Bosch, J., Navasa, M., Silva, G., Kravetz, D., Bruix, J., Viola, C., and Rodés, J.,** Effects of continuous infusion and bolus injection of somatostatin on azygos blood flow and hepatic and systemic hemodynamics in patients with portal hypertension. Comparison with vasopressin, *J. Hepatol.,* 3 (Abstr.), 53, 1986.

45. **Bosch, J., Bordas, J. M., Mastai, R., Kravetz, D., Silva, G., Navasa, M., Viola, C., and Rodés, J.,** Measurement of wedge hepatic venous pressure (WHVP) accurately reflect the effects of vasoactive drugs on the pressure of the esophageal varices in alcoholic cirrhosis, *Hepatology,* 6, 1190, 1986.

46. **Bosch, J., Bordas, J. M., Rigau, J., Viola, C., Mastai, R., Kravetz, D., Navasa, M., and Rodés, J.,** Non invasive measurement of the pressure of esophageal varices using an endoscopic gauge: comparison with measurements by variceal puncture in patients undergoing endoscopic sclerotherapy, *Hepatology,* 6, 667, 1986.

47. **Zito, R. A., Diez, A., and Groszmann, R. J.,** Comparative effects of nitroglycerin and nitroprusside on vasopressin-induced cardiac dysfunction in the dog, *J. Cardiovasc. Pharmacol.,* 5, 586, 1983.

48. **Corlis, R. J., McKenna, D. H., Sailer, S., O'Brien, G. S., and Rowe, G. G.,** Systemic and coronary hemodynamic effects of vasopressin, *Am. J. Med. Sci.,* 256, 293, 1968.

49. **Conn, H. O., Ramsby, G. R., Storer, E. H., Mutchnik, M. G., Joshi, P. H., Phillips, M. M., Cohen, G. A., Fields, G. N., and Petrovski, D.,** Intraarterial vasopressin in the treatment of the upper gastrointestinal hemorrhage: a prospective controlled trial, *Gastroenterology,* 68, 211, 1975.

50. **Fogel, M. R., Knauer, C. M., Andres, L. L., Mahal, A. S., Stein, D. E. T., Kemeny, J., Rinki, M. M., Walker, J. E., Siegmund, D., and Gregory, P.,** Continuous intravenous vasopressin in active upper gastrointestinal bleeding, *Ann. Intern. Med.,* 96, 565, 1982.

51. **Kravetz, D., Bosch, J., Teres, J., and Rodés, J.,** Comparison of intravenous somatostatin and vasopressin infusion in the treatment of acute variceal hemorrhage, *Hepatology,* 4, 442, 1984.

52. **Greenwald, R. A., Rheingold, O. J., Chiprut, R. O., and Royers, A. I.,** Local gangrene: a complication of peripheral pitressin therapy for bleeding oesophageal varices, *Gastroenterology,* 74, 744, 1978.

53. **Grant, P. J., Davies, J. A., Tata, G. M., Boothby, M., and Prentice, C. R. M.,** Effects of physiological concentrations of vasopressin on haemostatic function in man, *Clin. Sci.,* 69, 471, 1985.

54. **Chojkier, M., Groszmann, R. J., Atterbury, C. E., Mar-Meir, S., Blei, A. T., Frankel, J., Glickman, M. G., Kniaz, J. L., Schade, R., Taggart, G. J., and Conn, H. O.,** A controlled comparison of continuous intraarterial and intravenous infusions of vasopressin in hemorrhage from esophageal varices, *Gastroenterology,* 77, 540, 1979.

55. **Shaldom, S. and Sherlock, S.,** The use of vasopressin ("Pitressin") in the control of bleeding from oesophageal varices, *Lancet,* 2, 222, 1960.

56. **Merigan, I. C., Plotkin, G. R., Davidson, C. S.,** Effect of intravenously administered posterior pituitary extract on hemorrhage from bleeding esophageal varices. A controlled evaluation, *N. Engl. J. Med.,* 266, 134, 1962.

57. **Nusbaum, M., Baum, S., Kuroda, K., and Blakemore, W. S.,** Control of portal hypertension by selective mesenteric arterial infusion, *Arch. Surg.,* 97, 1005, 1968.

58. **Johnson, W. C., Widdrich, W. C., and Ansell, J. E.,** Control of bleeding varices by vasopressin: a prospective randomized study, *Ann. Surg.,* 186, 369, 1977.

59. **Mallory, A., Schaefer, J. W., Cohen, J. R., Holt, S. A., and Norton, L. W.,** Selective intraarterial vasopressin infusion for upper gastrointestinal tract hemorrhage, *Arch. Surg.,* 115, 30, 1980.

60. **Sirinek, K. and Thomfolrd, N.,** Isoproterenol in offsetting adverse effects of vasopressin in cirrhotic patients, *Am. J. Surg.,* 129, 130, 1975.

61. **Gelman, S. and Ernst, S.,** Nitroprusside prevents adverse haemodynamics effects of vasopressin, *Arch. Surg.,* 113, 1465, 1978.

61a. **Westaby, D., Gimson, A., Hayes, P. C., and Williams, R.,** Haemodynamic response to intravenous vasopressin and nitroglycerin in portal hypertension, *Gut,* 29, 372, 1988.

62. **Gimson, A. E. S., Westaby, D., Hegarty, J., Watson, A., and Williams, R.,** A randomized trial of vasopressin and vasopressin plus nitroglycerin in the control of acute variceal hemorrhage, *Hepatology,* 6, 410, 1986.

63. **Tsai, Y.-T., Lay, C.-S., Lai, K.-H., Ng, W.-W., Yeh, Y.-S., Wang, J.-Y., Chiang, T.-T., Lee, S.-D., Chiant, B. N.,** Controlled trial of vasopressin plus nitroglycerin vs. vasopressin alone in the treatment of bleeding esophageal varices, *Hepatology,* 6, 406, 1986.

64. **Rudinger, J., Pliska, V., and Krejci, I.,** Oxytocin analogues in the analysis of some phases of hormone action, *Res. Prog. Horm. Res.,* 28, 131, 1972.

65. **Blei, A. T.,** Vasopressin analogs in portal hypertension: different molecules but similar questions, *Hepatology,* 6, 146, 1986.

66. **Pliska, V., Chard, T., Rudinger, J., and Forsling, M. L.,** In vivo activation of systhetic hormonogens of lysine-vasopressin. *N*-glycil-glycil-glysil-(8-lysine) vasopressin in the cat, *Acta Endocrinol.,* 81, 474, 1976.

67. **Cort, J. H., Albrech, I., Navakova, J., Muller, J. L., and Jost, K.,** Regional and systemic hemodynamic effects of some vasopressins: Structural features of the hormone which prolongs activity, *Eur. J. Clin. Invest.,* 5, 165, 1975.

68. **Rabol, A., Juhl, E., Schmidt, A., and Winkler, K.,** The effect of vasopressin and triglycil-lysine vasopressin (glypressin) on the splanchnic circulation in cirrhotic patients with portal hypertension, *Digestion,* 14, 285, 1976.

69. **Valla, D., Lee, S. S., Moreau, R., Hadengue, R., Sayegh, R., and Lebrec, D.,** L'effects de la glypressine sur la circulation splanchnique et systemique chez les malades atteints de cirrhosis, *Gastroenterol. Clin. Biol.,* 9, 877, 1985.

70. **Prowse, C. U., Douglas, J. G., and Forsling, M. L.,** Haemostatic effects of lysine vasopressin and triglycil lysine vasopressin infusion in patients with cirrhosis, *Eur. J. Clin. Invest.,* 10, 49, 1980.

71. **Freeman, J. G., Lishman, A. H., Cobden, I., Record, C. O.,** Controlled trial of terlipressin ("glypressin") versus vasopressin in the early treatment of oesophageal varies, *Lancet,* 2, 66, 1982.

72. **Walker, S., Stiehl, A., Raedsch, R., Kommerell, B.,** Terlipressin in bleeding esophageal varices: a placebo controlled double-blind study, *Hepatology,* 6, 112, 1986.

73. **Brazeau, P., Vale, W., Burgus, R., Ling, N., Butcher, M., Ravier, J., and Guillemin, R.,** Hypothalamic polypeptide that inhibits the secretion of immunoreactive pituitary growth hormone, *Science,* 178, 77, 1973.

74. **Patel, Y. and Reichlin, S.,** Somatostatin in hypothalamus, extrahypothalamic brain and peripheral tissue of the rat, *Endocrinology,* 102, 523, 1978.

75. **Gerich, J. E.,** Somatostatin, in *Handbook of diabetes mellitus,* Vol. 1, Brown Lee, M., Ed., Garland STPM, New York, 1981.

76. **Bennett-Clarke, C., Romagno, M. A., and Joseph, S. A.,** Distribution of somatostatin in the rat brain: telencephalon and diencephalon, *Brain Res.,* 188, 473, 1980.

77. **Hökgelt, T., Johansson, O., Ljungdahl, A., Lundberg, J. M., and Schultzberg, M.,** Peptidergic neurones, *Nature,* 284, 515, 1980.

78. **Van Noorden, S., Polak, J. M., and Pearse, A. G. E.,** Single cellular origin of somatostatin and calcitonin in the rat thyroid gland, *Histochemistry,* 53, 243, 1977.

79. **Reichlin, S.,** Somatostatin, *N. Engl. J. Med.,* 309, 1495, 1983.

80. **Reichlin, S.,** Somatostatin, *N. Engl. J. Med.,* 309, 1556, 1983.

81. **Sheppard, M. C., Shapiro, B., Pimstone, B. L., Kronheim, S., Berelowitz, M., and Gregory, M.,** Metabolic clearance and plasma half-disappearance time of exogenous somatostatin in man, *J. Clin. Endocrinol. Metab.,* 48, 50, 1979.

82. **Schusdziarra, U., Harris, V., and Unger, R. H.,** Half-life of somatostatin like immunoreactivity in canine plasma, *Endocrinology,* 104, 109, 1979.

83. **Kastin, A. J., Coy, D. H., and Jacquet, Y.,** Central nervous system effects of somatostatin, *Metabolism,* 27 (Suppl. 1), 1247, 1978.

84. **Berelowitz, M., Kronheim, S., Pimstone, B., and Shapiro, B.,** Somatostatin-like immunoreactivity in rat blood. Characterization, regional differences and responses of oral and intravenous glucosa, *J. Clin. Invest.,* 61, 1410, 1978.

85. **Shapiro, B., Sheppard, M., Kronheim, M., Pimstone, B.,** Trans-renal gradient of serum somatostatin-like immunoreactivity in the rat, *Horm. Metab. Res.,* 10, 55, 1978.

86. **Polonsky, K. S., Jaspan, J. B., Berelowitz, M., Emmanouel, D. S., Dhorajiwala, J., and Moossa, A. R.,** Hepatic and renal metabolism of somatostatin-like immunoreactivity simultaneous assessment in the dog, *J. Clin. Invest.,* 68, 1149, 1981.

87. **Webb, S., Kravetz, D., Bosch, J., Wass, J. A. H., Evans, J., Gomis, R., Rees, L. H., Rodés, J.,** Splanchnic and hepatic metabolism of somatostatin: a study in cirrhotic patients with portocaval shunt, *Hepatology,* 3, 193, 1983.

88. **Sacks, H. and Terry, L. C.,** Clearance of immunoreactivity somatostatin by perfused rat liver, *J. Clin. Invest.,* 67, 419, 1981.

89. **Tyden, G., Samnegard, H., Thulin, L., Muhrbeck, O., and Effendic, S.,** Circulatory effects of somatostatin in anesthetized man, *Acta Chir. Scand.,* 145, 443, 1979.

90. **Samnegard, H., Thulin, L., Andreen, M., Tyden, G., Hallberg, D., and Effendic, S.,** Circulatory effects of somatostatin in anesthetized dog, *Acta Chir. Scand.,* 145, 209, 1979.

91. **Sonnenberg, G. E., Keller, V., Perruchoud, A., Burckhardt, D., and Gyr, K.,** Effects of somatostatin on splanchnic hemodynamic in patients with cirrhosis of the liver and normal subjects, *Gastroenterology,* 80, 526, 1981.

92. **Becker, R. H. A., Scholtholt, J., Schölkens, B. A., Jung, W., and Speth, O.,** A microsphere study on the effects of somatostatin and secretin on regional blood flow in anesthetized dog, *Regulatory Peptides,* 4, 341, 1982.

93. **Jaspan, J., Polonsky, K., Lewis, M., and Moosa, R.,** Reduction in portal vein blood flow by somatostatin, *Diabetes,* 28, 888, 1979.

94. **Tyden, G., Samnegard, H., Thulin, L., Friman, L., and Effendic, S.,** Treatment of bleeding oesophageal varices with somatostatin, *N. Engl. J. Med.,* 299, 1466, 1978.

95. **Thulin, L., Tyden, G., Samnegard, H., and Muhrbeck, O.,** Treatment of bleeding oesophageal varices with somatostatin, *Acta Chir. Scand.,* 145, 395, 1979.
96. **Jenkins, S. A., Devitt, P., Day, D. W., Baxter, J. N., and Shields, R.,** Effects of somatostatin on hepatic hemodynamics in the cirrhotic rat, *Digestion,* 33:126—134, 1986.
97. **Eriksson, L. S., Lan, D. H., Sato, Y., and Wahren, J.,** Influence of somatostatin on splanchnic hemodynamics in patients with liver cirrhosis, *Clin. Physiol.,* 4, 5, 1984.
98. **Merkel, C., Gatta, A., Zuin, R., Finucci, G. F., Nosadini, R., and Ruol, A.,** Effect of somatostatin on splanchnic hemodynamics in patients with liver cirrhosis and portal hypertension, *Digestion,* 32, 92, 1985.
99. **Price, B. A., Jaffe, B. M., and Zinner, M. J.,** Effect of exogenous somatostatin infusion on gastrointestinal blood flow and hormones in the conscious dog, *Gastroenterology,* 88, 80, 1985.
100. **Kravetz, D., Bosch, J., Arderiu, M. T., Pizcueta, M. P., Casamitjana, R., Rivera, F., Rodés, J.,** Effects of somatostatin on splanchnic hemodynamics and plasma glucagon in portal hypertensive rats, *Am. J. Physiol.,* in press.
101. **Sicuteri, F., Panconesi, A., Del Bianco, P. L., Franchi, G., and Anselmi, B.,** Venospastic activity of somatostatin in vivo in man. Naloxone reversible tachyphylaxis, *Int. J. Clin. Pharmacol. Res.,* 4, 253, 1984.
102. **Benoit, J. N., Barrowman, J. A., Harper, S. L., Kvietys, P. R., and Granger, D. N.,** Role of humoral factors in the intestinal hyperemia associated with chronic portal hypertension, *Am. J. Physiol.,* 247, E486, 1984.
103. **Benoit, J. N., Zimmerman, B., Premen, H. J., Go, V. L. W., Granger, D. N.,** Role of glucagon in splanchnic hyperemia of chronic portal hypertension, *Am. J. Physiol.,* 251, G674, 1986.
104. **Kravetz, D., Arderiu, M. T., Bosch, J., Fuster, J., Visa, J., Casamitjana, R., and Rodés, J.,** Hyperglucagonemia and hyperkinetic circulation following portocaval shunt in the rat, *Am. J. Physiol.,* 252, G257, 1987.
105. **Raptis, S. and Zoupas, C.,** Somatostatin not helpful in bleeding esophageal varices, *N. Engl. J. Med.,* 300, 736, 1979.
106. **Magnusson, I., Ihre, T., Johansson, C., Seligson, V., Torngren, S., and Uvnas-Moberg, K.,** Randomized double blind trial of somatostatin in the treatment of massive upper gastrointestinal haemorrhage,
107. **Limberg, B. and Kommerell, B.,** Somatostatin for cimetidine resistant gastroduodenal haemorrhage, *Lancent,* 2, 916, 1980.
108. **Jenkins, A., Baxter, J. N., Corbett, W., Devitt, P., Ware, J., and Shields, R.,** A prospective randomized controlled clinical trial comparing somatostatin and vasopressin in controlling acute variceal haemorrhage, *Br. Med. J.,* 20, 275, 1985.
109. **Bonfils, S.,** New somatostatin molecule for management of endocrine tumours, *Gut,* 26, 433, 1985.
110. **Wood, S. M., Kraenzlin, M. E., Adrian, T. E., and Bloom, S. R.,** Treatment of patients with pancreatic endocrine tumours using a new long-acting somatostatin analogue symptomatic and peptide response, *Gut,* 26, 438, 1985.
111. **Bauer, W., Briner, U., Doepfner, W., Haller, R., Huguenin, R., Marbach, P., Petcher, T. J., Pless, J.,** SMS 201-995: A very potent and selective octapeptide analogue of somatostatin with prolonged action, *Life Sci.,* 31, 1133, 1982.
112. **Wahren, J., Eriksson, L. S.,** The influence of long-acting somatostatin analogue on splanchnic haemodynamics and metabolism in healthy subjects and patients with liver cirrhosis, *Scand. J. Gastroenterol.,* 21 (Suppl. 119), 103, 1986.
113. **Jenkins, S. A., Baxter, J. N., Corbett, W. A., Shields, R.,** The effects of somatostatin analogue SMS 201-995 on hepatic haemodynamics in the cirrhotic rats, *Br. J. Surg.,* 72, 864, 1985.

CONCLUSIONS

The principal cardiovascular complication of chronic liver disease is portal hypertension. This involves not just the portal circulation, but initiates a unique sequence of events that affect the entire circulation. This is expressed as the hyperkinetic circulation of chronic liver disease. Historically, the hyperkinetic circulation of liver disease was defined as decreased blood transit time through the peripheral circulation due to arteriovenous shunting which led to a reduction in the total peripheral resistance and elevated cardiac output (and decrease in the arteriovenous oxygen difference).

Since the introduction of this definition in the 1950s and with recent advances in cardiovascular physiology, we asked if the definition of the hyperkinetic circulation was still apt. Our contributors have responded by identifying the cardiovascular changes in the various circulations, by describing the effect of the disease upon the regulatory systems of the cardiovascular system and clearly indicating that the major complications of portal hypertension, apart from encephalopathy, are associated with cardiovascular abnormalities.

Having done so, we can answer the questions, "Has the definition changed?" and "What do we really understand by the expression the hyperkinetic circulation of chronic liver disease?" The answer to the first question is no, because all the essential elements, namely, portal hypertension, decreased blood transit time, arteriovenous shunting, peripheral vasodilatation, and elevated cardiac output, are the constants in the definition or equation. What has changed are a number of variables that make up the equation because our understanding of basic cardiovascular physiology is greater. Hence, the answer to the second question is more difficult. First, in some instances our knowledge base still has gaps, and second, we do not always understand the significance of the constants. The onset of symptoms in cirrhosis takes many years and much of our information has been obtained from clinical observations. In view of the time course of the disease and our incomplete knowledge, it is often difficult to interpret the clinical findings. This in turn limits our ability to give an accurate prognosis and probably explains why therapeutically, we have sometimes been unsuccessful in the management of cirrhotic patients.

Investigators have attempted to resolve some of these problems using a variety of animal models of portal hypertension, in the presence and absence of chronic liver disease. These models reproduce most but not all of the cardiovascular complications of chronic liver disease in a relatively short period, usually a few months. The animal models clearly show a difference in the sequence of onset of the cardiovascular abnormalitites leading to development of cirrhosis and its complications. These animal studies have helped us to answer the second question by showing us that the sequence of events leading to portal hypertension is important in the expression of the hemodynamic abnormalities.

To summarize, we can confidently say that we do indeed have an improved definition or map of the hyperkinetic circulation. However, our map remains incomplete. So, where do we go if we have not yet graduated from this course in medical geography? In recent years, by sequential studies of patients with esophageal varices, we have learned much about factors that determine the onset of bleeding. Undoubtedly, the first port of call now is to sequentially study patients with cirrhosis of different etiologies, prior to the onset of complications. In this way, we may be able to learn more about why patients develop varices or why they start retaining sodium. In doing so, we will be able to interpret more accurately the clinical findings, and this, in turn, will improve our ability to give an accurate prognosis. From this point, we will also know if the different animal models truly reflect any of the clinical types of cirrhosis. Using this knowledge base, we can graduate from the course in medical geography and begin to develop more appropriate targets and therapeutic directions to protect the patient from the cardiovascular complications of chronic liver disease.

A. Bomzon, M.D.
L. M. Blendis, M.D.

INDEX

A

Absolute bradycardia, see Bradycardia
Acetaldehyde, as vasodilator, 304
Acetaminophen, 82
Acetate, 304—306
Acetylcholine
  blood vessel radius and, 210
  portal hypertension pathogenesis and, 213
  stimulation of endothelial-derived relaxation factor and, 214
  effect of, in liver, 153
ACTH, see Adrenocorticotropic hormone
Actin, 153
Adenine nucleotide, 180
Adenosine
  blood vessel radius and, 210
  role in organ blood flow, 218
  as vasodilator, 306
Adenosine deaminase, 180, 181
ADH, see Antidiuretic hormone
Adrenal cortex, 47
Adrenaline, 326
β_1-Adrenergic receptors
  renin release and, 30
  sympathetic neuropathy and, 70, 71
α-Adrenoceptor
  agonists, 320
  antagonists, 321
  sympathetic neuropathy and, 70, 71
β-Adrenoceptor
  agonists, 84, 321
  antagonists, 168, 321—328
Adrenocorticotropic hormone, 32
Adult respiratory distress syndrome, 228
Albumin, 3, 158
Alcohol, see Ethanol
Alcohol dehydrogenase pathway, 304
Alcoholic polyneuropathy, and vagus nerve degeneration, 64
Aldosterone, 342
  effect of, 32
  hypersecretion in ascitic cirrhosis, 45
  increase in drug-induced cirrhosis, 20
  levels in ascitic vs. nonascitic cirrhosis, 35
  metabolism of, 32
  synthesis of, 31
Aldosterone 18-glucuronide, 32
Almitrine biosynthesis, 116
Alzheimer's astrocytes, 246, 249
γ-Aminobutyric acid, 210, 213, 244, 248
Ammonia, 252
Ammonium salts, 252
Amyl nitrate, 110
Anesthesia, 320
  changes in circulatory response to β-blockade and, 327

effect after portal stenosis in rats, 18
effect on pressor response to angiotensin, 215
effect on cardiovascular function after ligation, 10, 13
role in reduction of ethanol metabolism, 311
ANF, see Atrial natriuretic factor
Angiomatoid lesions, in pulmonary hypertension, 108
Angiotensin, see also Angiotensin I; Angiotensin II; Angiotensin III
  effect of, 31
  inhibition of converting enzymes of, 338
  metabolism of, 30
  pressor effect in decompensated cirrhosis, 215
  vascular response to, in liver, 200
Angiotensin I, conversion to angiotensin II, 30, 129
Angiotensin II, 4
  adrenergic system and, 31
  blood vessel radius and, 210
  causative role in functional renal failure, 131, 135
  in drug-induced cirrhosis, 20
  effect on renal blood flow, 130
  effects on renal system, 31
  generation in kidney, 130
  levels in fulminant hepatic failure, 55
  pressor response in animal models, 215
  renin release and, 30
  as vasoconstrictor, 31, 130
Angiotensin II receptors, blockade by drugs, 338
Angiotensin III, conversion from angiotensin II, 31
Angiotensin converting enzymes, 30, 31
Angiotensinogen
  plasma levels, 37, 55
  stimulation by angiotensin and renin, 30
Animal models, 161, 227
  carbon tetrachloride effects on, 2, 19—21, 320
  dog, 10—15, 19
  pig, 19
  in pulmonary hypertension, 108
  rabbit, 11, 16, 19
  rat, 11, 12, 15, 16, 17—19
Antidiuretic hormone, 132, 275
  effect of angiotensin on release of, 31
  glomerular filtration rate and, 134
  elevation in cirrhosis, 133
  interaction with V-1 and V-2 receptors, 133
  in pathogenesis of functional renal failure, 135
  release of and sinusoidal portal hypertension, 139
  renal plasma flow and, 134
  renin release and, 30
  role in generation of cyclic AMP, 133
  role in water retention, 133, 134
  as vasoconstrictor system, 135
Antihypertensive drugs, 110, see also specific entries
Antimineralocorticoids, 338, 343

in drug-induced cirrhosis, 20, 21
hepatic endotoxin clearance and, 108
Positron emission tomography, 242, 254
Posthepatic portal hypertension, 189
Postsynaptic receptors; 65, 71—73, see also α-Adrenoceptor; β-Adrenoceptor
Posture; see also Neck-out water immersion; Head-out water immersion
changes in plasma volume and plasma renin activity and, 39
effect of change on renal function in ascitic cirrhosis, 266
effect on renin-angiotensin system, 30, 43
supine and release of atrial natriuretic factor, 284
Potassium
excretion, 53, 54, 264
ions, as vasoregulator, 180
plasma levels and effect on aldosterone, 32, 44
PRA, see Plasma renin activity
Prazosin, 165, 169, 321
Pressor agents, in dog model, 85
Pressor responsiveness, 14, 40, 210, 211
Progressive functional renal failure, see Hepatorenal syndrome
Prolactin, 270
Propranolol, 4, 5, 226
as β-adrenoceptor antagonist, 235—236, 322
-diuretic, 341
dose-related effects of, 338
effect on azygos blood flow, 323, 326
effect on cardiac output, 322, 323, 324, 339
effect on hepatic venous pressure, 323
effect on plasma renin activity, 339
effect on renal function, 339
hepatic blood flow and clearance of, 338
lack of response to, 322, 323
oxygen transport and, 226, 230, 232
as renin release inhibitor, 338
in treatment of recurring variceal hemorrhage, 168, 169
Prostacyclin, as pulmonary vasodilator, 110, see also Epoprostenol
Prostaglandin E, 4, 73
as antagonist of antidiuretic hormone, 279
effect of angiotensin II on, 31, 43, 73
Prostaglandins, see also Prostaglandin E
blood vessel radius and, 210
effect on glomerular filtration rate, 136
effect on renal blood flow, 135, 136
levels in portal hypertension, 196
maintenance of renal hemodynamics and, 137
as metabolites of arachidonic acid metabolism, 135
as modulators of splanchnic blood flow, 182
renal, effect on sodium retention, 270
renin release and, 30
role in pathogenesis of liver disease, 214
synthesis of, 135
Pulmonary abnormalities, and liver disease, 104
Pulmonary arterial pressure, measure of, 104
Pulmonary arteritis, 108

Pulmonary hypertension, 104—111
clinical features, 108—111
pathogenesis, 106—108
pathology, 108
prevalence, 104—106

R

Redox potential, measurement in liver cells, 302
Relative bradycardia, see Bradycardia
Renal blood flow, 3, 270
after bile duct ligation, 14, 274—275
in decompensated cirrhosis, 71
effect of angiotensin II on, 31
norepinephrine levels and, 72
renin-angiotensin system and, 41, 42
sympathetic nervous activity and, 72
Renal hemodynamics, relation to cardiac output in cirrhosis, 267
Renal hypoperfusion, 38
Renal ischemia, 33
Renal potassium excretion, 53, 54
Renin, see also Renin-angiotensin system
circadian rhythms of, 30
effect of bile duct ligation of activity of, 14
in fulminant hepatic failure, 55
plasma concentration, 30
release of, 30
factors affecting, 129
inhibition by drugs and, 338
Renin-angiotensin system, 3
activity of related to aldosterone, 47
arterial hypervolemia and, 130
in cirrhosis without ascites, 33
effect on sodium retention, 270
as factor in pathogenesis of functional renal failure, 129
inhibition, 130, 338—345
role in ascites formation, 131
as vasoconstrictor system, 135
Renin-angiotensin-aldosterone system, 33, 70—71

S

Saline, 263
Saralasin, 47, 339, see also Captopril
as antagonist of angiotensin II, 39, 42
in ascitic cirrhosis, 266, 267
effect on angiotensin II levels, 216
effect on blood pressure, 343
effect on renin-angiotensin system, 130
Sclerotherapy
effects on pulmonary vasculature, 117
in treatment of variceal hemorrhage, 166, 167, 170
Secretin, as modulator of splanchnic blood flow, 182, 198
Septic shock, 228
Serotonin, 200
antagonists of, 328
blood vessel radius and, 210